First Aid and Emergency Care

The sponsoring organization confers upon

this

Certificate of Completion

for satisfactorily completing _____ training hours and _____ college credits in First Aid and Emergency Care

_____
Date

_____
Sponsoring College/University

_____
Department

_____
Course Instructor

The above person has also successfully completed the Cardiopulmonary Resuscitation (CPR) training requirements of the American Heart Association and the American Red Cross.

_____
CPR Instructor

First Aid
and
Emergency Care
Workbook

For Colleges and Universities

Fourth Edition

By

Brent Q. Hafen, Ph.D.
Keith J. Karren, Ph.D.

BRADY
MORTON SERIES
Prentice Hall, Englewood Cliffs, NJ 07632

Previously published by Morton Publishing Company

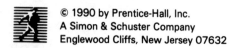 © 1990 by Prentice-Hall, Inc.
A Simon & Schuster Company
Englewood Cliffs, New Jersey 07632

Printed in the United States of America

10 9 8 7 6 5 4 3 2 1

ISBN   0-13-321183-5

Prentice-Hall International (UK) Limited, London
Prentice-Hall of Australia Pty. Limited, Sydney
Prentice-Hall Canada Inc., Toronto
Prentice-Hall Hispanoamericana, S.A., Mexico
Prentice-Hall of India Private Limited, New Delhi
Prentice-Hall of Japan, Inc., Tokyo
Simon & Schuster Asia Pte. Ltd., Singapore
Editora Prentice-Hall do Brasil, Ltda., Rio de Janeiro

PREFACE

Sudden illnesses, injuries, and accidents often happen with little or no warning. In many cases, prompt and efficient action on the part of the first person to help the victim may mean the difference between a speedy recovery and chronic disability (or even death).

Prompt and efficient action goes far beyond calling for an ambulance or a doctor. A certain amount of time lapses before professional medical help arrives; offering prompt, effective emergency care includes providing life support measures and stabilizing the victim while waiting for help to arrive. Therefore, everyone should be prepared to give first aid and emergency care.

The purpose of this text/workbook is to provide instruction in first aid and emergency care procedures.

The authors recognize that training and practice are the keys to efficiency. We have, therefore, organized each section of the text/workbook according to the following format:

1. Content — Well illustrated, precise and up-to-date.

2. Self-test — A two-page chapter evaluation that can be submitted to the instructor.

3. Problem scenario — Case situations which offer the opportunity to apply one's knowledge.

4. Practical skills check-off — Provides a record of the first aid skills the student has mastered.

This publication may be used without supplementary materials, and contains the information and procedures necessary for Advanced First Aid certification and CPR certification as stipulated by the American Heart Association.

The use of the pronouns "he" and "him" throughout this publication is for grammatical reasons only. The authors recognize and acknowledge the significant contributions and service which have been made and will continue to be made by women in First Aid and Emergency Care.

Words **BOLDED** in the text are defined in an extended glossary of key words contained in the back of this book.

ACKNOWLEDGMENTS

Photography and consultation was provided by Max Wilson with the assistance of the following individuals:

Ron Hammond
Steve Hawks
Kevin Crawford
Judy Berryessa
Chuck Tandy
Gary Jolley
Joe McRae

Appreciation is also expressed to the following for allowing us to use their color photographs — with special thanks to Blayne Hirsche, M.D.; James Clayton, M.D.; and Spenco Medical Corp. Companies and individuals that generously assisted with photographs are:

Dyna Med, Inc.
California Medical Products, Inc.
REEL Research & Development
Philip C. Anderson, M.D.
Paul S. Auerbach, M.D.
Cameron Bangs, M.D.
W. Henry Baughman, H.S.D.
Robert Biehn
John A. Boswick, Jr., M.D.
Jim Bryant
N. Branson Call, M.D.

Douglas C. Cox, Ph.D.
Drug Intelligence Publications, Inc.
Corine A. Dwyer
Larry Ford
Dyna Med Industries
Michael D. Ellis
Bruce Halstead, M.D.
Niles W. Herrod, D.D.S.
Glen R. Hunt, M.D.
Renner Johnson, M.D.
Arthur K. Kahn, M.D.
Thomas Morton, M.D.
Eugene Robertson, M.D.
Pat Sullivan
Lawrence Wolheim, M.D.
World Life Research Institute
Michael and Jacqueline Gelotte
Mark and Sharlene Sumison

Additional appreciation is expressed to Susan Strawn and Dennis Giddings for their outstanding artwork, to Bob Schram for cover design, and to Dianne Borneman and Joanne Saliger for their editorial, design, and typesetting expertise that brought the entire project together.

Finally, our special thanks to Doug Morton, our publisher, whose support has helped through the development of this book.

CONTENTS

CHAPTER ONE

OBJECTIVES

- Identify the need for properly prepared First Aiders.
- Identify the components of a functioning emergency medical services (EMS) system.
- Understand the roles, responsibilities, and functions of a First Aider.
- Understand the first aid and legal aspects of emergency medical care.
- Become familiar with AIDS and its connection with first aid.

INTRODUCTION TO FIRST AID AND EMERGENCY CARE

THE PROBLEM: EMERGENCIES IN AMERICA

One of the most critical and visible health problems in America today is the sudden loss of life and disability from catastrophic accidents and illnesses. While facts and figures are not essential to the preparation of emergency rescuers, they do paint a picture of the great need for properly prepared First Aiders at the accident site. Consider the following:

- Over 70 million Americans receive hospital emergency care each year. One American in three suffers a non-fatal injury.

- Over 150,000 people die each year from **TRAUMA**, and 400,000 permanent injuries occur, making trauma the fourth largest killer in the United States and the leading cause of death up to age fourteen.

- At least 1.4 million injuries occur on American highways, resulting in 51,900 traffic deaths and permanent disability to 150,000. Injury is the fourth leading cause of death among Americans,

preceded in order by heart disease, cancer, and stroke.

- Each year there are 2 million burn accidents, 1.5 million heart attack victims (50 percent of these victims dying within two hours of onset), and 5 million poisonings (90 percent of these victims being children).

- Every year, more than 80,000 Americans become permanently disabled because of injury to the brain or spinal cord (Figure 1-1).

NEED FOR EFFECTIVE CARE

Too often, those who arrive first at the scene of an accident, and even some ambulance personnel, are not trained sufficiently to give proper, on-the-scene emergency care or in-transit emergency assistance. Often, too much time passes after an accident before proper emergency care is given, and victims who might have been saved die due to lack of necessary care.

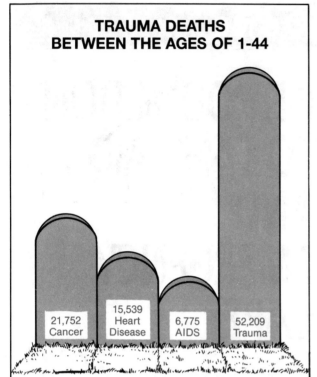

TRAUMA DEATHS BETWEEN THE AGES OF 1-44

21,752 Cancer

15,539 Heart Disease

6,775 AIDS

52,209 Trauma

Trauma can strike you at any minute of any day. Each year, more than 62 million people are injured. That's about one out of every five persons in the United States.

Trauma permanently disables more than 325,000 people each year. As Surgeon General C. Everett Koop stated in his address to the U.S. Senate, "There are no one-time costs associated with injuries. There are only *lifetime* costs." (1989)

Trauma most often strikes at the prime of life. This means children and young adults. Each year, 19 million children under the age of 15 — one child in every four — are injured seriously enough to need to visit a doctor.

Source: American Trauma Society, 1988

FIGURE 1-1. How trauma affects you.

NEED FOR WELL-TRAINED FIRST AIDERS

Remarkably, studies suggest that 15 to 20 percent of accidental highway deaths could be avoided if prompt, effective emergency care was available at the scene. The old philosophy of "load and go" is just not acceptable. The Maryland Institute for Emergency Medical Services describes the time immediately after an accident as the "Golden Hour," when lives that hang in the balance can be saved through administration of proper first aid and emergency care.

The first people on the scene, the First Aiders, can initiate lifesaving procedures, such as:

- Airway and respiratory intervention.
- Cardiopulmonary resuscitation.
- Bleeding control.
- Special wound care (such as head, chest, and abdominal wounds).
- Stabilization of spinal injuries.
- Splinting of fractures.

You will become an important part of the emergency care team as you properly prepare with the right knowledge and practical skills to render appropriate lifesaving care (Figure 1-2).

WHAT IS FIRST AID?

First aid is the temporary and immediate care given to a person who is injured or suddenly becomes ill. First aid also involves home care if medical assistance is delayed or not available. First aid includes recognizing life-threatening conditions and taking effective action to keep the injured or ill person alive and in the best possible condition until medical treatment can be obtained.

First aid does not replace the physician, nurse, or paramedic. One of the primary principles of first aid is to obtain medical assistance in all cases of serious injury. The principle aims of first aid are:

- To prepare properly so as to avoid errors and know what *not* to do as well as what *to* do.
- To care for life-threatening conditions.
- To minimize further injury and complications.
- To make the victim as comfortable as possible to conserve strength.
- To minimize infection.
- To transport the victim to a medical facility, when necessary, in such a manner so as not to complicate the injury or subject the victim to unnecessary discomfort.

A part of proper preparation is to become more safety conscious. This will help to reduce the number of accidents and potential first-aid situations. Three key terms in the promotion of safety awareness are *cause*, *effect*, and *prevention*.

The major cause of accidents is human failure. Mechanical or structural failures can also cause accidents. It is essential that every possible hazard be eliminated, controlled, or avoided.

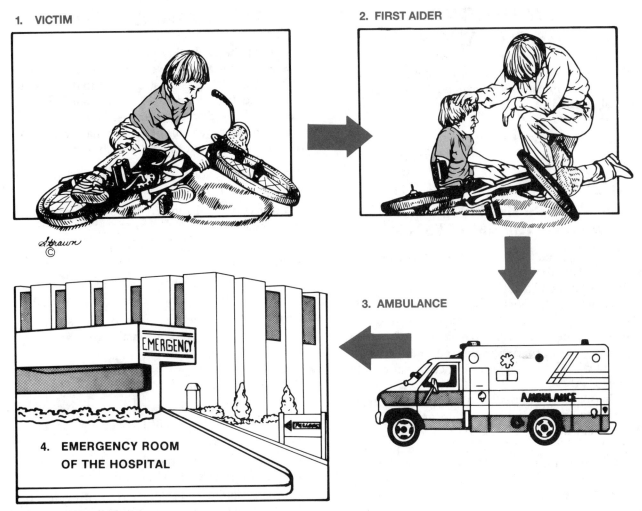

FIGURE 1-2. The emergency care team.

The effects of an accident or a sudden illness may change the function and structure of the body. The goal of first aid is to not allow these changes to cause death or permanent injury. The avoidance of untimely accidents and illnesses directly prevents suffering and loss of lives.

First Aiders should be able to recognize life-threatening problems, supply artificial ventilation and circulation, control bleeding, and protect injuries from infection and other complications. They should then be able to arrange for medical assistance and transportation. When first aid is administered properly, the victim's chances of recovery are increased greatly.

First Aiders must be able to take charge of a situation, keep calm while working under pressure, and organize others to do likewise. By demonstrating competence and using well-selected words of encouragement, First Aiders should win the confidence of others nearby and do everything possible to reassure the apprehensive victim.

GENERAL DIRECTIONS

The First Aider is generally involved in a sudden injury or illness situation that requires fast thinking and action. This necessitates a plan of action.

- Observe the accident scene as you approach it.
- If necessary, have others direct traffic and position safety flares, keep bystanders at a safe distance, make essential telephone calls, turn off engines that may be still running, etc.
- Provide basic life support to those whose lives are threatened. Give first aid to the most seriously injured victims first.

EVALUATING THE SITUATION

When a person is injured, someone must (1) take charge, (2) administer first aid, and (3) arrange for medical assistance.

ARRANGING FOR MEDICAL ASSISTANCE (ACTIVATING THE EMS SYSTEM)

During the first minutes after an accident, it is essential that the Emergency Medical Services (EMS) system be activated. If a victim has suffered a heart attack, the First Aider activates the EMS system as soon as the victim is found pulseless. In other situations where victims have a pulse and are breathing, they should be stabilized while another First Aider finds a telephone to activate the EMS system.

In the majority of urban and in some rural areas in the United States, the First Aider can activate the EMS system by telephoning 911. Other areas will have a local emergency number. If the emergency number is unknown, the First Aider should dial 0 (zero or operator). After the proper connection is made, the following information should be given to the dispatcher:

- The exact location, such as the correct and complete address, the number of the floor or office in the building, or any other information that will identify the exact location of the victim.

- A correct phone number where the First Aider may be reached.

- Any necessary information that will help the dispatcher send appropriate personnel and equipment.

If possible, the First Aider should send a responsible bystander to telephone with the above information. If the First Aider is alone, he should perform the ABC's (airway, breathing, circulation) of emergency care for one minute, then quickly telephone for help. If no telephone is available, the First Aider should continue giving emergency care until a bystander is available to activate the EMS medical system. First Aiders should take charge with full recognition of their own limitations and, while caring for life-threatening conditions, should briefly and clearly explain to others what they should do to obtain assistance.

FIRST AIDER SKILLS

Some of the skills that you have or will need to acquire as a First Aider have already been discussed. The following is a basic list of skills that forms the core of the first-aid course. Other skills may be added to the course by your instructors. You may want to check these skills off as you master them. At the conclusion of your course, you should be able to:

- Control the accident scene so that further injury will not occur.

- Gain access to victims in the easiest and safest ways possible.

- Effectively and quickly evaluate the accident scene for cause, and control it for safety.

- Obtain information about the accident or sudden illness from bystanders and the victim(s).

- Perform quick, effective primary and secondary surveys, including taking vital signs (breathing, pulse, skin temperature).

- Determine any diagnostic signs and relate those to possible injuries or sudden illnesses that require emergency care.

- Perform the necessary ABCBs of emergency care.
  A — Open airway.
  B — Breathing (breathlessness — provide artificial ventilation).
  C — Circulation (pulselessness — provide one- and two-rescuer cardiopulmonary resuscitation).
  B — Bleeding control (hemorrhage controlled by direct pressure and elevation, pressure points, and tourniquets).

- Detect any spinal injuries and immobilize accordingly.

- Detect and care for shock.

- Detect and care for soft-tissue and internal injuries, including performing basic dressing and bandaging techniques.

- Detect and care for open and closed fractures, sprains, strains, and dislocations, including providing cold treatment and basic splinting.

- Detect and care for poisoning, including alcohol and drug abuse.

- Detect and care for heart attack, stroke, diabetic coma, insulin shock, and epileptic or other seizures.

- Detect and care for facial and head injuries, neck and spinal injuries, and chest injuries, including fractured ribs, flail chest, and penetrating chest wounds.

- Detect and care for first-, second-, and third-degree burns and smoke inhalation.
- Detect and care for exposure to heat and cold, including heat cramps, heat exhaustion, heat stroke, hypothermia, and frostbite.
- Assist in childbirth and care of the newborn.
- Give psychological and proper first aid care to victims of crisis and disasters.
- Perform non-emergency and emergency moves and other proper transportation techniques.

LEGAL ASPECTS OF FIRST AID

It is natural for a First Aider to wonder if he can safely give a victim emergency care and be free from liability or litigation. Legally, you are not forced to give emergency care, but becoming a First Aider indicates that you choose to do so.

GOOD SAMARITAN LAWS

In certain instances, a victim may feel justified in (or may simply try to justify) suing a First Aider for the way in which the victim was handled during emergency care. In order to protect health-care personnel from being sued, states have enacted **GOOD SAMARITAN LAWS**. These laws indicate that the practitioner (First Aider) is not held liable for his actions as long as he does not do anything that can be defined as grossly negligent or that constitutes willful misconduct. Because of these laws, lawsuits against emergency medical personnel (such as First Aiders) have been extremely rare. Good Samaritan laws provide some guidelines for personnel rendering aid and make it difficult for one who is aided to sue.

If such a case *is* taken to court, the case is prosecuted as a tort proceeding — a civil court action designed to determine whether the natural rights of an individual have been violated. A tort action is not a criminal action or one involving a broken contract or failure to pay a debt.

In tort proceedings involving emergency medical personnel, the First Aider must be accused of negligence — carelessness, inattention, disregard, inadvertence, or oversight that was accidental but avoidable. In a tort proceeding, there are three categories of negligence:

1. *Nonfeasance:* The First Aider failed to perform his duty.
2. *Misfeasance:* The First Aider failed to perform his duty properly.
3. *Malfeasance:* The First Aider performed his duty without consent.

In order to establish negligence, the court must decide that:

- The victim was injured.
- The First Aider's actions or lack of action caused or contributed to the injury.
- The First Aider had a duty to act.
- The First Aider acted in an unusual, unreasonable, or imprudent way.

OBTAIN CONSENT

It is essential that the First Aider receive consent to care for a victim. The four types of consent are:

1. *Actual consent:* To be effective, the consent must be an informed one. Oral consent is valid. A consent form does not eliminate the need for conversation.
2. *Implied consent:* In a true emergency in which the risk of death, disability, or deterioration of condition is significant, the law assumes that the victim would give his consent.
3. *Minor's consent:* The right to consent is usually given to the parent or other person so close to the minor as to be treated as a parent.
4. *Consent of the mentally ill:* The situation is similar to that for minors.

THE RIGHT TO REFUSE CARE

A competent adult has the right to refuse emergency care and/or transportation for himself or a minor who is in need of such care. There may be religious or other reasons. In this situation, make every reasonable effort to influence the victim or guardian to give consent. If the victim or guardian refuses to consent, you may *NOT* give emergency care or forcibly transport the victim. Emergency care or transportation by force may result in an assault suit. If a refusal occurs and a life is at stake, summon the police.

"REASONABLE-MAN" TEST

Critical to the First Aider's defense is the "reasonable-man" test: Did the First Aider act the same way that a normal, prudent person would have acted under the same circumstances if that normal, prudent person had the First Aider's background and training? The First Aider usually has the support of expert witnesses who are called to testify about how a person with training and background would have acted under those circumstances. The jury then decides six critical issues:

1. Did the First Aider act, or fail to act?
2. Did the victim sustain physical, psychological, or financial injury?
3. Did the action or inaction of the First Aider cause or contribute to that injury?
4. Was the victim guilty of contributing to his own injury?
5. Did the First Aider violate his duty to care for the victim?
6. If the victim proves his case, what damages should be awarded?

In any court case of this kind, the burden of proof is on the victim. The only time that the First Aider *can* be prosecuted is when he is guilty of gross negligence, recklessness, willfull or wanton conduct, or intentional injury to the victim.

Basically, the First Aider's duty legally can be defined as follows:

■ The First Aider should not interfere with the first aid help being given by others.

■ The First Aider should follow the directions of a police officer and do what a reasonable First Aider would do under the circumstances.

■ The First Aider should not force his help on a victim unless the situation is life-threatening (such as severe bleeding, attempted suicide, poisoning, cardiac arrest, and so on). When the victim is unconscious, consent is automatic (by law). If the victim is not in a life-threatening situation and if he resists care, the First Aider can be charged with battery (physical contact of a person's body or clothing without consent) if care is forced on the victim without consent.

■ Once a First Aider has voluntarily started care, he should not leave the scene or stop the care until a qualified and responsible person relieves him; if he does, it constitutes abandonment.

■ The First Aider should follow accepted and recognized emergency care procedures taught in this and other first-aid texts.

AIDS AND FIRST AID

AIDS is a disease that renders the immune system ineffective. The AIDS virus (which has been named HIV by various groups of researchers) enters the body and affects the immune system's T-lymphocytes. The body can no longer recognize and respond to foreign cells, like viruses and cancer cells, and as a result can no longer fight disease.

The AIDS virus can be transmitted by a person who is ill with AIDS, by a person who has AIDS-related complex, or by a person who carries the AIDS virus (HIV) but does not have symptoms. HIV is extremely fragile and unable to survive very long outside the human body, so it cannot be transmitted casually. Researchers have confirmed that the only way AIDS can be transmitted is by intimate contact with the bodily fluids of an infected individual (even though the infected individual may not realize that he is sick).

AIDS cannot be transmitted by shaking hands, coughing, sneezing, sharing meals, sharing eating utensils, or any other casual contact. You cannot get AIDS from toilet seats, towels, office equipment, eating utensils, or other objects casually handled by infected persons. *AIDS transmission requires intimate contact with the bodily fluids (mostly semen, blood, and cervical secretions) of infected persons.* This contact usually occurs through sexual intercourse, infected needles, or infected blood and blood products.

Health-care workers are advised to protect themselves from HIV by wearing surgical gloves, masks, protective eyewear, and gowns. However, this is very impractical for First Aiders. You *should* take the following practical precautions:

■ Immediately wash your hands with soap and warm water if contaminated with blood or other bodily fluids.

■ Try to prevent injuries caused by any sharp instrument while giving first aid.

■ Use a pocket mask or mouthpiece, where possible, while administering mouth-to-mouth resuscitation.

Remember that the risk of contracting AIDS or other infections from a victim while giving first aid is very remote. Do not withhold first aid because of this unlikely possibility.

CONTROVERSIES IN FIRST AID CARE

The first aid and emergency-care procedures in this text are accepted practices in the United States. However, there are still some areas of controversy in first aid care. The most common and accepted procedures are presented in this text. When controversies exist, the student is advised to follow local protocol. [Follow the guidelines of your instructor.]

| **1** | **SELF-TEST** | **1** |

Student: _____ Date: _____

Course: _____ Section #: _____

PART I: True/False   If you believe that the statement is true, circle the T. If you believe that the statement is false, circle the F.

T (F) 1. Accidents are the leading cause of death among those from age one to thirty-eight, and twice as many women die from accidents as do men.

(T) F 2. An injured person should not be moved immediately unless a specific hazard — such as fire, spilled chemicals, or noxious fumes — is present.

(T) F 3. Two important words in a definition of first aid are immediate and temporary.

(T) F 4. Activating the EMS system is an important part of first aid.

T F 5. A First Aider should explain the victim's probable condition to concerned bystanders.

T (F) 6. The first thing to do for an injured person is to control bleeding.

(T) F 7. One of the main concerns of a First Aider is to prevent adding injury or death.

(T) F 8. It is as important to know what *not* to do as well as what *to* do.

(T) F 9. The First Aider should not worry about activating the Emergency Medical Services system until all possible emergency care has been given.

(T) F 10. An important part of first aid is to control the accident scene.

T (F) 11. A person who receives first-aid training is required by law to stop and help at an accident scene.

PART II: Multiple Choice   For each question, circle the answer that best reflects an accurate statement.

1. Accidents are the leading cause of death for which age group:
   - (a) 1 to 38 years old.
   - b. 40 to 45 years old.
   - c. 46 to 49 years old.
   - d. 70 to 90 years old.

2. First aid is the immediate action taken to:
   - (a) care for the injured until medical help is available.
   - b. supplement proper medical or surgical treatment.
   - c. preserve vitality and resistance to disease.
   - d. rescue and transport the injured.

3. When administering first aid, the condition that should be cared for first is:
   - a. the most painful one.
   - (b) the most life-threatening one.
   - c. the most obvious one.
   - d. bleeding.

4. Avoid moving an injured victim until all injuries are identified so that:
   - a. investigating authorities can know what happened.
   - b. the victim will not suffer unnecessary pain.
   - c. the victim can be stabilized before being moved.
   - (d) the victim will not suffer further injury.
   - e. it is not necessary to identify injuries before moving a victim.

5. By definition, first aid is:
   - (a) immediate care given to someone who is ill or injured.
   - b. care administered at home.
   - c. self help.
   - d. all of the above.

6. Which of the following is an immediate priority?
   - (a) determining the cause of injury.
   - b. controlling severe bleeding.
   - c. taking measures to keep the victim warm.
   - d. all of the above.

7. Under normal circumstances, the best first contact for help in case of accident is:
   - a. the hospital emergency room.
   - b. the fire department.
   - c. the police or highway patrol.
   - d. the Emergency Medical Services (EMS) system.

8. If the First Aider is alone, what should he do about telephoning for help?
   - a. he should telephone quickly and then begin emergency care.
   - b. he should perform the ABCBs of emergency care for one minute, then phone.
   - c. he should concentrate on emergency care and not take time to phone.
   - (d) he should stabilize the victim and then phone.

9. The "reasonable-man" test is:
   a. administered to a First Aider to test his skills in practical logic before he is allowed to begin victim care.
   b. administered to a normal, prudent person to determine what personality traits a First Aider should have.
   c. administered to the First Aider to ascertain if his actions during a given victim-care experience were fair, reasonable, and unbiased.
   d. to determine if the First Aider acted as a normal, prudent person with First Aider training would have acted.

10. What can the First Aider be charged with if he administers care when the victim is not in a life-threatening situation and refuses care?
    a. negligence.
    b. battery.
    c. abandonment.
    d. assault.

11. What has first priority in emergency care?
    a. open the airway.
    b. control hemorrhage.
    c. determine if there is a pulse.
    d. stabilize any possible head, neck, or back fractures.

PART III: Matching Match the following terms with their proper meaning.

_3_ Actual consent

_1_ Implied consent

_2_ Minor's consent

1. In a true emergency, the law assumes that the victim would give his consent.
2. The right to consent is given to the parent or guardian.
3. An informed consent.

PART IV: Practical Skills Check-Off The following is a list of first-aid and emergency-care skills. Read them through and indicate if you feel prepared to perform them by checking the appropriate column.*

FIRST AID SKILLS	At Beginning of Your Course Yes	No	At Conclusion of Your Course Yes	No
1. Control the accident scene so that further injury will not occur.				
2. Gain access to victims in the easiest and safest way possible.				
3. Effectively and quickly evaluate the accident scene for cause, and control the scene for safety.				
4. Obtain information about the accident or sudden illness from bystanders and the victim(s).				
5. Perform quick, effective primary and secondary victim surveys, including vital signs (breathing, pulse, skin temperature).				
6. Determine any diagnostic signs and relate those to possible injuries or sudden illnesses that require emergency care.				
7. Perform the necessary ABCBs of emergency care. A - Open Airway. B - Breathing (Breathlessness — provide artificial ventilation). C - Circulation (Pulselessness — provide one- and two-rescuer cardiopulmonary resuscitation). B - Bleeding Control (Hemorrhage controlled by direct pressure and elevation, pressure points, and tourniquets).				
8. Detect and care for shock.				
9. Detect and care for soft-tissue and internal injuries, including performing basic dressing and bandaging techniques.				
10. Detect and care for open and closed fractures, sprains, and dislocations, including providing cold treatment and basic splinting.				
11. Detect and care for poisoning, including alcohol and drug abuse.				

*Check this list again at the end of your course to measure improvement in your preparation.

CHAPTER TWO

OBJECTIVES

■ Understand the organization of a proper victim assessment.

■ Distinguish between signs and symptoms.

■ Learn how to establish rapport with the victim and control the scene.

■ Describe and conduct a primary survey, learn how to determine the chief complaint, and understand the significance of vital signs (pulse, respiration, blood pressure).

■ Know how to conduct a neuro exam.

■ Describe how to take a history.

■ Understand the sequence and practical application of the secondary survey.

VICTIM ASSESSMENT

The ability to assess a conscious or unconscious victim is one of the most important and critical parts of first aid. Without being able to assess at least roughly, you cannot possibly know where to begin or what care to give the victim. Another important skill critical to a life-threatening emergency is the ability to monitor vital signs.

Injury victims may have obvious, easy-to-see injuries or hidden, not-easy-to-see injuries. Some victims will be conscious and be able to direct you to their injuries. Others may be unconscious and of no help. Some easy-to-see injuries (e.g., a bleeding soft-tissue wound) may look threatening but not be nearly as life-threatening as an obstructed airway, which is harder to recognize.

To administer proper first aid, you must understand how to assess correctly. This chapter will teach you a routine that will cover all of the important points in an order that has been refined by the experience of many emergency-care providers. If you follow this order, you will not overlook important areas, and you will be able to establish priorities for emergency care.

Having a well-practiced routine also will help you maintain control during tense and disorienting situations (multiple injuries, grotesque or hemorrhaging

injuries) when you could become "rattled." You also will need to learn how to take a history in a certain order, asking questions that omit no vital points. Victim assessment and history taking have three main purposes:

1. To win the victim's confidence and thereby alleviate some of the anxiety contributing to discomfort.

2. To rapidly identify the victim's problem(s) and establish which one(s) require immediate care in the field.

3. To obtain information about the victim that may not be readily available later in the hospital (e.g., observations about the environment in which the victim was found).

SIGNS AND SYMPTOMS

Signs and symptoms are different, yet the terms are often used interchangeably by emergency medical personnel. They should *not* be. A **SIGN** is something that the First Aider observes or sees about a victim such as a deep arm laceration or a leg deformed by a fracture (Figure 2-1). A **SYMPTOM** is something that the victim feels and describes to the First Aider, such as pain in the abdomen or head, or a feeling of **NAUSEA** or dizziness (Figure 2-2).

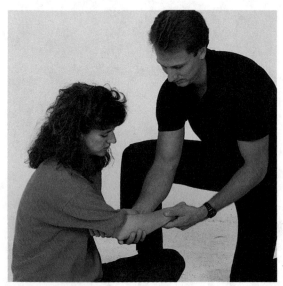

FIGURE 2-1. A victim exhibiting a sign, such as a deformed wrist.

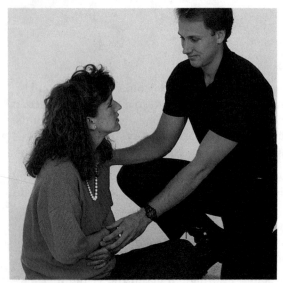

FIGURE 2-2. A victim describing a symptom, such as a stomach pain.

THE ROUTINE OF VICTIM ASSESSMENT

This chapter organizes the discussion on victim assessment in the order listed below. Remember — experience and the specific emergency situation will tell you when to adapt or change this sequence.

1. Arriving at the scene.
2. Establishing rapport and controlling the scene.
3. Conducting a primary survey.
4. Determining the chief complaint.
5. Assessing vital signs.
6. Looking for medical information devices.
7. Conducting a neuro exam.
8. Taking a history.
9. Conducting a secondary survey.

ARRIVING AT THE SCENE

As you arrive at the scene, quickly assess the environment and/or the victim(s). The accident or illness situation may indicate potential problems (e.g., the presence of police cars may be indicative of trauma or violence). Are any environmental dangers present (e.g., dangling power lines, icy roads, fuel spills)? Are the police present and in control of the traffic? Is the mechanism of injury (how the person was injured) observable? Take all appropriate safety precautions to protect yourself, bystanders, and victims at the scene.

ESTABLISHING RAPPORT AND CONTROLLING THE SCENE

When you arrive at an accident or illness situation, you may find the people hurt, frightened, anxious, and possibly angry and in shock. These are all high-intensity emotions. You will need to establish scene control by utilizing the three "C"s: competence, confidence, and compassion. If you convey these qualities, you will get better cooperation and have to deal with few irrational responses.

These three "C"s will be exhibited through your personal appearance and professional manner. If the victim is alert and no obvious life-threatening conditions are present, it may be appropriate to be briefed by a relative or someone who witnessed the accident or sudden illness. This need not take more than a minute. Look directly at the person and say, "I'm (your name), and trained in emergency care. Can you tell me what's happened here and what emergency care has been given?" However, if the victim is unconscious and life-threatening injuries are observed, go directly to the victim and ask bystanders questions while you give emergency care.

After the briefing, go directly to the victim. Observe any clues at the scene that may help you in assessment, such as:

■ Damage to a vehicle or other mechanism of injury.

- The victim's position.
- Pills or food in the environment.
- Warmth of the environment.
- Anything else that may help you better assess the victim's condition.

Introduce yourself to the conscious victim and ask for the victim's name. Be sure to also say, "I'm going to help you. Is that all right?" This is the important matter of receiving consent for emergency care discussed in Chapter 1. Continue to address the victim by name throughout the examination.

Maintain eye contact during these important first few seconds and be courteous. Speak calmly and deliberately. People who are under stress or in medical shock process information more slowly. Speak distinctly. Raise your voice only if the person is hard of hearing or disoriented. Otherwise, try to give orders quietly. People follow emotions, and emotions can escalate quickly in tense situations. Smooth, rather than jerky, movements also communicate competence and control.

Place yourself at a comfortable level in relation to the victim. If your eye level is above that of the victim, you are in a dominant position, denoting authority and control. If the eye levels are equal, so is the authority. Since you usually want the victim to remain immobile, position yourself so that he is not tempted to twist his neck or tip his head.

Victim assessment must be unhurried and systematic; a hasty, shotgun approach always leads to omissions. Learn to perform a victim assessment and take a history in a specific order so that no important information is missed. Let the urgency of the situation determine the detail of your questions.

The remainder of this chapter will discuss how to conduct a **PRIMARY SURVEY**, how to take **VITAL SIGNS**, how to take a **HISTORY**, and how to conduct a **SECONDARY SURVEY**(Figure 2-3). *In the field, the order will be dictated by circumstances.* You must always deal first with life-threatening emergencies like obstructed airways, cardiac arrest, and severe bleeding.

Some of the survey steps can be done simultaneously. You can take a pulse, notice skin color and temperature, and ask, "What happened?" all in the same few seconds. You may want to take the history while taking vital signs, conducting the secondary survey, or giving emergency care. Let judgment and experience dictate the best order of approach.

Be systematic but flexible. Remember — your victim's condition, or a change in that condition, warrants rearranging usual priorities. As you work

VICTIM ASSESSMENT PYRAMID

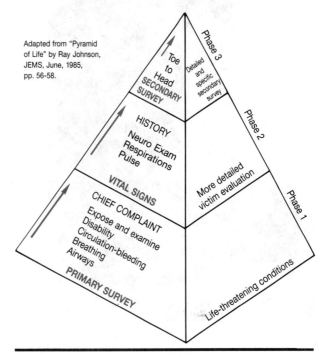

Adapted from "Pyramid of Life" by Ray Johnson, JEMS, June, 1985, pp. 56-58.

FIGURE 2-3.

through the evaluation, remember that your major concerns are:

- To identify and correct any life-threatening problems.
- To protect yourself from harm and injury.
- To render proper emergency care.
- To stabilize and prepare the victim for possible transportation.

CONDUCTING A PRIMARY SURVEY

The major goal of the primary survey is to evaluate for life-threatening problems. This is accomplished through the following steps.

- Ask, "What happened?" The victim's response will tell you the airway status, the adequacy of **VENTILATIONS**, and the level of consciousness. You may also find out the **MECHANISM OF INJURY** and information about other victims.
- Then ask, "Where do you hurt?" This question will identify the most likely points of injury (Figure 2-4).
- Visually scan the victim for general appearance, **CYANOSIS** (blueness from lack of oxygen), and sweating.

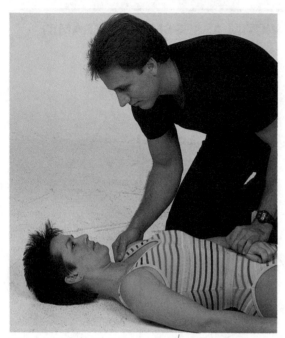

FIGURE 2-4. Ask, "What happened?" and, "Where do you hurt?"

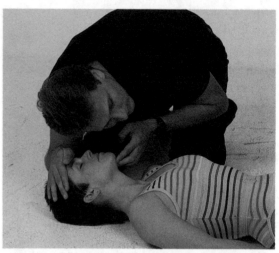

FIGURE 2-5. Establish an open airway, then check for adequate breathing by the look-listen-feel technique. Assure an adequate open airway by the head tilt/chin lift method.

You now have a very quick idea of your victim's overall condition. The rest of the primary survey consists of identifying conditions that may *become* life-threatening. The five steps of the primary survey are:

1. Airway and cervical spine.
2. Breathing.
3. Circulation — bleeding.
4. Disability.
5. Expose and examine.

You should be able to conduct this survey in *sixty seconds* unless you find life-threatening problems that must be treated immediately.

Airway and Cervical Spine

■ *Airway.* Is it open? (Figure 2-5) Are blood, secretions, etc. making it hard for the victim to breathe? Chapter 3 describes two methods for clearing the airway: (1) the **HEAD TILT/CHIN LIFT** and (2) the **MODIFIED JAW THRUST** (Figure 2-6).

■ *Cervical Spine.* The way in which the airway is opened will be determined by the potential for a cervical-spine injury. Movement of a fractured spine to establish an airway can cause **NEURO-LOGICAL** damage. Pay attention to the mechanism of injury, what the victim tells you, and any deformity. If there is a potential cervical spine

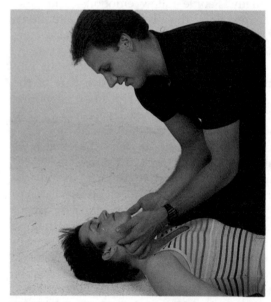

FIGURE 2-6. If a cervical spine injury is suspected, use a modified jaw thrust to open the victim's airway.

injury, the modified jaw thrust is used, and the victim's neck should be immobilized with the most efficient method available.

Breathing

Is the victim breathing? How? Is breathing absent or adequate? Check approximate rate, depth, regularity, and ease. *Look* and listen at the chest for open wounds (**SUCKING CHEST WOUNDS**), and at the diaphragm for normal breathing movements. *Listen* for breathing sounds at the mouth and nose, and *feel* whether air is passing in and out of the nose and/or mouth (Figure 2-7). Note the skin color. Is there any cyanosis? If you suspect chest injuries that may complicate breathing, give the proper emergency care.

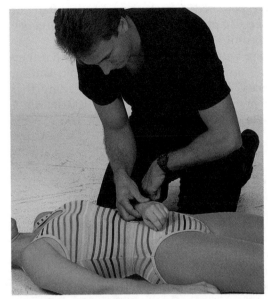

FIGURE 2-8. Palpate (feel) the radial pulse at the wrist.

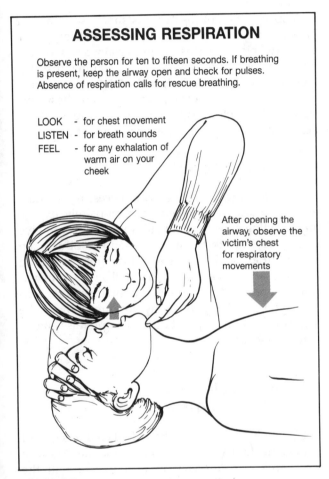

ASSESSING RESPIRATION

Observe the person for ten to fifteen seconds. If breathing is present, keep the airway open and check for pulses. Absence of respiration calls for rescue breathing.

LOOK - for chest movement
LISTEN - for breath sounds
FEEL - for any exhalation of warm air on your cheek

After opening the airway, observe the victim's chest for respiratory movements

FIGURE 2-7.

usually the last pulse to disappear if the victim goes into shock.) Is the pulse absent or adequate?

At the same time, check for serious or profuse bleeding. (If you can, put on a pair of latex or surgical gloves to protect yourself against possible contamination.) Is there major external hemorrhage? Cut clothing away quickly to see a bleeding site clearly. Check for bleeding by gently, but thoroughly and quickly, running your hands over and under the head and neck, upper extremities, chest and abdomen, pelvis and buttocks, and lower extremities (Figure 2-9). Use extreme care in case a spinal injury

If the victim is not breathing spontaneously, begin **ARTIFICIAL VENTILATION** immediately and continue until spontaneous breathing recurs or until you are relieved by trained personnel (see Chapter 3). If the victim is breathing adequately through an open airway, continue the primary survey.

Circulation — Bleeding

Now determine if heart action and blood circulation are present by palpating (feeling) the **RADIAL PULSE** at the wrist (Figure 2-8); or, if the victim is unconscious and the radial pulse is absent, palpate the **CAROTID PULSE** in the neck. (The carotid pulse is

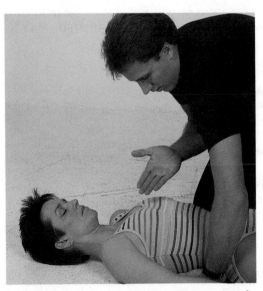

FIGURE 2-9. Perform a quick body sweep for bleeding, check your hands often for blood.

may have occurred. Check your hands often for blood. See Chapter 6 for the necessary emergency care to control bleeding.

Bleeding wounds can be misleading in that they sometimes are not as serious as they look. During the primary survey, only deal with bleeding that requires immediate action, such as **HEMORRHAGE** that is spurting or flowing freely.

Disability

After the airway, breathing, and circulation have been assessed, note any signs and/or symptoms that make you suspect damage to the central nervous system.

Check the level of consciousness (LOC) and responsiveness. (See "Conducting a Neuro Exam" later in this chapter for a more detailed discussion.) If the brain does not receive enough oxygen or glucose, it will not be able to control thought, speech, and skills. Changes in mental states may reveal a potential medical problem.

Assess the victim's level of consciousness by noting the quality of his response to the question, "Are you okay?" Observe if the victim's extremities move spontaneously. The victim's LOC or "mental state," can be described using the following memory device — AVPU:

A = Alert.
V = Voice commands bring responses.
P = Painful stimuli bring responses.
U = Unresponsive.

The victim is alert or **ORIENTED** to person, place, and date if he can focus on you and answer the following questions. If he cannot, he is **DISORIENTED**. Ask:

■ What's your name?

■ What's happened to you?

■ Where were you going, or where are you?

■ Can you tell me the date (day of the week, year, etc.)?

Document and record the victim's condition precisely, e.g., "disoriented to time." Do not ask yes-no questions; do not ask questions for which you do not know the answer; and if the victim cannot answer a specific question, get more general. The victim is **RESPONSIVE** if he seems to be unconscious but will:

■ Open his eyes if you speak to him or try to answer a question.

■ Respond to a light touch on the hand.

If you even suspect a head or neck injury, tell the victim to lie very still (**GROUND SPLINT**), immobilize the neck as best as you can, and call for medical assistance to transport the victim as soon as possible. Keep the head and neck in alignment at all times. Another First Aider can guard the stability of the spine. (See "Conducting a Neuro Examination" later in this chapter to learn how to check for neurological damage.)

A special type of disability is shock (see Chapter 7). Shock is an acute circulatory deficiency (inadequate blood perfusion in certain areas of the body). Shock often accompanies trauma (psychological as well as physical) and **ACUTE** illness. If the victim is likely to develop shock or manifests the signs and symptoms, give emergency care for shock before moving on to the next assessment step.

Expose and Examine

Expose as much of the body as necessary to examine for injuries and bleeding. Completely expose any bleeding sites so that you can examine and give emergency care to the whole wound. Clothing can hide injuries, so do not be afraid to remove clothing as necessary. It is a good idea to tell a conscious victim or concerned bystanders (family members, etc.) what you are doing and why you are doing it. Be cognizant of modesty, but do not compromise quality emergency care.

DETERMINING THE CHIEF COMPLAINT

Up to this point, you have looked for signs of immediate injury or illness to check the ABCs of emergency care. You were more concerned with the quality of the response when you asked the victim, "Are you okay?" Now it is time to ask specific questions and listen carefully to the victim's symptoms.

The answer you receive from the victim when you ask, "Can you tell me where you are hurt?" is the **CHIEF COMPLAINT**. In many instances, this will be obvious, such as the victim who lies bleeding in the street after being struck by an automobile. Even in this circumstance, however, it is useful to determine what is bothering the victim most, for his report may lead you to unexpected findings. For example, the victim who is struck by a car may have a dramatically obvious **OPEN FRACTURE** of the leg, yet his chief complaint may be, "I can't breathe," leading you to discover an unsuspected chest injury. Most chief complaints are characterized by pain, abnormal function, some change from a normal state, or an observation made by the victim.

If the victim is not conscious, the chief complaint may come from a "Can you tell me what happened?" question directed to a nearby relative or other bystander.

ASSESSING VITAL SIGNS

After the chief complaint has been investigated, the victim's vital signs (pulse, respirations, temperature, and skin color) should be assessed. Knowing how to read and interpret these signs correctly determines how successful your emergency care will be. Vital signs should be repeated at two- to five-minute intervals. Changes in vital signs reflect not only alterations in victim condition, but the effectiveness of your emergency care. You can monitor all of these vital signs with your senses (look, listen, feel, smell).

Pulse

Each time the heart beats, the arteries expand and contract with the blood that rushes into them. The pulse is the pressure wave generated by the heartbeat. It directly reflects the rhythm, rate, and relative strength of the contraction of the heart. It can be felt at any point where an artery crosses over a bone or lies near the skin. When you take a pulse, you should note the following:

▪ Its rate — slow or fast. This important reading is expressed in beats per minute. Normal resting rates are 60 to 80 beats per minute for an adult and 80 to 200 beats per minute for a child.

▪ Its strength — a normal pulse is full and strong. A **THREADY PULSE** is weak and rapid. A **BOUNDING PULSE** is unusually strong.

▪ Its rhythm — an **IRREGULAR PULSE** is one that is spaced irregularly. A normal pulse is regular. Irregularity of beats usually signifies cardiac disease.

As an example, you might express the pulse of a victim as "72, strong and regular." The rate, strength, and regularity of the pulse are relative indicators of cardiac function. They tell what the heart is doing at any given time. When taken in conjunction with other vital signs and observations of a victim's overall appearance, the pulse can help a First Aider to determine the *effectiveness* of circulation.

First Aiders most commonly take the pulse at the wrist where the radial artery crosses the **DISTAL** end of the **RADIUS**. This is the larger of the two major arteries that supply the hand. The other, not as easy

to palpate, is the **ULNAR ARTERY**, also named for the bone associated with it. To take the radial pulse:

▪ The victim should usually be lying down or sitting.

▪ Use the tips of two or three fingers, and examine the pulse gently by touch.

▪ You can count the number of beats for fifteen seconds and multiply by four to obtain the number of beats per minute.

▪ Always write down the pulse and any other vital signs immediately after taking them. Do not rely on your memory.

▪ Avoid using your thumb to take pulses, as the thumb has a prominent pulse of its own that may be palpated by mistake.

Another area where a pulse may be taken is the **CAROTID ARTERY** in the neck (Figure 2-10).

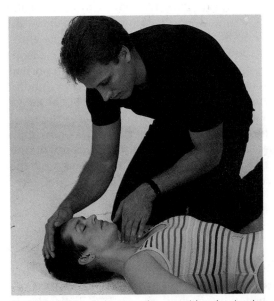

FIGURE 2-10. Palpating the carotid pulse in the neck.

A pulse rate should be taken as early as possible. Changes in rate and intensity are important, so take the pulse frequently. You can gauge what is happening to the victim by the pulse. A rapid pulse may indicate shock; a rapid, bounding pulse can occur with fright. Absence of pulse indicates that an artery has been blocked or injured, that the blood pressure is very low, or that the heart has stopped beating. A change in the pulse can mean changes in the heart (due to injury, alarm, or death), in the amount of blood circulating through the vessels, in the blood vessels themselves, or even in the effectiveness of respiration.

Respiration

The number of times per minute that a person breathes in and out can be a telltale sign of injury or illness. A respiration consists of one inhalation plus one exhalation. The normal number of respirations per minute varies with the sex and age of the victim, but the average is twelve to twenty times per minute. Normal respirations are easy and occur without pain or effort.

The depth of a victim's respirations gives a clue as to the *volume* of air that is being exchanged in a given amount of time; e.g., a minute. You can gauge depth of respiration by placing your hand on the victim's chest and feeling for chest movement. If the victim appears to be an **ABDOMINAL BREATHER** (the chest does not seem to move, but the abdomen does), simply feel the abdomen instead. Either way, you should note at least one inch of expansion in a forward direction.

How difficult does breathing seem to be for the victim? You can tell this in several ways. Normally, the work required by breathing is minimal; we do not even think about it. It does require some effort to inhale, but almost none to exhale. For this reason, normal inspiration takes slightly longer than normal exhalation. Prolonged expiration is seen frequently in victims with **CHRONIC OBSTRUCTIVE PULMONARY DISORDERS (COPD)** such as emphysema. Prolonged inspiration indicates an upper airway obstruction. Cardinal signs of respiratory distress include flaring of the nostrils, contracting of the trachea, and the use of accessory muscles in the neck and abdomen.

Temperature

The most common temperature taken by First Aiders in the field is **RELATIVE SKIN TEMPERATURE**, accomplished by touching the victim's skin with the back of the hand (Figure 2-11). It is useful as an indicator of abnormally low and high temperatures.

Normally, skin temperature rises as blood vessels near the skin **DILATE**, and it falls as blood vessels **CONSTRICT. FEVER** and high environmental temperatures cause vessels to dilate, while shock causes vessels to constrict under most circumstances. Normal skin is fairly dry. Stimulation of the sympathetic nervous system, as in shock, normally results in perspiration, **PALLOR**, and cool skin. Depression of the **SYMPATHETIC NERVOUS SYSTEM**, as may occur in cervical, thoracic, or lumbar spine injuries, can cause the skin in the affected areas to be abnormally dry and cool. Placing the back of your hand against the victim's forehead will give you some idea of skin temperature.

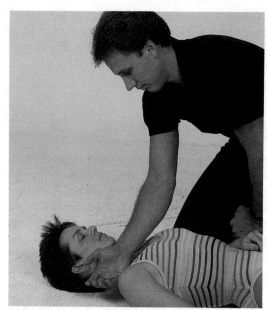

FIGURE 2-11. For relative skin temperature, touch the victim's skin with the back of your hand.

Changes in temperature can alert you to certain injuries and illnesses. A victim whose temperature is low may be suffering from shock, **HEAT EXHAUSTION**, or exposure to cold; a high temperature can result from fever in illness or **HEAT STROKE.**

The body temperature can change over a period of time or be different in various areas of the body. Circulatory problems may result in a cold **APPENDAGE**, while an isolated "hot" area may indicate a localized **INFECTION.**

LOOKING FOR MEDICAL INFORMATION DEVICES

While taking vital signs, be on the lookout for a **MEDIC ALERT** tag, necklace, or bracelet. This medical identification may give important information about the victim.

The Medic Alert system was credited directly with saving 2,000 lives during a recent twelve-month period. Medic Alert is a nonprofit, charitable, tax-exempt organization that provides a twenty-four-hour emergency information system for the one out of five people who have a hidden medical condition, such as a heart problem, **DIABETES, EPILEPSY,** or allergies to **PENICILLIN** and other medications. In case the victim is unable to speak or communicate due to an accident or sudden illness, the emblem on the tag can alert First Aiders to the possible problem (Figure 2-12).

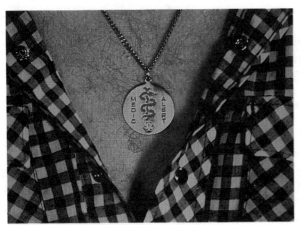

FIGURE 2-12. Medic Alert necklace.

The **VIAL OF LIFE PROGRAM** is a similar emergency medical information system being used extensively. The system uses a small, prescription-type bottle or vial that contains a medical information form filled out in advance by the victim. This vial usually is kept in the home refrigerator. Stickers near or on the front entrance of a victim's home and on the refrigerator tell First Aiders that the vial is present.

CONDUCTING A NEURO EXAMINATION

Conduct this examination anytime you suspect injury to the **NERVOUS SYSTEM**. Local protocol may place it normally during the primary or secondary exam. This exam checks three areas:

1. Level of consciousness (orientation and responsiveness).
2. Motor functions, such as voluntary movement and response to pain.
3. Sensory functions: What can the victim feel? Can he identify the stimulus? How does he respond to pain?

See the discussion earlier on level of consciousness. Talk to the victim to determine whether he is alert or confused.

■ Is he oriented to time (time of day, day of week, date), to place, and to person?
■ Note the victim's speech. Progressive slurring of words or vagueness in answering questions, especially when the victim formerly spoke clearly and coherently, indicates a decreasing level of consciousness. Garbled words may indicate a

STROKE. (Determine whether a victim may be intoxicated. An alcohol effect may duplicate or cover up signs and symptoms of another medical problem.)

■ If the victim cannot speak, try to discover whether he can understand by giving a simple command (such as, "Squeeze my hand", or, "Push my hands up or down with your feet") (Figures 2-13–2-15).
■ Estimate the alertness of young children or infants by observing their voluntary movements and their interest in their surroundings.

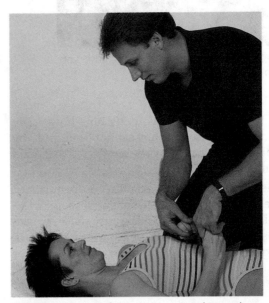

FIGURE 2-13. See if the victim can understand you by stating, "Squeeze my hand."

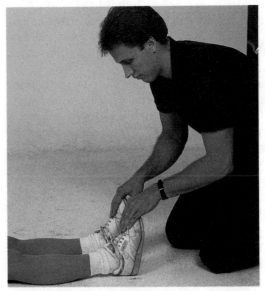

FIGURE 2-14. Assess the victim's alertness by having the victim push up your hands with the feet.

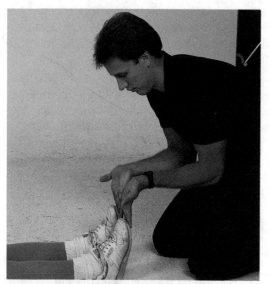

FIGURE 2-15. Then have the victim push your hands down with the feet.

- With unconscious victims, determine how easily they can be aroused. If they cannot be aroused by verbal stimuli, can they be aroused by a pain stimulus like a pinch?

- Is the victim restless, irritable, or combative? Restlessness can indicate general discomfort, a full bladder, a reaction to restraints, etc. However, restlessness is also one of the earliest signs of lack of oxygen in the blood, internal bleeding, or poisoning.

TAKING A HISTORY

Taking a history begins with scene assessment. What is the victim's position? Does the placement of the victim and any objects at the scene give clues about how the injury occurred?

Depending upon the urgency of the situation, either ask yes-no questions ("Have you eaten today?" "Does it hurt when you move your arm?") or open-ended questions ("When does the pain come on?" "Tell me about your last meal."). It is preferable to ask open-ended questions (if this is possible) so that you do not suggest answers to the victim. You might also get additional information that you did not think to ask about.

CONDUCTING A SECONDARY SURVEY

Once you have completed the quick primary survey, attended to life-threatening problems, and taken vital signs and the medical history, take a closer look at the victim and systematically examine him from head to toe for less obvious injuries or medical problems. This examination, called the secondary survey, consists of conducting a full-body assessment with your hands, checking for swelling, depression, deformity, bleeding, etc. (Figure 2-16).

Be very careful not to move the victim unnecessarily until you are sure that there are no neck or spinal injuries. The examination itself may cause the victim some discomfort, but it helps if you explain what you are going to do. Be very systematic in your approach; it will keep victim discomfort to a minimum.

Begin your examination at the head, and end it at the feet, checking all parts of the body in the following order.

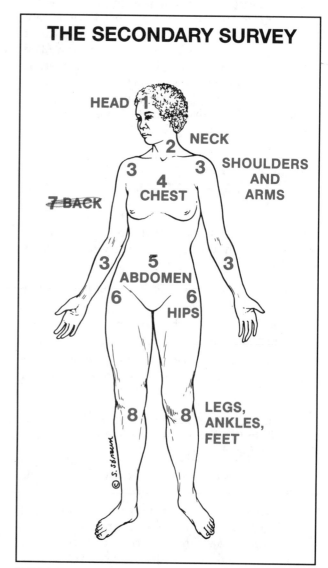

FIGURE 2-16.

Check the Facial Features

Run your fingers over the forehead, eye orbits, and facial structure to feel for abnormalities (Figure 2-17). Check the ears and nose for fluid and possible injury, the mouth for internal lacerations or unusual breath odor, and the eyes for **PUPILLARY** response and injuries (Figures 2-18 to 2-22). The face should be symmetrical, and the teeth should align well (Figure 2-23). No fluids should be coming from the ears, nose, or throat. The eyes should track a moving object smoothly and together into all four quadrants of their normal range of motion.

It may be necessary to remove contact lenses in an unconscious victim, but do not try to remove **FOREIGN OBJECTS** embedded in the eye. Place the contacts in a safe place in a container, and make sure that they are transported with the victim.

Feel the Head and Neck

Check for depressions and bruises that may indicate skull **FRACTURE** or **DISLOCATION** of **CERVICAL VERTEBRAE**. The **TRACHEA** should be in the **MIDLINE** of the neck. The neck veins should not be **DISTENDED** if the victim is sitting upright, except perhaps near the end of exhalation. The carotid pulses should be equal in intensity. The victim should be able to swallow without discomfort. The voice should not be hoarse, unless this is normal for the victim. Any tenderness in the **POSTERIOR** neck should be regarded as an indicator of cervical fracture until the victim has been examined *for that possibility* by a physician. **ANTERIOR** neck pain may indicate an injury that might **OCCLUDE** the airway or circulation to the brain (Figures 2-24–2-25).

CHECK THE FACIAL FEATURES

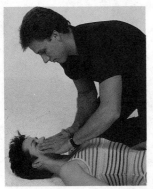

FIGURE 2-17. Run your fingers over the forehead, orbits of the eyes, and facial structure.

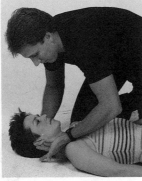

FIGURE 2-18. Check the nose and ears for blood or clear fluid (cerebrospinal fluid).

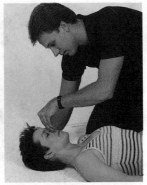

FIGURE 2-19. Gently check the nose for any possible injury.

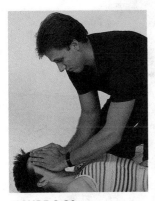

FIGURE 2-20.

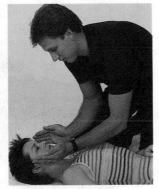

FIGURE 2-21.

Check the eyes for reactive pupils and for possible damage.

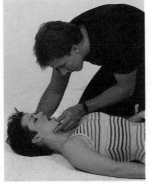

FIGURE 2-22. Check the mouth for lacerations or obstructions. Is any unusual breath odor present?

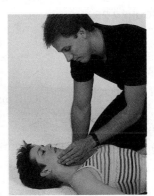

FIGURE 2-23. Check the face for symmetry and the teeth for alignment.

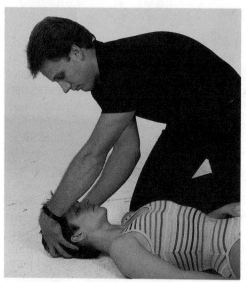

FIGURE 2-24. Gently palpate the skull for any depressions; bleeding; soft, hard or mushy lumps; etc.

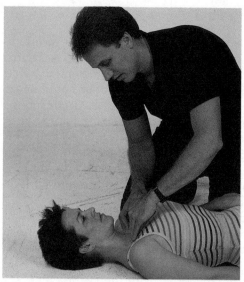

FIGURE 2-26. Palpate the clavicles and ask about any pain.

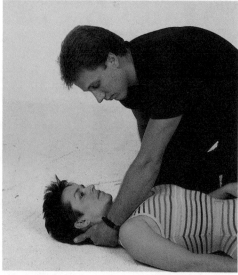

FIGURE 2-25. Gently palpate the neck to check for any abnormality of the cervical vertebrae.

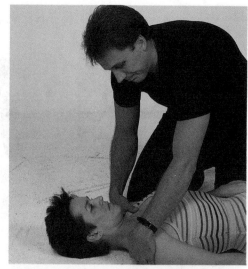

FIGURE 2-27.

If cervical-spine mechanism of injury, neck pain, or neurological deficit are *not* present, continue the survey. If they are, have a second First Aider maintain neutral or in-line immobilization of the head and neck.

Check the Clavicles and Arms

Feel the **CLAVICLES**, shoulders, and each arm. Note dislocations at the joints and any fractures. Have the victim grip your hands to see if he has equal strength in both hands (Figures 2-26–2-28).

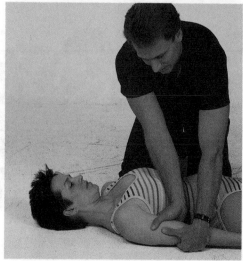

FIGURE 2-28.

Palpate each shoulder and arm.

Check the Chest

Check the chest for abnormalities, **SOFT-TISSUE** injuries, or apparent breathing problems. Be alert for cuts, bruises, and indentations, or other signs of fractures, **IMPALED OBJECTS**, or sucking chest wounds. Check for symmetry of respirations by placing the tips of your thumbs on the **XIPHOID PROCESS** (the lower tip of the breastbone) and spreading your hands over the lower rib cage. Both hands should move an equal distance with each breath. In injury victims, also feel for tenderness and instability over the ribs (Figure 2-29).

Place the ulnar edge of one hand or both hands on the sternum, one on top of the other, and push down gently (rib spring), checking for pain (Figure 2-30).

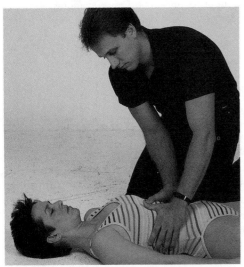

FIGURE 2-29. Apply compression to the rib cage to discover any rib-cage damage. At the same time, visually inspect the chest for deformities, wounds, and equal chest expansion.

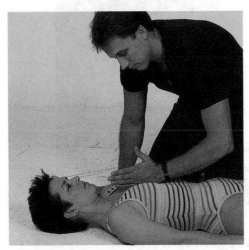

FIGURE 2-30. Gently press on the sternum for possible chest injury.

Check the Abdominal Region

Usually it is best to have the victim lying down. Keep him warm, and be sure that your hands are warm. Shivering will make the abdominal muscles tense. Be gentle, because sudden pokes will also tense the muscles.

Begin by visually examining the abdomen for protrusions, soft-tissue wounds, lumps, or swelling. Are there bruises over the **FLANK** (between the ribs and pelvis on the sides) or around the navel? If there are, the victim may be bleeding internally. Gently palpate the four quadrants of the abdomen separately, using the pads of your fingers and holding your hands almost parallel to the victim's abdomen (Figure 2-31). If you suspect injury in any area, check that region last. Gently feel for the presence of abnormal masses. Ask about abdominal pain. Pain plus a rigid (wooden or boardlike) abdomen indicates serious internal injury. The victim also will experience pain upon taking a deep breath, and he therefore may breathe shallowly. In such cases, do not put pressure on the tender area during palpation. Recognize this as a medical emergency and call for help immediately.

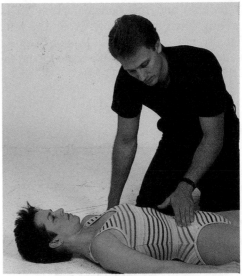

FIGURE 2-31. Visually inspect the abdomen, then palpate each quadrant for tenderness and deformity.

Check the Pelvic Region for Tenderness

Damage here can cause great pain, so be gentle. Tell the victim what you are doing and prevent embarrassment. First put your hands on each side of the hips and compress inward, checking for tenderness, **CREPITUS**, and instability (Figure 2-32). Put the

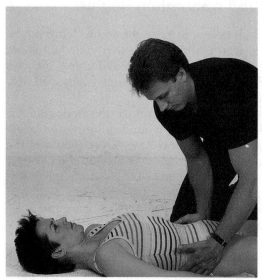

FIGURE 2-32. Put your hands on each side of the hips and compress inward, checking for tenderness, crepitus, and instability.

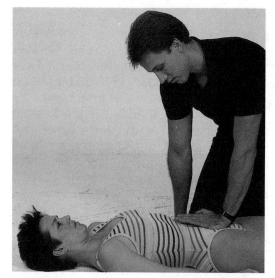

FIGURE 2-34. Apply gentle, then firmer, compression to check for pelvic fractures.

base of your hands on the **PUBIC BONES**, covering the **ILIAC CREST** (wings) and hip bones (Figure 2-33). Compress gently, then more firmly. Note any tenderness. Visually note any possible loss of bladder control, bleeding, or an erection in a male victim (a possible **CNS** injury) (Figure 2-34).

Check the Back

Without moving the victim, slip your hand beneath his back and feel for possible fractures, dislocations, or deformities.

If you need better access to the back, gently lift the victim's arm on the side that you are examining. Place the arm across his chest, with his hand toward the opposite shoulder. This will let you slip your hand down the full length of the spine. Do not lift more than is absolutely necessary (Figure 2-35). Ask

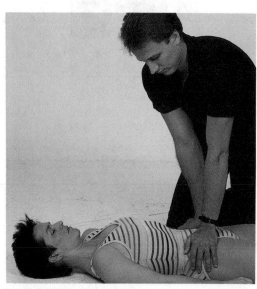

FIGURE 2-33. Put the base of your hands on the pubic bones, covering the iliac crest and hip bones.

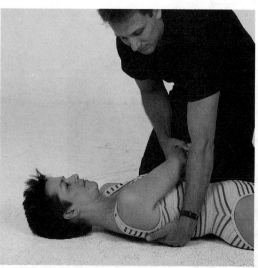

FIGURE 2-35. Check the back for point tenderness and deformity. Keep the head and neck in alignment, and be very careful of movement.

the victim to tell you if he experiences tenderness at any point. If he does, keep the victim immobile. Check simultaneously, with little or no spine movement, for bleeding in this area. Keep the victim quiet until ambulance personnel arrive, and immediately relay this information to them.

Check the Feet, Ankles, and Legs

Look for bruises, fractures, dislocations, or swelling. Check for abnormal positions of the legs. Signs of a fractured hip are a leg that is turned away, shortened, and/or rotated. Palpate the entire limb for protrusions, depressions, abnormal movement, and tenderness (Figures 2-36–2-39).

CHECK THE FEET, ANKLES, AND LEGS

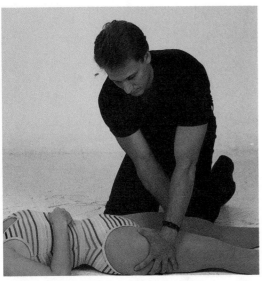

FIGURE 2-36. Check the upper leg for pain and deformity.

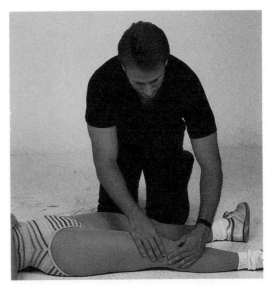

FIGURE 2-37. Palpate the knees and feel the patella (kneecap) for any pain or deformity.

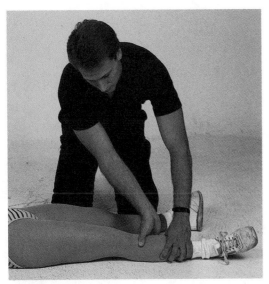

FIGURE 2-38. Feel the lower legs; palpate the tibia, ankles and feet.

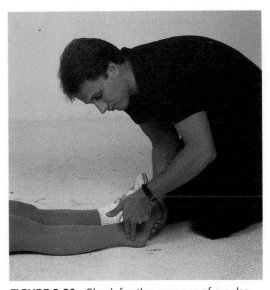

FIGURE 2-39. Check for the presence of a pulse.

Check for the presence of a pulse, sensation, and motion. Check the warmth of the limb as a circulation gauge.

PUTTING IT ALL TOGETHER

The *primary survey* (ABCDE) identified any life-threatening injuries for which you gave emergency care. The *chief complaint* helped to identify the major problem of the victim. The *vital signs* gave you a good indication of the victim's physical condition, and the *history* helped to clear the picture. The head-to-toe *secondary survey* identified any non–life-threatening problems that should have been cared for if time had allowed.

A key point is to identify and give emergency care for any life-threatening conditions and to activate the emergency-care system (ambulance) as quickly as possible. The amount of victim assessment and emergency care that you provide after the primary survey will depend upon the response time of ambulance personnel.

| **2** | **SELF-TEST** | **2** |

Student: _____   Date: _____

Course: _____ Section #: _____

PART I: True/False   If you believe that the statement is true, circle the T. If you believe that the statement is false, circle the F.

T   ~~F~~   1. Serious injuries are usually very obvious to the First Aider.

(T) F   2. It is important for a First Aider to know how an accident took place.

T (F)   3. A thready pulse is full and strong.

T (F)   4. The "B" in the "A-B-Cs" of first aid stands for "broken bones."

(T) F   5. The number-one treatment priority is an open airway.

(T) F   6. In a secondary survey, you begin at the head and usually work down the body.

T (F)   7. The normal breathing rate in the average adult is about twenty to twenty-five breaths per minute.

T (F)   8. The normal pulse rate in adults is 80 to 100 beats per minute.

PART II: Multiple Choice   For each question, circle the answer that best reflects an accurate statement.

1. In the order of priorities, which of the following are the three primary first-aid measures?
   - (a.) maintain breathing, stop bleeding, manage shock.
   - b. stop bleeding, maintain breathing, reduce shock.
   - c. prevent shock, stop bleeding, maintain breathing.
   - d. stop bleeding, prevent shock, avoid infection.

2. What should be looked for while conducting the body survey?
   - a. blood in the hair.
   - b. abdominal spasms and tenderness.
   - c. paralysis of the extremities.
   - (d.) all of the above.

3. During the course of the secondary survey, what should be done if a spinal injury is suspected?
   - a. stop the survey and call for more assistance.
   - b. stabilize the head.
   - c. continue the survey to find other problems.
   - d. stop the survey altogether.

4. How long should the First Aider spend on the primary survey?
   - a. ten to twelve minutes.
   - b. five to ten minutes.
   - c. two to three minutes.
   - (d.) one minute or less.

5. Medic Alert tags are worn:
   - a. to identify allergies.
   - b. to warn of hidden medical conditions, such as diabetes.
   - (c.) to provide pertinent information about a victim's special medical needs if he is unable to communicate due to an accident or illness.
   - d. all of the above.

6. Which step in emergency care should be taken first?
   - a. treat for shock.
   - (b.) remove victims from life-threatening situations.
   - c. summon police authorities to control bystanders and traffic.
   - d. determine the mechanism of injury.

7. The primary survey, a search for immediate life-threatening problems, is conducted in the following order:
   - a. check for bleeding, breathing, and pulse.
   - (b.) check for breathing, pulse, and bleeding.
   - c. check for pulse, breathing, and bleeding.
   - d. check for pulse, bleeding, and breathing.

8. The most common temperature taken by First Aiders in the field is the:
   - a. oral temperature.
   - (b.) relative skin temperature.
   - c. rectal temperature.
   - d. axillary temperature.

9. The secondary survey is:
   - a. a repetition of the primary survey, to locate anything that you may have missed.
   - (b.) a full-body assessment, head to toe.
   - c. an assessment of the extremities.
   - d. a check for internal injuries.

10. As you approach a conscious victim of an accident or illness, the first thing you should do is:
    - a. get close to the victim and introduce yourself.
    - b. start a victim survey without delay.
    - c. secure the scene; get bystanders to direct traffic.
    - (d.) get consent from the victim for you to treat him.

11. Level of consciousness is determined by the _____ method.
    - (a.) AVPU.
    - b. OPQRST.
    - c. BREATH.
    - d. ABCHN.

12. The first thing to do in history taking is:
    - a. assess the scene.
    - b. talk to bystanders.
    - c. take the primary survey.
    - (d.) obtain the victim's chief complaint.

13. Vital signs should be taken:
    - a. during the primary survey.
    - b. after all fractures are immobilized.
    - c. during the secondary survey.
    - (d.) after the chief complaint.

14. A First Aider involved in the look, listen, and feel process is:
    - a. securing the scene.
    - b. checking for bleeding.
    - c. checking the circulation.
    - d. checking for breathing.

15. The artery in the neck where First Aiders most commonly take a pulse on an unconscious victim is called the:
    - a. cranial.
    - b. subclavian.
    - c. brachial.
    - (d.) carotid.

PART III: Matching The AVPU method is helpful in determining level of consciousness. Match each letter with the proper description.

_____ A: 1. Responds to pain only.

_____ V: 2. Unresponsive.

_____ P: 3. Knows his name and where he is.

_____ U: 4. Is verbally responsive but does not know name.

Place yourself in the following accident situation: A young boy falls out of a tree onto a rock pile below. You are the first person to reach the boy, who is unconscious. In what order would you give this boy a victim survey? Using the list below rearrange the items in the correct order.

A • Check the head for lacerations.

B • Check clavicles and arms for fractures.

C • Check the neck for spinal injuries.

D • Check for an open airway.

E • Check for adequate breathing.

F • Check the chest for movement on both sides and for fractures.

G • Check for a pulse.

H • Check the back for abnormalities.

I • Check the pelvis for fractures.

J • Check for any severely bleeding injuries.

K • Check the legs, ankles and feet.

L • Check the abdomen for tenderness and spasms or rigidity.

The Primary Survey

1. _____

2. _____

3. _____

4. _____

The Secondary Survey

5. _____

6. _____

7. _____

8. _____

9. _____

10. _____

11. _____

12. _____

PART IV: What Would You Do If:

1. You are in a mall where an elderly woman has fallen. She says, "I'm dizzy," and she can't get up from the chair where she is slumped. Her lips are bluish and she is breathing in shallow gasps. When you ask her what day it is, she says, "I'm having a heart attack, aren't I?"

    • Which are signs and which are symptoms?
    • How would you pursue a victim assessment?
    • When would you decide to phone for an ambulance?

PART V: Practical Skills Check-Off _____has satisfactorily passed the following practical skills:
                                                                    Student's Name

	Date	Partner Check	Inst. Init.
1. Primary victim survey.	___/___/___	☐	_____
2. Survey of vital signs.	___/___/___	☐	_____
3. Secondary victim survey.	___/___/___	☐	_____

BASIC LIFE SUPPORT: ARTIFICIAL VENTILATION

The first priority in any emergency is to establish and maintain an adequate airway. Because breathing is vital, a First Aider's quick and efficient care will spell the difference between life and death for many victims of an emergency. In some instances, airway obstruction itself may be the emergency: a swimmer stays underwater too long and inhales water, a business executive at a banquet begins to choke on a piece of steak, or a woman carrying a bag of groceries trips on the curb, is knocked unconscious, and quits breathing. Such instances cause 3,900 avoidable deaths per year. By understanding the physiological process of breathing and the methods of care, you will be able to quickly initiate and maintain an adequate airway in cases of emergency.

UNDERSTANDING THE RESPIRATORY SYSTEM

Oxygen is essential to human life; all living tissue depends on the oxygen carried by the blood. Oxygen enters the body through **RESPIRATION**, the breathing process. Any interference with breathing produces oxygen depletion (**ANOXIA**) throughout the entire body. Knowledge of the respiratory system and the organs concerned with respiration will greatly aid in understanding artificial respiration.

During **RESPIRATION**, air is taken into the lungs (**INHALATION**) and forced out (**EXHALATION**). It passes through the nose, throat, and windpipe. The air is warmed and moistened in the nose, where much of the dust is also filtered out.

The throat is a continuation of the nose and mouth. At its lower end are two openings, one in front of the other. The opening in front is called the trachea or **WINDPIPE** and leads to the lungs. The one behind is called the **ESOPHAGUS** or food pipe and leads to the stomach.

At the top of the windpipe is a flap, the **EPIGLOTTIS**, which closes over the windpipe during swallowing to keep food or liquid from entering it. When a person is unconscious, the flap fails to respond; therefore, no solids or liquids should be given by mouth, because they may enter the windpipe or the lungs and cause strangulation or serious complications. The tongue of an unconscious person, especially if the person is lying on his back, is apt to fall against the back of the throat and interfere with air reaching the lungs. In some cases, it may block the throat entirely. When a person is unconscious or breathing with difficulty, the chin should always be extended. This brings the tongue forward.

The windpipe extends into the chest cavity, where it divides into two bronchial tubes, one going to each lung. Within the lungs, the tubes branch out like limbs of a tree, until they become very small. After subdividing into these small branches, the bronchial tubes end in a group of air cells (**ALVEOLI**) that resemble a small bunch of grapes (Figure 3-1). Around each of the air cells, which have thin walls, is a fine network of small blood vessels or **CAPILLARIES**. The blood in these capillaries releases carbon dioxide and other waste matter, the by-products of tissue activity from all over the body, through the thin air-cell wall and, in exchange, takes on a supply of oxygen from the air breathed into the air cells. The discarded carbon dioxide and waste matter leave the air cells in the exhaled air.

The lungs are two cone-shaped bodies that are soft, spongy, and elastic. Each lung is covered by a closed sac called the **PLEURA**; another layer of pleura lines the inside of the chest cavity. The small space between the two layers of pleura is called the **PLEURAL SPACE**. The inside of the lungs communicates freely with the outside air through the windpipe.

Breathing consists of two separate acts: inhalation and exhalation. During inhalation, the chest muscles raise the ribs, and the arch of the **DIAPHRAGM** falls and flattens, expanding the chest cavity so that the air pressure within becomes less than that outside. Air rushes to fill the vacuum, inflating the lungs. In exhalation, the ribs fall to their normal position, the arch of the diaphragm rises, decreasing the capacity of the chest cavity, and air is forced out (Figure 3-2).

If any air gets through the chest wall, or if the lung is punctured so that air from the outside can fill the pleural space, the lungs will not fill. This is because the air pressure is equal outside and inside the chest cavity. Thus, no suction is created on inhalation.

Breathing is usually automatic (controlled by the **BRAIN STEM**), and a person exerts only a certain degree of control. The amount of air breathed and the frequency of breathing vary according to whether the person is at rest or engaged in work or

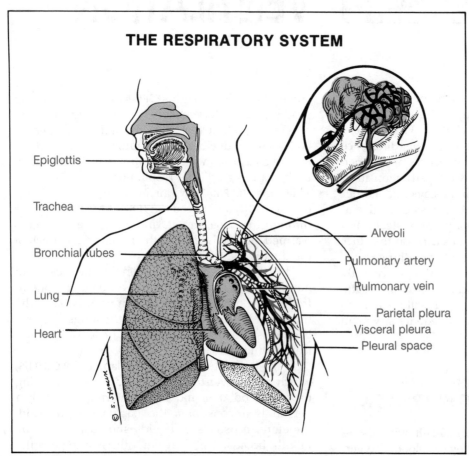

THE RESPIRATORY SYSTEM

Epiglottis

Trachea

Bronchial tubes

Lung

Heart

Alveoli

Pulmonary artery

Pulmonary vein

Parietal pleura

Visceral pleura

Pleural space

FIGURE 3-1.

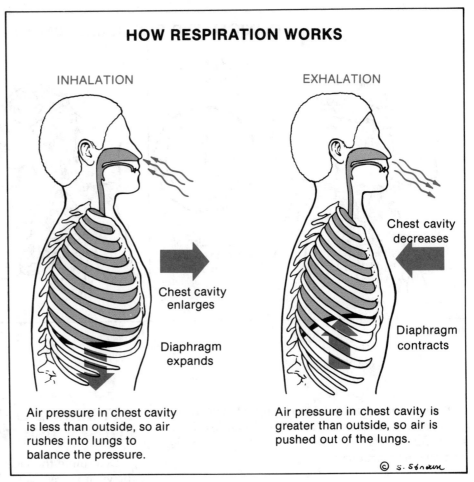

HOW RESPIRATION WORKS

INHALATION

EXHALATION

Chest cavity
enlarges

Diaphragm
expands

Air pressure in chest cavity
is less than outside, so air
rushes into lungs to
balance the pressure.

Chest cavity
decreases

Diaphragm
contracts

Air pressure in chest cavity is
greater than outside, so air is
pushed out of the lungs.

© S. Sorum

FIGURE 3-2.

exercise. At rest, a healthy adult breathes between twelve and fifteen times per minute and takes in twenty-five to thirty-five cubic inches of air per breath. During strenuous work, the breathing rate and amount inhaled may be increased several times.

THE NEED FOR OXYGEN

Without oxygen, cells cannot produce energy and, therefore, die. If the respiratory system fails to place oxygen in the blood, or if the **CIRCULATORY SYSTEM** fails to carry oxygen to the cells, then cells, tissue, organs, and finally the system (the victim) die. Time is critical.

Many victims die from failure of the respiratory and/or circulatory systems. When oxygen is cut off to the lungs, hence to the brain and heart, the heart gradually becomes weaker as the brain cells that send signals to the heart begin to die from lack of oxygen. When it does not receive signals from the

brain, the heart falters and stops, resulting in **CARDIAC ARREST**.

When respiration and heart action cease, the victim is classified as **CLINICALLY DEAD**, because the two essential systems that continue life have been shut down. However, cells have a residual oxygen supply and can survive for a short time. The brain cells are the first to die — usually four to six minutes after being deprived of oxygenated blood. Irreversible brain damage occurs, and the system dies. This is called **BIOLOGICAL DEATH**. The period between clinical and biological death is short, which means that the First Aider must act quickly to reoxygenate the blood and get it to flow to the brain (Figure 3-3).

CAUSES OF
RESPIRATORY ARREST

Breathing may stop due to a variety of serious accidents. The most common causes of **RESPIRATORY**

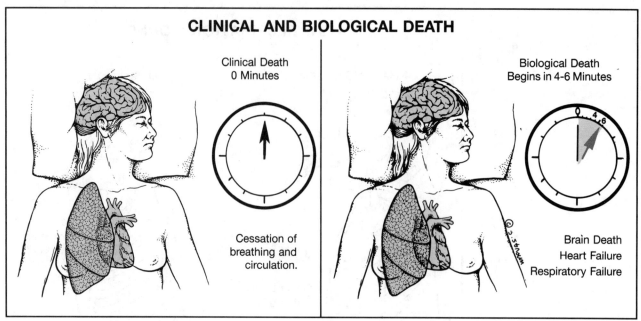

CLINICAL AND BIOLOGICAL DEATH

Clinical Death
0 Minutes

Cessation of
breathing and
circulation.

Biological Death
Begins in 4-6 Minutes

Brain Death
Heart Failure
Respiratory Failure

FIGURE 3-3.

ARREST are electric shock, drowning, **SUFFOCATION**, inhalation of poisonous gases, head injuries, heart problems, airway closure, stroke, drug overdose, and allergic reactions.

BASIC LIFE SUPPORT

The first crucial step in basic life support is assessment. All too often in **CPR** training, the complete assessment phase is overlooked. The American Heart Association has stated, "The assessment phases of basic life support are crucial. No victim should undergo any one of the more intrusive procedures of cardiopulmonary resuscitation (i.e., positioning, opening the airway, rescue breathing, and external chest compression) until the need for it has been established by the appropriate assessment."

VICTIM ASSESSMENT AND POSITIONING

The initial steps in victim assessment are:

1. Determine the level of consciousness.
2. Achieve control of the cervical spine.
3. Open the airway with the appropriate maneuver.

You may be able to accomplish all of these steps simultaneously upon arrival at the victim's side.

DETERMINE LEVEL OF CONSCIOUSNESS

Determine the victim's level of consciousness. (If the victim is responsive, your procedures will differ.) Tap the victim gently on the shoulder and ask loudly, "Are you okay?" You are not looking for an answer to the question as much as you are any kind of response — fluttering eyelids, muscle movement, turning from the noise, etc.

If the victim is unresponsive, follow the ABC procedure: **A**irway, **B**reathing, and **C**irculation (Figure 3-4). You need to implement basic life support as quickly as possible.

ACHIEVE CONTROL OF THE CERVICAL SPINE

It is critical that you assess for cervical-spine injury. The instructions in the remainder of this chapter assume that the neck and spine have *not* been injured. However, if you suspect such injuries, you must take precautions to protect the neck and spine. Assume cervical-spine injury if the victim has suffered injuries to the head or face; complains of neck pain, weakness, or tingling in the skin; or has

A,B,Cs of BASIC LIFE SUPPORT

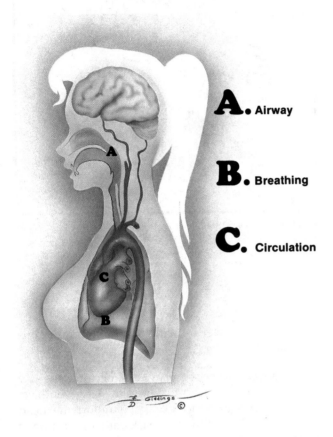

A. Airway

B. Breathing

C. Circulation

FIGURE 3-4.

an altered level of consciousness. Mechanism of injury alone frequently warrants assumption of a cervical-spine injury.

Maintain the head and neck in a neutral position, with the shoulders in line, then use the **JAW THRUST** to open the airway. This maneuver is safe if the head and neck are being maintained in neutral alignment.

OPEN THE AIRWAY

Next, open the airway. When unconsciousness causes the tongue to relax, it frequently will fall back and block the airway. The epiglottis can also relax and obstruct the **LARYNX** (voice box). Efforts to breathe will create negative pressure, which may draw the tongue, epiglottis, or both into the airway to block the trachea. Open the mouth with the **CROSSED-FINGER TECHNIQUE**.

1. Kneel above and behind the victim.
2. Cross the thumb and forefinger of one hand.
3. Place the thumb on the victim's lower incisors and your forefinger on the upper incisors.
4. Use a scissors motion or finger-snapping motion to open the mouth.

If you can see liquids like vomitus inside, quickly wipe the fluids away with your index and middle fingers, wrapped in cloth. If you can see solid foreign objects, such as broken teeth or dentures, hook them out with your index finger. Do this quickly.

Use one of the two methods described below to open the airway. Note that the general method is the **HEAD-TILT/CHIN-LIFT MANEUVER**. If a cervical-spine injury is suspected, use the jaw thrust.

Take special precautions with children. Hyperextending the head and neck can cause a child's supple trachea to collapse more easily than that of an adult. Never tilt an infant's head beyond neutral position. In older children, tilt it only slightly more than the sniffing position. A rolled towel under the shoulders may adjust the position enough.

Head-Tilt/Chin-Lift Maneuver

To accomplish this, do the following (Figure 3-5):

1. Place the tips of the fingers of one hand underneath the lower jaw on the bony part near the chin. Put the other hand on the victim's forehead, and apply firm backward pressure.
2. Bring the chin forward, supporting the jaw and tilting the head backward. Do not compress the soft tissues underneath the chin — they might obstruct the airway.
3. Continue to press the other hand on the victim's forehead to keep the head tilted backward.
4. Lift the chin so that the teeth are nearly brought together, but avoid closing the mouth completely.
5. The thumb is used rarely — only to keep the mouth slightly open.
6. If the victim has loose dentures, hold them in position, making obstruction by the lips less likely. If rescue breathing is needed, the mouth-to-mouth seal is easier when dentures are in place. But if the dentures are hard to manage in place, remove them.

HEAD-TILT/CHIN-LIFT MANEUVER

OPENING THE
AIRWAY BY THE
HEAD-TILT,
CHIN LIFT

In an uncon-
scious victim,
the tongue can
obstruct the
upper airway,
leading to
respiratory, then
cardiac
arrest.

Often, simply
opening the
airway will allow
resumption of
spontaneous
ventilation.

Tilt the head by
applying pressure
on the forehead
with one hand while
placing the
fingers of the
other hand
under the
mandible and
lifting the chin
upward. These
actions combine to
lift the tongue
base away from
the posterior
pharyngeal wall
and reestablish an
open airway.

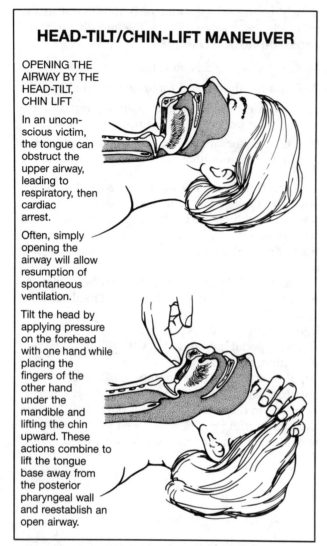

FIGURE 3-5. Apply pressure on the forehead with one hand (to extend the head) while placing the fingers of the other hand under the mandible and lifting the chin directly.

JAW-THRUST MANEUVER

If the head tilt/chin lift is unsuccessful, or if you suspect a cervical-spine injury, forward displacement of the jaw may be necessary. To do this (Figure 3-6):

1. Place your elbows on the surface on which the victim is lying, putting your hands at the side of the victim's head.
2. Grasp the jawbone on both sides where it angles up toward the victim's ears. Move the jaw forward and simultaneously tilt the head backward.

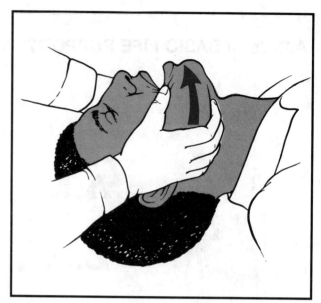

FIGURE 3-6. In the jaw-thrust maneuver, the First Aider places the fingers behind the angle of the victim's jaw and forcefully brings it forward.

3. Retract the lower lip with your thumb if the lips close.

If you suspect a neck injury, *first* perform the jaw thrust *without* the head tilt/chin lift. After you have displaced the jawbone forward, support the head carefully without tilting it backward or turning it from side to side.

CHECK FOR BREATHING

Now that the airway is opened, check to see if the victim is breathing. While maintaining an open airway, place your ear close to the victim's mouth and nose for three to five seconds, and:

LOOK for the chest rising.
LISTEN for breath sounds.
FEEL for breath against your cheek.

This process should take only three to five seconds. If the victim is breathing, *keep him in the present position* and go on with your evaluation. If the victim is not breathing and not lying on his back, he must be moved so that you can perform rescue breathing. **LOGROLL** the victim as a unit, taking care to keep the head and neck in alignment. Plan the move, perform it carefully, and only move the victim once if possible. Position the victim as the condition warrants it, *not* as an automatic basic-life-support step.

After positioning the victim, give two breaths using the method described next.

PROVIDE RESCUE BREATHING

You do not need any equipment to start rescue breathing (Figure 3-7). Use the best method, delivering about twelve breaths per minute (faster for infants and children). The most efficient method, if you can use it, is **MOUTH-TO-MOUTH VENTILATION**.

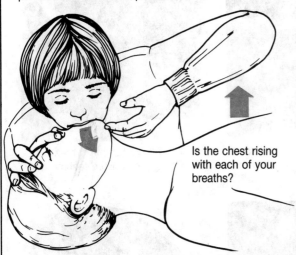

RESCUE BREATHING

Remove your hand from the victim's forehead and use it to pinch off the nostrils.

Apply your mouth tightly around the victim's mouth . . .

Deliver two rescue breaths, allowing 1-1.5 seconds for each inspiration.

As soon as you give these two breaths, move your eyes to the chest, which should begin to fall as exhalation occurs. Can you feel exhaled breath on your cheek? If you confirm these signs of effective rescue breathing, proceed to evaluate the pulses.

Is the chest rising with each of your breaths?

If breathing seems obstructed, repeat the airway-opening maneuver and the two rescue breaths. If signs of effective ventilation are still lacking, assume the victim has upper airway obstruction and proceed to the airway obstruction maneuvers.

FIGURE 3-7. Rescue breathing.

MOUTH-TO-MOUTH VENTILATION

The air that we breathe in contains about 21 percent oxygen. Of this 21 percent, only 5 percent is used by the body, and the remaining 16 percent is exhaled. Because the exhaled breath contains about 16 percent oxygen, a victim can be oxygenated using only the First Aider's breath.

After you have established that the victim is not breathing, use the hand engaged in the head tilt (forehead) to pinch together the victim's nostrils. Follow these basic procedures for mouth-to-mouth ventilation (Figures 3-8–3-15):

1. Open your mouth wide, take in a deep breath, and cover the victim's entire mouth with your mouth, forming a tight seal. Give two initial ventilations at 1 to 1.5 seconds per ventilation. Allow for full exhalations between ventilations and for completely refilling your own lungs after each breath. Use full, slow breaths. If you hurry or blow too hard, you will blow air into the stomach, a condition called **GASTRIC DISTENTION**, which will almost certainly cause vomiting and the risk of **ASPIRATION** (sucking vomitus into the lungs).

2. Remove your mouth and turn your head toward the victim's chest each time you take a breath. With your peripheral vision, watch the victim's chest rise, and with your head turned you can watch it fall.

3. Give these first ventilations in succession, allowing for deflation between ventilations. Remove your mouth, look at the victim's chest and abdomen, and let him exhale passively. The exhaled breath may be sensed on your cheek.

4. If you must use the jaw thrust, continue to hold the lower lip down with your thumb and forefinger; press your cheek against the victim's nostrils to seal them off. Form a tight seal over the mouth while you hold the lip down.

5. If you cannot blow air into the lungs, reposition the victim's airway and try again. The most common cause of difficulty with ventilation is improper positioning of the head and chin. If the second try also fails, assume that the airway is blocked by a foreign object and follow the instructions under "Emergency Care for Obstruction by a Foreign Object."

6. After the first successful ventilations, give one breath every five seconds, or approximately twelve per minute.

MOUTH-TO-NOSE VENTILATION

Use **MOUTH-TO-NOSE VENTILATION** (Figure 3-16) when the victim's mouth cannot be opened, when it is seriously injured, or when you cannot achieve a tight mouth-to-mouth seal.

RESCUE BREATHING

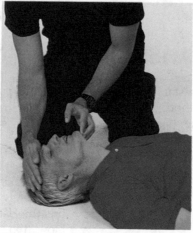

FIGURE 3-8. Position a victim who is not suspected of having a spinal injury on his back.

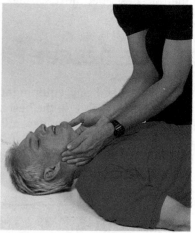

FIGURE 3-9. Open the airway by the head-tilt/chin-lift maneuver. Use two fingers just under the mandible, not on the soft part under the chin.

FIGURE 3-10. Opening the airway by the modified jaw thrust.

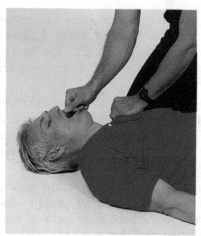

FIGURE 3-11. If the victim's mouth remains closed, open it with the cross-finger technique.

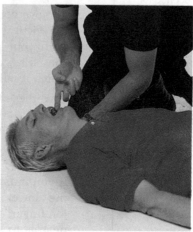

FIGURE 3-12. Remove any obstructions from the mouth if they are visible.

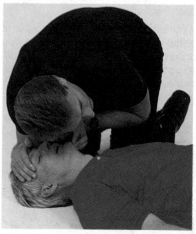

FIGURE 3-13. Establish breathlessness with the look-listen-feel method.

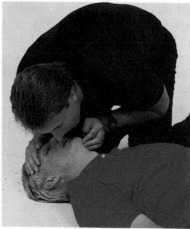

FIGURE 3-14. Mouth-to-mouth ventilation. Give two successive full breaths of air.

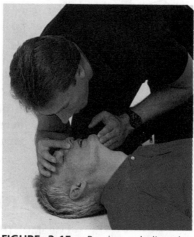

FIGURE 3-15. Passive exhaling by the victim.

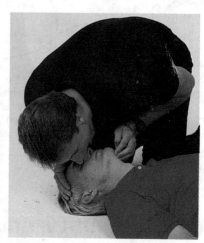

FIGURE 3-16. Mouth-to-nose ventilation.

1. Place one hand on the forehead, and tilt the victim's head backward. With your other hand, lift the lower jaw forward and seal the lips.

2. Take a deep breath, and place your mouth over the victim's nostrils, forming a tight seal.

3. Breathe slowly into the nostrils for 1 to 1.5 seconds until you feel the lungs expand or see the victim's chest rise.

4. Remove your mouth and make sure that air is escaping through the victim's nostrils; the chest should fall as exhalation occurs. If the victim is not exhaling enough, open the mouth to let air escape.

5. If you use the jaw thrust, keep the jaw in place with your hand, and seal the mouth with your cheek.

VENTILATING INFANTS AND CHILDREN

The technique for ventilating infants and children varies only slightly. If the victim is an infant or a small child:

1. Gently open the airway. Tilt the head to the neutral + position or only as much as necessary since you can actually obstruct (kink) a child's airway (Figure 3-17).

2. Cover the victim's nose and mouth with a tight seal during inhalation (Figure 3-18).

3. Deliver only small breaths or puffs of air — just enough to make the chest rise.

4. The breathing rate for infants (one month to one year) is once every three seconds; for a child (one to eight years), once every four seconds; and for a child above eight years, once every five seconds, the same as for an adult.

A child's smaller air passages provide a greater resistance to airflow; therefore, your blowing pressure will probably be greater than you would assume.

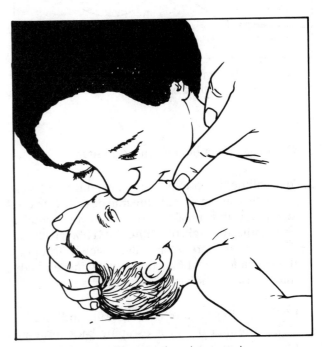

FIGURE 3-18. Mouth-to-mouth and nose seal.

MOUTH-TO-STOMA VENTILATION

Some people have all or part of their larynx removed through surgery (**LARYNGECTOMY**). A victim who has had a laryngectomy has a permanent opening (**STOMA**) in his neck and breathes through the stoma. The stoma is usually in the center, in front, and at the base of the neck. Sometimes there will be other openings in the neck, depending on the kind of surgery done on the victim, but the stoma is the only one pertinent to artificial ventilation. To perform artificial ventilation (Figure 3-19):

1. Remove all coverings (i.e., scarves, ties, etc.) from the stoma area.

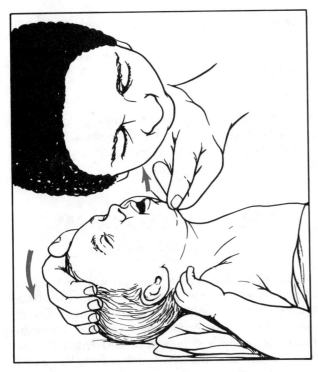

FIGURE 3-17. Head tilt/chin lift.

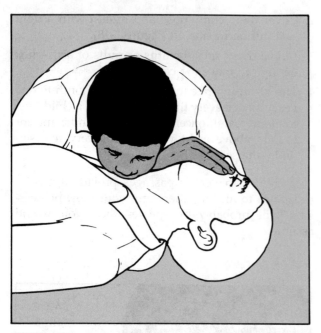

FIGURE 3-19. Performing mouth-to-stoma ventilation. Head does *not* need to be tilted backward.

2. Clear the stoma of any foreign matter.

3. You will not need to perform a head tilt on a victim with a stoma. Simply breathe directly into the stoma, forming a seal around it with your mouth, or breathe through the **TRACHEOSTOMY TUBE** in the stoma if there is one. Blow slowly through the stoma for 1 to 1.5 seconds, using just enough force to cause the victim's chest to rise.

4. Watch for the victim's chest to fall, and feel to make sure that the air is escaping back through the stoma during the exhalation.

5. If the chest does not rise, suspect a **PARTIAL NECK BREATHER**. Seal the nose and mouth with one hand so that air will not leak out the mouth or nose, and repeat the process. Pinch off the nose between the third and fourth fingers; seal the lips with the palm of the hand; place the thumb under the chin, and press upward and backward. Repeat ventilations.

GASTRIC DISTENTION

During artificial ventilation, it is common for air to get into the esophagus and, therefore, into the stomach. Gastric distention (inflation) happens most often in children and in airway-obstructed victims when you have exerted excessive pressure while blowing air into the victim's mouth or nose. If the distention is slight, you can safely ignore it. However, a larger quantity is dangerous because it can make the victim vomit and force up the diaphragm, limiting the amount of air that the lungs can hold.

You can minimize gastric distention by stopping ventilation when the chest rises, thus not blowing hard enough to open the esophagus. Also, reposition the head and neck to make sure that the airway is open.

The American Heart Association recommends *not* relieving gastric distention by pressing on the abdomen because of the danger of the victim aspirating stomach contents into the lungs. Aspirated vomitus can cause a severe chemical pneumonia. Attempt **DECOMPRESSION** only if the distention is so great that it interferes with ventilation. Follow these procedures for relieving gastric distention:

1. Turn the victim's body to one side.

2. Use the flat of your hand to exert moderate pressure on the victim's abdomen between the navel and rib cage.

3. Guard against the common mistakes in administering ventilation:
   - Ventilating the victim too forcefully.
   - Not keeping the head tilted, when appropriate.
   - Not allowing deflation between the first two ventilations.

4. If you can hear any gurgling or bubbling while you are ventilating a victim, stop resuscitation immediately or you will blow the gastric material into the lungs.

5. Logroll the victim onto his side.

6. After the vomiting has occurred, quickly wipe the mouth out with 4 × 4 gauze pads, wipe off the face, and return to resuscitation.

OBSTRUCTED AIRWAY EMERGENCIES

Any agent that causes upper airway obstruction occludes either the nasal passages, the **OROPHARYNX**, or the **LARYNGOPHARYNX**. Lower-airway obstruction can be caused by breathing in foreign materials or by a severe **BRONCHOSPASM** (Figure 3-20). In any case, the airway will need to be cleared so that the victim can breathe efficiently.

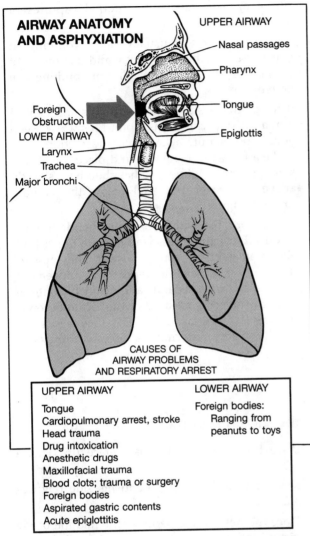

AIRWAY ANATOMY AND ASPHYXIATION

UPPER AIRWAY

Nasal passages

Pharynx

Tongue

Epiglottis

Foreign Obstruction

LOWER AIRWAY

Larynx

Trachea

Major bronchi

CAUSES OF AIRWAY PROBLEMS AND RESPIRATORY ARREST

UPPER AIRWAY	LOWER AIRWAY
Tongue	Foreign bodies:
Cardiopulmonary arrest, stroke	Ranging from
Head trauma	peanuts to toys
Drug intoxication	
Anesthetic drugs	
Maxillofacial trauma	
Blood clots; trauma or surgery	
Foreign bodies	
Aspirated gastric contents	
Acute epiglottitis	

FIGURE 3-20. The structure most commonly responsible for upper airway obstruction is the tongue. The type of foreign object that most frequently causes upper airway obstruction is food. Another common cause of obstruction is acute epiglottitis, which is more frequently seen in children than in adults. Do not overlook nasal obstruction as a cause of upper airway obstruction in infants who are nasal breathers rather than mouth breathers.

CAUSES OF AIRWAY OBSTRUCTION AND GENERAL EMERGENCY CARE

If the victim is unresponsive, try ventilating the lungs first. If a foreign object is present, it will become evident when your efforts to ventilate the lungs fail.

The most common source of upper-airway obstruction is the tongue. (If it partially blocks the

airway, your victim will make snoring sounds while breathing.) Reposition the head and neck with the head-tilt/chin-lift maneuver or jaw-thrust technique, and attempt to ventilate.

Foreign bodies may also obstruct the upper airway. According to the National Safety Council, an annual estimated 3,100 people choked on a foreign object and died in 1984. The typical victim of the so-called **CAFE CORONARY** is middle-aged or elderly and is commonly a denture wearer. He has usually had a few drinks, which both **DEPRESS** his protective reflexes and adversely affect his judgment about the size of bites he is taking. (The largest piece of meat extracted from the throat of a victim who choked was over eight inches long!) When the piece of solid food, often a chunk of meat, lodges in the airway, the victim becomes completely **APHONIC** (unable to talk, breathe, groan, cough, or cry out). He may try to get up and walk from the table or may pitch forward, all in complete silence, and is usually **CYANOTIC** (blue).

Other causes of upper-airway obstruction include **BLOOD CLOTS** that are the result of trauma or surgery, cancerous conditions of the mouth or throat, **TONSIL** enlargement, injury to the face or jaw, acute **EPIGLOTTITIS**, aspirated vomitus, and broken dental bridges. Nasal-passage obstruction may be a cause of upper-airway obstruction in infants who can breathe only through their noses.

When possible, educate people to prevent choking by following these steps:

- Avoid excessive intake of alcohol before and during meals.

- Cut food into small bite-size pieces.

- Denture wearers especially should chew slowly and thoroughly.

- Avoid talking and laughing during chewing and swallowing.

- Teach children not to put foreign objects in their mouths.

- Do not allow children to run about when they are eating.

SIGNS AND SYMPTOMS OF AIRWAY OBSTRUCTION

Sudden respiratory failure can be caused by conditions other than choking — for instance, fainting, stroke, heart attack, epilepsy, an obstructing **TUMOR**, or drug overdose — but these emergencies are managed differently. It is important to recognize foreign-body airway obstruction quickly. The following signs will help you:

- Audible, noisy breathing, or no breath sounds.
- Labored use of muscles required in breathing; nostrils are flared; neck and facial muscles are strained.
- Progressive restlessness, anxiety, and confusion.
- Cyanosis — lips and skin turn blue from lack of oxygen.
- Victim becomes unresponsive.

EMERGENCY CARE FOR PARTIAL OBSTRUCTION

A foreign body may cause a partial or complete airway obstruction. If the obstruction is partial, the victim may get some air exchange. If the victim can cough forcefully, air exchange is occurring. Allow the victim time to remove the obstruction himself. Encourage him to cough. Do not interfere with his attempts to expel the foreign object, but do *not* leave him. Monitor him closely, looking for signs of reduced air passage: a weak, ineffective cough, a high-pitched wheeze during inhalation, increased strain in breathing, clutching the throat, and the beginning of cyanosis.

EMERGENCY CARE FOR COMPLETE OBSTRUCTION

If the Victim is Conscious

1. Recognize the obstruction, either from your observations or, if you have just arrived, by asking the victim, "Are you choking?" If the victim cannot make a sound, and has one or two hands over his throat, the airway may be blocked (Figure 3-21). If the victim is having a heart attack or another problem, he will be able to speak or whisper.

2. Use the **HEIMLICH MANEUVER** (also called **SUBDIAPHRAGMATIC ABDOMINAL THRUSTS** or abdominal thrusts) to clear the airway. When this maneuver thrusts the diaphragm quickly upward, it can force enough air from the lungs to create an artificial cough that can dislodge and expel the foreign object.

3. It may take six to ten thrusts to succeed. If your hands are too high (on the lower edges of the rib cage), you can cause internal ruptures or lacerations.

4. This maneuver will usually cause vomiting. If you place your hand correctly and use the right amount of force, the possibility of vomiting will be reduced.

5. If the victim is standing or sitting, stand behind him and wrap your arms around his waist. Keep your elbows out, away from the victim's ribs. Make a fist with one hand, and place the thumb side on the midline of the abdomen slightly above the navel and well below the xiphoid process (Figure 3-22).

6. Grasp your fist with your other hand, thumbs toward the victim. Press your fist into the victim's abdomen with a quick, inward and upward thrust. If you need to repeat this movement, make each thrust separate and distinct. Continue until the object is released or the victim becomes unconscious (Figures 3-23–3-24). (See Figure 3-25 for the victim performing abdominal thrusts on himself.)

If the Victim Becomes Unconscious

1. Place the victim on his back, face up (Figure 3-26).

2. Kneel astride his thighs or to his side (Figures 3-27–3-28).

3. Place the heel of one hand on the midline of the victim's abdomen, between the xiphoid process and **UMBILICUS** (navel). Put your second hand directly over the first.

4. Lock your elbows and, exerting pressure from the shoulders, press downward and forward with a quick thrust. Your body weight will make the thrust more energetic. (Take care to avoid the xiphoid process. Putting pressure on it may lacerate vital organs.)

5. If this action does not dislodge the foreign body, open the victim's mouth by gripping the tongue and lower jaw between the thumb and fingers of one hand, and shift the jawbone forward. This will draw the tongue away from the back of the throat and may partially relieve the obstruction.

6. Insert the index finger of your other hand along the cheek and deep into the throat to the base of the tongue with a slow, careful hooking motion. (Use this maneuver only on an unconscious victim. A conscious victim will gag.)

7. Be careful not to force the object deeper into the airway. You may have to push the object against

EMERGENCY CARE FOR OBSTRUCTION BY A FOREIGN OBJECT

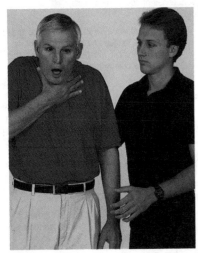

FIGURE 3-21. The universal sign of choking. Ask the victim, "Are you choking?"

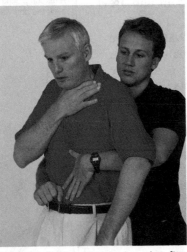

FIGURE 3-22. Positioning the fist, thumb side in, for the abdominal thrust.

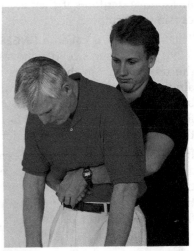

FIGURE 3-23. Administering the abdominal thrust on a standing victim.

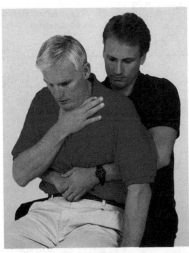

FIGURE 3-24. Administering the abdominal thrust to a sitting victim.

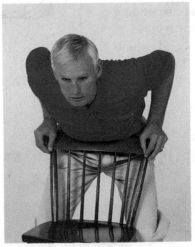

FIGURE 3-25. The choking victim performing an abdominal thrust on self.

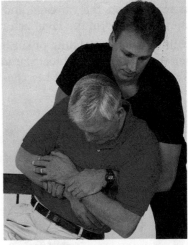

FIGURE 3-26. Remove an unconscious, sitting victim from the chair, and lie him face-up on the floor.

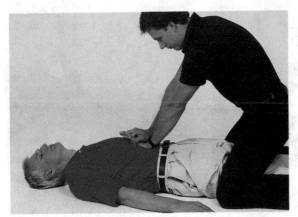

FIGURE 3-27. Performing abdominal thrusts on an unconscious victim while straddling the victim.

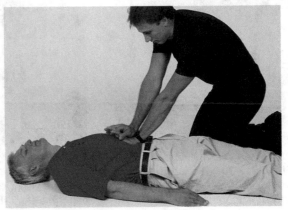

FIGURE 3-28. Performing abdominal thrusts while kneeling beside the victim.

the opposite side of the throat to dislodge it. Hook it up into the mouth where you can remove it. Remove dentures if they are present and are causing difficulties.

8. This maneuver is called a **FINGER SWEEP** (Figure 3-29). The finger sweep removes material from the oropharynx so that it does not reenter the airway during subsequent attempts at rescue breathing. Never use it on a baby, since the foreign body may be pushed farther back in the throat and cause further obstruction.

9. If the foreign object is still not expelled, open the airway and perform mouth-to-mouth resuscitation. If you cannot succeed in providing ventilation, repeat the cycle of abdominal thrusts, the finger sweep, and resuscitation again.

If the Victim is Pregnant or Obese and Conscious

1. In the advanced stages of pregnancy, there is no room between the rib cage and the expanding uterus to perform the Heimlich maneuver.

2. With the victim standing or sitting, stand behind her with your arms directly under her armpits. Wrap your arms around her chest (Figure 3-30).

FINGER SWEEPS

After completing the sequences of abdominal thrusts, clear the pharynx of debris.

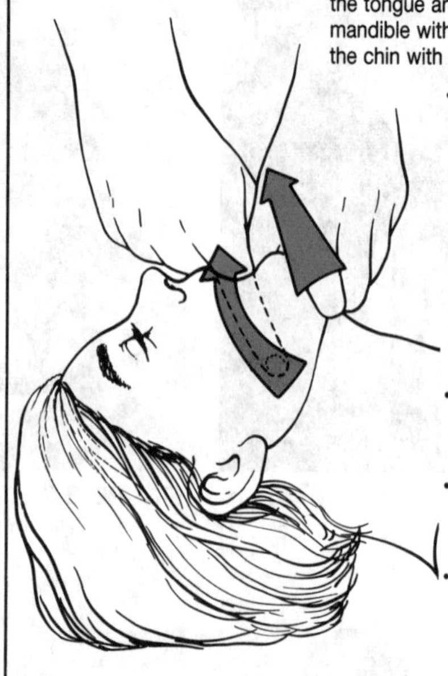

Perform a jaw lift with one hand, grasping the tongue and inner aspect of the mandible with the thumb and holding the chin with the other fingers.

- Now, using the index finger of the opposite hand, sweep any foreign material from deep in the throat toward you and up the pharyngeal wall and cheek to the mouth. Be careful about grasping foreign material between the fingers, as it may be very slippery.

- Once the airway is cleared, rescue breathing is continued.

- If the airway remains obstructed, repeat the airway maneuvers.

- After two successful ventilations in succession, check the carotid pulse.

FIGURE 3-29.

CHEST THRUSTS ON A PREGNANT VICTIM

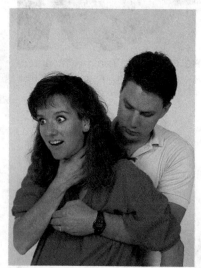

FIGURE 3-30. Position the thumb side of your fist on the middle of her breastbone (sternum).

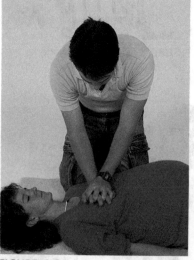

FIGURE 3-31. For an unconscious, pregnant victim, kneel at her side and perform a chest thrust.

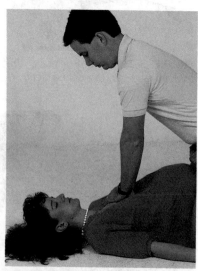

FIGURE 3-32. You may also straddle the pregnant victim to perform the chest thrusts.

3. Position the thumb side of your fist on the middle of the breastbone. If you are near the margins of the rib cage, you are too low.

4. Seize your fist firmly with your other hand, and thrust backward sharply.

5. Repeat until the object is expelled or the victim becomes unresponsive.

If the Victim Is or Becomes Unresponsive

1. Place the victim on her back and kneel beside her (Figures 3-31–3-32).

2. Place the heel of your hand directly over the *lower* one-half of the breastbone.

3. Give distinct, separate thrusts downward and forward.

After the foreign object is removed, call an ambulance to transport the victim to the emergency room. Her airway may close again from edema. She should also be evaluated routinely for a fractured rib or sternum, or a ruptured **LIVER** or **SPLEEN**. All of the above are possible complications of the Heimlich maneuver. See Figure 33-33 for performing chest thrusts on an obese victim. [The American Heart Association method of performing chest thrusts is shown in Figures 3-31 and 3-32 on page 40.]

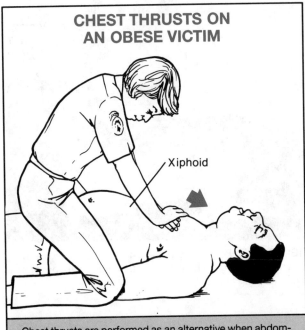

CHEST THRUSTS ON AN OBESE VICTIM

Xiphoid

Chest thrusts are performed as an alternative when abdominal thrusts are contraindicated, such as in victims with advanced pregnancy or in markedly obese victims.

Administer six to ten chest compressions with the hands well above the xiphoid.

FIGURE 3-33.

Obstructed Airway in the Infant

More than 90 percent of the **PEDIATRIC** fatalities resulting from foreign bodies occur in children under the age of five. Sixty-five percent occur in infants. Remember that, compared to an adult, an infant has a proportionally larger tongue, a larger and stiffer glottis, and concave vocal cords. Infants under the age of eight months breathe only through their noses.

The narrowest part of a child's airway is not at the level of the vocal cords, but the **CRICOID CARTILAGE** below the cords. This is true of children up to age twelve. Below the vocal cords, the airway is lined with a loose mucous membrane that can be inflamed or bruised easily, with resultant swelling.

Overextension of the neck can occlude the trachea in a child more easily than in an adult. Tilt an infant's head to neutral position or neutral + (tilt until breaths go in easily). In older children, tilt it only slightly more than sniffing position.

For partial obstruction and assuming no cervical or spinal injuries, place the child on his right side so that secretions, blood, and vomit can drain out to the mouth. The jaw will also fall forward, bringing the tongue and epiglottis away from the airway.

For the Conscious Choking Infant Under Twelve Months

1. Assess the airway. Only perform the following procedures if the obstruction is a foreign body. If obstruction is caused by airway swelling from infection or disease, have the victim transported immediately to a medical facility. Also have the victim transported if he is still conscious but is having difficulty breathing. *If the infant is choking and coughing but still breathing, allow him an attempt to expel the foreign object before commencing the following steps.*

2. Deliver four back blows within three to five seconds. First, "straddle" the infant over one arm with the face down and the head lower than the trunk at about a sixty-degree angle. With the heel of your other hand, deliver four **BACK BLOWS** rapidly and forcefully between the shoulder blade, but remember that this is an infant (Figure 3-34).

3. Next, deliver four **CHEST THRUSTS** within three to five seconds. While supporting the infant's head, sandwich the body between your hands and turn the victim on his back, with the head lower than the trunk. Lay the infant on your thigh or over your lap with the head supported. Deliver four slow, firm thrusts in the midsternal region in the

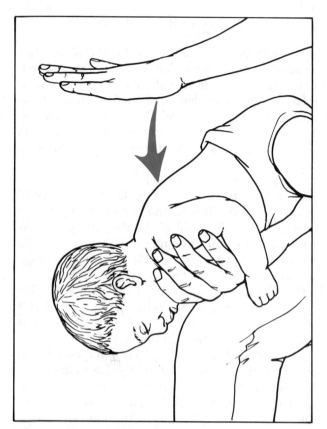

FIGURE 3-34. Back blow in infant.

same manner as for external chest compressions (Figure 3-35).

4. Repeat steps 2 and 3 until the obstruction is expelled or the infant becomes unconscious.

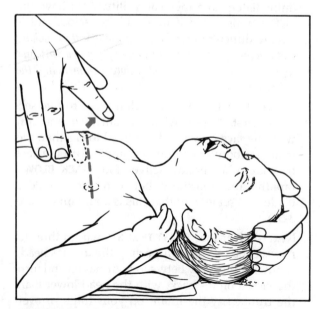

FIGURE 3-35. Locating the finger position for chest thrusts in infant.

For the Unresponsive, Nonbreathing Infant

1. Open the airway.
2. Attempt ventilation. If unsuccessful, reposition the head and try again.
3. Deliver four back blows within three to five seconds.
4. Deliver four chest thrusts within three to five seconds.
5. Perform a jaw-thrust maneuver to check for a foreign body. Do *not* perform a blind finger sweep. Remove the foreign body only if visible.
6. Reattempt ventilation and repeat steps 2 to 5 as necessary.

In a child over one year, use the same techniques as for an adult with the following modifications:

1. Kneel beside, not astride, a child lying down. Use one hand, rather than both hands (Figure 3-36).
2. Be sure to direct the thrusts at the midline of the abdomen, and not to either side. (See Chapter 16 for more information on pediatric breathing difficulties.)

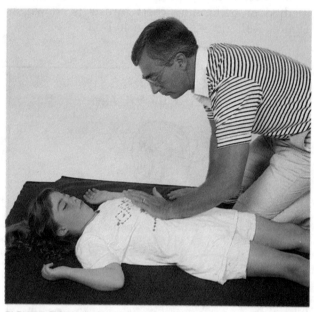

FIGURE 3-36. Performing abdominal thrusts on a child lying down. For a larger child, place other hand on top of first hand, as in an adult.

SUMMARIES

Figures 3-37 and 3-38 provide excellent summaries for this chapter. It is recommended that the student study these figures to gain a complete understanding of airway emergency care.

FIRST-AID FOR CHOKING

OBSTRUCTED AIRWAY TECHNIQUES FOR ADULTS (AGES 9 AND OVER)

Fitnus For Life

Conscious Victim Standing

1 Recognize choking signs.

Choking victim will have severe difficulty speaking, breathing, coughing and may be clutching throat between thumb and fingers (Universal Distress Signal). Ask if he or she is choking. If able to speak or cough effectively, do not interfere.

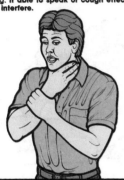

2 If choking— Give 6-10 abdominal thrusts.

Stand behind victim and wrap arms around his or her waist. Make a fist with one hand. Place thumb side of fist into abdomen above navel and below rib cage. Grasp fist with other hand and press inward and upward with 6-10 quick thrusts.

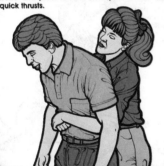

3 If pregnant or obese— Give 6-10 chest thrusts.

Stand behind victim, placing your arms under victims armpits, and encircle chests. Place thumb side of fist on the middle of the breastbone. Grasp fist with other hand and press backward with 6-10 quick thrusts.

Victim Lying Conscious or Unconscious

1 Check if conscious or unconscious.

Gently tap and shake shoulders to determine if victim is ok. If unresponsive call out for "Help!"

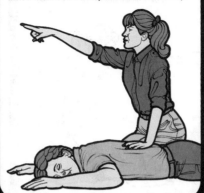

2 Position victim carefully on back.

If lying face down, roll victim flat onto back. Supporting head, neck, and torso carefully turn victim as a unit without twisting.

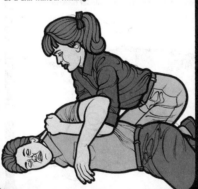

3 Open airway. Check for breathing.

Apply downward pressure with hand on forehead and gently lift with other hand just under chin. Place ear close to victim's mouth and nose. **LOOK** for rise and fall of chest. **LISTEN** and **FEEL** for breathing.

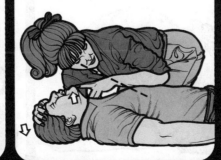

4 Attempt to ventilate.

Keeping head tilted and airway open, pinch victim's nose with thumb and index finger. Cover victim's mouth and attempt to get air into the lungs.

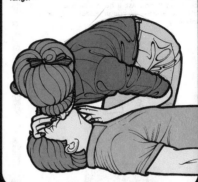

5 If unsuccessful— Give 6-10 abdominal thrusts.

Kneeling close to victim's hips, place heel of hand on victim's abdomen above navel and below rib cage. Put other hand on top of first, and press into abdomen with 6-10 quick inward and upward thrusts.

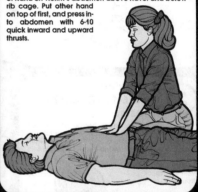

6 Finger sweep for foreign object.

Open victim's mouth by grasping tongue and lower jaw, and lift. Insert index finger of other hand deep into mouth along the cheek. Using hooked finger try to dislodge object.

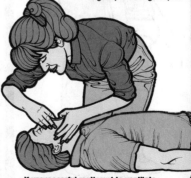

▪ If unsuccessful reattempt to ventilate ▪

Fitnus' For Life 3125 19th Street, Suite 305 • Bakersfield, CA 93301 • (805) 861-1100 · Algra, Inc. 1986

FIGURE 3-37. First aid for a choking adult.

FIRST-AID FOR CHOKING
OBSTRUCTED AIRWAY TECHNIQUES FOR CHILDREN (AGES 1 TO 8)

Fitnus® For Life

Conscious Victim Standing

1 Recognize choking signs.

Choking victim will have severe difficulty speaking, breathing, coughing and may be wheezing with a high-pitched noise clutching throat. Ask if he or she is choking. If able to speak or cough effectively, do not interfere.

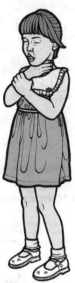

2 If choking— Give 6-10 abdominal thrusts.

Stand or kneel behind victim and wrap arms around child's waist. Make a fist with one hand. Place thumb side of fist into abdomen above navel and below rib cage. Grasp fist with other hand and press inward and upward with 6-10 quick thrusts.

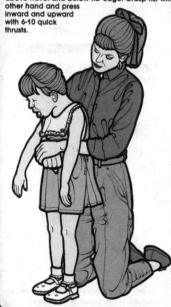

Victim Lying Conscious or Unconscious

1 Check if conscious or unconscious.

Gently tap and shake shoulders to determine if child is ok. If unresponsive call out for "Help!"

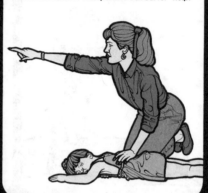

2 Position victim carefully on back.

If victim is lying face down, roll child flat onto back. Supporting head, neck, and torso carefully turn child as a unit without twisting.

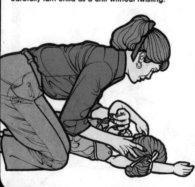

3 Open airway. Check for breathing.

Apply downward pressure with hand on forehead and gently lift with other hand just under chin. Place ear close to child's mouth and nose. **LOOK** for rise and fall of chest. **LISTEN** and **FEEL** for breathing.

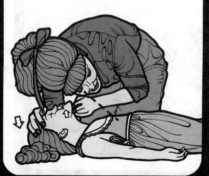

4 Attempt to ventilate.

Keeping head tilted and airway open, pinch child's nose with thumb and index finger. Cover child's mouth and attempt to get air into the lungs.

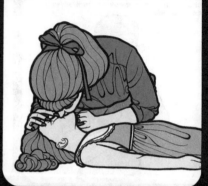

5 If unsuccessful— Give 6-10 abdominal thrusts.

Kneeling over child's legs, place heel of one hand on child's abdomen above navel and below rib cage. Put other hand on top of first, and press into abdomen with 6-10 quick inward and upward thrusts.

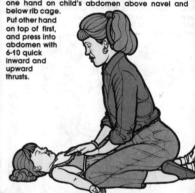

6 Finger sweep for foreign object.

Open child's mouth by grasping tongue and lower jaw, and lift. If foreign object can be seen, insert index finger of other hand along cheek deep in mouth. Using hooked finger try to dislodge object.

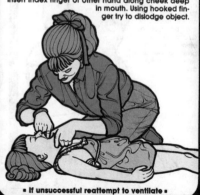

▪ If unsuccessful reattempt to ventilate ▪

Fitnus® For Life 3125 19th Street, Suite 305 • Bakersfield, CA 93301 • (805) 861-1100 Algra, Inc. 1986

FIGURE 3-38. First aid for a choking child.

| 3 | SELF-TEST | 3 |

Student: _____ Date: _____

Course: _____ Section #: _____

PART I: True/False   If you believe that the statement is true, circle the T. If you believe that the statement is false, circle the F.

T F   1. If a choking person is unable to speak, you should assume that the emergency is life-threatening.

T F   2. When resuscitating infants or small children, use more frequent, less powerful puffs of air into both the nose and mouth simultaneously.

T F   3. To check effectiveness of artificial respiration, you should watch to make sure that the stomach is bulging.

T F   4. If you suspect that the heart has stopped beating, you should not attempt artificial respiration.

T F   5. An adult victim should be provided with one breath every eight to nine seconds.

T F   6. The average person may die in six minutes or less if his oxygen supply is cut off.

T F   7. You should only do artificial ventilation for thirty minutes; longer than that will do no good if the victim has not already responded.

T F   8. Mouth-to-mouth is the most effective method of artificial respiration.

T F   9. When giving mouth-to-nose resuscitation, you keep the mouth tightly closed through the *complete* process.

PART II: Multiple Choice   For each question, circle the answer that best reflects an accurate statement.

1. The purpose of artificial ventilation is to:
   a. prevent the tongue from being swallowed.
   b. provide a method of air exchange.
   c. clear an upper-air-passage obstruction.
   d. clear a lower-air-passage obstruction.

2. The first priority in an emergency is:
   a. call the police.
   b. check for a pulse.
   c. establish and maintain an airway.
   d. get consent to treat.

3. A major sign of a respiratory emergency is:
   a. no rising of the chest.
   b. distended abdomen.
   c. hot, flushed skin.
   d. constricted pupils.
   e. all of the above.

4. You can tell that you are performing mouth-to-mouth ventilation correctly if you can:
   a. see the victim's chest rise and fall.
   b. feel resistance as you blow air in.
   c. feel air escaping from the victim's mouth as he exhales.
   d. all of the above.

5. When you are giving mouth-to-mouth resuscitation, you should:
   a. hold the victim's nostrils closed while breathing into his mouth.
   b. avoid touching the nostrils unless cardiopulmonary resuscitation is being given at the same time.
   c. pinch the nostrils as you lift your mouth from his mouth.
   d. keep nostrils pinched all the time.

6. Clinical death occurs:
   a. after biological death.
   b. when respiration and heart action cease.
   c. when brain cells are irreversibly damaged.
   d. 4 to 6 minutes after respiration ceases.

7. Brain cells die after _____ without oxygen:
   a. 1 to 2 minutes.   c. 6 to 8 minutes.
   b. 4 to 6 minutes.   d. after 10 minutes.

8. The preferable method of opening the airway is the:
   a. jaw thrust.   c. head tilt/jaw thrust.
   b. neck lift/jaw thrust.   d. head tilt/chin lift.

9. The three facets of basic life support are:
   a. primary survey, secondary survey, transport.
   b. assess the airway, breathing, and circulation.
   c. maintain life, prevent injury, get medical attention.
   d. treatment for ABCs, shock, bleeding.

10. When ventilating nonbreathing adult victims by the mouth-to-mouth method, the First Aider should provide breaths approximately:
    a. every sixty seconds, or about sixty times a minute.
    b. every two seconds, or about thirty times a minute.
    c. every five seconds, or about twelve times a minute.
    d. every ten seconds, or six times a minute.

11. The artificial ventilation rate for an infant is:
    a. once every three seconds.
    b. once every second.
    c. once every five seconds.
    d. about ten breaths per minute.

12. The most common source of upper-airway obstruction is:
    a. fluid-mucous.   c. tongue.
    b. food.   d. swollen trachea.

13. To avoid airway obstruction:
    a. cut food into small pieces.
    b. avoid talking and laughing during chewing and swallowing.
    c. don't allow children to run about when they are eating.
    d. all of the above are correct.

14. The universal distress sign of choking is:
    a. cyanosis.
    b. pointing at the throat with a finger.
    c. inability to speak.
    d. clutching the throat with the thumb on one side and fingers on the other.

15. The most reliable indication of a blocked airway in a conscious person is:
    a. the inability to speak.
    b. a compression accident.
    c. partially digested food in mouth.
    d. cherry-red skin color.

PART III: Matching

1. A basic understanding of the respiratory system is essential to understand the problems and complications that may occur. Fill in the anatomical names in the blanks from the list provided.

Choose from this list

Heart	Pulmonary Vein
Lung	Pleura
Bronchial Tube	Trachea
Alveoli	Epiglottis
Pulmonary Artery	

2. **The Need for Oxygen**

   When respiration and heart action cease, the victim is classified as _____. The brain cells die from four to six minutes after being deprived of _____. When irreversible brain damage occurs and the system dies, it is called _____. Proper care may keep brain cells alive and keep the victim from _____. The key is knowing _____ the status of the respiratory and circulatory systems.

3. **Opening the Airway**

   The airway may be opened by two proper techniques. Place the name of each of these techniques under the proper diagram.

   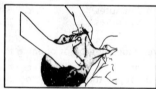   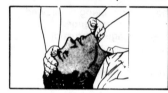

   List the three major ways you can recognize adequate breathing:

   Looking: *Chest rising*

   Listening: *sounds of breathing*

   Feeling: *breathing on face*

PART IV: What Would You Do If:

You are eating at a restaurant. Suddenly, a man at the next table stands up, knocks over his chair, and places both hands over his throat. His face has an alarmed look and his mouth is open.

1. What is the probable cause of this emergency situation?

2. What emergency care would you give for this situation?

3. What would you do if the victim still wasn't breathing after you performed the proper emergency care in question 2?

PART V: Practical Skills Check-Off

_____ has satisfactorily passed the following practical skills:

Student's Name

	Date	Partner Check	Inst. Init.
1. Obstructed airway; conscious adult.	__/__/__	☐	_____
2. Obstructed airway; unconscious adult.	__/__/__	☐	_____
3. Obstructed airway; conscious infant.	__/__/__	☐	_____
4. Obstructed airway; unconscious infant.	__/__/__	☐	_____
5. Mouth-to-mouth resuscitation.	__/__/__	☐	_____
6. Mouth-to-mouth and nose resuscitation.	__/__/__	☐	_____

CHAPTER FOUR

OBJECTIVES

- Understand the components and function of the circulatory system.
- Identify the differences between clinical and biological death.
- Describe the specific signs of cardiac arrest.
- Define cardiac arrest and identify its causes.
- Understand and practically apply cardiopulmonary resuscitation (CPR) on adults, children, and infants.
- Identify possible complications of CPR and know when to terminate CPR.

BASIC LIFE SUPPORT: CARDIOPULMONARY RESUSCITATION (CPR)

HEART ATTACKS and associated **HEART DISEASE** are America's number-one killer. Fortunately, hospitals have perfected a number of techniques that help to reverse cardiac disease and its crippling effects. Still, life-saving techniques exercised in the field by First Aiders are critical to saving lives.

CARDIOVASCULAR DISEASE takes the lives of approximately 980,000 Americans each year. This killer does not just occur in the older population, but also incapacitates people in their thirties and forties. Most people who die of a heart attack die before they ever reach a hospital. Ten percent of all heart-attack patients could be saved by immediate, efficient cardiopulmonary resuscitation (CPR), followed by advanced medical care, including **DEFIBRILLATION**, within eight to ten minutes.

THE HEART

The heart is a hollow, muscular organ about the size of a fist. It lies in the lower central region of the chest between the lungs and under the lower half of the breastbone. The heart is protected in the front by the ribs and breastbone and in the back by the backbone.

The heart contains four chambers. The two upper chambers are the left and right **ATRIA**, and the two lower chambers are the left and right **VENTRICLES**. The **SEPTUM** divides the right side of the heart from the left side. The heart also contains several one-way valves that keep blood flowing in the correct direction.

Two blood receptacles are located just below the heart — the liver to the right and center, and the spleen to the left (Figure 4-1). It is important to know the location of these organs to each other, because improper **CARDIAC COMPRESSIONS** may cause a fractured sternum or ribs. A piece of splintered or jagged bone could lacerate the lungs or liver, which could prove fatal to the victim.

THE HEART ACTION

By the heart's pumping action, blood is kept under pressure and in constant circulation throughout

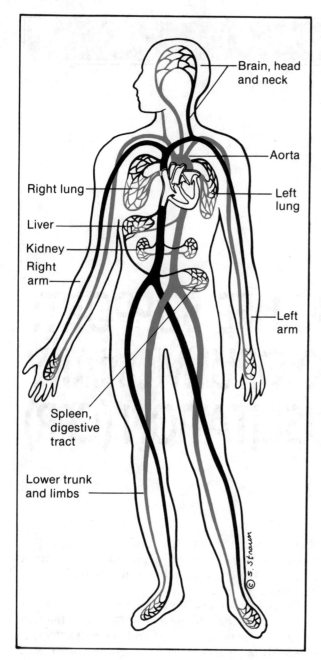

FIGURE 4-1. The heart pumps blood through the pulmonary and systemic circulation.

of the heart receives blood from all parts of the body and pumps it to the lungs to be reoxygenated (Figure 4-2). The effect of these contractions can be noted by means of the **PULSE** — the pressure exerted against the arterial wall during each contraction. Each time the heart pumps, a pulse can be felt throughout the **ARTERIAL SYSTEM**. The pulse can be felt most easily where a large artery is close to the skin surface, such as:

▪ The radial pulse in the wrist.

▪ The carotid pulse in the neck.

▪ The femoral pulse at the upper thigh (Figure 4-3).

The pulse is felt most easily over the carotid artery on either side of the neck, or on the thumb side of the inner surface of the wrist (radial). The radial pulse is generally the first pulse that the First Aider

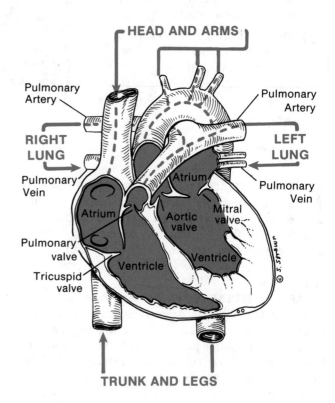

RIGHT HEART:
receives blood from the body and pumps it through the pulmonary artery to the lungs where it picks up fresh oxygen.

LEFT HEART:
Receives oxygen-full blood from the lungs and pumps it through the aorta to the body.

FIGURE 4-2.

the body. In a healthy adult at rest, the heart contracts between sixty and eighty times per minute; in a child, eighty to one hundred times per minute.

The heart may be likened to a four-cylinder pump, except that the "cylinders" of the heart do not discharge into a common outlet. The left side of the heart receives oxygenated blood from the lungs and pumps it to all parts of the body. The right side

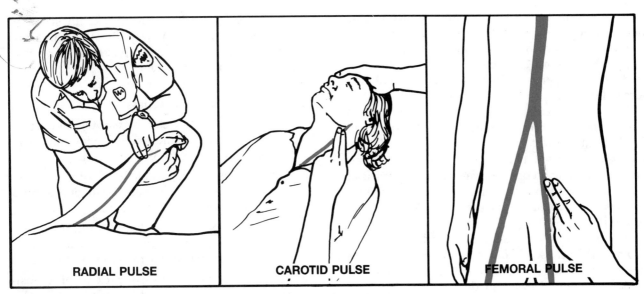

RADIAL PULSE | CAROTID PULSE | FEMORAL PULSE

FIGURE 4-3. Taking the radial pulse, the carotid pulse, and the femoral pulse.

palpates. If no radial pulse is found, the carotid pulse is palpated.

Three vital organs of the body — the heart, the lungs, and the brain — have a close relationship in sustaining life within the body because they are closely intertwined in function. When one of the organs cannot perform properly, the other two are handicapped in performing their functions. For example, a motorcycle accident victim is thrown against the motorcycle bars, crushing his trachea. This results in respiratory arrest. As the seconds tick by, the blood becomes deprived of oxygen because the oxygen in the lungs has been depleted. Therefore, the blood carries less and less oxygen to the brain, seriously impairing brain function. The cardiac control centers stop sending signals to the heart, which begins beating improperly, then stops beating (cardiac arrest). Within four to six minutes, the brain cells begin to die. The smooth functioning of each organ is crucial to the other two, and ultimately to the whole system. If one organ fails, the other two will follow.

See Chapter 3 for signs and emergency care of respiratory arrest.

CLINICAL AND BIOLOGICAL DEATH

Clinical death occurs when a victim is not breathing and the heart is not beating. Proper emergency care — namely, immediate, effective CPR — may reverse clinical death and possibly restore the victim to an undamaged state. Once the victim remains in clinical death for a certain time (typically four to six minutes), brain cells begin to die. The victim then experiences biological death, which is *not* reversible. (For more information on clinical and biological death, see Chapter 3.) Your goal is to become involved in giving emergency care while the victim is still in the clinical-death state. Immediate, effective CPR by a First Aider and early **ADVANCED CARDIAC LIFE SUPPORT (ACLS)** performed by EMT-Paramedics may be successful in saving a victim's life.

The key principles of CPR are to oxygenate and circulate the blood of the cardiopulmonary-arrest victim until definite corrective measures (advanced cardiac life support) can be given. Any delays in initiation of CPR increase the possibility of neurological impairment and reduce the victim's chance of survival. Survival rates improve with shorter time intervals between the onset of the cardiopulmonary arrest and the delivery of defibrillation and other ACLS measures.

CARDIOPULMONARY RESUSCITATION

You should immediately assess all unconscious victims for airway, breathing, and circulation. Assume that an unconscious person has experienced respiratory or cardiac arrest or both (**CARDIOPULMONARY ARREST**) until proven otherwise. Obvious cases where assistance is needed include trauma accidents, electric shock, suffocation, and near-drowning.

It is important to closely monitor an unconscious person who is breathing, because respiratory arrest can occur at any time. The heart muscle, being incapable of storing oxygen, is severely affected by lack of oxygen and loses its ability to contract forcefully.

Proper emergency care involves airway management, efficient artificial ventilation, and correct artificial circulation by cardiac compressions. Cardiopulmonary resuscitation (CPR) consists of opening and maintaining an open airway, providing artificial ventilation through rescue breathing, and providing artificial circulation by means of external cardiac compression.

It was formerly thought that cardiac compressions work because the blood is pumped out of the heart as the heart is squeezed between the sternum and backbone. Newer evidence indicates that **CLOSED-CHEST COMPRESSION** produces a generalized rise in **INTRATHORACIC** (inside the chest cavity) pressure that is applied to the pulmonary-**VASCULAR** bed, as well as to the heart. Because of this evidence, it is essential that you pay as much attention to the duration of the chest compression as you do to the rate of closed-chest compression. Compression should last at least 50 percent of the cycle. While study continues, you should rigorously follow the current CPR protocol of the American Heart Association described here and stay current on new CPR developments.

CPR must begin as soon as possible and continue until:

- The first aider is exhausted and is unable to continue.
- A qualified medical person takes over.
- The victim is resuscitated.
- Or the victim has been declared dead by a proper authority.

The key to the survival of a cardiac-arrest victim is:

- Early access to the victim by rescuers (including First Aiders trained in CPR).
- Early CPR.
- Early defibrillation by EMT-Paramedics or other medical personnel.

STEPS PRECEDING CPR

A victim of cardiac arrest will be unconscious, will have no pulse, will not breathe, and will have a deathlike appearance (grayish-blue skin and dilated and nonreactive pupils). The major factor, however, is the absent pulse.

In a case of cardiac arrest, take these steps (remember — A, B, C: **A**irway, **B**reathe, **C**irculate) (Figures 4-4–4-12). Quickly survey the scene and begin doing a primary survey.

1. **Establish unresponsiveness.**
   - Try to rouse the victim by tapping him gently on the shoulder and loudly asking him, "Are you okay? Are you okay?"
   - If he does not respond to touch or your voice, he is unresponsive. This evaluation should take no more than ten seconds.

2. **Call for help.** Call out "HELP!" You may have to send someone to call for the ambulance (alert the EMS system) and/or to help you do CPR.

3. **Position the victim on his back (supine position) on a hard, flat surface** (floor, sidewalk, etc.). If the victim is on his side or stomach, roll him as a unit into the supine position. A victim with a suspected neck injury *must have his neck stabilized* during the roll onto his back (See Chapter 3).

4. **Open the victim's airway and establish breathlessness** by the head-tilt/chin-lift or modified-jaw-thrust (in the case of a suspected neck injury) maneuver. The tongue often obstructs the upper airway, and many times, simply opening the airway will allow spontaneous resumption of breathing (see Chapter 3). Apply pressure on the forehead with one hand to extend the head while placing the fingers of the other hand under the mandible and lifting the chin upward. Take three to five seconds to look, listen, and feel for breathing.

5. **Give two full breaths.** If the victim is not breathing, deliver two successive breaths by mouth-to-mouth ventilation at 1 to 1.5 seconds per ventilation (see Chapter 3). Pinch off the victim's nostrils with the "forehead" hand, and seal your mouth over the victim's mouth. Allow full exhalation between breaths. This minimizes the chance of gastric distention. Watch the victim's chest to be sure that it inflates and deflates properly.

6. **Clear an obstructed airway.** If the victim's chest does not rise and fall with the ventilation, open his mouth and check for foreign matter. If you see nothing, reposition the head for an open airway. If that is unsuccessful, take the necessary steps to clear the obstructed airway. Then reattempt rescue breathing (see Chapter 3).

7. **Establish pulselessness.** Find the carotid pulse by placing two fingers on the larynx (**ADAM'S APPLE**), then slide them distally into the groove

STEPS PRECEDING CPR

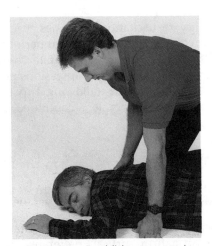

FIGURE 4-4. Establish unresponsiveness and call for help.

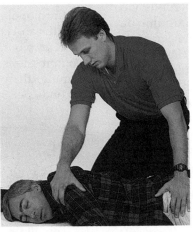

FIGURE 4-5. Position the victim on his back on a hard, flat surface.

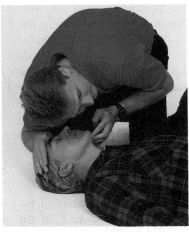

FIGURE 4-6. Open the airway with the head-tilt/chin-lift maneuver.

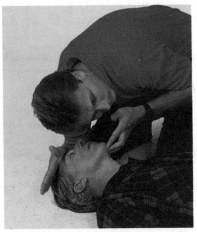

FIGURE 4-7. Establish breathlessness with the look-listen-feel method.

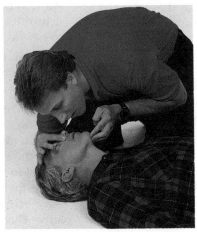

FIGURE 4-8. Perform mouth-to-mouth ventilation. Give two full breaths of air within five seconds.

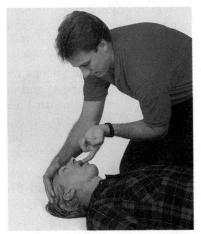

FIGURE 4-9. Clear an obstructed airway.

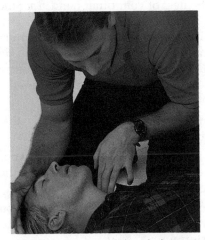

FIGURE 4-10. Establish pulselessness by palpating the carotid artery.

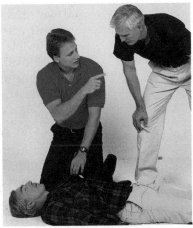

FIGURE 4-11. Send someone to activate the Emergency Medical Services system (e.g., 911).

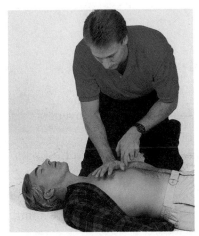

FIGURE 4-12. Bare the chest, landmark properly, and perform cardiopulmonary resuscitation.

between the larynx and the **STERNO-CLEIDOMAS-TOID MUSCLE** (large muscle in the neck). Palpate the carotid pulse for five to ten seconds (see Figure 2-10 in Chapter 2). Keep your thumb out of the way, and *do not* rest your hand across the trachea. If you feel no pulse, quickly try the opposite side. If a victim has a pulse, even a weak or irregular one, do *not* begin chest compressions — you could cause serious complications by doing so. Continue rescue breathing until spontaneous ventilation resumes or until paramedics take over to perform more definitive airway management. If you cannot detect a pulse, begin CPR.

8. **If no one has responded to your call for help previously, perform CPR for one minute, continually calling "HELP!", then try to get help by getting to a phone as quickly as possible.**

9. **Activate the Emergency Medical Service (EMS) system** by calling an ambulance or the emergency number 911. The victim of cardiac arrest needs to receive advanced life support as soon as possible. The reason for waiting until this point is to be sure of what is wrong. Unresponsiveness, breathlessness, and pulselessness are evidence of cardiac arrest. Call the ambulance yourself if you are alone, or send someone else. You should not leave the victim for more than thirty seconds. If possible, quickly return to the victim.

10. **If the victim's heart is not beating, continue with CPR.** Effective CPR is essential if the victim is to survive.

If in doubt about the assessment of cardiorespiratory arrest, assume that an arrest has occurred, and begin resuscitative procedures immediately.

SUMMARY OF STEPS PRECEDING CPR

1. Check for unresponsiveness.
2. Shout for help.
3. Position the victim on his back.
4. Open the airway.
5. Look, listen, and feel for breathing.
6. If the victim is not breathing, give two full breaths.
7. Check the carotid pulse.
8. Have someone phone the EMS system for help.
9. If there is no pulse, begin CPR.

PERFORMING CPR

Cardiopulmonary resuscitation combines rescue breaths and chest compressions. When you perform CPR by yourself, deliver fifteen consecutive chest compressions at a rate of 80 to 100 compressions per minute, then two rescue breaths (allowing 1 to 1.5 seconds per inspiration). This cycle is continued.

ONE-PERSON CPR

As you read this section, refer to the photo series "One-Person CPR," Figures 4-13–4-16.

1. The victim should already be lying horizontally on his back on a firm surface, preferably the ground or the floor. His legs should be elevated.

2. Remove the victim's shirt or blouse. (Do not waste time unbuttoning it — rip it open or pull it up). Cut a woman's bra in two, or slip it up to her neck.

3. Kneel on the firm surface *close* to the side of the victims shoulders. Have your knees about as wide as your shoulders.

4. Locate the lower tip (xiphoid process) of the victim's breastbone (sternum) by feeling the lower margin of his rib cage on the side nearest you with the middle and index fingers of your hand closest to the victim's feet. Then run your fingers along the victim's rib cage to the notch where the ribs meet the sternum in the center of the lower chest (Figure 4-17).

5. Place your middle finger on this notch, and put your index finger of the same hand on the lower end of the victim's sternum or breastbone.

6. Now place the heel of your other hand *above* the two fingers. When you apply pressure at that point with the heel of your hand, the sternum is flexible enough to be compressed.(If you do not position your hand properly, compression can fracture the sternum or the ribs, lacerating the heart, the lungs, and/or the liver.)

7. Another way of positioning your hands that does not require locating the xiphoid process is:

   ▪ With the index and middle fingers of your hand closest to the victim's feet, locate the lower border of the rib cage closest to you.

   ▪ Put your fingers along the rib cage until you find the **SUBSTERNAL NOTCH** (where the ribs meet the sternum).

   ▪ Keep your index finger on the lower end of the sternum and your middle finger on the notch.

ONE-PERSON CPR

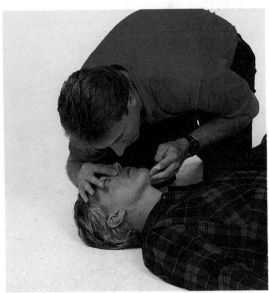

FIGURE 4-13. Establish breathlessness with the look-listen-feel method, open the airway, and perform mouth-to-mouth resuscitation.

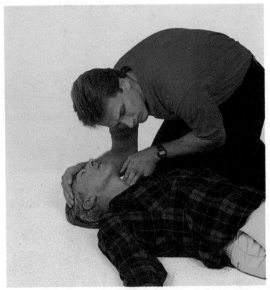

FIGURE 4-14. Establish pulselessness by checking the corotid artery in the neck.

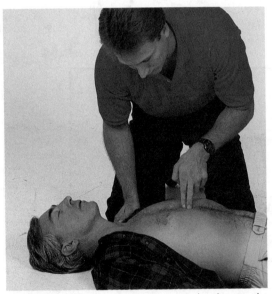

FIGURE 4-15. If you detect no pulse locate the xiphoid process, or sternal notch, and measure two finger widths above it.

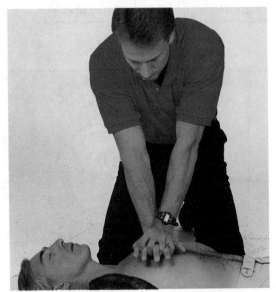

FIGURE 4-16. Compress 1½ to 2 inches on an adult at the rate of 80 to 100 per minute.

■ Now move your free hand to the midline of the sternum and place the thumb side against the index finger of your lower hand, making sure that the heel of your free hand is on the midline of the sternum. If you compress the xiphoid, you may lacerate the liver and cause severe internal bleeding (Figure 4-18).

8. Place your second hand on top of your first, bringing your shoulders directly over the victim's sternum.

9. Interlace your fingers. The fingers should be held off the chest wall (Figure 4-19).

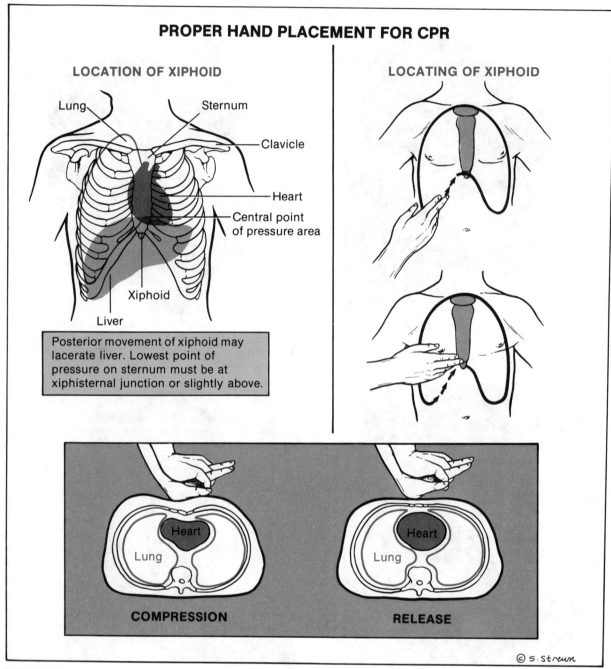

PROPER HAND PLACEMENT FOR CPR

LOCATION OF XIPHOID

Lung
Sternum
Clavicle
Heart
Central point of pressure area
Xiphoid
Liver

Posterior movement of xiphoid may lacerate liver. Lowest point of pressure on sternum must be at xiphisternal junction or slightly above.

LOCATING OF XIPHOID

COMPRESSION

Heart
Lung

RELEASE

Heart
Lung

© S. Streun

FIGURE 4-17.

10. Keeping your arms straight and your elbows locked, thrust from the shoulders and apply firm, heavy pressure so that you depress the sternum about one and one-half to two inches (four to five centimeters) on an adult (Figure 4-20). Do not make sudden, jerking movements. Even this amount of effective compression provides only one-fourth to one-third of normal blood flow, so anything less is ineffective. Use the weight of your upper body as you lean down over the victim to deliver the compressions. If necessary, add additional weight with your shoulders, but never with your arms — the force is too great, and you may fracture the sternum. Compression duration should occupy 50 percent of the pumping cycle.

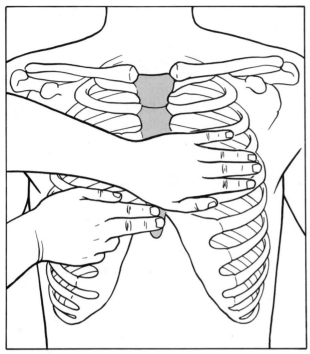

FIGURE 4-18 Place heel of hand on breastbone.

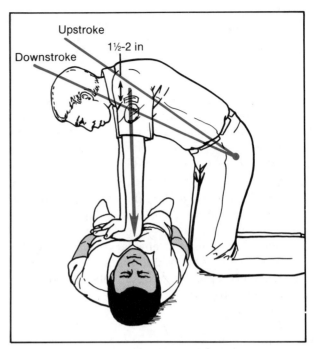

FIGURE 4-20. Proper positioning of the First Aider to perform chest compressions.

chest. If your fingers stay on the chest, the pressure from your compressions increases the possibility of fracture or rib-joint separation (Figure 4-21).

11. After each compression, completely relax the pressure so that the sternum returns to its normal

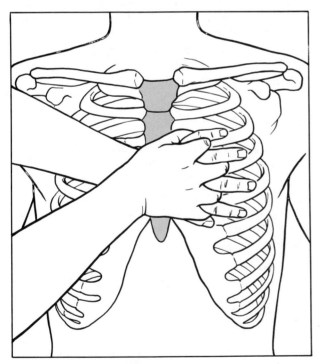

FIGURE 4-19. Interlace fingers.

▪ An acceptable alternative for those who have hand or wrist problems is to grasp the wrist of the hand lying on the chest with the hand that has been locating the lower end of the sternum. Pull your *fingers* upward, off the

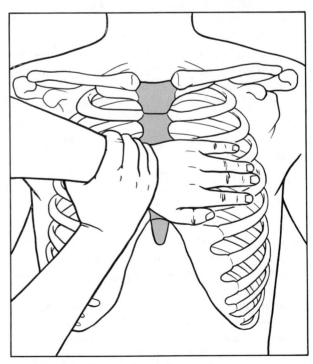

FIGURE 4-21. Alternate hand placement.

position, but do not remove your hands from the victim's chest or you will lose the proper positioning. The heel of your bottom hand should continue to touch the chest even during relaxation.

12. Your compressions should be regular, smooth, and uninterrupted, with compressions and relaxation time being about equal. Jabs make the blood spurt but do not increase the volume of flow, and they enhance the risk of injury.

13. Count as you administer compressions. It should take a little less than two seconds from the time you say "one" and compress the first time until you say "two" and compress the second time. This will enable you to administer eighty compressions per minute. Time yourself. Fifteen compressions should take between nine and eleven seconds.

One — push down
and — let up
two — push down
and — let up, etc.

14. Beware of becoming **HYPERVENTILATED**. It will be natural for you to breathe with the same rhythm you are counting, but this pattern is very deep and quick. You could easily hyperventilate. Learn to breathe at a regular tempo that is different from the rhythm that you are using for the compression/ventilation cycle. It is more important that the compressions be at least 50 percent of the cycle than that there be exactly eighty compressions per minute, since it is the compression that moves the blood.

15. Make sure that you administer pressure directly from above, not from the side. Deliver compressions at the rate of 80 to 100 per minute for an adult or child, and at least 100 per minute for an infant.

16. Give the two lung inflations within five seconds (1 to 1.5 seconds per lung inflation).

17. Never try to relieve gastric distention by pressing on the victim's abdomen at the same time you are doing CPR. The combined sources of pressure could rupture the liver.

18. After the first minute (four cycles of fifteen compressions and two ventilations) of CPR, and periodically thereafter, palpate the carotid artery (within five seconds) to check for the return of a spontaneous, effective heartbeat. Do this pulse check regularly in four- to five-minute intervals, or every few minutes thereafter, but do not interrupt CPR for more than a few seconds.

If A Second Rescuer Takes Over One-Person CPR

If another rescuer trained in CPR is at the scene, this person should do two things: first, phone the EMS system for help if this has not been done; second, take over CPR when the first rescuer is tired. Here are the steps for entry of the second rescuer:

1. The second person should first identify himself as a CPR-trained rescuer who is willing to help.

2. If the EMS system has been called and if the first rescuer is tired and asks for help, then:

   ■ The first rescuer should stop CPR after the next set of two breaths.

   ■ The second rescuer should kneel next to the victim opposite the first rescuer, tilt the head back, and feel for the carotid pulse for five seconds.

   ■ If there is no pulse, the second rescuer should give two breaths and continue CPR.

   ■ The first rescuer should then check the adequacy of the second rescuer's breaths and chest compressions. This is done by watching the victim's chest rise and fall during rescue breathing, and by feeling the carotid pulse for an artificial pulse during chest compressions. This artificial pulse will tell you that blood is moving through the body.

TWO-PERSON CPR

All professional rescuers should learn both the one-rescuer technique and the two-rescuer coordinated technique, which is less fatiguing. Your instructor will tell you whether you will become trained in two-person CPR. As you read this section, refer to the photo series "Two-Person CPR," Figures 4-22–4-29.

1. If two trained First Aiders are present, you should kneel at the victim's side and perform cardiac compressions while the other First Aider kneels on the *opposite side* near the victim's head and delivers artificial ventilation.

2. In this case, the ventilation should be delivered during a pause after every fifth cardiac compression so that ventilation is at the rate of twelve per minute.

3. Use an audible count of "one and two and three and four and five and pause," so that you achieve five compressions every three to five seconds.

4. The compression First Aider counts the sequence aloud. Compressions occur on each number (one, two, etc.).

TWO-PERSON CPR

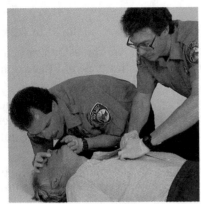

FIGURE 4-22. After establishing breathlessness, one rescuer gives two breaths while the other rescuer bares the chest and gets into position to perform chest compressions.

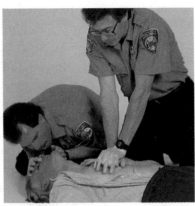

FIGURE 4-23. After establishing pulselessness, one rescuer gives a ventilation. The other rescuer then begins chest compressions.

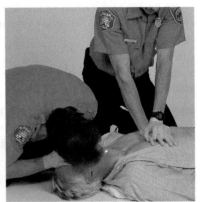

FIGURE 4-24. CPR continues at a ratio of five compressions to one ventilation, during which the rescuer performing the compressions pauses.

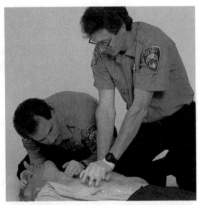

FIGURE 4-25. Stop CPR to assess the carotid pulse after the first minute, and every few minutes thereafter.

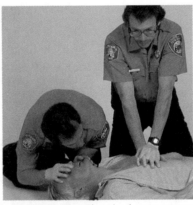

FIGURE 4-26. The tired compressor requests a switch.

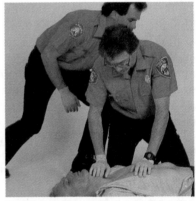

FIGURE 4-27. Changing positions in two-rescuer CPR. The rescuer ventilating delivers a breath as usual, then moves into position to assume cardiac compressions while the other rescuer checks the carotid pulse and positions himself to ventilate.

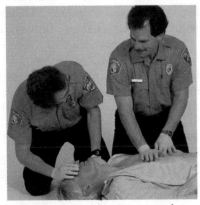

FIGURE 4-28. The rescuer performing the compressions quickly moves to the victim's head and checks the carotid pulse and breathing for five seconds. The other rescuer readies for compressions.

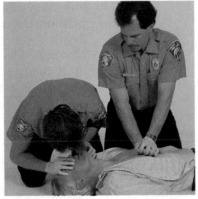

FIGURE 4-29. Completing the change. If no pulse is found, the rescuers continue CPR.

> **If possible, the second rescuer should be on the OPPOSITE side of the victim. Both rescuers in this series were photographed on the same side of the victim for reader clarity.**

5. The ventilation First Aider takes a deep breath on "three and," positions himself to ventilate on "four and," and begins breathing into the victim after "five." The compressor pauses for 1 to 1.5 seconds so that the victim receives a full breath.

6. Always stop CPR to assess the carotid pulse (five to ten seconds) after the first minute, and every few minutes thereafter.

7. The ventilator rescuer should occasionally check the carotid pulse *during* the chest compression to be sure that the **"FLUTTER" PULSE** is there. This indicates that blood is being moved from the heart satisfactorily.

Changing Positions in Two-Person CPR

When the rescuer performing cardiac compressions gets tired, he should switch with the one who is delivering ventilations. Here is the seven-second method:

1. The rescuer doing compressions calls for a switch at the end of the compression cycle by substituting "change" for "one." The audible count remains the same for the remaining four compressions. (Any mnemonic that satisfactorily accomplishes the change is acceptable. Another popular technique uses as the count, "Change, on, the, next, breath.") A similar phrase can also be used to "call" for the move of the victim or to "call" for a pulse check. It simply involves substituting:

"1-and	2-and	3-and	etc."
"CHANGE-and	2-and	3-and	etc."
"Lift-and	2-and	3-and	etc."
"Pulse-and	2-and	3-and	etc."

2. After the fifth compression, the rescuer performing the ventilations gives the full breath, then moves to the chest, locates the landmark notch, and gets into position for compressions.

3. The rescuer performing the compressions moves quickly to the victim's head after the fifth compression and checks the carotid pulse and breathing for a maximum of five seconds.

4. If no pulse is found, the rescuer at the head gives a breath and announces, "No pulse; continue CPR."

5. The rescuer at the chest is in position and begins compressions.

6. If the compressor becomes short of breath and cannot give the full count out loud, at least say the "four and, five and," count so that the ventilator will know when to breathe.

If one rescuer is performing CPR and a second rescuer or other rescuer becomes available, follow this procedure:

1. He should identify himself as qualified in CPR.

2. The first rescuer nods as compressions are continued and he completes the cycle of fifteen compressions and two ventilations.

3. At the end of the cycle (15-2), the first rescuer checks the carotid pulse for five seconds, then gives one ventilation. The second rescuer gets into position and becomes the compressor.

4. Compressions resume. A ventilation should be given during a pause after each fifth chest compression.

5. Continue CPR until pulses resume or until ACLS can be initiated!

SIGNS OF SUCCESSFUL CPR

- Each time that the sternum is compressed, you should feel a pulse (it will feel like a flutter) in the carotid artery.
- The lungs should expand.
- The pupils *may* react, or appear normal.
- A normal heartbeat *may* return.
- A spontaneous gasp of breathing *may* occur.
- The victim's skin color *may* improve or return to normal.
- The victim *may* move his arms or legs on his own.
- The victim *may* try to swallow.

Remember that "successful" CPR does not mean that the victim lives. "Successful" means that you performed it correctly. Very few victims will survive, despite the best CPR, if they do not receive advanced life support, defibrillation, oxygen, and drug therapy. The goal of CPR is to prevent biological death in a clinically dead person for a few crucial moments in hopes that advanced life support will reach him quickly.

CPR IN INFANTS AND CHILDREN

Infants (up to one year) and children (one to eight years) require slightly different procedures for evaluation and performance of CPR.

Cardiac arrest in children is rarely caused by heart problems. The heart nearly always stops beating because of oxygen deprivation due to injuries, suffocation, smoke inhalation, **SUDDEN INFANT DEATH SYNDROME (SIDS)**, or infections.

As you read this section, refer to the photo series "Infant and Child CPR," Figures 4-30–4-38.

ESTABLISHING UNRESPONSIVENESS OR RESPIRATORY DIFFICULTY

- No **BRACHIAL PULSE**.
- No chest movements.
- No audible heart sounds.
- Blue or pale skin.
- No response when shaken or gently tapped.
- Gasps, muscular contractions, and seizure-like convulsive activity.

An infant or child with breathing difficulty but who is not blue probably has an adequate airway and should be transported immediately to an advanced-life-support facility.

OPENING THE AIRWAY

1. Open the airway using the head-tilt/chin-lift maneuver.
2. Make sure that the mouth is open, that the tongue is not blocking the airway, and that your fingers are not pressing the soft tissue underneath the jaw. Be gentle!
3. Do not overextend the neck. A neutral position is best. An overextended neck may collapse the trachea in an infant.

BREATHING

Often, an infant will resume breathing when the airway is open. If the child gasps or struggles to catch his breath after the airway is open, let him breathe on his own if the lips are pink. Have the victim transported immediately. If the lips are blue (cyanotic), the victim is not getting adequate oxygen.

1. If the victim does not breathe, begin ventilations by giving two gentle breaths at 1 to 1.5 seconds per ventilation. Allow deflation between breaths.
2. Force and volume used should be that of a puff from the cheeks. Do not overinflate. Use only enough air to make the chest rise.
3. Watch the motion of the chest wall with each breath to be sure that air is getting in and out.

GASTRIC DISTENTION

Getting air into the infant's stomach may interfere with emergency breathing by elevating the diaphragm, thereby decreasing lung volume. You can cut down the incidence of gastric distention by limiting ventilation volumes to the point at which the chest rises. *Do not* attempt to press the abdomen to relieve gastric distention unless ventilation is ineffective. The risk of the infant aspirating vomitus is too great. See Chapter 3.

AIRWAY OBSTRUCTION

Airway obstruction is very common in infants and children. If any airway is obstructed by an **INFECTIOUS** disease (e.g., **CROUP**, epiglottitis), the infant should be transported immediately. Typically, this is a child who has been ill with a fever, barking cough, and progressive airway obstruction.

If a foreign object causes partial or complete airway obstruction and the child is attempting to expel it, do not interfere immediately. If poor air exchange is shown by an ineffective cough, increased respiratory difficulty, high-pitched noises when inhaling, and blueness of the lips, nails, and skin, relieve the obstruction by a combination of back blows and chest thrusts. *Do not use abdominal thrusts in infants, because the abdominal organs are injured too easily.*

1. Straddle an infant over your arm, with his head lower than his trunk.
2. Support the infant's head by placing your hand around his jaw and chest. Rest his thigh on your forearm.
3. Deliver four back blows in rapid succession with the heel of your hand between the infant's shoulder blades.
4. Immediately after you deliver the back blows, place your free hand on the infant's back so that he is sandwiched between your two hands, one hand supporting the back, the other supporting the neck, jaw, and chest.
5. Now turn the infant, and place him on your thigh, with his head lower than his trunk.
6. Deliver four chest thrusts in rapid succession in the same way that you perform external chest compressions in the infant (Figure 4-39).
7. Avoid blind finger sweeps, because they are likely to push the obstruction farther inward. If you can see a foreign object, remove it with your finger and thumb.
8. After your attempts, try ventilations again. If the chest does not rise, repeat the obstruction procedures to relieve the obstruction.

INFANT AND CHILD CPR

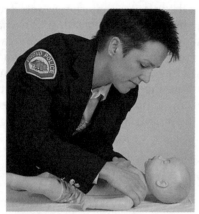

FIGURE 4-30. Determine unresponsiveness in the infant by a GENTLE "shake and shout" method. You may also try flicking the soles of the baby's feet.

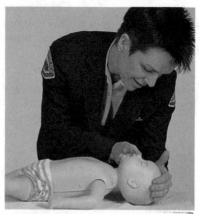

FIGURE 4-31. Gently open the airway using the head-tilt/chin-lift maneuver. Do NOT tilt the head back very far.

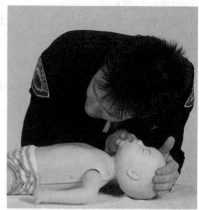

FIGURE 4-32. Establish breathlessness by the Look-Listen-Feel method.

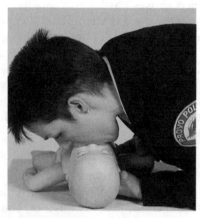

FIGURE 4-33. Infant mouth-to-mouth and nose ventilation. The rescuer covers the baby's mouth and nose with a good seal, then gives two ventilations.

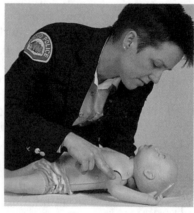

FIGURE 4-34. Check the infant for pulselessness by gently palpating the brachial artery.

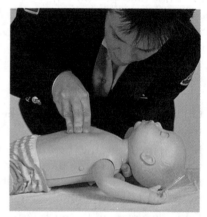

FIGURE 4-35. Perform cardiac compressions in an infant by placing the middle and ring fingers in the midline, one finger's breadth below the intermammary line.

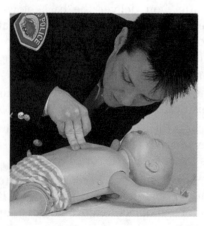

FIGURE 4-36. The lower sternum is depressed ½ to 1 inch at a minimum compression rate of 100 per minute.

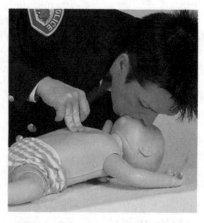

FIGURE 4-37. A gentle puff of air is given after each fifth compression.

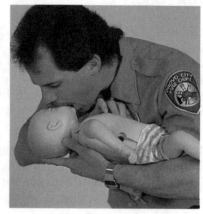

FIGURE 4-38. Performing infant CPR while carrying the baby.

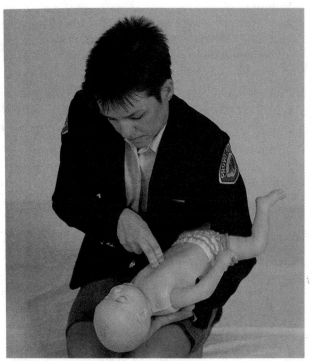

FIGURE 4-39. For an airway obstruction, place the infant on your thigh, with the head lower then the trunk, and deliver four chest thrusts in rapid succession.

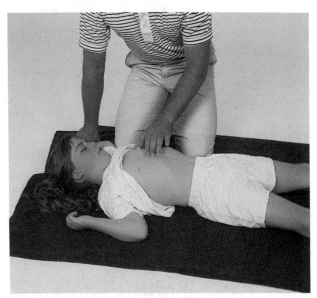

FIGURE 4-40. Proper finger position on a child.

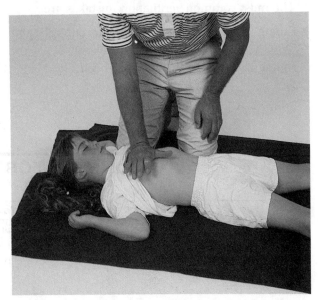

FIGURE 4-41. For a larger child, compress the sternum one to one and one-half inches with the heel of one hand.

CIRCULATION

1. After you are successful in delivering the two consecutive breaths, *check the carotid pulse in a child*, but *check the brachial pulse in the infant.*

2. If there is no pulse, begin performing ventilations and chest compressions.

   ■ Make sure that the victim is lying on a firm surface.

   ■ The correct area of compression in the infant is one finger width below an imaginary line between the nipples.

   ■ Use the flat part of your second and third fingers to compress the infant's sternum one-half to one inch. For a larger child, compress the sternum one to one and one-half inches with the heel of one hand (Figures 4-40–4-41).

   ■ The compression rate for infants is at least 100 per minute; for children, it is 80 to 100 compressions per minute.

   ■ The ratio of compressions to respirations is five to one in both infants and children.

   ■ In one-person CPR, breathe once for the victim after each fifth compression.

   ■ With two-person CPR on a child, ventilate during a pause after each fifth compression. Count compressions at this rhythm:

   Infant — one, two, three, four, five, breathe.
   Child — one and two and three and four and five and breathe.

SIGNS OF SUCCESSFUL CPR

The methods of checking for successful CPR in infants or children are almost the same as for adults.

1. Check the brachial pulse periodically.
2. Check the dilated pupils to see if they regain activity or constrict.
3. Watch for a spontaneous heartbeat, spontaneous breathing, and consciousness. See Figure 4-42 for a summary of pediatric CPR.

COMPLICATIONS OF CPR IN CHILDREN

One of the most common complications in trauma and sudden illness in children is **HYPO-THERMIA**. Keep the child or infant warm.

MISTAKES IN PERFORMING CPR

The most common ventilation mistakes are:

■ Failing to tip the head back far enough and thereby not giving adequate ventilations.
■ Failing to maintain an adequate head tilt.

■ Failing to pinch the nose or maintain the pinched nose during ventilations, allowing air to escape, and not covering the mouth *and* nose during infant ventilations.
■ Not giving full breaths.
■ Completing a cycle in fewer than five seconds.
■ Failing to watch and listen for exhalation.
■ Failing to maintain an adequate seal around the victim's mouth, nose or both during ventilation. (The seal should be released when the victim exhales.)

Some common chest compression mistakes:

■ Elbows bent instead of straight.
■ Shoulders not directly above sternum of the victim.
■ Heel of bottom hand not in line with the sternum, or too low; not depressing the chest (sternum) one-half to two inches.
■ Fingers touching the victim's chest.
■ Pivoting at knees instead of at hips.
■ Incorrect compression rate.

SUMMARY FOR PEDIATRIC C.P.R.

Child's age	Less than 1 year	1-7 years	8 years and over
Ventilation force	blow until chest rises	blow until chest rises	blow until chest rises
Ventilation rate	20/min	15/min	12/min
Sternal compression site	midsternum, 1 finger width below nipple line	2 finger widths up from xiphoid process (on sternum at nipple line)	2 finger widths up from xiphoid process (lower half of sternum)

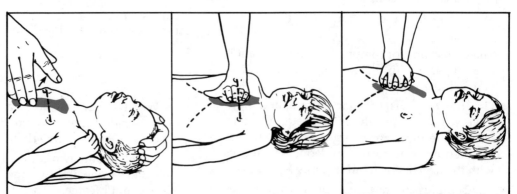

Compression delivery	2 or 3 fingers	heel of one hand	heels of both hands, using body pressure
Compression depth	½-1 inch	1-1½ inches	1½-2 inches
Compression rate	100-120/min	80-100/min	80-100/min

FIGURE 4-42.

- Compressions given in jerky movements rather than smoothly.
- Hand not remaining on victim's chest between compressions.

COMPLICATIONS CAUSED BY CPR

Even properly performed, CPR may cause rib fractures in some victims. Other complications that may occur with properly performed CPR include fracture of the sternum, **PNEUMOTHORAX**, **HEMO-THORAX**, lung **CONTUSIONS**, and lacerations of the liver. You can minimize these complications by giving careful attention to performance — but remember, effective cardiopulmonary resuscitation is necessary even if it results in complications, since the alternative is death.

The rib cartilage in elderly victims will often separate easily. You will hear it crunch as you compress. Be sure that your hand is positioned correctly and that you are compressing to the correct depth, but do not stop.

WHEN TO TERMINATE CPR

First Aiders, as they recognize cardiac arrest, must administer CPR to the best of their ability and knowledge and should not be held liable for failure to initiate CPR if that decision is consistent with current American Heart Association standards. They should continue resuscitation efforts until one of the following occurs:

- Effective spontaneous ventilation and circulation have been restored.
- Another responsible or professional person assumes responsibility for life support.
- A physician, physician-directed individual, or physician-directed team assumes responsibility for life support.

- The victim is transferred to an appropriate emergency-medical-service facility.
- The rescuer is exhausted and unable to continue life support.
- The victim is declared dead by a physician.

WHEN TO WITHHOLD CPR

You are legally required to begin CPR on any victim who needs it for whom "there is no legal or medical reason to withhold it," according to the 1986 American Medical Association guidelines. For all practical purposes, there is no way you can tell if such a legal or medical reason exists, and you should simply initiate CPR under all reasonable conditions.

The medical reasons for not beginning CPR are "irreversible cessation of all functions of the entire brain, including the brain stem." You, of course, have no way of determining whether the condition is irreversible until you try to reverse it. Only in the presence of **RIGOR MORTIS**, **DECAPITATION**, obviously **MORTAL** wounds, severe crushing of the chest and/or head, or established **LIVIDITY** (signs of death) could you be absolutely sure that resuscitation would not be possible.

As a practical matter, however, long-term survival decreases dramatically if the patient has not been resuscitated after thirty minutes (exceptions are drowning and hypothermia cases).

Several studies have shown that CPR technical skills deteriorate rapidly without frequent practice and retraining. Retraining in CPR skills should occur quarterly, and recertification should occur every one to two years.

FOR FURTHER STUDY

It is recommended that the student study Figures 4-43–4-45 for an excellent review of this chapter.

CPR

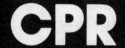

CARDIOPULMONARY RESUSCITATION FOR INFANTS (YOUNGER THAN 1 YEAR)

Fitnus® For Life

1 Check if conscious or unconscious.

Gently tap and shake shoulders to determine if infant is conscious. If unresponsive, call out for "Help!" Infant must be lying on his or her back on a hard flat surface (table or floor). If positioning is necessary, support head and neck and turn infant as a unit onto back.

4 Check for pulse.

Place thumb on outside of upper arm between elbow and shoulder. Put index fingers on the inside and gently press to find pulse.

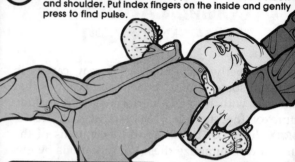

PULSE FOUND	**NO PULSE**
Give 1 breath every 3 seconds until breathing resumes (DO NOT GO TO STEPS 5 AND 6)	Landmark and begin chest compressions (GO TO STEPS 5 AND 6)

2 Open airway. Check for breathing.

Place one hand on forehead and tilt head gently back. Place index finger just under chin and lift gently until nose, mouth, and chin are in horizontal position. Do not close infant's mouth completely. Put ear close to infant's mouth and nose. **LOOK** for movement of chest and stomach. **LISTEN** and **FEEL** for breathing.

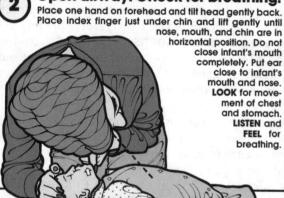

5 Landmark for finger position.

Place 3 fingers on breastbone with index finger just below imaginary line between nipples. Location for compression being one finger's width below line, use middle and ring fingers to compress breastbone.

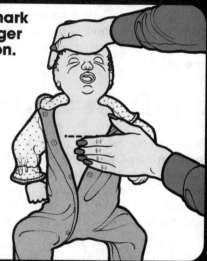

3 If not breathing—Give 2 slow breaths.

Keeping airway open, take a deep breath and cover infant's mouth and nose with your mouth making a tight seal. Give 2 slow breaths with a pause between for you to take a breath.

6 Chest compressions.

Using fingertips of middle and ring fingers compress breastbone ½-1 inch with smooth and even movements at a rate of 100 compressions per minute. Give 5 compressions counting: "one, two, three, four, five." Follow 5 compressions with 1 breath and repeat.

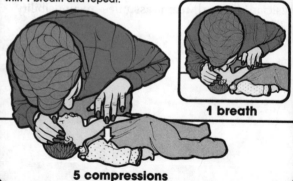

1 breath

5 compressions

Fitnus® For Life 3125 19th Street, Suite 305 ▪ Bakersfield, CA 93301 ▪ (805) 861-1100 ▪ Aigra, Inc. 1986

FIGURE 4-43.

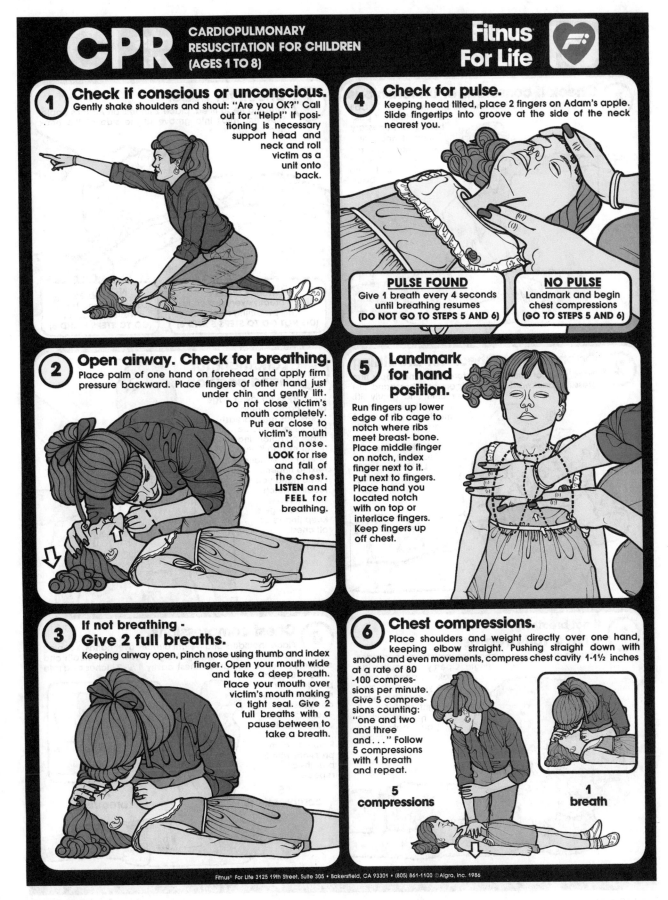

FIGURE 4-44.

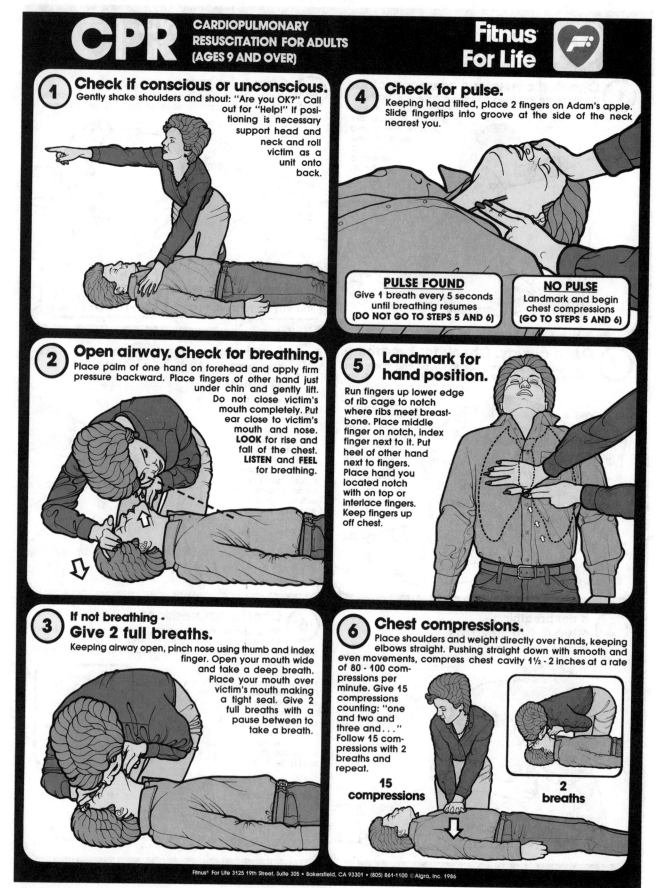

CPR
CARDIOPULMONARY RESUSCITATION FOR ADULTS (AGES 9 AND OVER)

Fitnus For Life

① Check if conscious or unconscious.
Gently shake shoulders and shout: "Are you OK?" Call out for "Help!" If positioning is necessary support head and neck and roll victim as a unit onto back.

② Open airway. Check for breathing.
Place palm of one hand on forehead and apply firm pressure backward. Place fingers of other hand just under chin and gently lift. Do not close victim's mouth completely. Put ear close to victim's mouth and nose. **LOOK** for rise and fall of the chest. **LISTEN** and **FEEL** for breathing.

**③ If not breathing -
Give 2 full breaths.**
Keeping airway open, pinch nose using thumb and index finger. Open your mouth wide and take a deep breath. Place your mouth over victim's mouth making a tight seal. Give 2 full breaths with a pause between to take a breath.

④ Check for pulse.
Keeping head tilted, place 2 fingers on Adam's apple. Slide fingertips into groove at the side of the neck nearest you.

PULSE FOUND	**NO PULSE**
Give 1 breath every 5 seconds until breathing resumes **(DO NOT GO TO STEPS 5 AND 6)**	Landmark and begin chest compressions **(GO TO STEPS 5 AND 6)**

⑤ Landmark for hand position.
Run fingers up lower edge of rib cage to notch where ribs meet breastbone. Place middle finger on notch, index finger next to it. Put heel of other hand next to fingers. Place hand you located notch with on top or interlace fingers. Keep fingers up off chest.

⑥ Chest compressions.
Place shoulders and weight directly over hands, keeping elbows straight. Pushing straight down with smooth and even movements, compress chest cavity 1½ - 2 inches at a rate of 80 - 100 compressions per minute. Give 15 compressions counting: "one and two and three and..." Follow 15 compressions with 2 breaths and repeat.

15 compressions

2 breaths

Fitnus® For Life 3125 19th Street, Suite 305 ▪ Bakersfield, CA 93301 ▪ (805) 861-1100 ©Algra, Inc. 1986

FIGURE 4-45.

| **4** | **SELF-TEST** | **4** |

Student: _____   Date: _____

Course: _____   Section #: _____

PART I: True/False   If you believe that the statement is true, circle the T. If you believe that the statement is false, circle the F.

T   F   1. Cardiac compressions on a male adult should depress the sternum four to five inches.

T   F   2. The best way to find out if a person has stopped breathing is to check the carotid pulse.

T   F   3. Even though a person's heart stops beating, he may keep breathing for awhile.

T   F   4. Biological death can be reversed.

T   F   5. You should begin CPR immediately after you find that the victim is not breathing.

T   F   6. For adult CPR, proper hand placement on the chest is two finger widths above the xiphoid process.

T   F   7. One rescuer should give compressions at the rate of sixty per minute.

T   F   8. The compression rate for infants is at least 100 per minute.

T   F   9. Heartbeat in an infant should be checked by palpating the brachial pulse.

T   F   10. A First Aider should terminate CPR if the victim doesn't respond within fifteen minutes.

PART II: Multiple Choice   For each question, circle the answer that best reflects an accurate statement.

1. The correct hand position for administering CPR to an infant is:
    a. two fingers above the sternal notch.
    b. at the base of the sternum.
    c. in the lower one-third of the sternum.
    d. two fingers, one finger width below the intermammary line.

2. After each chest compression during CPR, your hands should:
    a. come completely off the chest.
    b. apply small amount of pressure on the chest.
    c. rest on the chest in normal CPR position.
    d. none of the above.

3. If you are alone, giving CPR, you should give _____ inflations after each _____ compressions.
    a. 2, 15.   c. 1, 2.
    b. 15, 2.   d. 1, 4.

4. Basic life support consists of:
    a. recognition of cardiac arrest and providing artificial ventilation and circulation.
    b. checking for breathing and applying rescue breathing.
    c. checking for heartbeat and applying artificial circulation.
    d. checking for heartbeat and applying rescue breathing.

5. CPR must begin when a need for it is recognized and continue until *all but one* of the following occurs:
    a. the patient is declared dead by the First Aider.
    b. the patient is resuscitated.
    c. the rescuer can no longer go on.
    d. a qualified medical person takes over.

6. To check the carotid pulse for circulation:
    a. use your thumb.
    b. take the pulse on the opposite side of the trachea so that you can feel air exchange in the trachea.
    c. check the pulse with your fingertips after you give two full breaths.
    d. none of the above.

7. You should periodically stop and check to see if the heartbeat has returned by:
    a. checking the pupils.
    b. checking the pulse.
    c. listening for a heartbeat with a stethoscope.
    d. never stop CPR unless the patient is obviously revived.

8. Which of the following is *not* a sign of successful CPR?
    a. improvement of skin color.
    b. reactive pupils.
    c. perceptible pulse when the chest is compressed.
    d. vomiting by the victim.

PART III: Matching

1. **Clinical and Biological Death**

    Quick action is needed before the victim experiences clinical, then biological death. Identify those two terms by completing the following table:

Lapsed Time	Type of Death (Clinical or Biological)	Possibility of Brain Damage
0-4 minutes	C	Small, but brain cells are being weakened by lack of fuel.
4-6 minutes	C	Brain cells are dying rapidly.
6-10 minutes	B	Extensive irreversible brain damage has occurred and death is imminent.
over 10 minutes	B	Too many brain cells have usually been destroyed for life to continue.

2. **Circulation**

You can identify whether the heart is beating by trying to locate a pulse. Match the two types of pulses with the proper diagram.

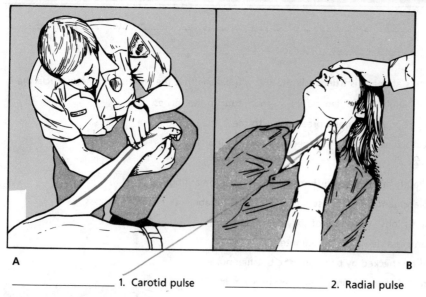

A   B

_____ 1. Carotid pulse   _____ 2. Radial pulse

PART IV: What Would You Do If:

You are eating at a restaurant with your family when a middle-aged man at another table clutches at his chest and collapses on the floor. You hear the commotion and come on the scene. You ask, "Is he choking?" No one can tell you. People are crowded around the body, the man's wife is shaking him and screaming, but no one is in charge.

1. What signs and symptoms would tell you that the man is suffering a heart attack?

2. What first-aid step would you perform first?

3. Identify the steps you would perform under each category.

   A - Airway

   B - Breathing

   C - Circulation

PART V: Practical Skills Check-Off   _____ has satisfactorily passed the following practical skills:
                                                             Student's Name

	Date	Partner Check	Inst. Init.
1. One-Rescuer CPR: Adult.	___/___/___	☐	_____
2. One-Rescuer CPR: Child-Infant.	___/___/___	☐	_____
3. Two-Rescuer CPR: (if applicable)	___/___/___	☐	_____

OBJECTIVES

■ Understand the significance of bleeding and how it affects various aspects of the circulatory system.

■ Describe and demonstrate how to control external bleeding using direct pressure, elevation, pressure points, splints, air splints, tourniquets, and cryotherapy.

■ Identify the most common sites and signs and symptoms of internal bleeding.

■ Describe and demonstrate the general procedures for controlling internal bleeding.

CONTROL OF BLEEDING

CIRCULATORY SYSTEM

The life processes depend on an adequate and uninterrupted blood supply. An understanding of what blood is and how it is circulated will help explain why and how blood loss must be stopped quickly and effectively.

In order to function, a person's body must receive a constant supply of nourishment (such as oxygen), which is distributed by the blood. If the supply of blood is cut off, the tissues in the body will die for want of nourishment.

The circulatory system, by which blood is carried to and from all parts of the body, consists of the heart and blood vessels. Through the blood vessels, blood is circulated to and from all parts of the body under pressure supplied by the pumping action of the heart (Figure 5-1).

BLOOD

Blood is composed of **SERUM** or **PLASMA**, **RED CELLS**, **WHITE CELLS**, and **PLATELETS**. Plasma is a fluid that carries the blood cells and transports nutrients to all tissues. It also transports waste products resulting from tissue **METABOLISM** to the organs of excretion. Red cells give color to the blood and carry oxygen. White cells aid in defending the body against infection. Platelets are essential to the formation of blood clots, which are necessary to stop bleeding. Clotting normally takes six to seven minutes.

The process whereby body cells receive oxygen and other nutrients and wastes are removed is called **PERFUSION**. An organ is perfused if blood is entering

DISTRIBUTION OF BLOOD IN THE BODY

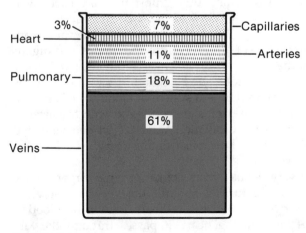

FIGURE 5-1.

through the **ARTERIES** and leaving through the **VEINS**.

One-twelfth to one-fifteenth of the body weight is blood. A person weighing 150 pounds will have approximately ten to twelve pints of blood. If the blood supply is cut off from the tissues, they will die from lack of oxygen. The loss of two pints, 8 to 10 percent of the body's blood, by an adult, usually is serious, and the loss of three pints may be fatal if it occurs over a short time, such as one to two hours. At certain points in the body, fatal hemorrhages may occur in a very short time. The cutting of the principal blood vessels in the neck, in the arm, or in the thigh may cause hemorrhage that will prove fatal in one to three minutes or less if uncontrolled. **RUPTURE** of the main blood vessels of the chest and abdomen may cause fatal hemorrhage in less than thirty seconds.

The loss of blood causes a state of physical **SHOCK**. This occurs because there is insufficient blood flowing through the tissues of the body to provide food and oxygen. All processes of the body are affected. When a person is in shock, vital bodily functions slow down. If the conditions causing shock are not reversed, death will result.

BLOOD VESSELS

Oxygenated blood is carried from the heart by a large artery called the **AORTA**. Smaller arteries branch off from this large artery, and those arteries in turn branch off into still smaller arteries. These arteries divide and subdivide until they become very small, ending in threadlike vessels known as capillaries, which extend into all the organs and tissues. Through the very thin capillary walls, oxygen, carbon dioxide, and other substances are exchanged between body cells and the circulatory system.

After the blood has furnished the necessary nourishment and oxygen to the tissues and organs of the body, it takes on waste products, particularly carbon dioxide. The blood returns to the heart by means of a different system of blood vessels known as veins. The veins are connected with the arteries through the capillaries. Veins collect deoxygenated blood from the capillaries and carry it back to the heart.

Very small veins join, forming larger veins, which, in turn, join until the very largest veins return the blood to the heart. Before the blood is returned to the heart, it passes through the **KIDNEYS**, where certain waste products are removed.

When the blood from the body reaches the heart, carbon dioxide and other waste products contained in the blood but not removed by the kidneys must be eliminated, and the oxygen used by the body replaced. The heart pumps the blood delivered to it by the veins into the lungs, where it flows through another network of capillaries. There, the carbon dioxide and other waste products are exchanged for oxygen through the delicate walls of air cells, called alveoli. Thus, the blood is oxygenated and ready to return to the heart, which recirculates it throughout the body. The time taken for the blood to make one complete circulation of the body through miles and miles of blood vessels is approximately seventy-five seconds in an adult at rest.

HEMORRHAGE OR BLEEDING

SEVERITY OF BLEEDING

Generally, hemorrhage is considered more severe as the breathing rate increases, the pulse quickens, the blood pressure drops, and the level of consciousness falls (Figure 5-2). The severity of hemorrhage depends on a number of factors:

- How fast the blood is flowing from the vessel (the size of the vessel).
- Whether bleeding is arterial or venous.
- Whether blood is flowing freely or into an enclosed body cavity.
- Where the bleeding originated.
- How much blood has already been lost.
- The victim's age and weight.
- The victim's general physical condition.
- Whether bleeding is a threat to respiration (Figure 5-3).

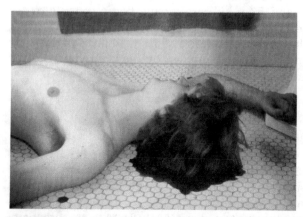

FIGURE 5-2. Detecting and controlling profuse bleeding are part of the primary survey.

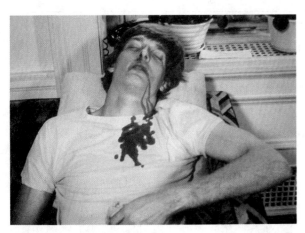

FIGURE 5-3. Bleeding from the mouth and/or nose in an unconscious victim can be a serious threat to respiration if proper precautions are not taken for drainage.

EFFECTS OF HEMORRHAGE

Hemorrhage causes the following effects:

- The loss of red blood cells causes a lack of oxygen to the body systems.
- A decrease in **BLOOD VOLUME** causes a decrease in **BLOOD PRESSURE**.
- The heart's pumping rate increases to compensate for reduced blood pressure.
- The force of the heartbeat is reduced, since there is less blood to pump.

If hemorrhage goes uncontrolled, it will lead to the following signs (see Figure 5-4):

- Moderate shock (follows loss of 15 percent of blood volume, or two pints in the average male).
- Severe or fatal shock (follows loss of 30 percent or more of blood volume, or four pints in the average male).

BLEEDING FROM AN ARTERY

When bright red blood spurts from a wound, an artery has been cut. The blood in arteries comes directly from the heart and spurts with each heart contraction. Because the blood has a fresh supply of oxygen, it is bright red in color (Figure 5-5). Blood loss from an artery is often rapid and profuse. Unless the artery is very small, blood in an artery usually will not clot, because the flow is too rapid; even if a clot forms, it can be forced out by the pressure of the blood flow. A completely severed artery can constrict and seal itself off, as often happens in cases of traumatic **AMPUTATION**.

BLEEDING FROM A VEIN

When dark bluish-red blood flows from a wound in a steady stream, a vein has been cut (Figure 5-5). The blood in veins, on its way back to the heart, flows more slowly than arterial blood. Having given up its oxygen and received carbon dioxide and waste products in return, the blood is dark in color. While bleeding from a vein can be profuse, it is usually easier to control than bleeding from an artery. The danger from venous bleeding is the tendency of the vein to suck in air and debris, creating potentially fatal air **EMBOLISMS** that can lodge in the lung, heart, or brain. This generally occurs only in the large veins, such as the jugular.

BLEEDING FROM CAPILLARIES

When dark red blood oozes slowly from a wound, capillaries have been cut (Figure 5-5). There is usually no danger from the bleeding, since little blood can be lost. Blood drips steadily from the wound until clotting occurs; direct pressure with a **COMPRESS** applied over the wound is usually enough to cause clotting. Bleeding from capillaries often clots spontaneously, without any treatment. When a large skin surface is involved, the threat of infection is of much greater concern than the loss of blood.

"BLEEDERS"

HEMOPHILIACS, sometimes called "**BLEEDERS**," are people whose blood will not clot due to congenital abnormalities in the clotting mechanisms. Even a slight wound that cuts a blood vessel can cause a hemophiliac to bleed to death. In addition to aggressive measures to control bleeding through direct pressure, you should administer oxygen and transport a wounded hemophiliac to the hospital as quickly as possible, as you would any victim with significant bleeding.

GENERAL PROCEDURES FOR CONTROLLING BLEEDING

The following are *general* procedures for control of bleeding (see Figure 5-18, Summary — Control of External Bleeding, page 79):

- Conduct a quick assessment to determine the cause and source of bleeding and the general condition of the victim.

THE FOUR STAGES OF HEMORRHAGE

STAGE 1	STAGE 2	STAGE 3	STAGE 4
Up to 15% blood loss*	Up to 30% blood loss	Up to 40% blood loss*	More than 40% blood loss

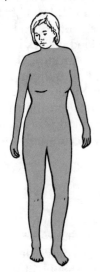 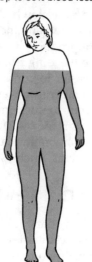 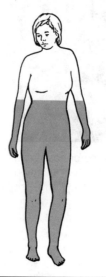 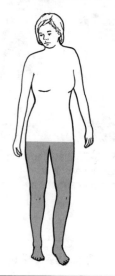

HOW THE BODY RESPONDS

Compensatory mechanisms (essentially sympathetic nervous system responses such as vasoconstriction) maintain homeostasis.

EFFECT ON VICTIM

- Victim remains alert.
- Blood pressure stays within normal limits.
- Pulse stays within normal limits or increases slightly; pulse quality remains strong.
- Respiratory rate and depth, skin color and temperature all remain normal.

*The average adult has 5 liters (1 liter = approximately 1 quart) of circulating blood; 15% is 750 ml (or about 3 cups). With internal bleeding, 750 ml will occupy enough space in a limb to cause swelling and pain. With bleeding into the body cavities, however, the blood will spread throughout the cavity, causing little, if any, initial discomfort.

- Vasoconstriction continues to maintain adequate blood pressure, but with some difficulty now.
- Blood flow is shunted to vital organs, with decreased flow to intestines, kidneys, and skin.

EFFECT ON VICTIM

- Victim may become confused and restless.
- Skin turns pale, cool, and dry because of shunting of blood to vital organs.
- Systolic blood pressure starts to fall.
- Diastolic pressure may rise or fall. It's more likely to rise (because of vasoconstriction) or stay the same in otherwise healthy victims with no underlying cardiovascular problems.
- Pulse pressure (difference between systolic and diastolic pressures) narrows.
- Sympathetic responses also cause rapid heart rate (over 100 beats per minute). Pulse quality weakens.
- Respiratory rate increases because of sympathetic stimulation.

- Compensatory mechanisms become overtaxed. Vasoconstriction, for example, can no longer sustain blood pressure, which now begins to fall.
- Cardiac output and tissue perfusion continue to decrease, becoming potentially life-threatening. (Even at this stage, however, the victim can still recover with prompt treatment.)

EFFECT ON VICTIM

- Victim becomes more confused, restless, and anxious.
- Classic signs of shock appear – rapid heat rate, decreased blood pressure, rapid respiration and cool, clammy extremities.

- Compensatory vasoconstriction now becomes a complicating factor in itself, further impairing tissue perfusion and cellular oxygenation.

EFFECT ON VICTIM

- Victim becomes lethargic, drowsy, or stuporous.
- Signs of shock become more pronounced. Blood pressure continues to fall; pulse pressure continues to narrow (although if diastolic pressure "drops out," pulse pressure may actually widen).
- Lack of blood flow to the brain and other vital organs ultimately leads to organ failure and death.

FIGURE 5-4.

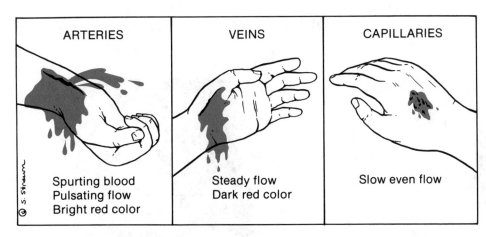

ARTERIES	VEINS	CAPILLARIES
Spurting blood Pulsating flow Bright red color	Steady flow Dark red color	Slow even flow

FIGURE 5-5.
Bleeding characteristics.

■ Place the victim in a position in which he will be least affected by the loss of blood. If possible, have him lie down with the legs elevated in a semi-flexed position (to prevent aggravation of spinal injury and breathing impairment).

■ Control the bleeding with **DIRECT PRESSURE** or use of **PRESSURE POINTS**.

■ Maintain an open airway.

■ Prevent the loss of body heat by putting blankets over and underneath the victim; do not overheat.

■ Take vital signs every five minutes; repeat victim assessment every fifteen minutes.

■ Keep the victim at rest to prevent increased heart action, which interferes with clot formation and causes the blood to flow faster.

■ Remain alert for complications of blood loss.

SPECIFIC METHODS OF CONTROLLING BLEEDING

DIRECT PRESSURE

The best method of controlling bleeding — and the one that should be tried first — is applying pressure directly to the wound. Direct pressure is best applied by placing **STERILE GAUZE** or the cleanest material available (such as a handkerchief, sanitary napkin, or bed sheet) against the bleeding point and pressing firmly with the heel of your hand until a **BANDAGE** can be applied. (A **DRESSING** is a sterile covering for a wound, while a bandage holds the dressing in place.) Check the dressing every few minutes; if it soaks through with blood, do not remove it — simply place another dressing on top of it and resume pressure (Figures 5-6–5-9).

To bandage, wrap the dressing firmly with a self-adherent **ROLLER BANDAGE**; cover the area both above and below the dressing. Tie the bandage knot over the wound unless otherwise indicated. Do not remove the bandage or the dressing once they have been applied; bleeding may restart if the bandage is disturbed.

When **AIR SPLINTS** or **PRESSURE BANDAGES** are available, they can be used over dressings to supply direct pressure. See the section on air splints later in this chapter.

A blood pressure cuff can also be used to create a pressure bandage; use only slight pressure, and monitor it frequently to avoid damage from too much pressure (Figure 5-10).

Pressure dressings must remain undisturbed for at least ten minutes; earlier removal can disrupt the clot and cause bleeding to start again. If bleeding continues after the pressure bandage has been applied, it is not tight enough; either tighten the bandage or apply more pressure with the heel of your hand.

In cases of severe hemorrhage, do not waste time trying to find gauze or some other material; use your hand to apply direct pressure.

ELEVATION

Elevation of the injured limb should be used in conjunction with direct pressure to stop bleeding. Elevating the bleeding part above heart level slows the flow of blood and speeds clotting.

Do not elevate an injured limb if you suspect that a fracture, dislocation, impaled object, or spinal injury has occurred.

CONTROL OF BLEEDING FROM LACERATED WOUND

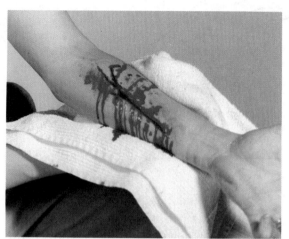

FIGURE 5-6. Bleeding from a lacerated wound on the forearm.

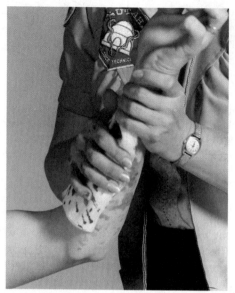

FIGURE 5-7. Control bleeding with direct pressure and elevation. If necessary, use your bare hand.

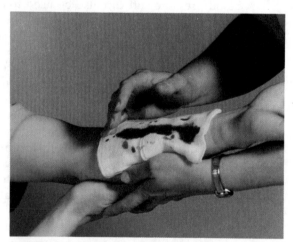

FIGURE 5-8. If bleeding soaks through the dressing, do not remove the original dressing.

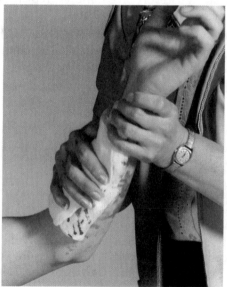

FIGURE 5-9. Add a new dressing on top of the original and continue with direct pressure and elevation. After bleeding is under control, bandage the dressing in place.

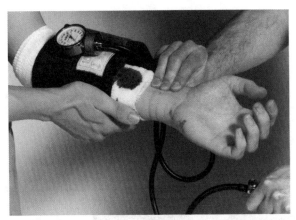

FIGURE 5-10. A blood pressure cuff can be used to apply pressure and control bleeding in an extremity.

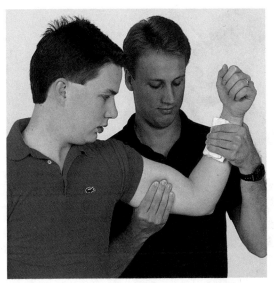

FIGURE 5-11. Applying direct and indirect pressure to control bleeding.

INDIRECT PRESSURE

Arterial bleeding can be controlled by digital thumb or finger pressure applied at any of twenty-two pressure points. Pressure points are places where an artery is close to a bony structure and also near the skin surface; pressing the artery against the underlying bone can control the flow of blood to the injury. Use of pressure points requires skill and a knowledge of the exact location of each point.

In severe bleeding that is not being controlled by direct pressure and elevation, digital pressure can be used. Do not substitute indirect pressure for direct pressure — both kinds of pressure should be used simultaneously (Figures 5-11–5-12). The wound is probably supplied by more than one major blood vessel, so using the pressure point alone is rarely enough to control severe bleeding. Hold the pressure point only as long as necessary to stop the bleeding; reapply indirect pressure if bleeding recurs.

Pressure points should be used with caution, since indirect pressure can cause damage to the limb due to inadequate blood flow. Never use indirect pressure if the bone below the artery may be injured.

Pressure points on the arms (brachial pressure points) and in the groin (femoral pressure points) are the ones most often used (Figures 5-13–5-14). The location of these pressure points should be identified thoroughly and the method to occlude them practiced until the technique can be applied quickly and effectively. Pressure on the arterial pulse points (Figure 5-15) may also be used to help slow bleeding when direct pressure is inadequate.

Do not exert pressure on the carotid pressure point because it can cause cardiac **DYSRHYTHMIA** or cardiac arrest. If one vessel is partially occluded,

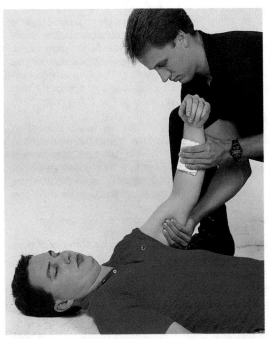

FIGURE 5-12. Applying direct and indirect pressure to control bleeding.

pressure on the other one can cause **CEREBROVASCU-LAR ACCIDENT** (stroke). If pressure is applied to both carotid arteries simultaneously, the occlusion may restrict blood flow to the brain, with lethal results.

Brachial Artery

Pressure on the brachial artery (see Figures 5-11–5-12) is used to control severe bleeding from a

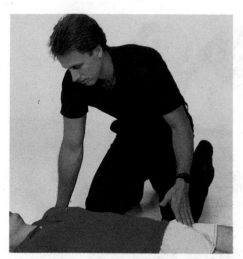

FIGURE 5-13. Locating the femoral artery.

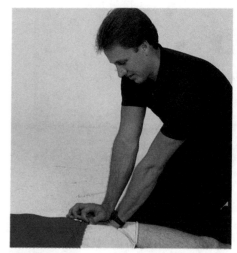

FIGURE 5-14. Applying pressure to the femoral artery.

ARTERIAL PULSE POINTS

Arterial pulse points are areas in the circulatory system where an artery lies close to the skin or passes over a bony prominence, facilitating arterial palpation (the ability to feel an underlying artery with gentle fingertip pressure). Palpation of these pulse points makes it possible for you to determine whether the heart is still beating, whether circulation is sufficient to various parts of the body, and whether arteries that are distal to the pulse point have been damaged.

While direct pressure is still the best way of controlling hemorrhage, compression of the arterial pulse points can sometimes be used in addition to direct pressure to help control severe bleeding. (Use of arterial pressure points alone is rarely sufficient in controlling hemorrhage, since most parts of the body are supplied by more than one artery.)

Major arterial pulse points include the following:

■ Carotid arteries, located on each side of the neck next to the larynx, supply blood to the head. Do not exert pressure on the carotid pressure points.

■ The external maxillary artery supplies much of the blood to the face; one can be palpated on each side of the face on the inner surface of the lower jaw.

■ The temporal artery supplies part of the blood supply to the scalp; one can be palpated on each side of the face just above the upper portion of the ear.

■ The brachial artery, located on the inner arm just above the elbow, supplies blood to the arms.

■ The radial and ulnar arteries, located in the wrist, also supply blood to the arms and hands.

■ The femoral arteries, which pass through the groin, supply blood to the legs.

■ The posterior tibial artery, which passes through the ankle, and the dorsalis pedis artery, on the front surface of the foot, can determine circulation to the feet. While the dorsalis pedis pulse cannot always be felt, it is easy to find and feel when it is.

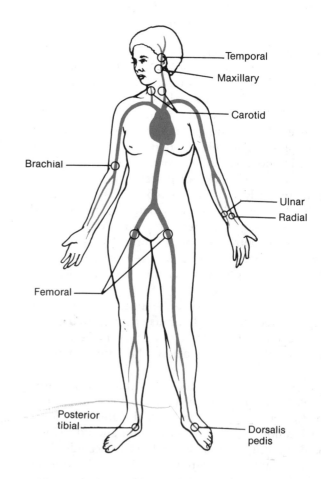

FIGURE 5-15.

wound on the upper extremity. The pressure point is located in a groove on the inside of the arm between the armpit and the elbow. To apply pressure:

1. Grasp the middle of the victim's arm with the thumb on the outside of the arm and the fingers on the inside.

2. Press the fingers toward the thumb.

3. Use the flat, inside surface of the fingers, not the fingertips. This inward pressure closes the artery by pressing it against the humerus.

Femoral Artery

The femoral artery (Figures 5-13–5-14) is used to control severe bleeding from a wound on the lower extremity. The pressure point is located on the front center part of the crease in the groin area. This is where the artery crosses the pelvic basin on the way into the lower extremity. To apply pressure:

1. Position the victim flat on his back, if possible.

2. Kneeling on the opposite side from the wounded limb, place the heel of one hand directly on the pressure point, and lean forward to apply the small amount of pressure needed to close the artery.

3. If bleeding is not controlled, it may be necessary to press directly over the artery with the flat surface of the fingertips and apply additional pressure on the fingertips with the heel of the other hand.

SPLINTS

Significant bleeding may accompany fractures, since the jagged bone end may lacerate skin, muscle, and underlying tissue, causing bleeding. Left unsplinted, the bone ends can continue to irritate surrounding tissue, with continued bleeding. In cases of fracture, splinting the bone can help control bleeding. Specific instructions on splinting are given in Chapters 10 and 11.

AIR SPLINTS

If air splints are available, they can be used to create a pressure bandage and control bleeding in an extremity (Figure 5-16).

To use an air splint:

1. Cover the wound with a thick sterile dressing; use several layers of thick sterile gauze, a sanitary napkin, or some other thick material.

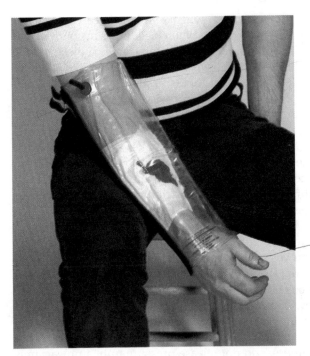

FIGURE 5-16. Air splints can be used to apply pressure and control bleeding from an extremity.

2. Slip the splint over the dressing, without moving the dressing.

3. Inflate the splint. Take care not to overinflate; you should be able to depress the surface of the air splint at least one-half inch with your fingertips.

4. Check distal pulses frequently if they are not covered by the splint, and look for mottled skin or blanched fingernails or toenails.

5. Do not deflate the air splint once you have applied it, and do not let any air out of it until a physician is present.

TOURNIQUET

A **TOURNIQUET** is a device used to control severe bleeding. It is used *only as a last resort* after all other methods of control have failed and is used only on the extremities. Before you use a tourniquet, you should thoroughly understand the dangers and limitations of its use. Improper use by inexperienced, untrained persons can cause severe tissue injury or loss of a limb. The tourniquet may completely shut off the blood supply to a limb, killing all tissue below the tourniquet. The pressure from a tourniquet can crush underlying tissue, causing permanent damage to skin, nerves, and muscles. As a general rule, consider a tourniquet only when a large artery has been severed, when a limb has been partially or totally severed, and when bleeding is uncontrollable.

The standard tourniquet is usually a piece of web belting about thirty-six inches long, with a buckle or snap device that holds it tightly in place when applied. You can improvise a tourniquet from a strap, belt, suspender, handkerchief, towel, necktie, cloth, or other suitable material; a triangular bandage that has been folded makes a good tourniquet. Never use wire, cord, or anything that will cut into the flesh; ideally, the tourniquet should be at least three inches wide to distribute pressure evenly over the tissues.

With some cautions, you can use a blood-pressure cuff as a tourniquet. Secure it well so that the Velcro does not pop open as a result of the pressure. Continually monitor the pressure so that it does not drop; the pressure should be maintained in the 150 mmHg range for as long as the tourniquet is in place. A blood-pressure cuff used as a tourniquet can be left inflated safely for up to thirty minutes; do not release pressure until a physician is present.

The procedure for applying a tourniquet is as follows (Figure 5-17).

1. While the proper pressure point is being held to control the bleeding temporarily, place the tourniquet between the heart and the wound; leave approximately two inches of uninjured flesh between the tourniquet and the wound.

2. Apply a thick pad over the artery or area to be compressed.

3. *Never* use a clamp on a blood vessel; it will impair the surgeon's ability to repair the vessel.

4. If using an improvised tourniquet, fold the material so that it is three to four inches wide and, ideally, six or seven layers thick. Wrap the material tightly around the limb twice, and tie it in a half-knot on the upper surface of the limb.

5. Place a short stick or similar stout object at the half-knot, and tie a square knot.

6. Twist the stick to tighten the tourniquet *only* until the bleeding stops; do not make any additional turns.

7. Secure the stick in place with the base ends of the tourniquet, another strip of cloth, or some other suitable material; smooth the wrapping.

8. *Never* cover a tourniquet; leave it in full view.

9. Make a written note of the tourniquet location, the time it was applied, and the vital signs at the time of application. Attach the note to the victim's clothing. Using lipstick or a red marker, make a "T" or "TK" on the victim's forehead and indicate the time the tourniquet was applied.

10. Activate the EMS system as soon as possible.

Once the tourniquet is tightened, it should not be loosened or removed except by or on the advice of a physician. The loosening or removal of a tourniquet may dislodge clots and result in sufficient loss of blood to cause severe shock and death.

Refer to Figure 5-18 for a summary of emergency care for control of external bleeding.

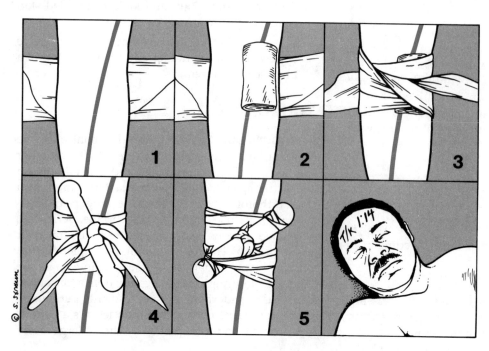

FIGURE 5-17.
Application of a tourniquet.

SUMMARY — CONTROL OF EXTERNAL BLEEDING

Type & Nature of Bleeding

CAPILLARY   Oozing, most common type of external hemorrhage. This type of bleeding is expected in all minor cuts, scratches, and abrasions. Dark bluish-red color.

VENOUS   Slow, even blood flow. Occurs when a vein is punctured or severed. Venous blood is dark in color (maroon). Danger in venous bleeding from neck wound is that an air bubble may be sucked into the wound.

ARTERIAL   Occurs when an artery is punctured or severed. Less common than venous bleeding because arteries are located deep in the body and are protected by bones. Arterial bleeding is characterized by spurting of bright red blood. Common arteries injured in accidents: carotid, brachial, radial, femoral.

Emergency Care

External bleeding is bleeding that can be seen coming from a wound. Excessive external bleeding can create a crisis situation; the platelets, which usually help the blood clot, aren't effective in cases of severe bleeding or when the blood vessels have been damaged.

Serious blood loss is defined as one liter in an adult and half a liter in a child. If the bleeding remains uncontrolled, shock and death may result.

Elevate Extremity

Direct Pressure

1.   Apply direct pressure against the bleeding site.

2.   Use a dressing; if necessary, even your bare hand. If dressing soaks through do not remove it — put another on top and continue applying pressure.

3.   Maintain firm pressure until the bleeding stops or until the victim reaches the hospital.

4.   If the wound is on an extremity, elevate it while you apply direct pressure.

Pressure Points

The most important arteries used in pressure-point control include:

Brachial Artery   Along the inside of the upper arm midway between the elbow and the shoulder; compression will stop or control bleeding below the pressure point. See Figures 5-11, 5-12, and 5-15.

Femoral Artery   In the groin, slows bleeding in the leg on the appropriate side. See Figures 5-13–5-15.

Splints & Counterpressure Devices

In cases of open fractures, splintered bone ends can damage tissue and cause external bleeding. Properly applied splints can immobilize the fracture and lessen the chance of further injury. Air splints can aid in controlling bleeding, particularly in the upper extremities.

Tourniquet

Use of a tourniquet is rarely warranted, because control of external bleeding can almost always be achieved by using some other means. Tourniquets should be used as a *last resort only,* and only after trying all other methods of control.

FIGURE 5-18.

CRYOTHERAPY

CRYOTHERAPY, the use of cold packs to reduce bleeding, is not effective on its own but can be effective when used in combination with direct pressure and/or elevation. In addition to slowing the flow of blood, cold packs relieve pain and reduce swelling.

When using cold packs, never let the ice or cold pack come into direct contact with the victim's skin; guard against **FROSTBITE** by placing a layer of gauze or other suitable material between the cold pack and the skin. Never use a cold pack for longer than twenty minutes at a time. If prolonged treatment is needed, use the cold pack for twenty minutes, wait ten minutes, then use it again for twenty minutes.

INTERNAL BLEEDING

Internal bleeding generally results from **BLUNT TRAUMA** or from certain fractures (such as pelvic fracture); though internal bleeding is not visible, it can be very serious — even fatal. A victim of internal bleeding can develop life-threatening shock before you even realize that he is bleeding. And diagnosis is not easy: many times you will need to assume that a victim has internal bleeding based on the mechanism of injury (such as a fall, a **DECELERATION INJURY**, severe blunt trauma, and so on) and on signs and symptoms.

Assume that a victim has internal bleeding if he has a bone fracture (especially of the hip or pelvis), a rib fracture, or a penetrating wound of the skull, chest, or abdomen (see Figures 5-19 and 5-20).

Signs and symptoms of internal bleeding include the following:

- Bruises or contusions.
- Pain, tenderness, swelling, or discoloration at the site of suspected injury.
- Bleeding from the mouth, rectum, or other body openings; blood or bloody fluid in the nose or ears.
- Nonmenstrual bleeding from the vagina.

COMMON SITES OF INTERNAL BLEEDING

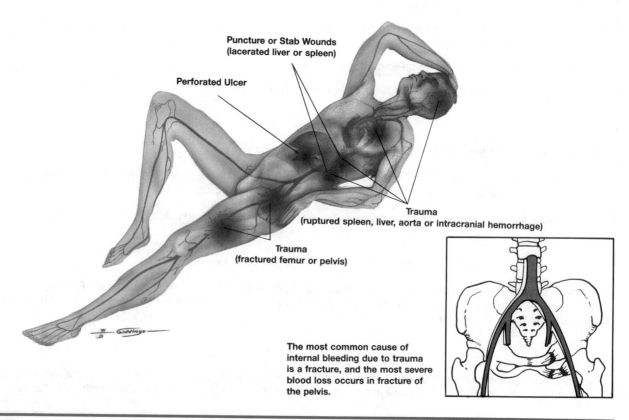

Puncture or Stab Wounds
(lacerated liver or spleen)

Perforated Ulcer

Trauma
(ruptured spleen, liver, aorta or intracranial hemorrhage)

Trauma
(fractured femur or pelvis)

The most common cause of internal bleeding due to trauma is a fracture, and the most severe blood loss occurs in fracture of the pelvis.

FIGURE 5-19. Internal bleeding.

- Dizziness in the absence of other symptoms (dizziness when going from lying to standing may be the only early sign of internal bleeding).
- Cold and clammy skin.
- Profuse sweating.
- Dull eyes, clouded vision, dilated pupils that are slow to respond to light.
- Severe respiratory distress.
- Restlessness, combativeness, and anxiety.
- Feeling of impending doom.
- Weak, rapid pulse.
- Nausea and vomiting.
- Abdominal bruising, pain, rebound tenderness, rigidity, spasms, or distention.

- Lower back pain.
- Blood in the urine or d
- Shallow, rapid breathir
- Thirst.
- Weak, helpless feeling.
- Dropping blood pressu
- Altered levels of consc

Serious internal blee tures. As an example, a f (thigh bone) can lacerate the femoral artery and result in an internal loss of one liter of blood. One of the most serious causes of internal blood loss is pelvic fracture.

The victim with a history of gastrointestinal **ULCER** or one who reports having vomited blood or passed

blood by th
amount o
bright r
ance

SUMMARY — EMERGENCY CARE FOR INTERNAL BLEEDING

Internal bleeding is an extremely serious condition. It is just as dangerous as external bleeding and, when uncontrolled, can lead to death due to shock. It may be caused by a tearing or bruising force that actually ruptures or tears apart one of the internal organs or tissues. Pressure on nerves from internal bleeding can cause great pain or paralysis. The most common cause of internal bleeding due to trauma is a fracture. The most severe blood loss occurs in fracture of the pelvis. Extensive swelling can cut off blood circulation to a limb. Internal bleeding is often hard to assess and can prove rapidly fatal. The signs of internal bleeding are similar to those of shock — look for restlessness, anxiety, cold, clammy skin, weak, rapid pulse, rapid breathing, and, ultimately, a drop in blood pressure. In addition, the victim may cough up or vomit bright red blood, vomit dark blood (the color of coffee grounds), pass dark stools, pass bright red blood, or have a tender, rigid abdomen that enlarges.

Common Causes	Signs and Symptoms	Emergency Care
Hard blow to any part of the body will cause contusions and/or rupturing of internal organs.	A fractured bone, hard blow, or other force may cause internal bleeding and swelling. A closed fracture may cause loss of blood internally.	Internal bleeding usually requires surgical correction. 1. Activate the EMS system immediately.
Fractured ribs, causing puncture of lungs. Fractured sternum from too vigorous CPR.	Bright red frothy blood coughed up usually means bleeding from the lungs. Pale, moist skin; weak, rapid pulse; shallow, rapid respiration.	2. If bleeding originates in an extremity, elevate it.
Bleeding ulcer. Ingestion of a sharp object, i.e., glass.	Vomiting bright red blood may indicate stomach bleeding. Blood which has been in stomach a longer time will resemble coffee grounds.	3. Application of a splint or pressure dressing may also help.
Disease corroding intestines, tapeworms, blow to abdominal area, appendicitis.	Slow bleeding in the intestinal tract above the sigmoid colon will cause the stools to be jet black (tar color). Hardness or spasm of abdominal muscles accompanies.	
Blockage of urethra may result in rupture of bladder, causing internal bleeding; multiple trauma may cause fractured pelvis, which may puncture kidneys.	Blood in urine may indicate bladder rupture or injury to the urinary tract. Urine may be a smoky color.	

FIGURE 5-20.

...e rectum may have lost a significant ... blood internally. Vomited blood can be ...d, dark red, or blackened, with the appear-... of coffee grounds.

...he highest priorities in terms of treatment are internal bleeding into the chest cavity and into the abdominal cavity.

To treat victims of internal bleeding:

1. Check for fractures; splint if appropriate.

2. Secure and maintain an open airway.

3. Keep the victim quiet; position and treat for shock. Loosen restrictive clothing at the neck and waist. Unless you suspect spinal injuries, elevate the feet six to twelve inches.

4. Monitor vital signs every five minutes.

5. Anticipate vomiting; if you do not suspect spinal injuries, position the victim on his side with his face pointing downward, to allow for drainage.

6. Activate the EMS system as soon as possible.

If the internal bleeding is into an extremity, use a pressure bandage or air splint to apply pressure; pressure will tend to close off the ends of the bleeding vessels. Elevate the limb after it has been immobilized. If you suspect a fracture, use extreme caution in applying any kind of pressure bandage — application directly over the fracture could further injure tissue or complicate the fracture.

NOSEBLEEDS

NOSEBLEEDS are a relatively common source of bleeding and can result from an injury, disease, activity, the environment, or other causes. Generally, they are more annoying than serious, but enough blood may be lost to cause shock. Bleeding from the nose can be caused by the following:

- Hemophilia or other bleeding disorders.
- Facial injuries, including those caused by a direct blow to the nose.
- A cold, **SINUSITIS**, infections, or other abnormalities of the inside of the nose.
- High blood pressure.
- Strenuous activity.
- Exposure to high altitudes.
- Fractured skull.
- Chronic colds or allergies that prompt a victim to wipe or abrade nasal mucosa.

If a fractured skull is suspected as the cause of the nosebleed, *do not* attempt to stop the bleeding — to do so might increase pressure on the brain. Cover the nasal opening loosely with a dry, sterile dressing to absorb blood; do not apply pressure. Treat the victim for skull fracture as outlined in Chapter 12.

Nosebleed from other suspected causes may be treated as follows:

1. Keep the victim quiet and in a sitting position, leaning forward to prevent aspiration of blood. If a sitting position is made impossible because of other injuries, have the victim lie down with head and shoulders elevated.

2. If there is no nasal fracture, apply pressure by pinching the nostrils together (Figure 5-21) or by placing rolled gauze between the victim's upper lip and gum; press with your fingers if necessary.

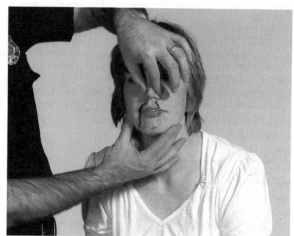

FIGURE 5-21. Apply pressure by pinching the nostrils and, if necessary, apply cold compresses to the nose and face.

3. Apply cold compresses to the nose and face.

4. If this does not control the bleeding, insert a small clean pad of gauze into one or both nostrils and apply pressure again, pinching the nostrils. Make sure that a free end of gauze extends outside the nostril to facilitate removal later.

5. If the victim is conscious, apply pressure beneath the nostril above the upper lip.

6. Instruct the victim to avoid blowing his nose for several hours, as this could dislodge the clot.

7. If bleeding continues, take the victim to a physician, or, if severe enough, activate the EMS system.

| 5 | **SELF-TEST** | 5 |

Student: _____   Date: _____

Course: _____   Section #: _____

If you believe that the statement is true, circle the T. If you believe that the statement is false, circle the F.

T   F   1. Indirect pressure is a good substitute for direct pressure.

T   F   2. The brachial and the femoral pressure points are the ones most often used.

T   F   3. The carotid pressure points are a safe and convenient way of controlling bleeding in the head.

T   F   4. Pressure on the arterial pulse points may help slow bleeding when direct pressure is inadequate.

T   F   5. Blood from a vein flows in spurts with each heartbeat.

T   F   6. Bleeding from capillaries rarely clots spontaneously.

T   F   7. A victim of internal bleeding can develop life-threatening shock before the bleeding is apparent.

T   F   8. A completely severed artery can sometimes constrict and seal itself off.

T   F   9. The most severe fracture-related blood loss occurs in fractures of the femur.

T   F   10. Internal bleeding usually results from blunt trauma or fractures.

PART II: Multiple Choice   For each question, circle the answer that best reflects an accurate statement.

1. Which of the following is the best method for controlling severe bleeding (and should therefore be applied first)?
   a. elevation.
   b. pressure point.
   c. direct pressure.
   d. tourniquet.

2. List the four methods of controlling bleeding in order of preference: (1) elevation; (2) direct pressure at the wound; (3) indirect pressure (pressure points); (4) tourniquet.
   a. 2, 1, 3, 4.
   b. 2, 3, 1, 4.
   c. 1, 2, 3, 4.
   d. 3, 2, 1, 4.

3. Which pressure points are used most often?
   a. brachial, femoral.
   b. ulnar, carotid.
   c. subclavian, axillary.
   d. temporal, dorsalis pedis.

4. Severe bleeding from the upper arm may be controlled by finger pressure on the:
   a. femoral artery.
   b. temporal artery.
   c. radial artery.
   d. brachial artery.

5. One of the greatest dangers in bleeding from a neck wound is:
   a. an air bubble that may be sucked into the wound.
   b. shock.
   c. you cannot apply a tourniquet or use pressure points.
   d. later infection

6. When a dressing becomes saturated with blood, you should:
   a. remove it and apply a new dressing.
   b. apply a tourniquet.
   c. leave the dressing in place and apply an additional dressing on top of it.
   d. tie the knot on the bandage tighter.

7. Which of the following is *not* an effect of hemorrhage?
   a. increased heart pumping rate.
   b. force of heartbeat reduced.
   c. irregular heartbeat.
   d. lack of oxygen to body systems.

8. How long does clotting take in most instances?
   a. one to two minutes.
   b. six to seven minutes.
   c. ten to twelve minutes.
   d. eighteen to twenty minutes.

9. What component of blood is essential for the formation of blood clots?
   a. platelets.
   b. white blood cells.
   c. red blood cells.
   d. plasma.

10. What condition may cause a person to bleed to death from a minor wound?
    a. anemia.
    b. leukemia.
    c. hypochondria.
    d. hemophilia.

11. Do *not* try to stop a nosebleed in the case of:
    a. broken nose.
    b. fractured skull.
    c. fractured jaw.
    d. high blood pressure.

12. A victim with a nosebleed should:
    a. sit quietly and then pinch the nostrils to apply pressure.
    b. blow the nose until the bleeding stops.
    c. tilt the head back or lie flat while applying pressure to the bridge of the nose.
    d. lean forward, pack the nostrils, and apply heat.

13. Which of the following is *not* a component of blood?
    a. platelets.
    b. capillaries.
    c. white cells.
    d. plasma.

14. Perfusion means:
    a. the process of blood clotting.
    b. manufacture of red blood cells.
    c. another word for transfusion.
    d. circulation of blood within an organ.

15. Which of the following characterizes arterial bleeding?
    a. dark red color and spurting flow.
    b. bright red color and spurting flow.
    c. dark red color and steady flow.
    d. bright red color and steady flow.

16. What is a pressure point?
    a. a point where the blood pressure drops low enough to stop bleeding.
    b. a place where the artery is protected on all sides by bone and muscle.
    c. a place where an artery is close to the skin surface and over a bone.
    d. a point where an artery is near the wound.

17. Use a tourniquet only if:
    a. there is severe hemorrhage.
    b. bleeding cannot be controlled by direct pressure.
    c. bleeding cannot be controlled by pressure at the appropriate pressure point.
    d. bleeding cannot be controlled by any other means.

18. Which of the following may *not* be sign of internal bleeding:
    a. vomiting of bright, red blood.
    b. pale, moist skin.
    c. strong, bounding pulse.
    d. dizziness.

PART III: Matching

1. Tourniquets should only be used for severe life-threatening hemorrhage that cannot be controlled by any other means. Order the following procedures for the proper application of a tourniquet (1, 2, 3, etc.).

   _____ Secure the stick in place.

   _____ Wrap the tourniquet around the limb twice and tie in a half-knot on the limb's upper surface.

   _____ Do not cover a tourniquet.

   _____ Twist the stick to tighten the tourniquet only until bleeding stops.

   _____ Place the tourniquet between the heart and the wound.

   _____ Activate the EMS system.

   _____ Place a short stick at the half-knot and tie a square knot.

   _____ Make a written note of the location and the time the tourniquet was applied.

PART IV: What Would You Do If:

1. You arrive at the scene of an auto/bicycle accident and find a teenager who has a large laceration on the lower leg and is bleeding profusely.

2. A college student loses control of a chainsaw and sustains a large laceration of his left arm. The bleeding is severe.

PART V: Practical Skills Check-Off

_____ has satisfactorily passed the following practical skills:
Student's Name

	Date	Partner Check	Inst. Init.
1. Demonstrate how to control bleeding by direct pressure and elevation.	_/_/_	☐	_____
2. Locate the brachial and femoral pressure points and demonstrate how to apply indirect pressure.	_/_/_	☐	_____
3. Demonstrate how to apply a tourniquet.	_/_/_	☐	_____
4. Demonstrate appropriate care (position and pressure) for a nosebleed.	_/_/_	☐	_____

CHAPTER SIX

OBJECTIVES

- Understand the basic causes and physiology of shock.
- Understand the factors that may influence the severity of shock.
- Recognize the various types of shock.
- Identify the signs/symptoms and stages of shock.
- Describe and demonstrate the management of shock.

SHOCK

In 1852, shock was defined as "A rude unhinging of the machinery of life." Probably no better definition exists to describe the devastating effects of this process on a victim, but a more recent definition calls shock "the collapse and progressive failure of the cardiovascular system." Shock, left untreated, is fatal — and it may well be the First Aider's worst enemy. In the field, shock must be recognized and treated immediately, or the victim may die.

The definition of shock does not involve low blood pressure, rapid pulse, or cool clammy skin — these are merely the signs. Simply stated, shock results from inadequate **PERFUSION** of the body's cells with oxygenated blood.

WHEN DOES SHOCK OCCUR?

Basically, shock occurs when the heart does not pump adequate amounts of blood to fill the arteries at great enough pressure to provide oxygen to the organs and tissues.

Every cell in the body requires oxygen to function. Oxygen is delivered to the cells through the bloodstream, is taken in by the cells, and undergoes a complicated physiologic process (metabolism) that produces energy and waste by-products. Simply stated, oxygen and **GLUCOSE** produce energy and waste products such as carbon dioxide. Long-term survival requires delivery of nutrients — most important, oxygen and glucose — to body cells. The cells most sensitive to a lack of oxygen are those in the heart, brain, and lungs; they can be irreparably damaged in just four to six minutes without oxygen and glucose. Skin and muscle cells can last for three to six hours; the contents of the abdominal cavity can last for forty-five to ninety minutes. (See Figure 6-1, which depicts the continuous cycle of traumatic shock.)

CAUSES OF SHOCK

There are three primary ways in which inadequate perfusion might occur; i.e., there are three basic causes of shock (Figure 6-2):

1. Fluid is lost from the circulatory system (**HYPOVOLEMIC SHOCK**). This loss usually results from injury that causes hemorrhage, from burns (which lead to loss of plasma), or through **DEHYDRATION** (which is the loss of fluids). In response, the brain releases signals and hormones that cause increased cardiac output and that cause the vessels to increase the resistance. A person can lose 25 percent of his total blood volume and be in moderate shock; if he loses 30 to 35 percent of his total volume, he is considered to be in serious shock.

CONTINUOUS CYCLE OF TRAUMATIC SHOCK*

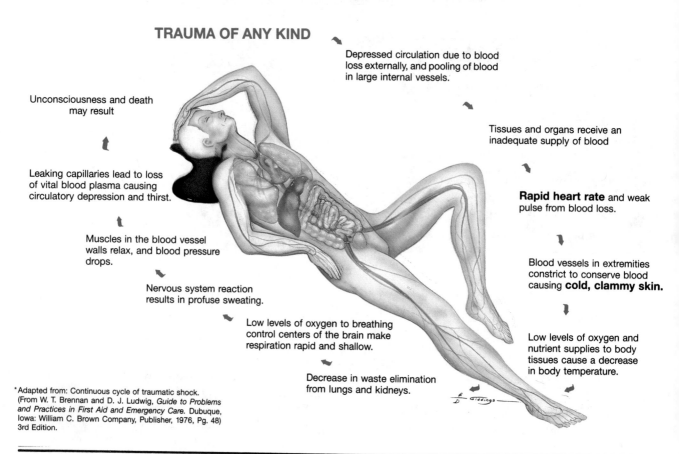

TRAUMA OF ANY KIND

Depressed circulation due to blood loss externally, and pooling of blood in large internal vessels.

Tissues and organs receive an inadequate supply of blood

Rapid heart rate and weak pulse from blood loss.

Blood vessels in extremities constrict to conserve blood causing **cold, clammy skin.**

Low levels of oxygen and nutrient supplies to body tissues cause a decrease in body temperature.

Decrease in waste elimination from lungs and kidneys.

Low levels of oxygen to breathing control centers of the brain make respiration rapid and shallow.

Nervous system reaction results in profuse sweating.

Muscles in the blood vessel walls relax, and blood pressure drops.

Leaking capillaries lead to loss of vital blood plasma causing circulatory depression and thirst.

Unconsciousness and death may result

*Adapted from: Continuous cycle of traumatic shock. (From W. T. Brennan and D. J. Ludwig, *Guide to Problems and Practices in First Aid and Emergency Care.* Dubuque, Iowa: William C. Brown Company, Publisher, 1976, Pg. 48) 3rd Edition.

FIGURE 6-1.

2. The heart fails to pump enough blood (cardiogenic shock). Shock is a vicious cycle: the heart fails to pump enough blood, which makes the blood flow diminish. This, in turn, lowers the blood pressure, which weakens the heart — and a weakened heart fails to pump enough blood.

3. The blood vessels dilate or constrict, causing blood to pool away from vital areas (peripheral shock, which includes **SEPTIC** and **NEUROGENIC SHOCK**). There can be many reasons for this, including head injury.

FACTORS INFLUENCING THE SEVERITY OF SHOCK

Some degree of shock occurs from all injuries; its severity depends on certain factors. What might cause a mild case of shock in one person could cause a severe case in another.

Certain people are at higher risk for developing shock and are more devastated by its progression. You should be especially alert to the possibility of shock when assessing these victims. These people include:

▪ The elderly.

▪ Infants (children may mask shock well for a long time, then suddenly "crash").

▪ Persons with known hemorrhage or trauma, especially trauma victims with multiple injuries.

▪ Victims with massive **MYOCARDIAL INFARCTION**.

▪ Pregnant women (in shock, the body quickly diverts blood from the abdomen and, therefore, from the fetus in an attempt to maintain the mother's blood pressure; the fetus may die rapidly).

CAUSES AND RESULTS OF SHOCK

Some of the major causes of shock are as follows:

- Allergic reactions
- Bites or stings of poisonous snakes or insects
- Poisons
- Exposure to extremes of heat and cold
- Emotional stress
- Myocardial infarction
- Spinal injuries

- Severe trauma
- Severe pain
- Loss of blood
- Severe burns
- Electrical shock
- Gas poisoning
- Certain illnesses

Resulting in one or more of:

- Failure of heart to pump sufficient blood
- Severe blood or fluid loss so that there is insufficient blood in the system
- Enlargement: dilation of blood vessels so that there is insufficient blood to fill them
- Breathing problems result in insufficient oxygen traveling through the system

RESULT: No matter what the reason, the result is the same: all normal bodily processes are affected. There is insufficient blood flow (perfusion) to provide nourishment and oxygen to all parts of the body. The key to managing shock is adequate ventilation and oxygenation.

FIGURE 6-2.

The following factors may have a significant effect on the degree of shock induced by trauma and disease:

- **Pain.** Pain can produce or increase the severity of shock.

- **Physical condition.** People who have been starved, deprived of water, or exposed to extremes of cold or heat go into shock very easily.

- **Fatigue.** Excessive fatigue can increase the severity of shock.

- **Disease.** As a general rule, people who have any kind of **CHRONIC** illness go into shock more easily than healthy people.

- **Individual reaction.** Some unexplained differences exist between individuals regarding their resistance to shock. An injury that might cause serious, perhaps even fatal, shock in one person may cause only mild shock in another.

■ **Improper evaluation/care/movements.** Shock may be increased by rough handling and by delay in treatment.

TYPES OF SHOCK

Any injury that results in a decrease in the amount of blood that is effectively circulating will produce symptoms of shock. There are many different types of shock (**HEMORRHAGIC**, respiratory, **NEUROGENIC**, **PSYCHOGENIC**, cardiac, etc.), but the result is the same: perfusion of organ systems fails and the victim is in a serious emergency. Study Figure 6-3, which provides a summary of the descriptions and causes of the different types of shock. Also, study Figure 6-4, which depicts the progressive circle of hemorrhagic shock and summarizes the emergency care.

STAGES OF SHOCK

Shock is progressive — it passes through three stages and, if left untreated, ends in death. The three basic stages of shock include the following (Figure 6-5):

COMPENSATORY SHOCK

In **COMPENSATORY SHOCK**, the first stage, the body uses its normal defense mechanisms to try to maintain normal function. There are minimal signs and symptoms at this stage. As the victim's blood pressure begins to drop, the heart rate increases and the blood vessels constrict in an attempt to restore normal blood pressure. If no further complications occur, the body corrects the condition within twenty-four hours. Signs and symptoms of compensatory shock include pale skin, rapid heart rate, and normal blood pressure.

SUMMARY — TYPES OF SHOCK	
TYPE	**DESCRIPTION AND CAUSE**
Hemorrhagic (Hypovolemic or Traumatic)	Loss of blood resulting in not enough blood going to tissues, i.e., wounds, internal bleeding. Possible causes — multiple trauma and severe burns. There is insufficient blood in the system to provide adequate circulation to all body parts.

Respiratory	There is an insufficient amount of oxygen in the blood because of inadequate breathing or respiratory arrest due to:
	    a) spinal injury resulting in damage to respiratory-controlled nerves
	    b) obstruction of airways — mucous plug, foreign body
	    c) chest trauma, flail chest, punctured chest, etc.

Neurogenic	Spinal or head injury resulting in loss of nerve control and thus **integrity** of blood vessels. The nervous system loses control over the vascular system — the blood vessels dilate and there is insufficient blood to fill them.
Psychogenic	Something psychological affects the victim, i.e., the sight of blood, loved one injured, etc.; blood drains from the head and pools in the abdomen, person faints due to lack of blood in the brain because of a temporary dilation of blood vessels.
Cardiac	Cardiac muscle not pumping effectively due to injury or previous heart attack. The heart muscle no longer imparts sufficient pressure to circulate the blood through the system.
Metabolic	Loss of body fluids with a change in biochemical equilibrium. Example: insulin shock or diabetic coma, vomiting, diarrhea.
Septic	Severe infection. Toxins cause pooling of blood in capillaries with dilation of blood vessels; not enough blood to tissues. Bacteria attack small blood vessel walls so that they lose blood and plasma and can no longer constrict.
Anaphylactic	Severe allergic reaction of the body to sensitization by a foreign protein, such as insect sting, foods, medicine, ingested, inhaled or injected substances. It can occur in minutes or even seconds following contact with the substance to which the victim is allergic.

FIGURE 6-3.

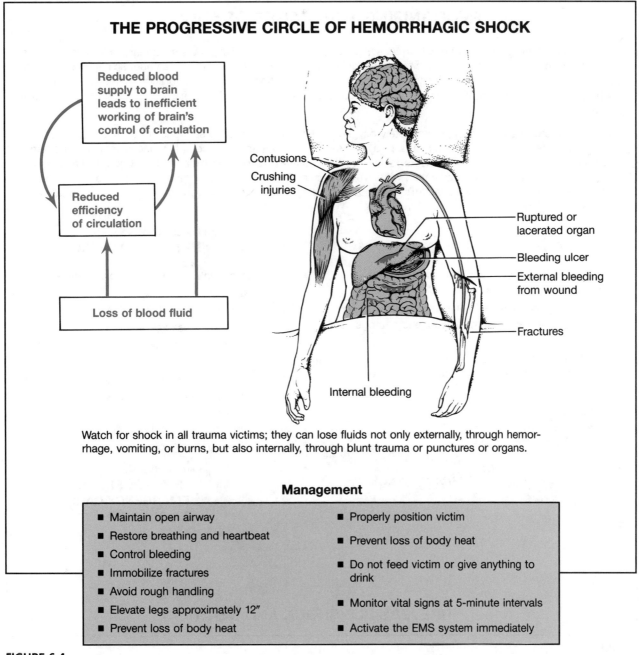

THE PROGRESSIVE CIRCLE OF HEMORRHAGIC SHOCK

Reduced blood supply to brain leads to inefficient working of brain's control of circulation

Reduced efficiency of circulation

Loss of blood fluid

Contusions
Crushing injuries

Ruptured or lacerated organ
Bleeding ulcer
External bleeding from wound
Fractures

Internal bleeding

Watch for shock in all trauma victims; they can lose fluids not only externally, through hemorrhage, vomiting, or burns, but also internally, through blunt trauma or punctures or organs.

Management

- Maintain open airway
- Restore breathing and heartbeat
- Control bleeding
- Immobilize fractures
- Avoid rough handling
- Elevate legs approximately 12"
- Prevent loss of body heat

- Properly position victim
- Prevent loss of body heat
- Do not feed victim or give anything to drink
- Monitor vital signs at 5-minute intervals
- Activate the EMS system immediately

FIGURE 6-4.

PROGRESSIVE SHOCK

When bleeding is uncontrolled, the body's mechanisms can compensate only so much. Then the victim progresses to the second stage, or **PROGRESSIVE SHOCK**. In an attempt to keep the vital organs perfused with oxygenated blood, the body shunts away blood from the extremities and the abdomen to the heart, brain, and lungs. As a result, the tissues in the extremities and the abdomen produce toxic by-products. At this stage, the body cannot correct the shock itself; without medical intervention, further decline occurs. Signs and symptoms include cyanotic or mottled skin, decreased blood pressure, and major changes in level of consciousness.

IRREVERSIBLE SHOCK

There are no clear immediate signs and symptoms of **IRREVERSIBLE SHOCK**, which is the final stage. Damage usually begins to manifest itself

RECOGNIZING THE STAGES OF SHOCK

Shock is inadequate perfusion of bodily tissues. It is not a disease in itself but occurs secondary to trauma or illness. Shock may develop when serious injury causes significant blood loss, pump (heart) damage, spinal cord injury, or pulmonary injury, or when serious illness causes peripheral vasodilation or severe dehydration. Remember — in order for blood to circulate properly there must be adequate blood volume, a good working pump, and an intact vascular system.

When the cells of the body are not adequately oxygenated and/or nourished, a sequence of events may occur that, if left uncorrected, will result in death. The body will set in motion a series of complex mechanisms in an attempt to achieve homeostasis and compensate for shock. If the state of shock is severe or prolonged, it may become irreversible. If this occurs, no intervention will save the victim. Recognizing the signs and symptoms of each stage of shock will help you classify the victim's condition according to its severity so you can intervene appropriately.

COMPENSATORY STAGE

- Restlessness, anxiety, irritability, apprehension
- Slightly increased heart rate
- Pale and cool skin in hypovolemic shock, warm and flushed skin in septic, anaphylactic, and neurogenic shock
- Slightly increased respiratory rate
- Slightly decreased body temperature (except fever in septic shock)

PROGRESSIVE (UNCOMPENSATED) STAGE

- Listlessness, apathy, confusion, slowed speech
- Rapid heart rate
- Slowed, irregular, weak, thready pulse
- Decreased blood pressure
- Cold, clammy, cyanotic skin
- Rapid breathing
- Severely decreased body temperature
- Confusion and incoherent, slurred speech, possibly unconsciousness
- Dilated pupils slow to react
- Slow, shallow, irregular respirations

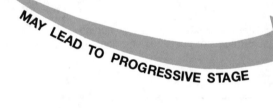

MAY LEAD TO PROGRESSIVE STAGE

IF APPROPRIATE EMERGENCY CARE IS NOT GIVEN

IRREVERSIBLE SHOCK AND DEATH

FIGURE 6-5.

several days later, when organs die and stop functioning. In this last stage, blood is shunted away from the liver and kidneys to the heart and brain; the liver and kidneys then die. Blood vessels are no longer able to sustain the pressure needed to feed the heart and brain; blood begins to pool away from the vital organs, and death occurs.

Even with treatment, damage to the vital organs is permanent; untreated, this stage of shock leads to death.

SIGNS AND SYMPTOMS OF SHOCK

Remember — the most obvious changes in vital signs occur late in the shock process. If you are "fooled" by normal early vital signs and wait to begin emergency care until vital signs start to deteriorate, you may reduce the overall effectiveness of the emergency care rendered.

The signs and symptoms of shock should not be studied merely as a means of identifying shock, but are of tremendous value in helping to determine what will be required in caring for the condition. The clinical picture of shock depends on what is occurring in the body. Decreased blood flow to the skin causes it to become pale, clammy, and cyanotic. When cardiac output decreases, the pulse will be more rapid as the heart tries to compensate. As blood pressure drops, the pulse will become shallow. Inadequate perfusion of the brain will cause anxiety, confusion, apathy, and loss of consciousness. Inadequate perfusion to the stomach will cause nausea and/or vomiting.

SIGNS AND SYMPTOMS COMMON TO ALL BUT ANAPHYLACTIC SHOCK

Signs and symptoms *that are common to all but anaphylactic shock* include the following (Figure 6-6):

- Restlessness, anxiety, fear, disorientation, mental confusion, and an anxious or dull expression.
- Feeling of impending doom.
- Cold, clammy, moist skin.
- Profuse sweating.
- Extreme thirst.
- Nausea and/or vomiting.
- Initial dull, chalklike appearance to the skin; later cyanosis. (See Figure 6-7 for determining shock in a dark-skinned victim.)
- Shallow, irregular breathing; may also be labored, rapid, or gasping.
- Dizziness.
- Loss of consciousness or altered levels of consciousness.
- Closed or partially closed eyelids; dilated pupils; dull, lusterless eyes.
- Weak, rapid pulse.
- Rarely, shaking and trembling of the arms and legs, as if chilled, or trembling of the entire body.

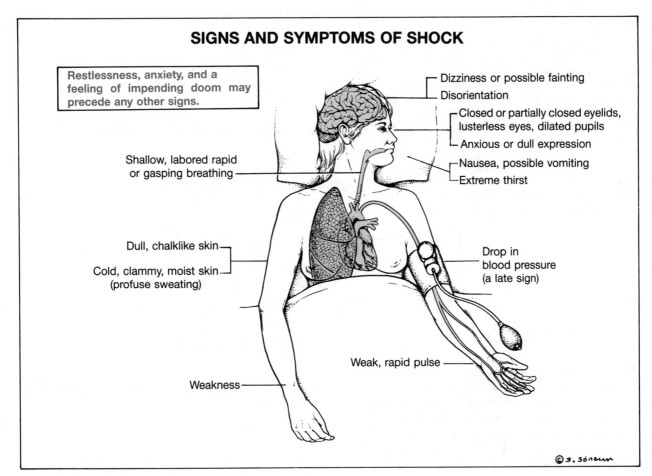

SIGNS AND SYMPTOMS OF SHOCK

Restlessness, anxiety, and a feeling of impending doom may precede any other signs.

Dizziness or possible fainting

Disorientation

Closed or partially closed eyelids, lusterless eyes, dilated pupils

Anxious or dull expression

Nausea, possible vomiting

Extreme thirst

Shallow, labored rapid or gasping breathing

Dull, chalklike skin

Cold, clammy, moist skin (profuse sweating)

Drop in blood pressure (a late sign)

Weak, rapid pulse

Weakness

©S. Sörzen

FIGURE 6-6.

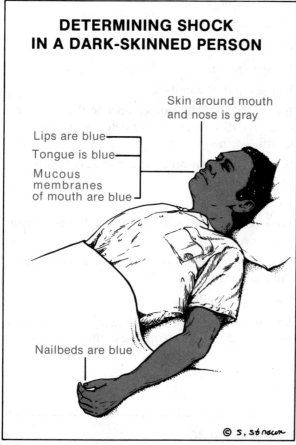

DETERMINING SHOCK IN A DARK-SKINNED PERSON

Skin around mouth and nose is gray

Lips are blue

Tongue is blue

Mucous membranes of mouth are blue

Nailbeds are blue

© S. Sброжин

FIGURE 6-7. A healthy person with dark skin will usually have a red undertone and show a healthy pink color in the nailbeds, lips, mucous membranes of the mouth, and tongue. However, a Black victim in shock from a lack of oxygen does not exhibit the marked skin color changes. Rather, the skin around the nose and mouth will have a grayish cast, the mucous membranes of the mouth and tongue will be blue (cyanotic), and the lips and nailbeds will have a blue tinge. If shock is due to bleeding, the mucous membranes in the mouth and tongue will not look blue but will have a pale, graying, waxy pallor. Other landmarks include the tips of the ears, which may be red during fever.

ANAPHYLACTIC SHOCK

ANAPHYLACTIC SHOCK results from a severe allergic reaction of the body to a foreign protein, such as an insect sting, food, medicine, pollen, or some other inhaled, ingested, or injected substance. The most common causes of anaphylactic shock are bee stings and drugs; at least 1 percent of the general population is at risk for developing anaphylactic shock from bee stings alone. The reaction can occur within minutes — or even seconds — following a sting or other exposure, and immediate treatment is required to prevent death.

Anaphylactic shock should be considered a grave medical emergency. The severity of the reaction is inversely related to the time elapsing between exposure and the onset of symptoms: the shorter the time before symptoms appear, the greater the risk of a fatal reaction.

Anaphylactic shock may result in any combination of the following signs and symptoms (Figure 6-8):

1. **Signs and symptoms involving the skin:**
   - Itching and burning of the skin with flushing, especially around the face and chest.
   - Blueness (cyanosis) around the lips.
   - Raised, hivelike patches with severe itching.
   - Swelling of the face and tongue.
   - Paleness.
   - Swelling of the blood vessels just underneath the skin.

2. **Signs and symptoms involving the heart and circulation:**
   - Weak, rapid pulse.
   - Low blood pressure.
   - Dizziness.
   - Restlessness.
   - Diminished **STROKE VOLUME** and cardiac output.

3. **Signs and symptoms involving the respiratory tract:**
   - Spasm of the bronchioles.
   - A painful, squeezing sensation in the chest.
   - Difficulty in breathing.
   - Coughing; bronchial obstruction.
   - Swelling of the larynx.
   - Swelling of the epiglottis.
   - Respiratory wheezes.

4. **Signs and symptoms involving the gastrointestinal tract:**
   - Nausea.
   - Vomiting.
   - Abdominal cramps.
   - Diarrhea.

ANAPHYLACTIC SHOCK

Anaphylactic shock is a severe allergic reaction of the body to sensitization by a foreign protein, such as insect sting; foods; medicine; ingested, inhaled, or injected substances. It can occur in minutes or even seconds following contact with the substance to which the victim is allergic. This is a grave medical emergency.

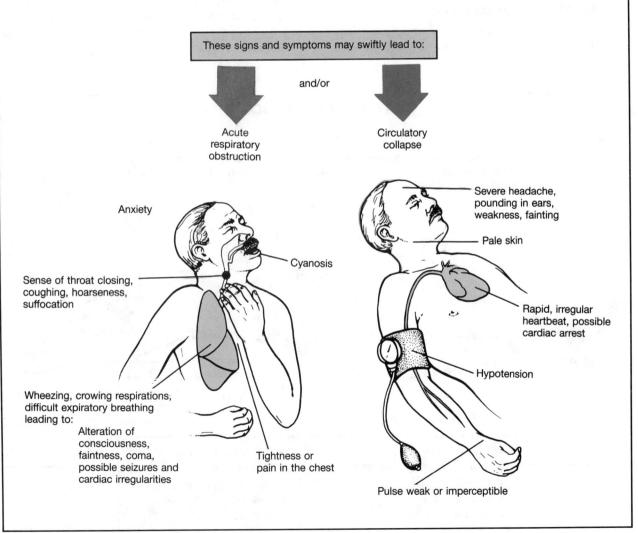

Rapidity of onset

As a rule, anaphylactic reactions occur more frequently and rapidly when the antigen is injected (seconds to minutes). By the oral route, they may be delayed (up to hours), although immediate, catastrophic progression is also a possibility with oral ingestion.

Common early symptoms and signs

Flushing, itching

Sneezing, watery eyes and nose

Skin rash, airway swelling

'Tickle' or 'lump' in the throat which cannot be cleared, cough

Gastrointestinal complaints

These signs and symptoms may swiftly lead to:

and/or

Acute respiratory obstruction

Circulatory collapse

Anxiety

Cyanosis

Sense of throat closing, coughing, hoarseness, suffocation

Wheezing, crowing respirations, difficult expiratory breathing leading to:

Alteration of consciousness, faintness, coma, possible seizures and cardiac irregularities

Tightness or pain in the chest

Severe headache, pounding in ears, weakness, fainting

Pale skin

Rapid, irregular heartbeat, possible cardiac arrest

Hypotension

Pulse weak or imperceptible

FIGURE 6-8.

MANAGEMENT OF SHOCK

The following steps should be taken to manage shock (Figure 6-9).

1. Secure an open airway. (Give extra attention to victims with an obvious airway compromise, with respiratory rates over twenty per minute, with noisy respiration, or to those not breathing.)

2. Control any obvious bleeding; use direct pressure, pressure points, elevation, an air splint, a blood-pressure cuff, or a tourniquet if indicated.

3. Elevate the lower extremities and maintain a head-low position except when other wounds or discomfort do not make this possible.

4. Splint any fractures. This can help reduce shock by slowing bleeding and helping to relieve pain.

5. Keep the victim warm by conserving his body heat, but do not overheat.

   ■ If possible, remove any wet clothing.

   ■ Place the victim on a blanket and cover him with blankets, but do not overheat.

   ■ A victim with a head, neck, or spinal injury should not be moved onto a blanket; instead, wrap him as well as possible by placing blankets on top of him.

   ■ Move the victim to a warm environment; if you cannot move the victim, erect some kind of barrier to protect him from wind, drafts, or other cold-weather elements.

   ■ If you do not have access to blankets, use plastic garbage bags or plastic sheeting that retains heat well.

6. Keep the victim quiet and still; shock is aggravated by rough and/or excessive handling.

7. Give the victim nothing by mouth because of the possible need for surgery, because of possible injury to the digestive system, and because it may cause vomiting. If the victim complains of intense thirst, it may help to wet his lips with a wet towel.

8. Activate the EMS system immediately.

9. Monitor the victim's state of consciousness and pulse, and record at five-minute intervals. Keep checking vital signs every five minutes until the emergency team arrives.

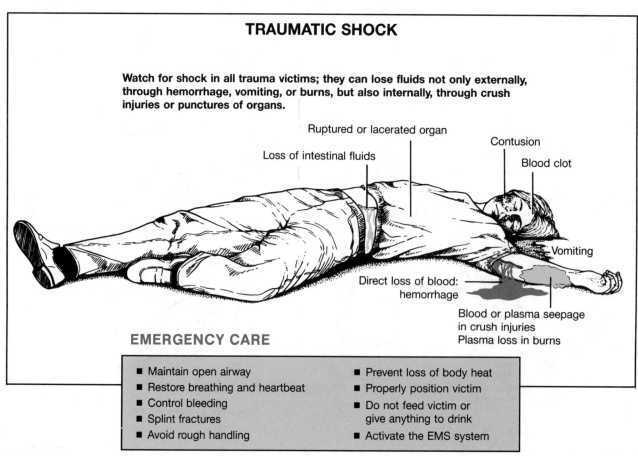

TRAUMATIC SHOCK

Watch for shock in all trauma victims; they can lose fluids not only externally, through hemorrhage, vomiting, or burns, but also internally, through crush injuries or punctures of organs.

Ruptured or lacerated organ

Loss of intestinal fluids

Contusion

Blood clot

Vomiting

Direct loss of blood: hemorrhage

Blood or plasma seepage in crush injuries
Plasma loss in burns

EMERGENCY CARE

■ Maintain open airway
■ Restore breathing and heartbeat
■ Control bleeding
■ Splint fractures
■ Avoid rough handling

■ Prevent loss of body heat
■ Properly position victim
■ Do not feed victim or give anything to drink
■ Activate the EMS system

FIGURE 6-9.

MANAGEMENT OF ANAPHYLACTIC SHOCK

1. Secure an open airway and maintain ventilations.
2. Begin CPR if indicated.
3. If the reaction is due to an insect sting or injection, place a constricting band between the injection site and the heart if possible. See Chapter 20.
4. Help the victim administer his medication (usually **EPINEPHRINE** and/or **ANTIHISTAMINES**).
5. Activate the EMS system. The victim should be transported immediately to a medical facility for further life-saving treatment.

PREVENTING SHOCK

The following preventive measures should be carried out in all cases of impending shock except those in which the specific measure would be against the best interests of the victim (Figures 6-10–6-17).

1. Control bleeding. Use direct pressure, elevation, pressure points, or a tourniquet if appropriate.
2. Assure adequate breathing. This may involve:
   - Merely observing the victim's breathing.
   - Using your finger to sweep his mouth and clear it of foreign matter.
   - Giving artificial ventilation.
   - Positioning the victim to assure adequate drainage of any fluid obstructing his air passages.
   - Giving cardiopulmonary resuscitation.
3. Loosen restrictive clothing, especially at the neck, waist, and any other place where it binds the victim.

4. Reassure the victim; remain calm and in control. Be receptive and accessible, but initiate conversations only to give instruction or warnings or to get necessary information. Answer the victim's questions in a brief but straightforward manner.
5. Splint and immobilize fractures.
6. Relieve pain with proper dressing, bandaging, splinting, and positioning of the victim.
7. Position the victim.
   - Use small pieces of padding so that bony prominences (like the cheek, elbow, shoulder, hip, or knee) do not press against the stretcher, the ground, or any other unyielding support.
   - Use the semi-prone position for victims who are unconscious; who have injuries of the face, head, neck (except fracture), or chest; or when vomiting is likely.
   - Use the head-dependent position (supine with feet elevated approximately six inches) for a conscious victim who has no external injury or injury only of the extremities; do not use the head-dependent position in victims with neck or spinal fractures or with any of the conditions listed under the semi-prone position.
8. Keep the victim warm, but do not overheat.
   - If possible, remove wet clothing.
   - Tuck blankets next to the victim's skin.
   - Watch closely for signs of overheating (such as perspiration) or cooling (such as chilling).
   - In hot weather, shade the victim from direct sunlight.
9. Continually monitor for the possibility of vomiting.

BODY POSITIONING AND CARE FOR PREVENTING SHOCK

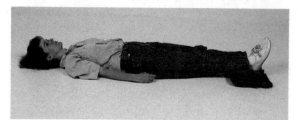

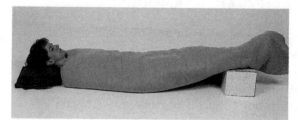

FIGURE 6-10.   Normally, the lower extremities should be elevated. By gravity this will reduce the blood in the extremities and may improve the blood supply to the heart. If the victim has leg fractures, the legs should not be elevated unless they are well splinted.   **FIGURE 6-11.**

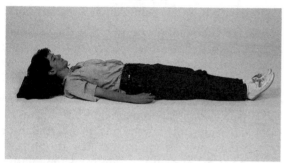

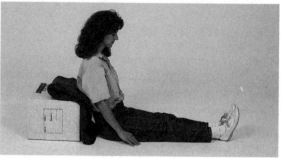

FIGURE 6-12. If there are indications of head injuries, the head could be raised slightly to reduce pressure on the brain. The feet may also be elevated. The head should not be elevated if there is mucus in the throat.

FIGURE 6-13. If there are breathing difficulties, the victim may be more comfortable with the head and shoulders raised, that is, in a semi-sitting position.

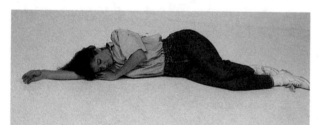

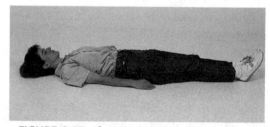

FIGURE 6-14. If the victim is unconscious, she should be placed on her side in coma position.

FIGURE 6-15. If circumstances indicate, the individual should be left in the position found.

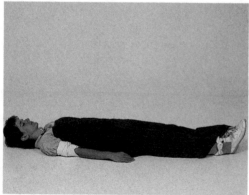

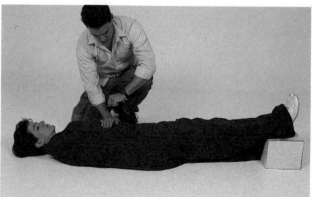

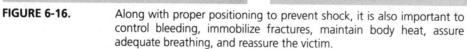

FIGURE 6-16.   Along with proper positioning to prevent shock, it is also important to control bleeding, immobilize fractures, maintain body heat, assure adequate breathing, and reassure the victim.   **FIGURE 6-17.**

| **6** | **SELF-TEST** | **6** |

Student: _____   Date: _____

Course: _____   Section #: _____

PART I: True/False   If you believe that the statements about shock are true, circle the T. If you believe that the statement is false, circle the F.

T   F   1.   Normally the lower extremities should be elevated.

T   F   2.   If there are possible head injuries, always raise the feet.

T   F   3.   During shock, the oxygen supply is decreased because the heart needs less oxygen.

T   F   4.   Respirations may increase and become shallow and irregular during shock.

T   F   5.   One common cause of shock is the failure of the heart to pump enough blood.

T   F   6.   Losing fluid from the circulatory system is one of the primary causes of shock.

T   F   7.   One of the causes of most cases of shock is the pooling of blood in the vital areas.

T   F   8.   Give a shock victim fluids if he is conscious.

T   F   9.   Keep the victim dry and attempt to raise his body temperature above normal to compensate for lack of blood flow to the extremities.

T   F   10. If the victim is unconscious, put him in a semi-reclining position.

PART II: Multiple Choice   For each question, circle the answer that best reflects an accurate statement.

1.   Management of *all but one* of the following emergencies should precede shock:

    a.   bleeding.
    b.   burns.
    c.   cardiac arrest.
    d.   breathing stoppage.

2.   Which of the following are signs of anaphylactic shock?

    a.   strong, bounding pulse; heavy breathing; dizziness.
    b.   weak pulse, itching or burning skin; swelling of the tongue and face.
    c.   fever, sweating, chest pain, pale coloring.
    d.   increased blood pressure; rapid, strong pulse; convulsions.

3.   The body's response to shock can be observed by summarizing the general signs and symptoms of shock. *All but which one* of the following are signs and symptoms of shock?

    a.   restlessness and anxiety.
    b.   weakness.
    c.   feeling of impending doom.
    d.   bounding pulse.

4.   Anaphylactic shock should be considered:

    a.   a true medical emergency.
    b.   an emergency only in a sensitized person.
    c.   an emergency only if the person has been stung on the face or hand.
    d.   a non-emergency situation.

5.   Shock can occur:

    a.   even though only one area of the body may be impaired.
    b.   only when large amounts of blood are lost.
    c.   when the extremities do not get enough blood.
    d.   in conjunction with severe cases of high blood pressure.

6.   Which of the following shock processes occurs first?

    a.   brain loses its ability to function.
    b.   vital organs and brain do not receive enough blood.
    c.   blood rushes to the brain and vital organs, thus depriving other body cells nutrients.
    d.   internal organs and brain cells begin to die.

7.   In what order should the First Aider care for the following emergencies: (1) cardiac arrest; (2) shock; (3) respiratory failure; (4) bleeding.

    a.   3, 1, 4, 2.
    b.   1, 2, 3, 4.
    c.   1, 3, 4, 2.
    d.   2, 3, 1, 4.

8.   What is the first event in the ongoing cycle of shock?

    a.   the brain loses its ability to function.
    b.   blood rushes to the brain, depriving other organs of oxygen.
    c.   blood flow in the entire body is disrupted.
    d.   the internal organs and brain cells start to die.

9.   The most important single requirement in management of shock is to:

    a.   reassure the victim so neurogenic shock does not complicate the victim's condition.
    b.   establish an airway, stop bleeding, and prevent loss of body heat.
    c.   arrest and reverse progressive deterioration and restoration of the circulatory system.
    d.   treat the injuries quickly and efficiently.

10. Which of the following is *not* an emergency-care technique for anaphylactic shock?

    a.   elevate the lower extremities and maintain a head-lowered position.
    b.   if the reaction is due to an insect sting, place a constricting band above the site.
    c.   assist the victim in administering his medication if legally advisable.
    d.   establish an airway.

11. Which of the following is *not* a means of preventing shock?

    a. keep the victim's body temperature above normal.
    b. reassure the victim.
    c. loosen constrictive clothing.
    d. control hemorrhage by direct pressure, elevation, or pressure points.

12. Which of the following is *not* a type of shock?

    a. hypothermic.
    b. neurogenic.
    c. septic.
    d. cardiogenic.

13. Which of the following is *not* an indication of shock?

    a. dull, lackluster eyes.
    b. constricted pupils.
    c. cold, clammy, moist skin.
    d. shallow respiration, possibly irregular or labored.

14. In anaphylactic shock, the shorter the time before symptoms appear:

    a. the greater the chance of a recovery in a short time.
    b. the greater the chance of swelling of the larynx.
    c. the greater the risk of a fatal reaction.
    d. the greater the chance of an antigen-antibody reaction.

15. A person may be in anaphylactic shock from which preceding event?

    a. sight of a bloody accident.
    b. eating berries.
    c. head injury.
    d. severe illness.

16. The major objective in treating shock is to:

    a. maintain the victim's body temperature.
    b. improve and/or maintain circulation.
    c. help the victim stay conscious.
    d. keep the victim's head elevated.

17. Shock that is caused by blood loss is called:

    a. hemorrhage.
    b. anaphylactic.
    c. respiratory.
    d. cardiac.

18. Which of the following procedures for management of shock comes first?

    a. prevent loss of body heat.
    b. establish an airway.
    c. monitor the victim's state of consciousness.
    d. elevate lower extremities except when contraindicated.

PART III: Matching Match the following types of shock with the correct definition of each.

Types	Definitions
_____ 1. Septic	A. Spinal or head injury resulting in loss of nerve control and thus integrity of blood vessels.
_____ 2. Hemorrhagic hypovolemic	B. Loss of body fluids with a change in biochemical equilibrium.
	C. Toxins cause pooling of blood in the extremities.
_____ 3. Nonhemorrhagic hypovolemic	D. Allergic reaction of the body to sensitization by a foreign protein.
	E. Loss of blood resulting in not enough blood going to tissues.
_____ 4. Cardiogenic	F. Something psychological affects the victim; blood drains from the head and pools in the abdomen.
_____ 5. Neurogenic	
_____ 6. Anaphylactic	G. Cardiac muscle not pumping efficiently.
_____ 7. Psychogenic	

PART IV: What Would You Do If:

1. An elderly woman has been in an auto accident and has several lacerations on her head and face. The bleeding is not severe, but she is disoriented, has cold, clammy skin, and a weak, rapid pulse. She is very anxious and her breathing is shallow and rapid.

2. Your neighbor is stung by a bee and did not think too much about his flushed, itching skin, sneezing, and watery eyes, but now he is complaining about a tightness in his chest. He is coughing, sounds hoarse, looks cyanotic, and feels like his throat is closing.

PART V: Practical Skills Check-Off _____ has satisfactorily passed the following practical skills:
Student's Name

	Date	Partner Check	Inst. Init.
1. Demonstrate how to position a shock victim who has no external injuries.	__/__/__	☐	_____
2. Demonstrate how to position a victim who is in shock and has a head injury.	__/__/__	☐	_____
3. Demonstrate how to maintain body heat in a shock victim.	__/__/__	☐	_____

SOFT - TISSUE INJURIES

WHAT IS A SOFT-TISSUE INJURY?

In the injured victim, the skin not only reflects blood circulation but may itself (as well as underlying structures) be the site of damage. The entire surface of the body must therefore be inspected for soft-tissue injuries. Although this type of injury may be the most obvious and dramatic, it is seldom the most serious unless it compromises the airway or is associated with massive hemorrhage. Thus, the First Aider must search systematically and thoroughly for other injuries or life-threatening conditions before treating the soft-tissue trauma.

Soft-tissue injuries involve the skin and underlying **MUSCULATURE**. An injury to these tissues is commonly referred to as a **WOUND**. More specifically, a wound is a traumatically caused injury to the body that disrupts the normal **CONTINUITY** of the tissue, organ, or bone affected.

Wounds may be classified generally as **CLOSED** or **OPEN**, single or multiple. They are also classified according to anatomical location (position on the body). These include head wounds (subdivided into skull, face, and jaw wounds); abdominal wounds; chest wounds; wounds of the limbs (arms and legs); wounds of the joints; and spinal and pelvic wounds.

The part of the body most severely injured determines the subclassification of multiple wounds.

CLOSED WOUNDS

In a closed injury, such as a **BRUISE**, or contusion, soft tissues beneath the skin are damaged but the skin is not broken (Figure 7-1). Contusions are

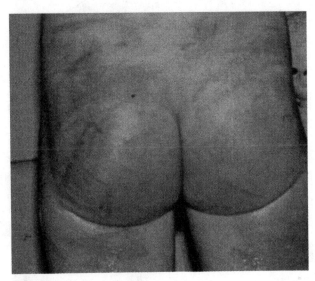

FIGURE 7-1. Contusions.

marked by local pain and swelling. If small blood vessels beneath the skin have been broken, the victim will also exhibit **ECCHYMOSIS** (black and blue discoloration); blood and fluid will leak into the damaged tissue. If large vessels have been torn beneath the bruised area, a **HEMATOMA** — a collection of blood beneath the skin — will be evident as a lump with bluish discoloration. Generally, closed wounds are characterized by pain at the injury site, ecchymosis, and swelling.

Small bruises generally require no treatment. For larger bruises, apply ice or cold compresses to help relieve pain and reduce swelling. (To guard against frostbite, never apply ice directly to the skin.) With large contusions, apply ice to relieve pain and reduce swelling, use pressure (manual compression) to help stop internal bleeding, and splint to decrease pain and limit mobility. Elevate the affected limb to help reduce pain and swelling.

In a closed injury, treat for internal bleeding if you are in doubt. If large bruised areas are present, assess carefully for fracture, especially if any swelling or deformity is present.

CHAPTER 9

OPEN WOUNDS

In an open wound, the skin is broken and the victim is susceptible to external hemorrhage and wound **CONTAMINATION**. An open wound may be the only surface evidence of a more serious injury, such as a fracture. Open wounds include **ABRASIONS, INCISIONS, LACERATIONS, PUNCTURES, AVULSIONS, BITES,** and **AMPUTATIONS** (Figure 7-2).

In general, you should transport a victim of an open wound to a physician or activate the EMS system if:

■ The wound has spurted blood (even if you have been able to control the bleeding).

■ The wound is deeper than the outer skin layer.

■ There is uncontrolled bleeding.

■ There is embedded debris or an embedded object, or extensive contamination.

■ The wound involves nerves, muscles, or tendons.

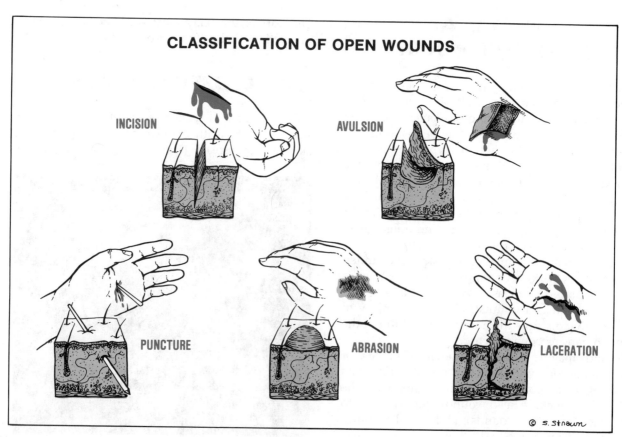

CLASSIFICATION OF OPEN WOUNDS

INCISION

AVULSION

PUNCTURE

ABRASION

LACERATION

© S. Straum

FIGURE 7-2.

- The wound involves the mouth, tongue, face, genitals, or a place where a scar would be noticeable and/or disfiguring.
- The wound is a human or animal bite.

ABRASIONS

An abrasion is a superficial wound caused by rubbing or scraping (friction) in which part of the skin layer — usually the epidermis and part of the dermis — has been lost (Figure 7-3). Blood may ooze from the abrasion, but bleeding is usually not severe. All abrasions, regardless of size, are extremely painful because of the nerve endings involved. Abrasions can pose a threat if large areas of skin are involved (as can happen in a motorcycle accident when the rider is thrown against the road).

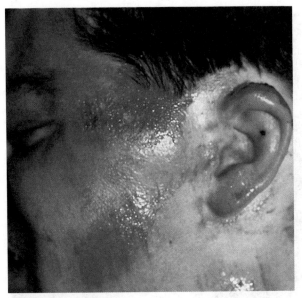

FIGURE 7-3. Abrasions.

Emergency Care

Provide the following care for abrasions:

1. Cleaning wounds should be left to medical personnel. However, some EMS areas recommend rinsing abrasions under cold running water. *Follow local protocol.*
2. Cover the abrasion with a sterile dressing of nonadherent material, and bandage in place.
3. Leave the cleaning of embedded debris to a physician. If you cannot transport the victim, however, bathe the abrasion with clean water and gently remove debris from around the wound. Loosely cover with a sterile dressing and bandage in place. *Follow local protocol.*

INCISIONS

Incisions are sharp, even cuts with smooth edges that tend to bleed freely because the blood vessels and tissue have been severed (Figure 7-4). Incisions are caused by any sharp, cutting object, such as a knife, razor blade, or broken glass. The greatest dangers with incisions are severe (often profuse) bleeding and damage to **TENDONS** and **NERVES**. Incisions usually heal better than lacerations because the edges of the wound are smooth and straight.

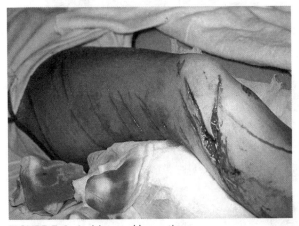

FIGURE 7-4. Incision and lacerations.

Emergency Care

Provide the following care for incisions:

1. The first priority is to control bleeding by direct pressure.
2. Draw the wound edges together, apply a sterile pressure dressing, and bandage in place. See Chapter 9.
3. Give emergency care for shock.
4. Transport the victim to a physician, or, if serious enough, activate the EMS system.

LACERATIONS

A laceration is a tear inflicted by a sharp, even instrument (such as a broken glass bottle) that produces a ragged incision through the skin surface and underlying tissues (Figures 7-5 and 7-6). A laceration can also result from blunt trauma to tissue overlying a bone.

Lacerations can cause significant bleeding if the sharp instrument also cuts the wall of a blood vessel, especially an artery. This is particularly true in

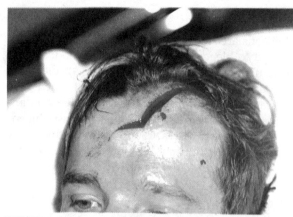

FIGURE 7-5. Laceration of the forehead and scalp.

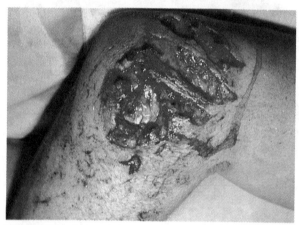

FIGURE 7-6. Deep abrasions and lacerations.

areas where major arteries lie close to the skin surface, such as in the wrist. Because the edges of the wound are jagged, healing is not as good as in incisions; skin and tissue may be torn away partly or completely, and the laceration may contain foreign matter that can lead to infection.

Emergency Care

Provide the following care for lacerations:

1. Control bleeding with direct pressure and elevation; if possible, use sterile gauze over the wound.

2. Once bleeding is controlled, remove surface dirt and loose debris. Wound cleaning should be left to medical personnel. *Follow local protocol.*

3. Cover with a sterile dressing, and bandage in place. See Chapter 9.

4. Elevate the affected part to help control pain and bleeding.

5. Splinting and immobilizing the injured part may also help control bleeding.

6. Give emergency care for shock.

7. Transport the victim to a physician or activate the EMS system.

PUNCTURES

A puncture wound is caused by the penetration of a sharp object (such as a nail) through the skin and underlying structures (Figure 7-7). Even though the opening in the skin may appear very small, the puncture wound may be extremely deep, posing a serious threat of infection.

Internal organs may also be damaged by punctures. In some cases, the object that causes the injury remains embedded in the wound.

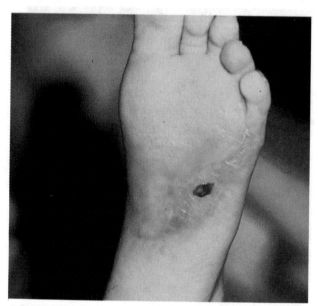

FIGURE 7-7. Puncture wound of the foot.

A puncture usually does not cause a bleeding problem unless it is located in the chest or abdomen (where resultant bleeding can be rapidly fatal). In a puncture wound, always assess for an exit wound as well. (See pages 114-116 for discussion of stab and gunshot wounds.)

Emergency Care

Provide the following care for a puncture wound:

1. Let the wound bleed freely for a few minutes to help wash out bacteria.

2. Clean the area around the wound with soap and water, and soak the puncture for ten to fifteen

minutes in a combination of warm water and **BACTERICIDE** (the warm water will encourage a small amount of bleeding). *Follow local protocol.*

3. Cover the wound with a light, sterile dressing and bandage in place.

4. Give the victim emergency care for shock.

5. Transport the victim to a physician; immobilize the injured part in a comfortable position.

If there is an impaled object in the wound, do *not* remove it — efforts to do so can cause underlying tissue damage and severe hemorrhage. See Chapter 8.

AVULSIONS

An avulsion is the tearing loose of a flap of skin, which may either remain hanging or be torn off altogether (Figures 7-8 and 7-9). **SCARRING** is often extensive, and avulsions usually bleed profusely. If the avulsed skin is still attached by a flap of skin and the skin is folded back, circulation to the flap can be compromised severely; always make sure that the

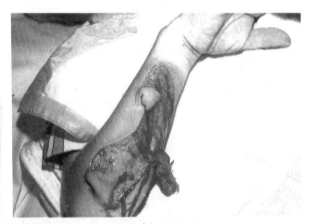

FIGURE 7-8. Forearm avulsion.

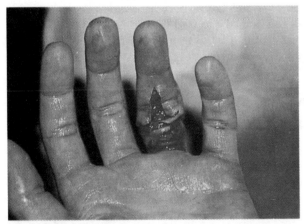

FIGURE 7-9. Ring avulsion.

flap is lying flat and that it is aligned in its normal position.

The most commonly avulsed skin on the body is that on the fingers and toes, hands, forearms, legs, feet, ears, nose, and penis. Most often, the patient with an avulsion works with machinery — home accidents involving lawnmowers and power tools are especially increasing in number. Avulsions also occur commonly in automobile or motorcycle accidents.

Emergency Care

To care for an avulsion:

1. Clear the wound surface. *Follow local protocol.*

2. Fold the skin flap back into normal position.

3. Control bleeding by direct pressure.

4. Apply a bulky, dry, sterile or compression dressing once the bleeding has been controlled.

5. Give the victim emergency care for shock.

6. Transport the victim to a physician or activate the EMS system.

   - If the avulsion is complete, send all avulsed parts with the victim.

   - Rinse the part with clean water to remove gross debris.

   - Wrap the part in dry sterile gauze, seal it in a plastic bag, and transport it on ice in another container. Do not use dry ice.

   - Prevent freezing of the tissue; never submerge the plastic bag in the ice.

BITES

More than two million domestic animal bites and more than two thousand snakebites occur in the United States each year. The number of human bites is not recorded but probably would be staggering if known. Nine out of ten animal bites are inflicted by dogs; 10 percent require suturing; and 1 percent require hospitalization (Figures 7-10 and 7-11). Complications can include infection (greatest in those under the age of four or over fifty), **CELLULITIS**, **TETANUS**, **SEPTICEMIA**, and **HEPATITIS**.

A domestic animal wound that does not involve an actual bite is **CAT-SCRATCH FEVER**, caused by an unknown **PATHOGEN** on a cat's claws. While it is not commonly seen in the field, cat-scratch fever can result in fever and swollen glands, and in swelling, warmth, drainage, streaking, and redness at the wound site.

Although bites and other domestic-animal–related wounds are handled similarly as any other

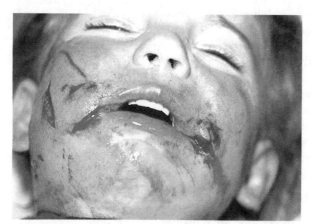

FIGURE 7-10. Dog bite.

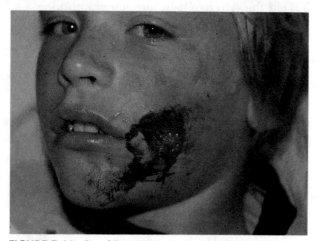

FIGURE 7-11. Dog bite.

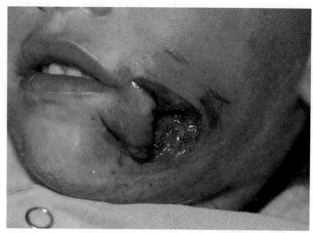

FIGURE 7-12. Horse bite.

Emergency Care

When you encounter a victim with a dog bite:

1. If the neck or face are involved, manage the airway to ensure adequate breathing.
2. Control hemorrhage with direct pressure.
3. Immediately and thoroughly wash the wound with large amounts of soapy water.
4. Some EMS areas recommend irrigating the bite with a disinfectant. However, *never* use alcohol on a bite. *Follow local protocol.*
5. Apply a dry sterile dressing and bandage in place.
6. Transport the victim to a physician with the limb elevated, or activate the EMS system.

Do not kill the dog unless absolutely necessary to prevent a full-scale, crippling attack. If you do kill the dog, call an animal control officer and request that the corpse be examined for **RABIES**, a viral infection that affects the nervous system. If you do not kill the dog, try to trap it in some kind of enclosure so that it can be examined for rabies; remember to guard your own safety. Take care not to injure the animal's head.

The bites of other animals should be cared for in the same manner as dog bites. Care for snakebite is more specific and is discussed in Chapter 20.

The most difficult bite is the human bite because of the high infection rate associated with it. Human bites usually involve the ears, nose, and fingers. They are inflicted most frequently by children involved in play or fights, or by people of all ages confined in mental institutions or involved in sexual assault and fights. Self-inflicted bites can result from

wound of the same type, these wounds have some peculiarities (Figure 7-12).

Of all domestic animal bites, dog bites are the most common. Most bites are inflicted by family pets or familiar dogs, with stray dogs inflicting only 6 percent of the bites. The most common victims are young children, with two times as many boys as girls being bitten. Most dog bites occur in the afternoon and early evening on cool summer or warm winter days. Among victims of all ages, 30 percent of the bites occur on the hands and arms, 30 to 50 percent on the legs, 10 percent on the torso, and 10 percent on the head and neck; children under the age of twelve are bitten most frequently on the face.

The worst dog bites are those that leave puncture wounds and those that occur in low vascular areas. The power of a dog's jaws can cause a severe crushing injury: a large breed can bite with the estimated force of 400 pounds per square inch. (See Figures 7-13, 7-14 and Table 7-1.)

DOG BITES

Over 1 million people suffer dog bites in the United States annually. The typical victim is male, under 20 years of age, and bitten by his own pet or some "familiar" large dog between 1 and 9 PM during the summer. Facial wounds occur predominantly in young children and teenagers.

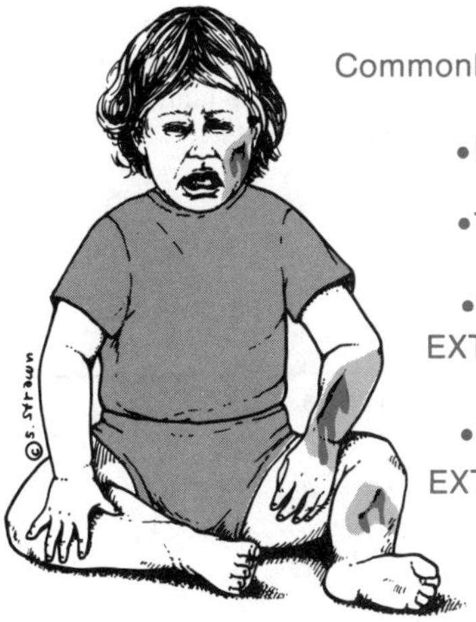

If possible, ascertain where the dog can be located: If an address is not possible, obtain a description of the dog, where it was encountered, and if the attack was provoked.

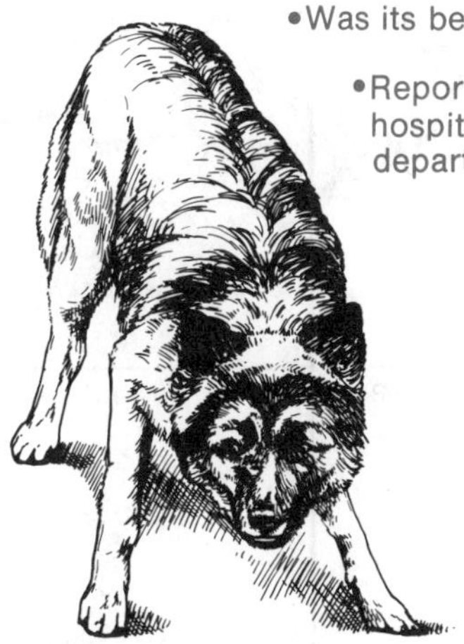

Commonly Bitten Areas:

- •FACE 11%

- •TRUNK 7%

- •UPPER EXTREMITIES 28%

- •LOWER EXTREMITIES 31%

- •Was its behavior unusual?

- •Report immediately to hospital and/or health department.

EMERGENCY CARE

- Wash wound thoroughly with soap and warm water and rinse well.
- If soap is not available, rinse bite thoroughly with warm water.
- In bites of the head, neck and face be sure airway is clear and position for drainage or suctioning.
- Cover wound with a thick dressing and apply gentle firm pressure.
- If wound is deep leave original dressing in place and add more gauze and then bandage in place.
- Immobilize injured part.
- The victim is usually frightened — calm him/her by talking to him while you are giving necessary care.
- If wounds are severe, monitor for shock, and maintain body heat.
- Always have a dog bite victim go to a hospital.

FIGURE 7-13.

vigorous gum chewing, ill-fitting dentures, broken teeth, the rough edges of decayed teeth, or seizures. It is common for police to be bitten while breaking up disturbances or trying to apprehend suspects.

Human bites should be considered serious. Even though the wound may look minor, the tissue may be badly lacerated. More serious than the tissue damage, however, is the threat of infection. The human mouth harbors millions of bacteria, in a greater variety than found in the mouths of animals, and massive contamination may result. Human bites on fingers have sometimes resulted in loss of the fingers involved and, in some cases, the entire hand.

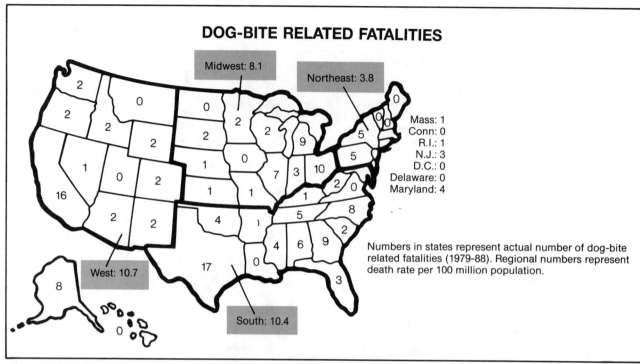

DOG-BITE RELATED FATALITIES

Source: Jeffrey J. Sacks, et. al., "Dog Bite–Related Fatalities", *Journal of the American Medical Association,* Vol. 262, No. 11, pg. 49.

FIGURE 7-14.

TABLE 7-1.
Breeds of dogs
responsible for fatal single-dog attacks
over a fourteen-year period.
(Other breeds involved in fatal pack attacks include boxers, collies, rottweilers, Labrador retrievers, and Yorkshire terriers.)

German shepherd	10
Husky	8
St. Bernard	7
Bullterrier (pit bull)	4
Great Dane	4
Malamute	5
Golden retriever	2
Dachshund	2
Doberman pinscher	2
Basenji	1
Chow chow	1
Mixed breed	5
Unknown breed	4

Reprinted with permission from: N. L. McGaffey, *Family Practice Recertification*, MRA Publications, Inc.

To treat a human bite:

1. Wash the bite with copious amounts of warm, soapy water. *Follow local protocol.*

2. Check the wound for any tooth fragments before applying a sterile dressing.

3. Transport the victim as soon as possible to a physician, where the wound can be cleaned in a sterile, controlled atmosphere, where unhealthy tissue can be removed, and where a **CULTURE** can be taken.

4. If you cannot transport a victim for some time, wash the wound immediately with an **ANTISEPTIC** soap. If such a soap is not available, rinse the wound continously with clean, running water. Cover the wound with a sterile dressing; bandage in place, and immobilize the injured area.

TRAUMATIC AMPUTATIONS

The ripping, tearing force of industrial and automobile accidents is great enough to tear away or crush limbs from the body. The victims are usually young males, and the effects can be tragic. There-fore, the initial emergency management of the vic-tim and of the dismembered limb is critical. New techniques in microreconstructive surgery make it possible to save many amputated limbs or digits, so care of the amputated part has become almost as crucial as care of the victim.

There are three general types of amputation:

1. Complete or total amputation, in which the body part is completely severed.

2. Partial amputation, in which more than 50 per-cent of the body part is severed.

3. Degloving amputation, in which skin and **ADIPOSE TISSUE** are torn away, but underlying tissue is left intact.

Because blood vessels are elastic, they tend to spasm and retract into surrounding tissue in cases of complete amputation; therefore, complete ampu-tations usually cause less bleeding than partial or degloving amputations, in which lacerated arteries continue to bleed profusely.

The most common sites of amputations include:

▪ Digits (Figures 7-15 and 7-16).

▪ Hands.

▪ Forearms.

▪ Ears.

▪ Toes (Figure 7-17).

▪ Below the knee.

▪ Through the knee.

▪ Above the knee.

▪ Penis.

▪ Nose.

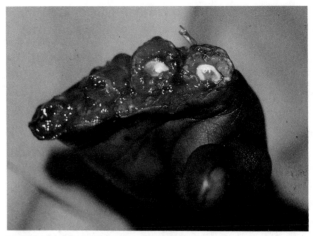

FIGURE 7-16. Finger amputation.

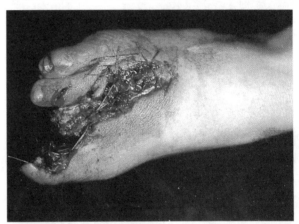

FIGURE 7-17. Toe amputation.

Emergency Care

Proper sequence of care for the amputation victim is as follows:

1. Establish and maintain the victim's vital func-tions (the ABCs of emergency care). Remember that trauma great enough to cause an amputation may also cause other bodily injury.

2. The limb, if crushed, may not bleed a great deal. Any hemorrhage should be controlled by direct pressure and elevation; use a tourniquet *only* as a lifesaving last resort. *Never* clamp blood vessels in an attempt to control bleeding; preserve the injured blood vessels as much as you can in case the amputated part can be reconstructed.

3. After bleeding has been controlled, apply a dressing to the amputated stump and wrap the end of the stump with an elastic bandage to replace hand pressure. Monitor the wound for a recurrence of bleeding.

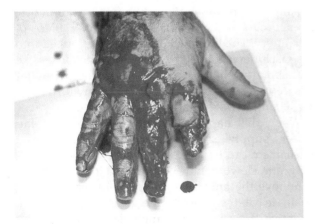

FIGURE 7-15. Finger amputation.

4. If the amputation was a degloving injury, apply a water-soaked dressing held in place with a bandage; never apply ice.

5. Treat the victim for shock.

6. Transport the victim to a hospital emergency department or activate the EMS system.

Try to locate amputated parts (*follow local protocol*), but do not neglect victim care in search of amputated parts. If you can find them quickly, or if someone you assign to the task can find them, handle them in the following manner (Figure 7-18):

1. Separate the severed part from dirt and other foreign matter; rinse with clean water, but do *not* immerse in liquid. Dry the part with sterile dressings or other absorbent material.

2. Wrap the part in dry, sterile gauze, a clean towel, or a clean sheet.

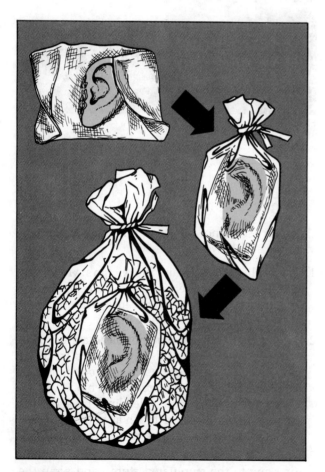

FIGURE 7-18. Emergency care for amputated parts consists of the following: (1) Wrap part completely in gauze or towel; wet the wrapping; (2) Place in plastic bag and seal shut; (3) Place bag inside an outer bag filled with ice; seal.

3. Place the severed part in a plastic bag and seal it shut; place the first plastic bag in a second plastic bag, and seal it shut. (The second bag provides added protection against moisture.)

4. Place the sealed bags in a container of ice or ice water. *Never* use dry ice.

5. Transport the part with the victim.

Proper handling of a severed part may allow it to be reattached up to twenty-four hours after the injury, although reattachment is best within six hours. In handling the severed part:

DO NOT:

▪ Freeze the part.

▪ Apply a tourniquet to the severed part.

▪ Make a judgment and throw the part away.

▪ Immerse the part in solution bath, soapy water, antiseptic solution, or water of any type.

Occasionally, you may find a victim whose limb has been lacerated or mangled severely but not completely amputated. The limb may be attached by a few strands of soft tissue and a small piece of skin. *Do not complete the amputation.* An important consideration in amputation is to preserve as much as possible of the original length of the limb. Even if a limb has been mangled severely and will eventually require amputation, the flap of skin holding the limb together may be used by the surgeon to cover the end of the stump, thereby allowing him to preserve a significant amount of limb length. In addition, the strands of soft tissue connecting the limb might contain nerves or blood vessels that, with proper surgical management, might allow the limb to survive.

Care for the open wound as described previously. Make sure that the skin bridge is not twisted or constricted by the pressure dressing.

Amputation, especially of the upper extremities, often occurs when a limb is caught in a piece of machinery. The limb will continue to be pulled into the machinery until some major obstruction — like the elbow or shoulder joint — is encountered. At this point, the limb will not progress any further — it will simply be ground up in the machine.

When this happens, immediately shut off the power supply to the machine. If the drive mechanism can be reversed, reverse the gears manually, and slowly remove the limb. If it is impossible to remove the limb, or if the piece of machinery is small, leave the limb in the machinery and disassemble the machinery. Immediately activate the EMS system.

BLUNT TRAUMA

Blunt trauma is caused by a sudden blow or force that has a crushing impact. This type of injury is treacherous, because the crushing force can result in serious internal injuries that initially display few, if any, external signs. A victim of an accident or other injury can look fine when first assessed by a First Aider, providing a false sense of security. The victim may then quickly decompensate, resulting in deep shock and/or death. For this reason, always suspect hidden internal damage in victims with injuries involving force.

GENERAL EMERGENCY CARE FOR OPEN WOUNDS

The chief duties of a First Aider in caring for an open wound are to stop bleeding and to prevent contamination from entering the wound. If germs do not enter, there will be much less chance of infection, and the wound will heal quickly (Figure 7-19).

All open wounds are contaminated to some extent; proper care can reduce the chances for further contamination and enhance the prospect for complete healing.

1. Completely assess the wound; tear or cut away clothing so that you can see the entire wound. Do not undress the victim in the conventional manner, since the motion of undressing can aggravate the wound or cause increased bleeding.

2. If there is severe bleeding from an artery, always control it by direct pressure using your hand or a dry, sterile compression dressing. A roller bandage can provide further pressure, and elevation of the affected limb can also help to control hemorrhage. Use a pressure point only if necessary. Use a tourniquet *only* as a last-resort, lifesaving measure.

3. Shock usually follows open wounds, especially if a considerable amount of blood was lost. Give emergency care promptly.

4. Never use harsh cleansing agents, soaps, or alcohol on an open wound.

5. If loose foreign particles are present around the wound, wipe them away with clean material. Always wipe away from the wound, not toward it (Figure 7-20). *Follow local protocol.*

6. Do not attempt to remove a foreign object embedded in the wound, since it may aid the

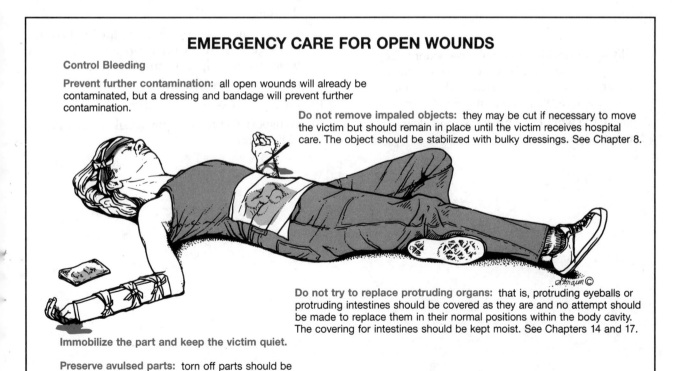

EMERGENCY CARE FOR OPEN WOUNDS

Control Bleeding

Prevent further contamination: all open wounds will already be contaminated, but a dressing and bandage will prevent further contamination.

Do not remove impaled objects: they may be cut if necessary to move the victim but should remain in place until the victim receives hospital care. The object should be stabilized with bulky dressings. See Chapter 8.

Do not try to replace protruding organs: that is, protruding eyeballs or protruding intestines should be covered as they are and no attempt should be made to replace them in their normal positions within the body cavity. The covering for intestines should be kept moist. See Chapters 14 and 17.

Immobilize the part and keep the victim quiet.

Preserve avulsed parts: torn off parts should be saved, and flaps of skin may be folded back to their normal position before bandaging.

FIGURE 7-19.

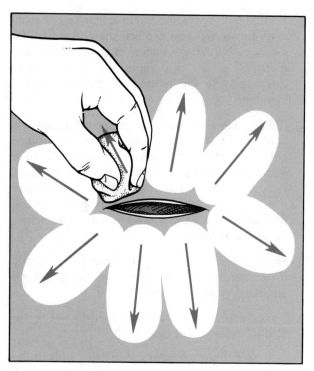

FIGURE 7-20. Use separate strokes and wipe away from edges when cleaning the area around a wound.

physician in determining the extent of the injury. Serious bleeding and other damage may occur if the object is removed. Stabilize the object with a bulky dressing. See Chapter 8.

7. Leave the work of complete wound cleansing to medical personnel.

8. Do not touch the wound with your hands, clothing, or anything that is not clean, if possible, and do not pour liquid into or on the wound.

9. Immobilize the injured part by splinting to prevent further bleeding. See Chapters 10 and 11.

10. Keep the victim quiet; keep him lying still, if possible.

11. Place a bandage compress or dressing over the wound, and tie or tape it in place. See Chapter 9.

12. All dressings should be wide enough to completely cover the wound and the area around it.

13. The dressing and bandage should be applied firmly and snugly but should not be so tight as to affect the blood supply to the injured part.

14. The bandage should be tied or fastened securely in place so that it will not move.

15. There should be no loose ends that could get caught on any other object while the victim is being moved.

16. Protect all bandages, compresses, or gauze dressings by an outer bandage made from a roller or triangular bandage, except dressings for wounds of the eye, nose, chin, finger, and toe, or **COMPOUND** (open) fractures of the hand and foot when splints are applied. If a bandage is used, open it enough to cover the entire dressing.

17. Unless otherwise specified, tie the knots of the bandage over the wound on top of the compress pad to help in controlling bleeding.

18. Preserve all avulsed parts.

19. Calm and reassure the victim.

20. Transport victim to a physician or activate the EMS system.

| **7** | **SELF-TEST** | **7** |

Student: _____ Date: _____

Course: _____ Section #: _____

PART I: True/False If you believe that the statement is true, circle the T. If you believe that the statement is false, circle the F.

T F 1. Clean most open wounds with alcohol.

T F 2. All bandages should be applied loosely so as not to do further damage.

T F 3. A laceration can result from blunt trauma to tissue overlying a bone.

T F 4. Elevating a leg that has a wound would seldom help in the control of bleeding.

T F 5. All dressings should be wide enough to cover the wound and the area around it.

T F 6. Always thoroughly clean a wound before dressing and bandaging.

T F 7. Avulsed parts or flaps of skin should not be folded back into place; this causes more contamination.

T F 8. Splinting and immobilizing an injured body part can help control bleeding.

T F 9. Nine out of ten animal bites are inflicted by dogs.

T F 10. Most dog bites of children under twelve occur on the face.

T F 11. Collies are responsible for most dog bites.

T F 12. Do not attempt to remove objects embedded in a wound.

T F 13. Proper handling of a severed body part may allow it to be reattached up to twenty-four hours after the injury.

T F 14. The chief duties of a first aider in caring for open wounds are to stop bleeding and to prevent contamination from entering the wound.

PART II: Multiple Choice For each question, circle the answer that best reflects an accurate statement.

1. Ecchymosis means:
   a. a lump beneath the skin.
   b. edema.
   c. black-and-blue coloring.
   d. external hemorrhage.

2. The soft-tissue injury resulting from the impact of a blunt object is called:
   a. a laceration.
   b. an avulsion.
   c. a contusion.
   d. an abrasion.

3. What type of wound has as its greatest danger severe bleeding and cut tendons and nerves?
   a. an incision.
   b. a laceration.
   c. a contusion.
   d. a puncture.

4. A type of open wound characterized by jagged skin edges and free bleeding is known as:
   a. a laceration.
   b. an incision.
   c. a contusion.
   d. a puncture.

5. What type of wound has the greatest danger of infection?
   a. an incision.
   b. a laceration.
   c. a contusion.
   d. a puncture.

6. When a puncture wound is caused by an impaled object:
   a. remove the object and cover with a sterile dressing.
   b. do not remove the object – stabilize it with a bulky dressing.
   c. apply slight pressure on the impaled object to stop bleeding.
   d. shorten the object for ease in transport.

7. A serious injury in which large flaps of skin and tissue are torn loose or pulled off is called an:
   a. abrasion.
   b. amputation.
   c. avulsion.
   d. incision.

8. To prevent contamination of a deep wound that is bleeding heavily and to help control bleeding, the First Aider should:
   a. replace dressings as soon as they become soiled.
   b. clean the area with an antiseptic solution.
   c. immediately remove any foreign object.
   d. leave the initial dressing in place.

9. Proper handling of a severed part includes:
   a. cleaning the part with an antiseptic solution.
   b. wrapping the part in gauze or a clean towel.
   c. freezing the part as quickly as possible.
   d. applying a tourniquet to the severed part to preserve fluids.

10. To control bleeding in a victim with traumatic amputation, first use:

    a. tourniquet.
    b. pressure dressing.
    c. pressure points.
    d. direct pressure.

11. Which of the following is a general guideline for emergency care of dog bites?

    a. pack the area in ice or with a cold compress.
    b. Apply indirect pressure to the wound to stop bleeding.
    c. wash the area with soapy water.
    d. do not cover the wound.

12. In cases where flaps of skin have been torn away but not cut off, the First Aider should:

    a. cut off any loose skin, then apply a dressing.
    b. gently fold the skin back to near-normal position and apply a dressing.
    c. place a cold, wet dressing over the loose flap.
    d. none of these answers.

13. When an amputation has occurred, which of the following is *not* true?

    a. soak the avulsed part in sterile antiseptic solution and put it in a plastic bag.
    b. place the bag with the avulsed part in a second bag filled with ice or cold water.
    c. never apply a tourniquet to the severed part.
    d. wrap the avulsed part in sterile material.

14. The chief duties of a First Aider in caring for open wounds are:

    a. to aid in proper healing of the wound and to treat for shock.
    b. to cleanse the wound and to apply bandages correctly.
    c. to calm and reassure the victim and to immobilize the injured part.
    d. to stop bleeding and to prevent germs from entering the wound.

15. A serious disease carried in the saliva of infected animals is called:

    a. lockjaw.
    b. rabies.
    c. tetanus.
    d. convulsions.

16. The danger with human bites is:

    a. infection.
    b. rabies.
    c. excessive bleeding.
    d. lawsuits.

17. What is the first step in the sequence of care for the amputation victim?

    a. apply a dressing to the stump.
    b. establish and maintain vital functions.
    c. treat for shock.
    d. control hemorrhage.

PART III: Matching   Match the following types of wounds and terms with the appropriate descriptions, emergency care, and/or definition.

_____ 1. Always assess for an exit wound.

_____ 2. Tearing loose of a flap of skin.

_____ 3. Degloving injury.

_____ 4. Rabies may be a concern.

_____ 5. Black-and-blue discoloration.

_____ 6. Most common victims are small children.

_____ 7. Greatest danger — severe bleeding and damage to tendons and nerves.

_____ 8. Wound edges usually jagged.

_____ 9. Smooth edges that tend to bleed freely.

_____ 10. Fold skin flap back into normal position.

_____ 11. Caused by rubbing or scraping.

_____ 12. Collection of blood beneath the skin.

A. Ecchymosis

B. Hematoma

C. Abrasion

D. Incision

E. Laceration

F. Puncture

G. Avulsion

H. Dog bites

I. Amputations

PART IV: What Would You Do If:

1. A three-year-old boy is bitten several times about the face by a large dog. The lacerations are deep and extensive.

2. A construction worker gets his arm caught in some roadway machinery, and his left arm is amputated at the elbow.

3. A warehouse worker gets his right arm caught between some large crates that are being moved and sustains a very painful crushing injury.

PART V: Practical Skills Check-Off   _____ has satisfactorily passed the following practical skills:

Student's Name

	Date	Partner Check	Inst. Init.
1. Demonstrate how to care for amputated body parts.	__/__/__	☐	_____
2. Describe general emergency care for open wounds.	__/__/__	☐	_____

CLAMPING AND PENETRATING INJURIES

A number of soft-tissue injuries involve foreign objects. Broken glass, sheet metal, knives, bullets, and power tools cause the worst and most extensive damage. To care for such injuries, use common sense, and inspect each wound to determine the following:

■ How did the injury occur?

■ What object caused the injury?

■ How much force was involved?

■ What kind of underlying tissue damage might have resulted?

■ What are the possibilities of contamination?

■ Could a foreign object (or part of one) be left behind in the wound?

Foreign bodies damage soft body tissues in four ways:

1. By clamping onto or around skin.

2. By penetrating the skin.

3. By becoming embedded in skin.

4. By penetrating the skin on one end and protruding from the other.

CLAMPING OBJECTS

Most **CLAMPING INJURIES** involve the hand (Figure 8-1) — more specifically, a finger, which can be

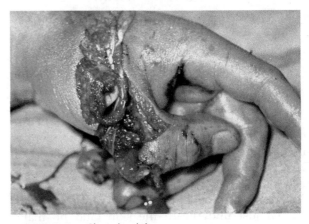

FIGURE 8-1. Clamping injury.

strangled when it is stuck into a hole and cannot be pulled out. Try to remove the finger as quickly as possible. The longer the finger is stuck, the harder it will be to remove, because the swelling will become more severe by the minute.

EMERGENCY CARE

Give the following emergency care:

1. Apply a lubricant such as green soap, and slowly but firmly wiggle the finger until it is loose.

2. If possible, elevate the hand above the victim's head while you remove the finger from the object.

3. If you are unable to loosen the finger, transport the victim immediately to a hospital emergency center or activate the EMS system. Keep the hand elevated above the victim's head during transport.

Another kind of **STRANGLING INJURY** occurs when a ring (or some other constricting object) strangles the finger or other body part due to severe constriction caused by inflammation from an injury. Remove the ring from the finger immediately. If you are unable to remove the ring, bend it so that the blood supply to the finger will resume. Transport the victim immediately.

A third kind of strangling injury occurs when an object is wound around a body part, cutting off circulation. Swelling is sometimes so bad that you will not be able to easily detect what is causing it (a rubber band, string, or hair).

Give the following care:

1. Examine the area closely. Find the cause of the swelling, and remove it promptly.

2. Elevate the body part to help reduce swelling.

3. Apply a cold pack.

4. Transport the victim to a physician or activate the EMS system immediately.

Use your judgment in deciding if you should care for the clamping injury at the site of the accident or first arrange transport of the victim to the hospital. Usually, livesaving measures must be taken in the field prior to transport because time is essential. However, a clamping injury that involves only skin and fat just underneath the skin (and no major blood vessels or nerves) is less serious and the victim can be transported first. Medical personnel can then separate the victim from the clamping mechanism.

If you decide to care for the injury in the field, observe and assess the injury carefully. If the clamp is restricting blood flow, it is best to attempt removal. While waiting for emergency personnel:

1. Apply a cold pack.

2. Elevate the injured area as high as possible.

3. Keep it well supported.

4. Never cool the injured area for longer than fifteen to thirty minutes at one time.

5. Treat for shock.

STAB WOUNDS

Knife and stab wounds are dangerous — and oftentimes fatal — and you must develop an efficient method of evaluation and emergency care. Because knife wounds are easier to detect than internal wounds, First Aiders too frequently concentrate only on the superficial wound to the skin. Remember — the superficial skin wound is almost never fatal. The fatalities all relate to the injured organs that lie beneath the skin wound (Figure 8.2).

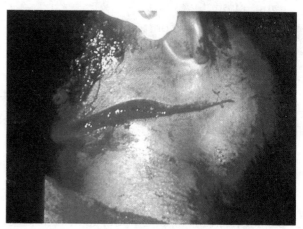

FIGURE 8-2. Knife wound of the neck.

EMERGENCY CARE

1. Do not concentrate only on the skin wound; deeper injuries with internal bleeding are much more critical.

2. Stabilize (with bulky dressings), and leave impaled knives in place.

3. Shock is usually caused by hemorrhage and breathing problems. Check for sucking chest wounds.

4. Use local pressure to control external bleeding. Do not use tourniquets unless bleeding cannot be controlled in any other way.

5. Maintain an adequate airway. Poor respiratory exchange and failure to maintain an adequate airway are the leading causes of death from stab wounds to the head, face, and neck.

6. Be alert for vomiting and blood in the mouth. Prevent aspiration by properly positioning the victim for drainage.

7. Maintain open airway, and administer artificial ventilation if necessary.

8. Cover all open wounds with a sterile dressing.

9. Seal any sucking chest wounds. See Chapter 16.

10. Immobilize extremities that have been injured, including the neck (fractures may have occurred).

11. Activate the EMS system immediately. Survival is directly related to the length of time that elapses between injury and surgery. Continuously monitor vital signs.

5. Immobilize injured extremities. If possible, place the victim on a **BACKBOARD** or rigid support, and apply a cervical collar if you suspect spinal or cervical damage.

6. Treat for shock.

7. Keep the victim as quiet as possible, and activate the EMS system immediately, monitoring vital signs while waiting for emergency personnel.

8. If you suspect that a crime has been committed, take care not to disturb potential crime-scene evidence; contact the police.

GUNSHOT WOUNDS

More than 30,000 people die of gunshot wounds each year in the United States, with thousands more being wounded either intentionally or accidentally.

Damage from a bullet is directly related to its velocity: a high-velocity bullet causes much more damage than a low-velocity one. Gunshot wounds can also cause both entrance and exit wounds. The entrance wound is generally much smaller and may be surrounded by powder burns if the victim was shot at close range, while the exit wound is generally two to three times larger and tends to bleed heavily. Assess the victim carefully — many have multiple gunshot wounds. Examine regions that may disguise a wound, such as under the arms. See Figures 8-3–8-8 for examples of gunshot wounds.

Do not enter the scene of a gunshot incident until the area has been secured by the police. Follow local protocol for reporting gunshot wounds (names, addresses, license numbers, and so on) to police.

EMERGENCY CARE

1. Make sure that the victim has an open airway, and assess for breathing.

2. If the victim is not breathing, administer artificial ventilation.

3. Check the victim's pulse. If he has no pulse, commence CPR.

4. Examine all wounds carefully; apply pressure or compression dressings to control external bleeding.

IMPALED OBJECTS

Objects that both penetrate and protrude are said to be impaled. The object may be a stick, glass, arrow, knife, steel rod, etc., that penetrates any part of the body.

This type of injury requires careful immobilization of the victim and the injured part. Any motion of the impaled object can cause additional damage to the surface wound, and particularly the underlying tissues.

EMERGENCY CARE

The only time an impaled object should be removed in the field is when it is impaled in the cheek: profuse bleeding into the mouth and throat can impair breathing (Figure 8-9). To remove an object impaled in the cheek:

1. Feel inside the victim's mouth to determine whether the object has penetrated completely.

2. Remove the object in the direction in which it entered.

3. Control bleeding on the cheek, and dress the wound.

4. If the object penetrated completely, pack the inside of the cheek (between the cheek wall and the teeth) with sterile gauze to control bleeding.

5. Activate the EMS system.

If you encounter too much resistance in trying to remove the object from the cheek, maintain the airway and activate the EMS system immediately. Stabilize the penetrating object while waiting for emergency personnel.

GUNSHOT WOUNDS

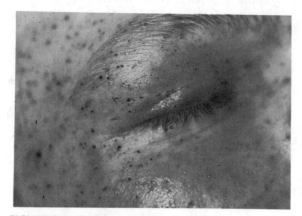

FIGURE 8-3. Powder burns from gunshot.

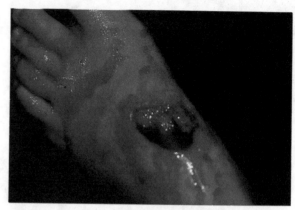

FIGURE 8-4. Gunshot wound to foot.

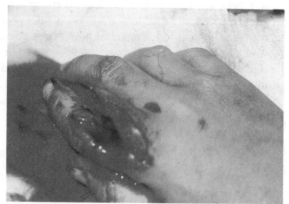

FIGURE 8-5. Gunshot wound to finger.

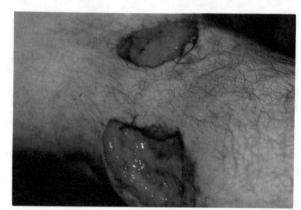

FIGURE 8-6. Gunshot entrance and exit wound to lower leg.

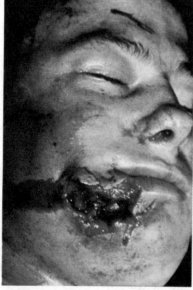

FIGURE 8-7. Gunshot wound to chin.

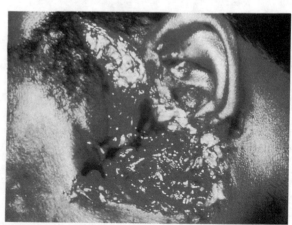

FIGURE 8-8. Gunshot wound to side of head.

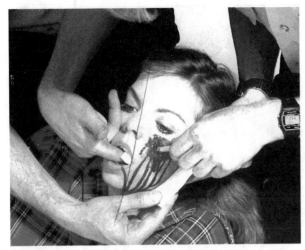

FIGURE 8-9. Impaled objects in the cheek may be removed. Dress outside of wound and put dressing on inside wound between cheek and teeth. Hold in place if necessary.

In cases of other impaled objects, provide the following emergency care (Figures 8-10–8-12):

1. Do not move or remove the impaled object; to do so may cause added bleeding and damage to underlying tissues (muscle, nerves, blood vessels, bones, organs, and so on).

2. Remove clothing so that the wound is exposed. Cut it away so that the impaled object is not disturbed.

3. Control bleeding with direct pressure, but do not exert any pressure on the impaled object or on the tissue margins around the cutting edge of the object.

4. Stabilize the impaled object with bulky dressings and bandage in place. The impaled object itself must be stabilized completely by bulky dressings;

IMPALED OBJECT INJURY

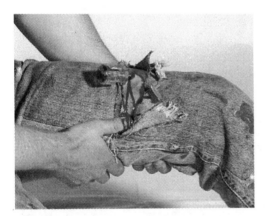

FIGURE 8-10. Impaled object injury.

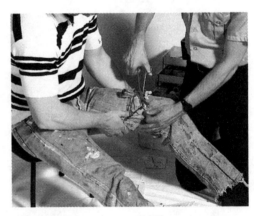

FIGURE 8-11. Cut away clothing.

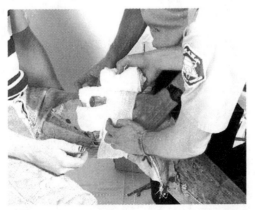

FIGURE 8-12. Stabilize and bandage impaled object in place.

the objective is to pack dressings around the object and tape them securely in place so that motion is reduced to a minimum. If possible, at least three-fourths of the object must be covered by dressings. The use of a "doughnut"-type ring pad may also help in stabilization (Figure 8-13).

5. Calm and reassure the victim as you monitor for shock.

6. Keep the victim at rest and administer artificial ventilation if necessary.

7. Do not attempt to cut off, break off, or shorten an impaled object unless transportation is not possible with it in place. If the object must be cut off, stabilize it securely before cutting. Remember — any motion is transmitted to the victim and can cause additional tissue damage and shock.

8. Activate the EMS system immediately, or, if necessary, promptly but carefully transport the victim to the hospital, avoiding as much movement as possible. *Follow local protocol.*

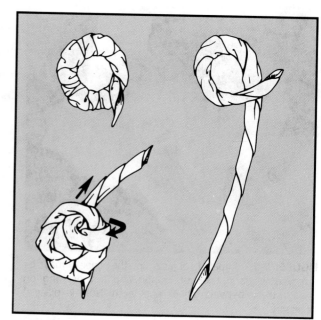

FIGURE 8-13.

| **8** | **SELF-TEST** | **8** |

Student: _____ Date: _____

Course: _____ Section #: _____

PART I: True/False   If you believe that the statement is true, circle the T. If you believe that the statement is false, circle the F.

T   F   1. Always break or cut off an impaled object before the victim is transported.

T   F   2. Objects impaled in the neck should be removed before the victim is transported.

T   F   3. Stabilize the impaled object with bulky dressings.

T   F   4. Control bleeding with direct pressure.

T   F   5. Use a "doughnut" ring pad to stabilize an impaled object.

T   F   6. Objects impaled in the cheek should rarely be removed.

T   F   7. When removing an impaled object in the cheek, remove the object in the opposite direction in which it entered.

T   F   8. Pressure points should always be used when controlling bleeding from an impaled object.

T   F   9. A clamping injury that involves only skin and fat just underneath the skin should always be cared for at the scene before transporting.

T   F   10. More than 30,000 people die of gunshot wounds each year in the U.S.

T   F   11. High velocity bullets cause less damage than low velocity bullets.

T   F   12. Objects that both penetrate and protrude are said to be impaled.

T   F   13. Even if you encounter resistance when trying to remove an impaled object in the cheek, continue to remove.

T   F   14. Be patient with clamping injuries of the finger — the longer a finger is stuck the easier it will be to remove.

T   F   15. If you are unable to remove a strangulating ring, bend it to aid blood flow.

T   F   16. Poor respiratory exchange and failure to maintain an adequate airway are the leading causes of death from stab wounds to the head, face and neck.

PART II: Multiple Choice   For each question, circle the answer that best reflects an accurate statement.

1. If a victim has a gunshot wound to the extremity, a First Aider should:
   a. use pressure points to stop bleeding.
   b. immobilize the injured extremity.
   c. try to remove the bullet.
   d. bandage the area and have the victim transported.

2. Which of the following statements about gunshot wounds is *not* true:
   a. the victim should be transported immediately to a medical center.
   b. exit wounds are usually much smaller than entrance wounds.
   c. superficial skin wounds are almost never fatal.
   d. the greatest danger is internal bleeding or damage to internal organs.

3. Initial assessment of a victim with a suspected gunshot wound includes:
   a. examining for an exit wound.
   b. determining the location from where the gun was fired.
   c. determining the caliber of the gun.
   d. all of these answers.

4. What is the proper emergency care for an object impaled in the cheek?
   a. always leave it in and stabilize.
   b. fill the mouth with gauze pads to control bleeding.
   c. pull the object out part way to ensure an adequate airway.
   d. remove the object.

5. The only time an impaled object should be removed in the field is when it is impaled in the:
   a. head.
   b. leg.
   c. cheek.
   d. chest.

6. An impaled object should not be cut or broken off unless the object:
   a. prevents adequate care or transport.
   b. is larger than eighteen inches.
   c. is impaled in the chest.
   d. is impaled in the head.

7. Which of the following is *not* a true statement about the emergency care of impaled objects?

    a. remove clothing and expose the wound.
    b. control bleeding with direct pressure.
    c. stabilize the object with bulky dressings.
    d. attempt to remove objects impaled in the extremities.

8. Most clamping injuries involve:

    a. the hands.
    b. the feet.
    c. the arms.
    d. the legs.

9. In treating stab wounds, *all but one* of the following is correct:

    a. use local pressure to control external bleeding — do not use a tourniquet.
    b. cover all open wounds with a sterile dressing.
    c. concentrate first on the skin wound.
    d. leave impaled knives in place and stabilize with bulky dressings.

10. Gunshot wounds generally:

    a. have no exit wounds.
    b. have a smaller exit wound than an entrance wound.
    c. have identical entrance and exit wounds.
    d. have a larger exit wound than entrance wound.

PART III: What Would You Do If:

1. A patron at a local gas station is stabbed in the chest with a large screwdriver. When you arrive, the victim is unconscious, and the screwdriver is still in place.

2. You hear a gunshot in your apartment building. Upon investigation, you find a middle-aged man with a gunshot wound to the upper thigh of the right leg. His wife tells you that he was cleaning the gun when it accidentally discharged.

PART IV: Practical Skills Check-Off

_____ has satisfactorily passed the following practical skills:
Student's Name

	Date	Partner Check	Inst. Init.
1. Demonstrate how to stabilize an impaled object.	__/__/__	☐	_____

BANDAGING

Once heavy hemorrhaging from a wound has been controlled, the wound should be dressed and bandaged to manage further bleeding. Proper wound care enhances healing, adds to the comfort of the victim, and promotes more rapid recovery. Improper wound care can delay healing, cause infection, cause severe discomfort to the victim, and — in rare cases — result in the loss of a limb.

The basic purposes of dressing and bandaging are to:

■ Control bleeding.

■ Prevent further contamination of the wound.

■ Protect the wound from further damage.

■ Keep the wound dry.

■ Immobilize the wound site.

DRESSINGS

A dressing is a sterile covering for a wound. It should be **STERILE** (meaning that all **MICROORGANISMS** and **SPORES** have been killed) and **ASEPTIC** (meaning that it is free of bacteria). A bandage holds the dressing in place. The dressing should be held in place tightly enough to control external bleeding but not so tightly that it stops blood circulation.

The ideal dressing is layered and consists of coarse-mesh gauze and self-adhering roller material (such as **KLING** or **KERLIX**). It should be bulky enough to immobilize the tissues and to protect the wound; such protection cuts down on renewed bleeding and wound contamination. In an emergency, you can use *clean* handkerchiefs, towels, sheets, cloth, or sanitary napkins as dressings; never use elastic bandages (they have a tourniquet effect) or paper towels, toilet tissues, or other material that could shred and cling to the wound.

Types of wound dressings include (Figures 9-1–9-4):

■ Aseptic (a sterile dressing free from bacteria).

■ Wet (a moist dressing that may not be sterile).

■ Dry sterile (a sterile dressing free from moisture).

■ Petroleum gauze (sterile gauze saturated with petroleum to prevent the dressing from sticking to an open wound).

■ **OCCLUSIVE** (plastic wrap, aluminum foil, petroleum gauze, or other dressings that form an airtight seal).

■ Compress (a bulky, usually sterile, dressing intended to stop and control bleeding).

■ **UNIVERSAL** (made from a nine-by-thirty-six-inch piece of thick, absorbent material).

━ SPECIAL DRESSINGS ━

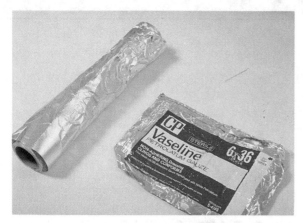

FIGURE 9-1. Petroleum and occlusive dressings.

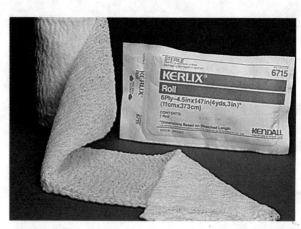

FIGURE 9-2. Nonelastic, self-adhering roller dressing and bandage.

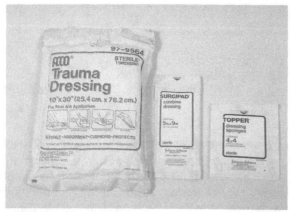

FIGURE 9-3. Sterile gauze pads.

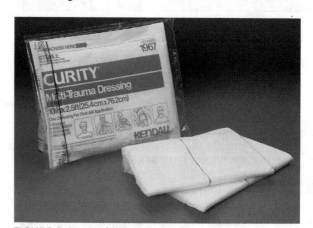

FIGURE 9-4. Multi-trauma dressing.

BANDAGES

A bandage holds a dressing in place over a wound, creates pressure over a bleeding wound for control of hemorrhage, helps wound closure (Figures 9-5 and 9-6), secures a splint to an injured part of the body, and provides support for an injured part. Properly applied, bandages promote healing, prevent severe complications, and help the victim remain comfortable during transport.

A bandage should not normally contact a wound; it should be used only to hold the dressing in place. A bandage should be applied firmly and fastened securely. It should not be applied so tightly that it stops circulation, or so loosely that it allows the dressing to slip. If bandages work themselves loose or become unfastened, wounds may bleed or become infected, and broken bones may become further displaced. It is essential, therefore, that bandages be properly applied and well secured.

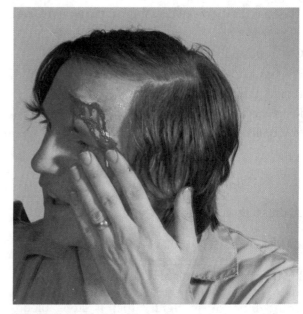

FIGURE 9-5.. Forehead laceration.

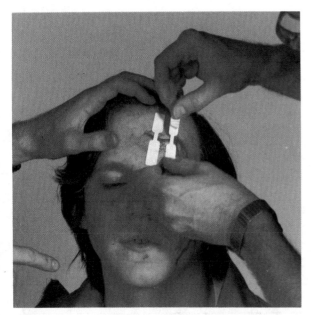

FIGURE 9-6. Butterfly strips (commercially prepared or improvised from adhesive tape) may be used to ensure wound closure.

Self-adhering, highly conforming roller bandages and **TRIANGULAR BANDAGES** are the most popular types and can be adapted to most situations. An air splint can also be used effectively to hold a dressing in place on an extremity, especially if a pressure dressing is needed to control profuse bleeding. However, air splints make palpation of distal pulses difficult.

Practice bandaging regularly; practice is the key to developing the skill. Avoid the two most common mistakes in bandaging: bandaging too loosely and bandaging too tightly.

Before you bandage a wound on the arm or hand, remove rings from the fingers and other jewelry that could restrict circulation as a result of swelling. Rings or hidden tape can cause pressure that may restrict circulation and could lead to **GANGRENE**.

If the bandaged part of the body is mobile, apply the bandage snugly to counter stretching. Make sure that the bandage is not too tight; loosen it slightly if signs of restriction occur. Signs that indicate an overtight bandage include:

- The skin around the bandage becomes pale or cyanotic (bluish).
- The victim complains of pain usually only a few minutes after you have applied the bandage.
- The skin is cold distally.
- The skin is tingling or numb distally.

If the pain or discomfort disappears after several hours, severe damage may have already occurred.

Permanent muscle paralysis may result. Improper bandaging can be defined in a court of law as negligence.

SPECIAL TYPES OF DRESSINGS AND BANDAGES

BANDAGE COMPRESS

A **BANDAGE COMPRESS** is a special dressing to cover open wounds (Figure 9-7). It consists of a pad made of several thicknesses of gauze attached to the middle of a strip of bandaging material. Pad sizes range from one to four inches. Bandage compresses usually come folded so that the gauze pad can be applied directly to the open wound with virtually no exposure to the air or fingers.

The strip of gauze at either side of the pad is folded back so that it can be opened up and the bandage compress tied in place with no disturbance of the sterile pad. The dressing portion of a bandage compress may be extended to twice its normal size by continued unfolding.

Unless otherwise specified, all bandage compresses and all gauze dressings should be covered with open triangular, cravat, or roller bandages.

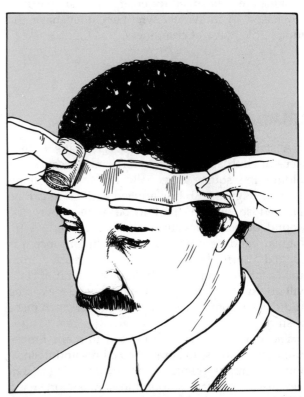

FIGURE 9-7. Ready-prepared bandage compresses, available in individual packages, are useful for larger wounds.

GAUZE PADS

Gauze is used several ways in applying dressings; plain gauze may be used in place of a bandage compress to cover large wounds. Plain gauze of various sizes is supplied in packets. Care should be taken not to touch the portion of the gauze that is to contact the wound.

Sterile gauze pads, two-by-twos, four-by-fours, and four-by-eights, are the most popular dressings that come individually wrapped. In cases of major multiple trauma, nonsterile bulk packages of four-by-four dressings are often used.

SPECIAL PADS

Large, thick-layered, bulky pads (some with waterproofed outer surfaces) are available in several sizes for quick application to an extremity or to a large area of the trunk (see Figure 9-4). They are used where bulk is required in cases of profuse bleeding. They are also useful for stabilizing embedded objects. These special pads are referred to as **MULTI-TRAUMA DRESSINGS**, **TRAUMA PACKS**, **GENERAL PURPOSE DRESSINGS**, **BURN PADS**, or **ABD DRESSINGS**.

Because of their absorbent properties, sanitary napkins are well suited for emergency-care work. If purchased in individual wrappers, they have the added advantage of cleanliness.

TRIANGULAR BANDAGE

A standard triangular bandage is made from a piece of cloth approximately forty inches square by folding the square diagonally and cutting along the fold (Figure 9-8). It is applied easily and can be handled so that the part to be applied over the wound or burn dressing will not be soiled. A triangular bandage does not tend to slip off once it is applied correctly. It is usually made from unbleached cotton cloth, although any kind of cloth will do. In emergencies, a triangular bandage can be improvised from a clean handkerchief or clean piece of shirt.

The triangular bandage is used to make improvised tourniquets, to support fractures and dislocations, to apply splints, and to form slings. If a regular-size bandage is found to be too short when a dressing is applied, it can be lengthened by tying a piece of another bandage to one end.

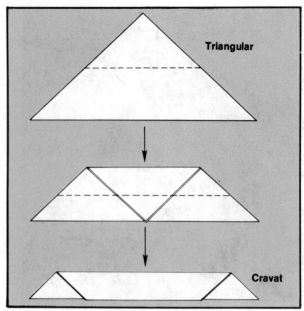

FIGURE 9-8. Triangular and cravat bandages.

CRAVAT BANDAGES

A triangular bandage may be used open or folded. When folded, it is known as a **CRAVAT** (Figure 9-8). A cravat bandage is prepared as follows:

1. Make a one-inch fold along the base of the triangular bandage.
2. Bring the point to the center of the folded base, placing the point underneath the fold; this makes a wide cravat bandage.
3. A medium cravat is made by folding lengthwise along a line midway between the base and the new top of the bandage.
4. A narrow cravat is made if folding is repeated.

This method has the advantage that all bandages can be folded to a uniform width, or the width may be varied to suit the purpose for which it is to be used. To complete a dressing, the ends of the bandage are tied securely.

ROLLER BANDAGES

The self-adhering (nonelastic), form-fitting roller bandage is the most popular and easy to use (Figures 9-9–9-17). It eliminates the need for much of the complex bandaging techniques required with regular gauze roller bandages or cravats.

This type of roller bandage is applied to hold a dressing securely in place over a wound. For this

— SELF-ADHERING ROLLER BANDAGES —

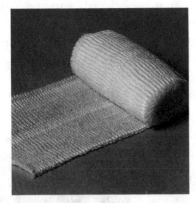

FIGURE 9-9. Self-adhering roller bandage.

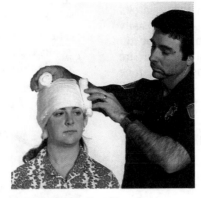

FIGURE 9-10. Head bandage.

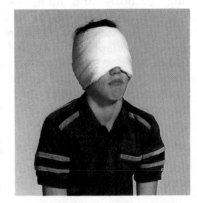

FIGURE 9-11. Head and/or eye bandage.

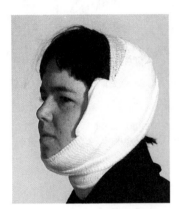

FIGURE 9-12. Cheek bandage (make sure the mouth will open).

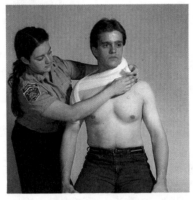

FIGURE 9-13. Bandage of neck and/or shoulder.

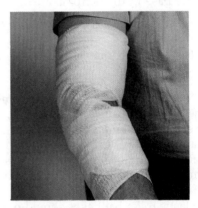

FIGURE 9-14. Elbow bandage.

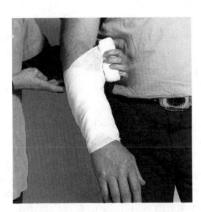

FIGURE 9-15. Lower arm bandage.

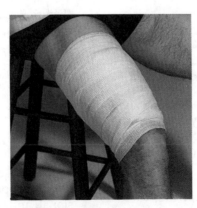

FIGURE 9-16. Thigh bandage.

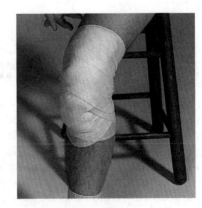

FIGURE 9-17. Knee bandage.

reason, it should be applied snugly, but not tightly enough to interfere with circulation. Fingers and toes should be checked periodically for coldness, swelling, cyanosis, and numbness. If symptoms occur, the bandage should be loosened immediately.

Self-adhering roller bandages are secured easily with several overlapping wraps and can then be cut and tied or taped in place. Commercial examples are Kerlix and Kling. Roller bandages of the head can be used to either hold a large dressing on a head wound or to encompass the complete cranial area. To apply (Figure 9-10):

1. Place the dressing over the wound.

2. Place the end of the roller bandage on the dressing, then wrap it around the head in a circular fashion.

3. Position the first wrap just above the eyebrows (unless it is necessary to cover the eyes — see Figure 9-11), and come down over the ears and the base of the occipital area.

4. Crisscross over the head until the complete area is covered.

5. Fasten the bandage in place with an adhesive strip.

Note: Another method to accomplish the same objective is to use two gauze rolls, wrapping alternately around and across the head until the head is wrapped completely.

Roller bandages of the cheek, shoulder, elbow, arm, thigh, and knee can also be applied, as illustrated in Figures 9-12–9-17).

Elastic roller bandages should not be used except in cases of profuse bleeding. (A tourniquet effect may result from an elastic bandage applied too tightly.) If you use an elastic roller bandage, take extreme care not to occlude blood flow beyond the bandage.

PRINCIPLES OF DRESSING AND BANDAGING

There are no hard-and-fast rules for dressing and bandaging wounds; often, adaptability and creativity are far more important ingredients of rescue than even the best-intentioned rules. In dressing and bandaging, use the materials you have on hand and the methods to which you can best adapt, as long as the following conditions are generally met:

- Material used for dressings should be as clean as possible (sterile, if you can obtain sterile materials).

- Bleeding is controlled. Generally, you should not bandage a dressing into place until bleeding has

stopped; the exception, of course, is a pressure bandage designed to stop bleeding.

- The dressing is opened carefully and handled in an aseptic manner; in other words, dirt and debris are kept off the dressing material.

- The original dressing is not removed. If blood soaks through, add another dressing on top of the original instead of removing it.

- The dressing adequately covers the entire wound (Figure 9-18).

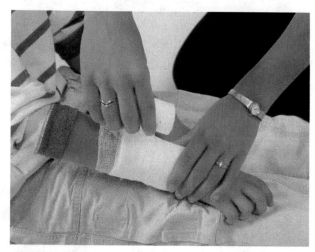

FIGURE 9-18. Dressings should cover wounds adequately, and bandages on extremities should cover a larger area than the wound.

- Wounds are bandaged snugly, but not too tightly.

- Bandages are not too loose; the bandage should not slip or shift and should not allow the dressing to slip or shift beneath it.

- Tie bandages in a square knot when possible (Figure 9-19).

- There are no loose ends of cloth, gauze, or tape that could get caught when the victim is moved or transported.

- All edges of the dressing are covered by the bandage.

- Tips of the fingers and toes are left exposed when arms and legs are bandaged so that you can check for circulation impairment.

- Loose ends are tucked in and the bandage is kept neat in appearance. You will look more professional, and the victim will have greater confidence in you, resulting in easier victim management.

- If you are bandaging a small wound on an extremity, cover a larger area with the bandage to avoid creating a pressure point and to distribute pressure more uniformly (Figure 9-18).

- Always place the body part to be bandaged in the position in which it is to remain. You can bandage across a joint, but do not try bending a joint *after* the bandage has been applied to it.

- Question the victim regarding how the bandage feels. If he complains that it is too tight, loosen it and make it comfortable, but snug.

APPLYING SPECIAL DRESSINGS AND BANDAGES

PRESSURE DRESSING

Apply a pressure dressing in the following way:

1. Cover the wound with a bulky, sterile dressing.

2. Apply hand pressure over the wound until bleeding stops.

3. Apply a firm roller bandage, preferably the self-adhering type; use an elastic bandage only in cases of profuse or difficult-to-control bleeding, and monitor constantly for signs of overtightness. An air splint or blood-pressure cuff may also be used to hold a pressure dressing in place. See Chapter 5.

4. If blood soaks through the original dressing and bandage, do not remove them — leave them in place and apply another dressing, securing it in place with another roller bandage.

SLINGS

SLINGS are used to support injuries of the shoulder, upper extremities, or ribs. In an emergency, they may be improvised from belts, neckties, scarves, or similar articles. Bandages, especially triangular bandages, should be used if available.

Tie a triangular bandage sling as follows (Figure 9-20):

1. Place one end of the base of an open triangular bandage over the shoulder of the injured side.

2. Allow the bandage to hang down in front of the chest so that its **APEX** will be behind the elbow of the injured arm.

3. Bend the arm at the elbow with the hand slightly elevated (four to five inches).

4. Bring the forearm across the chest and over the bandage.

5. Carry the lower end of the bandage over the shoulder of the uninjured side, and tie a square knot (Figure 9-19) at the uninjured side of the

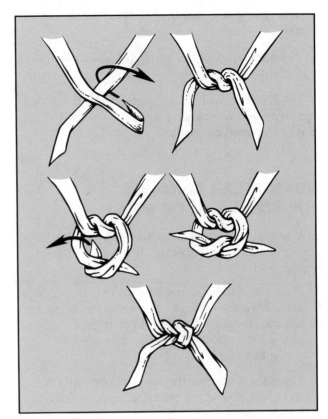

FIGURE 9-19. Tying a square knot.

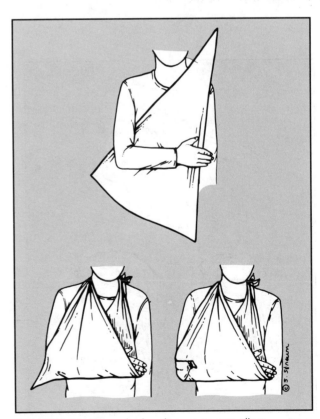

FIGURE 9-20. Triangular bandage as an arm sling.

neck, being sure that the knot is at the side of the neck.

6. Twist the apex of the bandage, and tuck it in at the elbow.

The hand should be supported with the fingertips exposed, whenever possible, to permit detection of impaired circulation.

TRIANGULAR BANDAGE FOR FOREHEAD OR SCALP

A triangular bandage can be used to hold dressings on the forehead or scalp. To apply the bandage (Figure 9-21):

1. Place the middle of the base so that the edge is just above the victim's eyebrows, and bring the apex backward, allowing it to drop over the back of the head (**OCCIPUT**). Bring the ends backward above the ears.

2. Cross the ends over the apex at the occiput; carry the ends around the forehead, and tie them in a square knot.

3. Turn the apex up toward the top of the head. Pin it with a safety pin, or tuck it in behind the crossed part of the bandage.

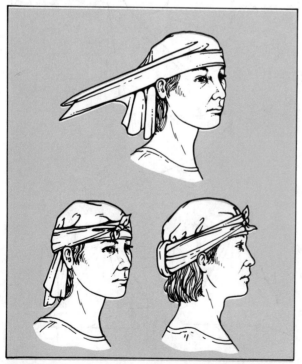

FIGURE 9-21. Triangular bandage for forehead or scalp.

TRIANGULAR BANDAGE FOR CHEST OR BACK

This bandage can be used to hold dressings on burns or on chest and back wounds. To apply the bandage (Figure 9-22):

1. Drop the apex over the shoulder on the injured side. Bring the bandage down over the chest (or back) to cover the dressing so that the middle of the base is directly below the injury. Turn up the cuff at the base.

2. Carry the ends around, and tie a square knot, leaving one end longer than the other.

3. Bring the apex down, and tie it to the long end of the first knot.

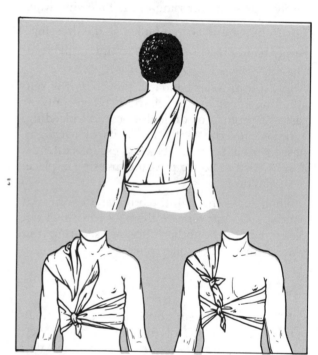

FIGURE 9-22. Triangular bandage for chest or back.

TRIANGULAR BANDAGE FOR SHOULDER

This bandage can be used to hold dressings on shoulder wounds. Two bandages are required: one a triangle; the other a cravat, roller bandage, or belt. Both bandages can be triangular bandages. To apply (Figure 9-23):

1. Place the center of the cravat, roller bandage, or belt at the base of the neck on the injured side, and fasten it just forward of the opposite arm.

2. Slide the apex of the open triangle under the cravat at the back of the neck, and place it over

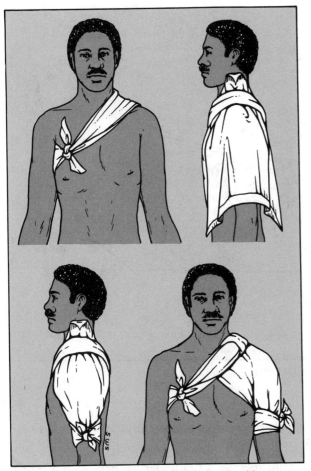

FIGURE 9-23. Triangular bandage for the shoulder.

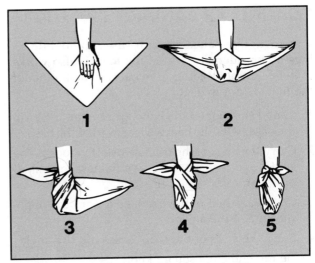

FIGURE 9-24. Triangular bandage for the hand.

TRIANGULAR BANDAGE FOR HIP

This bandage is used to hold dressings on the buttock or hip. It requires two bandages: one a triangle; the other a cravat, roller bandage, or belt. To apply (Figure 9-25):

1. Fasten the cravat, roller bandage, or belt around the waist.

2. Place the base of the triangle below the buttock, and slide the apex under the cravat at the waist. Fold the base upward to form a cuff, and carry the ends of the base around the thigh.

3. Tie the ends of the base with a square knot. Fasten the apex to the waist cravat with a safety pin or by tucking it under.

the dressing on the injured shoulder and upper arm. Turn up the cuff at the base.

3. Bring the ends around the arm, and tie them together.

4. Secure the apex to the cravat at the neck by tucking it in or by using a safety pin.

TRIANGULAR BANDAGE FOR HAND

The triangular bandage for the hand is used to hold dressings of considerable size on the hand. To apply (Figure 9-24):

1. Place the middle of the base well up on the **PALMAR** surface of the wrist.

2. Carry the apex around the ends of the fingers. Cover the back of the hand to the wrist, and tuck any excess fullness into the small pleats on each side of the hand.

3. Cross each half of the bandage toward opposite sides of the wrist.

4. Bring the ends of the triangle around the wrist.

5. Tie the ends in a square knot.

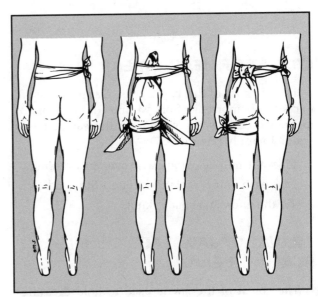

FIGURE 9-25. Triangular bandage for the hip.

TRIANGULAR BANDAGE FOR FOOT

A triangular bandage can be used to hold dressings of considerable size on the foot. It also works to help control bleeding from cuts on the bottom of the foot. To apply (Figure 9-26):

1. Center the foot on the bandage at right angles to the base, with the heel well forward of the base.
2. Carry the apex of the triangle over the toes to the ankle, and tuck any excessive fullness into small pleats on each side of the foot.
3. Cross each half of the bandage toward the opposite side of the ankle.
4. Bring the ends of the triangle around the ankle.
5. Tie the ends in a square knot.

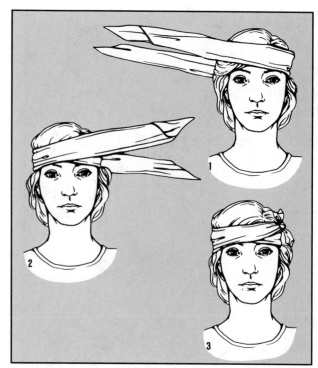

FIGURE 9-27. Cravat of head or ear.

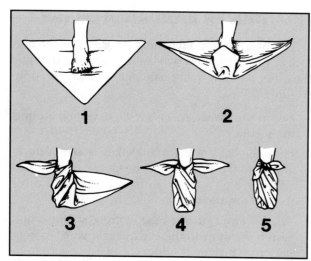

FIGURE 9-26. Triangular bandage for the foot.

CRAVAT OF HEAD OR EAR

The purpose of this bandage is to apply pressure to control hemorrhage from wounds of the scalp, or to hold dressings on wounds of the ear or lower scalp. To apply (Figure 9-27):

1. Place the middle of the cravat over the dressing.
2. Pass each end completely around the head.
3. Tie the ends in a square knot.

CRAVAT OF JAW, FACE, TEMPLE, SCALP, OR EAR

The cravat of the jaw is used to hold dressings on the chin, cheek, and scalp, and as a temporary

support to immobilize a fractured or dislocated jaw. To apply (Figure 9-28):

1. After making a triangular bandage into a cravat of proper width, place it underneath the chin, and carry the ends upward with one end longer than the other.
2. Bring the longer end over the top of the head. Cross both ends on the side of the head (ends should now be of equal length).
3. Pass the ends around the head in opposite directions, and tie them with a square knot on the other side of the head on the primary turn of the cravat.
4. If the victim vomits, a single cravat under the chin tied on top of the head with a bow knot is preferable for ease in removal.

CRAVAT OF EYE

The cravat of the eye is used to hold a dressing over the eye. Two cravats are required. To apply (Figure 9-29):

1. Place the center of the first cravat over the top of the head with the front end falling over the uninjured eye.
2. Bring the second cravat around the head, over the eyes, and over the loose ends of the first cravat. Tie the bandage in front.

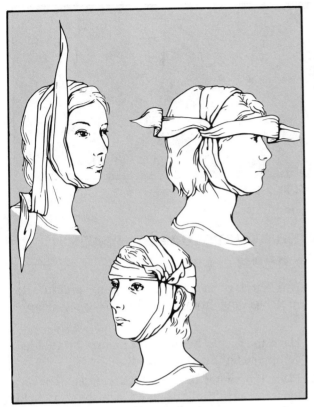

FIGURE 9-28. Cravat of jaw or cheek.

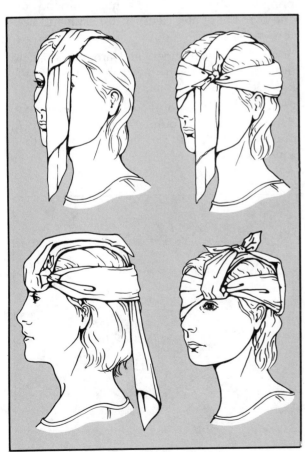

FIGURE 9-29. Cravat of eye.

3. Bring the ends of the first cravat back over the top of the head, tie them there, and pull the second cravat up and away from the uninjured eye.

CRAVAT OF ELBOW

The cravat of the elbow is used to hold dressings around the elbow. To apply (Figure 9-30):

1. Bend the arm at the elbow, and place the center of the cravat at the point of the elbow.

2. Bring the ends upward, and cross them in overlapping spiral turns.

3. Bring the ends to the front of the elbow, and tie them together.

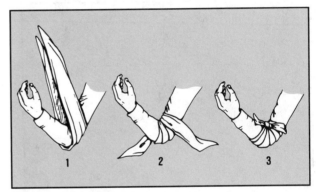

FIGURE 9-30. Cravat of elbow.

CRAVAT OF KNEE

The cravat of the knee is used to hold dressings around the knee. To apply (Figure 9-31):

1. Place the center of the cravat over the kneecap, and let the ends hang down on each side of the knee.

2. Cross the ends underneath, and continue several overlapping, descending turns down the calf and several overlapping, ascending turns up the thigh.

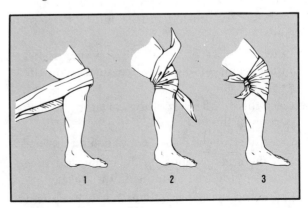

FIGURE 9-31. Cravat of knee.

3. Bring the ends together, and tie them under the knee.

CRAVAT OF LEG

The cravat of the leg is used to hold dressings on the leg. To apply (Figure 9-32):

1. Place the center of the cravat over the dressing.

2. Begin the ascending turns with the upper end and the descending turns with the lower end, with each turn covering two-thirds of the preceding turn until the dressing is covered.

3. Tie both ends together with a square knot.

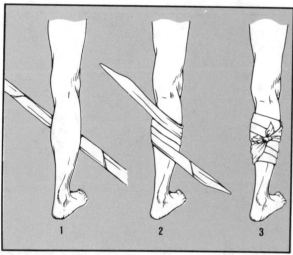

FIGURE 9-32. Cravat of leg.

CRAVAT ANKLE WRAP

This bandage has two important functions: (1) to give support and protection to an injured ankle; and (2) to place the leg in traction. The traction splint is fastened to the foot with the ankle wrap. This bandage must be put on the injured part securely if it is to serve its purpose. To apply (Figure 9-33):

1. Fold the triangular bandage into a three-inch cravat.

2. Leave the shoe on, especially if a sprain is suspected. Loosen the shoelace to accommodate swelling.

3. Place the middle part of the cravat in the instep portion of the foot.

4. Cross the two ends of the cravat behind the heel.

5. Pull the ends in opposite directions and downward, around and underneath the cravat.

6. Pull up on the cravat from each side to tighten it until the wrap is reasonably secure.

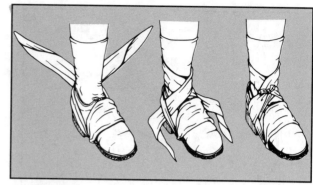

FIGURE 9-33. Cravat ankle wrap.

CRAVAT PRESSURE BANDAGE OF HAND

This bandage is used for applying pressure to control bleeding from the palm. To apply (Figure 9-34):

1. Have the victim hold a roll of gauze or a folded compress tightly in his hand.

2. Place the center of the folded bandage (cravat) over the inside of the wrist. The palm is held facing upward.

3. Bring the other end of the bandage around, up, and over the tightly clenched fist. Pull and hold this end securely.

4. Bring the other (longer) end around, up, and over the fist. Keep the bandage over the knuckles.

5. Cross the two ends of the bandage at the wrist, then wrap them around the wrist securely in opposite directions. Tie them together with a square knot.

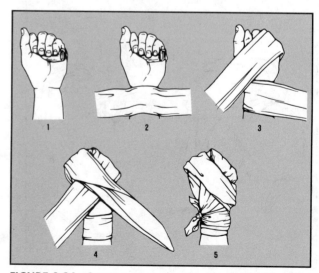

FIGURE 9-34. Cravat pressure bandage — palm of hand.

| **9** | **SELF-TEST** | **9** |

Student: _____   Date: _____

Course: _____ Section #: _____

PART I: True/False   If you believe that the statement is true, circle the T. If you believe that the statement is false, circle the F.

T   F   1. A bandage should normally contact a wound.

T   F   2. Bandages should be applied firmly and fastened securely.

T   F   3. The most popular and adaptable bandage is the cravat.

T   F   4. Never use an air splint to hold a dressing in place.

T   F   5. A bandage compress is a special dressing for creating a tourniquet effect.

T   F   6. Triangular bandages are usually made from cloth that is approximately twenty inches square.

T   F   7. You should always bandage a dressing in place before the bleeding has been controlled.

T   F   8. You should be careful enough when bandaging to cover the tips of the fingers and toes when an extremity has been injured.

T   F   9. Do not attempt to bandage an area any larger than the wound site.

T   F   10. If blood soaks through the original dressing, remove it and apply a new dressing.

T   F   11. Elastic roller bandages should not be used except in cases of profuse bleeding.

T   F   12. A sling should support the hand but leave the finger-tips exposed.

PART II: Multiple Choice   For each question, circle the answer that best reflects an accurate statement.

1. If the fingers or toes of an injured limb become cold, swollen, blue, or numb, the First Aider should:
    a. immediately loosen the bandage.
    b. elevate the affected limb.
    c. cover the limb with a warm blanket.
    d. treat the victim for shock.

2. The primary reason why elastic roller bandages are not recommended for use in emergency care is:
    a. they are difficult to remove.
    b. they tend to stretch after a period of time.
    c. they may seriously constrict blood flow if applied too tightly.
    d. they do not absorb moisture.

3. Which type of knot is most frequently used in bandaging?
    a. square knot.
    b. slip knot.
    c. half hitch.
    d. claw hitch.

4. Which of the following is *not* a principle for using a pressure dressing?
    a. apply hand pressure over the wound until bleeding is controlled.
    b. cover the wound with bulky sterile dressings.
    c. use an elastic bandage to hold it in place.
    d. do not remove the original dressing.

5. Which of the following is an example of an occlusive dressing?
    a. adhering gauze roller.
    b. petroleum gauze.
    c. butterfly bandage.
    d. gauze roller.

6. Which of the following statements about bandaging is *not* true?
    a. when applying a cravat bandage to the knee or elbow, the joint should be bent.
    b. a triangle bandage on the forehead or scalp should be applied so that it covers the victim's eyes.
    c. If the victim is likely to vomit, a single cravat under the chin tied on top of the head with a bow knot is preferable.
    d. a triangle bandage and a cravat are required for the triangle of the hip bandage.

7. Bandages should never:
    a. be applied directly over the wound.
    b. be applied tight enough to hinder circulation.
    c. be applied loosely.
    d. all of the above.

8. Which of the following statements about bandaging is *not* true?
    a. an air splint may be used to hold a dressing in place on an arm or leg.
    b. when in doubt, leave a bandage tied loosely.
    c. when bandaging the arm, leave the fingers uncovered.
    d. improper bandaging may be considered negligence in a court of law.

9. Which of the following is *not* a principle of bandaging?
    a. when bandaging the arm, leave the fingers uncovered.
    b. place the body part to be bandaged in the position in which it is to be left.
    c. leave no loose ends that could get caught on other objects.
    d. if in doubt, leave a bandage tied loosely.

10. Which of the following is *not* a guideline for use of an arm sling?
    a. it should cover the entire hand.
    b. the knot should not be tied in the middle of the back of the neck.
    c. bend the arm at the elbow and elevate it four to five inches.
    d. the apex of the bandage should be behind the elbow of the injured arm.

11. One of the primary purposes of a dressing is to:
    a. prevent the bandage from sticking to the wound.
    b. sterilize the wound.
    c. hold a bandage in place.
    d. prevent contamination of a wound.

12. Bandages should:
    a. have no loose ends that may be caught on other objects.
    b. be applied directly over any open wound.
    c. be applied loosely to allow air circulation.
    d. all of these answers.

13. Butterfly bandages are used for:
    a. abrasions.
    b. contusions.
    c. avulsions.
    d. minor incisions and lacerations.

14. Which of the following is *not* a recognized type of wound dressing?
    a. bacteriostatic dressing.
    b. aseptic dressing.
    c. petroleum gauze.
    d. dry sterile dressing.

15. All of the following are true statements about a triangle bandage of the hip *except*:
    a. the ends of the base are tied with a slip knot.
    b. both a cravat and a triangle bandage are needed.
    c. the apex of the triangle may be secured to the waist with a safety pin.
    d. the cravat is used around the waist.

PART III: Matching   Match the type of wound dressing with its description.

_____ 1. A dressing that may not be sterile.

_____ 2. A dressing that forms an airtight seal.

_____ 3. A sterile dressing.

_____ 4. Sterile gauze saturated with a substance to prevent the dressing from sticking to an open wound.

_____ 5. A dressing that is free of moisture.

_____ 6. A bulky, usually sterile dressing.

A. Aseptic

B. Compress

C. Wet

D. Dry sterile

E. Petroleum gauze

F. Occlusive

PART IV: What Would You Do If:

1. You were asked to describe the principles of dressing and bandaging wounds.

2. A pedestrian is hit by a car and sustains a large avulsion on the left thigh.

3. A motorcycle skids out of control on some gravel, and the driver sustains lacerations and abrasions of the shoulder and lower leg.

PART V: Practical Skills Check-Off   _____ has satisfactorily passed the following practical skills:
                                              Student's Name

	Date	Partner Check	Inst. Init.
1. Demonstrate the appropriate use of a sling.	__/__/__	☐	_____
2. Demonstrate the appropriate use of a triangular bandage on various parts of the body.	__/__/__	☐	_____
3. Demonstrate the appropriate use of a cravat bandage on various parts of the body.	__/__/__	☐	_____
4. Demonstrate the appropriate use of a roller bandage on various parts of the body.	__/__/__	☐	_____

CHAPTER TEN

OBJECTIVES

■ Understand the **ANATOMY** and **PHYSIOLOGY** of the musculo-skeletal system, including the major muscles and bones.

■ Describe the types and causes of musculoskeletal injuries.

■ Recognize and give emergency care for sprains, strains, and dislocations.

■ Learn how to examine and recognize a fractured bone.

■ Describe the two types and five classifications of fractures.

■ Learn the proper techniques of emergency care for fractures, including the various techniques of splinting.

MUSCULOSKELETAL INJURIES

I njuries to muscles, joints, and bones are some of the most common situations that First Aiders encounter. These injuries can range from the simple and non-life-threatening — such as a broken finger or sprained ankle — to the critical and life-threatening — such as a multiple break of the femur or a fracture of the neck or spine. Whether the injury is mild or severe, your ability to provide first aid efficiently and quickly may prevent further painful and damaging injury and may even keep the victim from suffering permanent deformity or death.

First aid for fractures, dislocations, and soft-tissue injuries within the first four hours following injury is critical in preventing permanent disabilities. An immediate assessment of the victim is essential so that concealed injury is not overlooked.

ANATOMY OF THE MUSCULOSKELETAL SYSTEM

The human **MUSCULOSKELETAL SYSTEM** is composed of 206 bones, 6 types of joints, and more than 600 muscles. The skeletal system (Figure 10-1) itself has four major functions:

1. It gives shape or form to the body.

2. It supports the body, allowing it to stand erect.

3. It provides the basis for **LOCOMOTION**, or movement, by giving muscles a place to attach, and it contains joints that allow movement (where bones are joined together by **LIGAMENTS**).

4. It forms protection for major body organs, such as the brain (skull), the heart and lungs

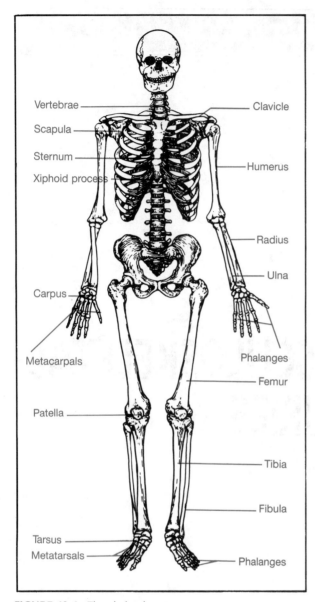

FIGURE 10-1. The skeletal system.

muscles that make up the arms, the legs, the upper back, and the hips, and they cover the ribs and the abdomen. Skeletal muscles are attached to the bones either directly or by tendons (tough, fibrous, **CONNECTIVE TISSUE**). When the voluntary muscle contracts through stimulation, it shortens and pulls on a part of the skeletal system, causing movement.

- **CARDIAC**, or heart **MUSCLE**, also known as **MYOCARDIUM**.

TENDONS

Tendons are highly specialized connective tissue. They allow for maximum strength because they are oriented in the direction of muscle pull (Figure 10-2). Tendons form a shiny, white band that attaches to the muscles and, through a network of tiny fibers, connects with a bone. If sharp, sudden force is applied, the tendon may pull loose from the bone and may even pull a small piece of bone away with it.

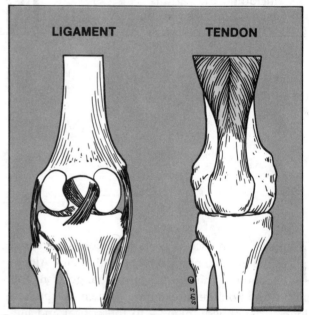

FIGURE 10-2. Ligaments connect bone to bone, while tendons attach muscles to bone.

(rib cage), pelvic organs, and the spinal cord (vertebrae).

MUSCLE

Muscle is a special type of tissue that **CONTRACTS**, or shortens, when stimulated. The three major types of muscle are:

- **INVOLUNTARY (SMOOTH) MUSCLES**, which are not under conscious control. They handle the work of the internal organs with the exception of the heart.
- **VOLUNTARY (SKELETAL) MUSCLES**, which are under conscious control. Voluntary muscles include

LIGAMENTS

Ligaments connect bone to bone (Figure 10-2). When a ligament is injured, the individual parts give way at different places along the entire ligament length. Skin lacerations are rarely involved.

Most **JOINTS** of the body have ligaments at the side located farthest from the center plane of motion. More complex joints (like the knee) feature ligaments that are attached to the **JOINT CAPSULE**. The ligament is often injured simultaneously with the joint, causing early joint swelling due to internal bleeding.

VICTIM ASSESSMENT

When you arrive on the scene of an accident or injury, do the following:

1. Conduct a primary survey of the airway, breathing, major bleeding, and circulation. A fracture may be the most obvious and dramatic of multiple injuries but is seldom life-threatening. Do the primary survey and manage any life-threatening conditions first. (Management of **ORTHOPEDIC** injuries is pursued during the secondary survey.)

2. Conduct a secondary evaluation to identify other less serious injuries.

3. Obtain the history of the injury and observe the scene carefully so that you can determine the mechanism of injury.

4. Treat all unconscious victims as if they had neck injuries. Most victims of musculoskeletal injuries will experience pain localized in the area of the injury. A fracture victim may complain of having felt something snap or of having heard a loud "pop."

5. Look for tissue bruising, deformity, unusual limb angulation, shortening of the extremity, and any lacerations or puncture wounds near the site of the fracture.

6. Palpate the length of the limb to detect deformities, swelling, etc. It is often difficult to distinguish between a severe sprain and a fracture unless the injury is X-rayed. If there is any question, treat the injury as a fracture by immobilizing, then get the victim to a medical facility.

TYPES OF INJURY TO MUSCLES, JOINTS AND BONES

The four major types of injuries that occur to the musculoskeletal system are (Figure 10-3):

1. **SPRAINS** — injuries in which ligaments are stretched and partially torn, usually due to sudden twisting of a joint beyond its normal range of motion.

2. **STRAINS** — soft-tissue injuries or muscle spasms around a joint.

3. Dislocations — displacement of a bone end from a joint.

4. Fractures — one or more breaks in a bone.

SPRAINS

EMERGENCY CARE

In most cases, it is best to care for the sprain as if it were a fracture and immobilize it accordingly. In the case of a sprained ankle, assume that the injury is a fracture, since without an X-ray, a sprain cannot be differentiated from a fracture. Most sprains (about 80 percent) are caused by the ankle turning outward, toward the outside of the body, with a popping or ripping sound.

Do not allow the victim to walk or stand on a sprained knee or ankle. Loosen the shoelaces so that you can remove the shoe if necessary.

Provide care based on the acronym RICE.[1]

R: Rest
I: Ice
C: Compression
E: Elevation

1. **Rest.** A severely sprained ankle may have torn tissues and even a fracture. If you suspect major tissue damage, give the sprained joint complete rest by splinting it. Do not allow the victim to walk on it. Make sure that the sprain is evaluated by a physician.

2. **Ice.** Cold reduces pain, bleeding, swelling, and muscle spasms in injured muscles. Put cold packs, crushed ice, or cold towels on the injured area, or immerse it in ice water. Protect against frostbite by putting towels or elastic wraps next to the skin and by applying the cold pack for fifteen to thirty minutes. This treatment will be continued in the emergency room. Some treatments recommend alternate hot-cold packs. The current recommendation is to use heat only after forty-eight hours when the swelling has gone down.

3. **Compression.** In a long emergency-care or transport situation, a compression bandage will limit internal bleeding and may also squeeze some fluid and debris out of the injury site. Wrap the

---

[1] Alton L. Thygerson, "Muscle Injuries," *Emergency* July 1985, pp. 50-51; Susanna Levin, "Sprains Are A Pain," *Walking Magazine*, June/July 1987, p. 75.

SIGNS AND SYMPTOMS OF COMMON ORTHOPEDIC INJURIES

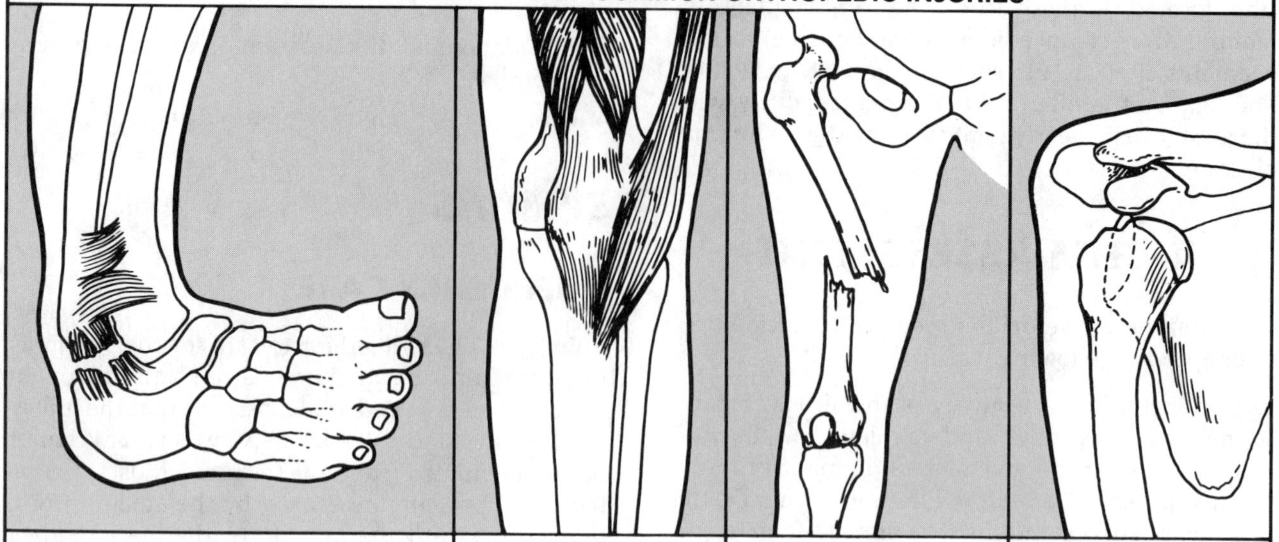

Sprain	Strain	Fracture	Dislocation
Pain on movement	Immediate, burning pain	Pain, tenderness	Pain
Tenderness	Little swelling	Deformity	Deformity
Painful movement, swelling	Little discoloration	Loss of use, swelling	Loss of movement
Redness		Bruising	Sprain
		Crepitus (grating)	
		Exposed bone ends	

FIGURE 10-3.

injured area with an elastic bandage, apply a cold pack, then wrap the pack to the sprained part with another layer of elastic bandage. Leave fingers and toes exposed so that you can check for color change or swelling that would indicate the bandage is too tight. Ask about pain, numbness, and tingling. A bandage that is too tight should be loosened.

4. **Elevation.** Raise the injured area, propped and supported with pillows, to about heart level, if possible. This will reduce circulation to the area and thus help to control internal bleeding.

5. **Apply an appropriate splint,** then transport to a medical facility or activate the EMS system. (See "Types of Splints" later in this chapter.)

For maximum benefit, begin the RICE treatment within ten to sixty minutes after the injury has occurred.

STRAINS

EMERGENCY CARE

Strains are best cared for by having the victim avoid stress on the injured area. In most cases, assume that a fracture may be involved and immobilize accordingly. If the exact nature of the injury is in question, immobilize the extremity and activate the EMS system.

Emergency care for the victim includes the following:

1. Place the victim in a comfortable position, such as in a reclining position with the knees drawn up to take pressure off of the back muscles.

2. If the victim does not have to be moved, apply heat directly to the strained area.

3. Have the victim get plenty of rest on a firm mattress, possibly with a board support beneath it.

DISLOCATIONS

The principle symptom of dislocation is pain or a feeling of pressure over the involved joint, as well as loss of motion of the joint. The principle sign of dislocation is deformity. If the dislocated bone end is pressing on a nerve, numbness or **PARALYSIS** may also occur below the dislocation. If a blood vessel is being compressed, loss of pulse may occur below the dislocation. In any victim with a fracture or dislocation, always check the strength of pulse and sensation on the side of the injury farthest from the heart. The absence of pulses means that the extremity is not receiving adequate blood. Activate the EMS system immediately, and check distal pulses and sensation after every immobilization and splinting.

1. To check distal pulses:
   - Palpate the pulse on the side of the injury away from the heart.
   - You may also check **CAPILLARY REFILL** by pressing a fingernail or toenail and observing how quickly color returns to the area. Normal refill time is two seconds or less.
   - Absence of pulses or a prolonged refill time means that either the injury itself or your splinting procedures are reducing circulation to the area. You must correct this situation immediately by straightening the fractured limb or loosening the splint.
2. To check distal sensations:
   - Ask the victim to wiggle his fingers and toes.
   - Touch a finger or toe and ask the victim if he can feel it.
   - If the victim is unconscious, gently probe or pinch the skin and note any reactions to this mild pain.

EMERGENCY CARE

Since dislocations involve the joints and are often accompanied by fractures, emergency care is to immobilize all suspected dislocations *in the position found* (Figure 10-4).

1. *Do not* try to straighten, or *reduce*, the dislocation. Check for a distal pulse.
2. Splint above and below the dislocated joint with an appropriate splint to maintain stability.
3. Give the victim care for shock, and keep him warm and quiet. The victim is often most comfortable sitting forward.
4. Place a cold pack of some type on the dislocation.
5. Transport the victim carefully to a medical facility, or activate the EMS system.

FRACTURES

TYPES OF FRACTURES

A fracture is a break in the continuity of a bone. It may be either closed, in which the overlying skin is intact, or open, in which the skin over the fracture site has been broken (Figures 10-5–10-8). Bone may or may not protrude through the wound. Open fractures are more serious than closed fractures because the risks of contamination and infection are greater.

Fractures may also be classified according to the position, number, and shape of the bone fragments (Figure 10-9).

- In a **TRANSVERSE FRACTURE**, the fracture line is more or less at right angles to the long axis of the bone. It usually is produced by an angulation force.
- An **OBLIQUE FRACTURE** is one in which the fracture line extends obliquely across the bone, and fragments of the bone tend to slip by each other. It usually is produced by a twisting force.

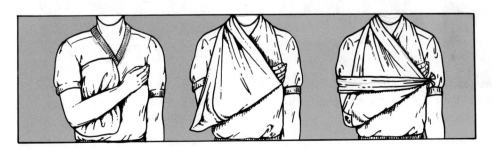

FIGURE 10-4. Immobilizing dislocation of shoulder. *Left:* position of cravat with pad; *Right:* position with sling. Cravat can be positioned over sling if desired.

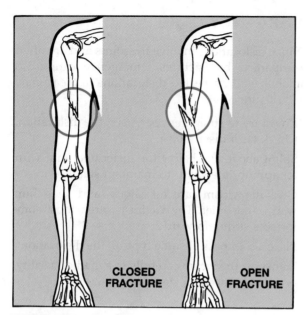

FIGURE 10-5. Closed and open fractures.

- In a **SPIRAL FRACTURE**, the fracture line is spiral or S-shaped. These fractures are produced by twisting injuries of the type seen among skiers or by torsion produced by muscular contraction.

- In a **LONGITUDINAL FRACTURE**, the fracture line splits the bone lengthwise.

- A **GREENSTICK FRACTURE** is an incomplete fracture by a compression force in the long axis of the bone. Usually the convex surface breaks, while the concave surface remains intact. This type of fracture is most common among children, whose bones are more elastic than those of adults.

- A **COMPRESSION FRACTURE** damages the bones with force from both ends. For example, one or more of the vertebrae of the spinal column may be compressed as a result of a blow or an **ACCELERATION-DECELERATION** accident.

- In **DEPRESSED FRACTURES,** a bone fragment is driven below the surface of the bone. This type of fracture occurs in flat bones, such as the skull.

- In an **IMPACTED FRACTURE**, the broken ends are violently jammed together so that one end telescopes into the other.

- In a **COMMINUTED FRACTURE**, which is produced by severe, direct violence, there are three or more fragments. Reduction is difficult to maintain in this type of fracture, and associated soft-tissue injuries frequently are severe.

- In an **AVULSION FRACTURE**, a piece of bone is pulled away from the rest — usually because a twisting injury pulls a ligament so forcefully that an attached piece of bone comes with it.

MECHANISMS OF INJURY

Bone fractures may result from a variety of mechanisms:

- Direct force — the bone breaks at the point of impact with a solid object, such as a dashboard or automobile bumper.

- Indirect force — this type of injury involves fracture or dislocation at some distance along the bone from the point of impact, such as a hip fracture caused by the knees forcefully striking the dashboard.

- Twisting force — this type of injury commonly occurs in football or skiing and results in fractures, sprains, and dislocations. Typically, the lower end of the limb remains fixed, such as when cleats or a ski hold the foot to the ground, while torsion develops in the upper end of the limb. The resulting forces cause shearing and fracture.

CLOSED AND OPEN FRACTURES

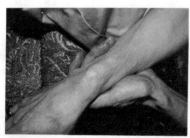

FIGURE 10-6. Closed fracture of the radius.

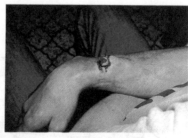

FIGURE 10-7. Open fracture of the radius.

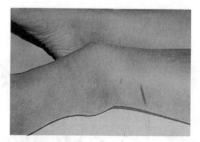

FIGURE 10-8. Closed fracture. Observe the deformity.

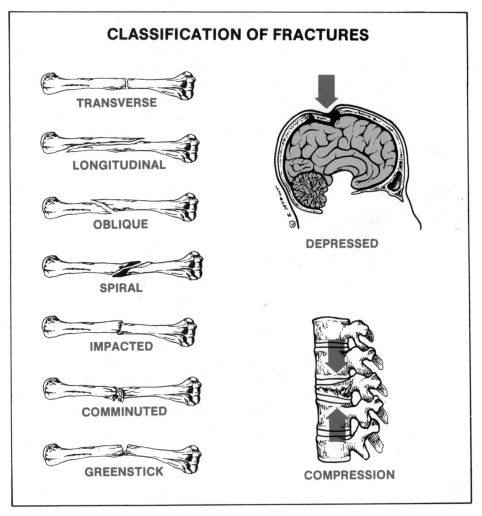

CLASSIFICATION OF FRACTURES

TRANSVERSE

LONGITUDINAL

OBLIQUE

SPIRAL

IMPACTED

COMMINUTED

GREENSTICK

DEPRESSED

COMPRESSION

FIGURE 10-9.

- Powerful muscle contractions — this type of injury, which occurs in seizures or tetanus, may tear muscle from bone or actually break away a piece of bone.
- Fatigue fractures — these are caused by repeated stress and most commonly occur in the feet after prolonged walking (**"MARCH** or **STRESS FRACTURES"**).
- High-energy forces — extreme forces slam into the body, causing destruction. Examples are multiple: vehicle accidents, trauma from blows with a blunt instrument (e.g., a baseball bat), gunshot wounds, and falls from heights.
- **PATHOLOGICAL FRACTURES** — these are seen in victims who have diseases that weaken areas of bone. These kinds of fractures occur with minimal force. The elderly also have weaker bones and are thus more prone to fracture, especially of the hip.

HISTORY

Ask specific questions, such as:

- When did the injury occur?
- What happened?
- Where does it hurt?
- What did you feel?

Most victims with significant musculoskeletal injury will complain of pain localized to the area of injury. The victim may also report feeling or hearing something snap. Try to determine the position of the limb when the injury occurred. In the case of a twisted ankle, for example, did the injury occur with the movement of the sole inward (**INVERSION**) or movement of the sole outward (**EVERSION**)? Does the victim have any serious illnesses (such as cancer) that might help to account for pathological fracture?

SIGNS OF FRACTURES

The primary signs of fractures are (Figure 10-10):

- Swelling and bruising (discoloration). Blood leaks from ruptured vessels in and about the fractured ends of bones.

- Deformity and/or shortening. Compare the injured extremity to the normal extremity. Is it in an unnatural position? Is its motion false or unnatural? Is there a difference in size or shape? In the case of the skull or rib cage, does any portion appear caved in?

- Point tenderness to touch. Press gently along the length of the bone to locate the area of the injury.

- Grating, or crepitus. Broken fragments of bone grind against each other with a grating noise. *Do not attempt to cause crepitus. You will only cause additional injury and pain.*

- Guarding and disability. The victim with a fracture will try to hold the injured area in a comfortable position and will avoid moving it. The victim with a dislocation will be unable to move the dislocated extremity.

- Exposed bone ends.

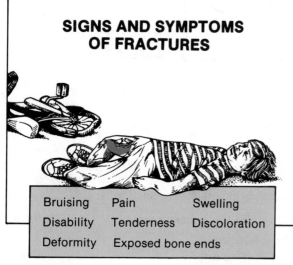

SIGNS AND SYMPTOMS OF FRACTURES

Bruising	Pain	Swelling
Disability	Tenderness	Discoloration
Deformity	Exposed bone ends	

FIGURE 10-10.

PHYSICAL ASSESSMENT

With rare exceptions, fractures and other orthopedic (bone) injuries are not life-threatening. In the multiple-injury victim, fractures may be the most obvious and dramatic injuries but may not necessarily be the most serious. Therefore, complete the primary survey and manage any life-threatening conditions first.

1. Establish an airway, protect the neck as needed, and control moderate to severe hemorrhage.

2. Never use a tourniquet on an open fracture unless a traumatic amputation has occurred, the limb has been mangled beyond all possibility of salvage, or all other methods to control bleeding have failed.

3. When life-threatening conditions have been cared for, identify and immobilize all fractures (during the secondary survey) in preparation for transport.

4. Priorities for treating fractures are:
   - Spinal fractures.
   - Fractures of the head and rib cage.
   - Pelvic fractures.
   - Fractures of the lower limbs.
   - Fractures of the upper limbs.

Remember, if there was enough force to damage the pelvis or cause severe head and facial injuries, assume that there are also injuries to the spine.

Although life-threatening injuries must be dealt with first, you must take time to examine the extremities for fractures. Use the signs of fracture previously listed to conduct your assessment.

EMERGENCY CARE

The most important emergency care is immobilization for suspected fracture or extensive soft-tissue injury. The following are important reasons for immobilizing:

- To minimize damage to soft tissue, muscle, or **PERIOSTEUM** (bone sheathing) that may become wedged between the fracture fragments. This complication may result in delayed healing that will require surgery.

- To prevent conversion of a closed fracture into an open one.

- To prevent more damage to surrounding nerves, blood vessels, and other tissues from the broken bone ends.

- To minimize bleeding and swelling.

- To diminish pain; this may help to control shock.

General principles for immobilizing fractures are as follows:

1. Remove clothing and jewelry around the injury site. Unless the victim objects strenuously, cut the clothing away with a pair of bandage scissors so that you will not move the fractured bone ends

and increase the victim's pain. Give any of the victim's jewelry to a confirmed family member, or bag it and put it with the victim so that it can be transported with the victim and turned over to the hospital staff with a receipt from the hospital.

2. Check the distal pulse of the suspected fracture site. If circulation is poor, immediately check for internal bleeding or pressure on a blood vessel (Figures 10-11 and 10-12).

3. Immobilize fractures involving joints in the position in which they are found.

4. Cover all wounds, including open fractures, with sterile dressings, then bandage gently. Do not attempt to push the bone ends back underneath the skin. Avoid excessive pressure on the wound. Support the fracture with your hand under the fracture site.

5. Apply minimal in-line **TRACTION**, preferably with a partner applying countertraction. Immobilize

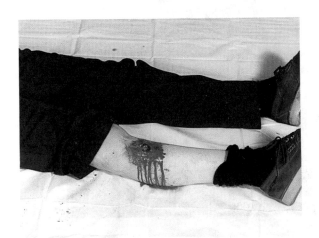

FIGURE 10-11. An open tibia fracture.

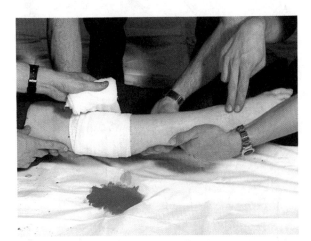

FIGURE 10-12. Support the limb, control bleeding, apply slight, in-line traction, locate a distal pulse, and splint. Brace the fracture with your hand under the fracture site.

the joints above and below the fracture. (If the radius is fractured, for instance, immobilize the wrist and elbow). Maintain traction until the splint has been applied and secured.

6. Wrap from the distal end of the splint to the proximal end. Splint firmly but not tight enough to stop circulation. Check pulses below the splint (or at its lower end) after your splint is in place to be certain that circulation is still adequate. If a pulse is absent, loosen your splint until you can again feel the pulse. Check and recheck splints to make certain that they are not compromising circulation.

REPOSITIONING OF FRACTURED OR DISLOCATED LIMBS

A number of complications may accompany the attempt to reposition fractured or dislocated limbs. Unnecessary manipulation, for instance, may create additional pain or injury. Sharp bone ends can cause trauma to ligaments or tendons, allow contamination of the fracture site, and damage tissues and blood vessels.

As a general rule, never straighten a wrist, elbow, knee, or shoulder. The major nerves and arteries near these joints mean that you would run a very high risk of causing further damage. Except for the wrist and shoulder, *make one attempt to straighten closed angulated fractures, if no distal pulse is found.* If pain, resistance, or crepitus increase, stop. Joints, however, should not be manipulated unless circulation is compromised.

Never apply emergency traction devices that must attach to the lower limb if there are possible fractures or dislocations about the ankle. *Never apply traction in the field to crushed injuries of the limbs.*

Severely angulated fractures at the shoulder, elbow, wrist, and knee should *not* be straightened because of the danger of crushing and lacerating the nerves or blood vessels in close proximity to the fractures.

SPLINTS

SPLINTS are used to support, immobilize, and protect parts with injuries such as known or suspected fractures, dislocations, or severe sprains. When in doubt, treat the injury as a fracture and splint it. Splints prevent movement at the area of the injury and at the nearest joints. Splints should immobilize and support the joints or bones above and below the break.

IMPROVISED SPLINTS AND SLINGS

First Aiders may have access to commercial splints in an emergency but should still be familiar with improvising; therefore, it is important to know how to make and apply improvised splints and slings (Figures 10-13 and 10-14). An effective improvised splint must be:

- Light in weight but firm and rigid.
- Long enough to extend past the joints and prevent movement on either side of the fracture (two splints may be tied together to reach the necessary length).
- As wide as the thickest part of the fractured limb.
- If cardboard, board, etc., is used, pad well so that the inner surfaces are not in contact with the skin. Pad hollows of the limbs well.

SELF-SPLINT

A simple emergency splinting technique is to tie the victim's injured leg to the uninjured one, or secure the injured arm to his chest if the elbow is bent or to his side of the elbow is straight. Always put padding between the legs and underneath the arm if possible.

FIXATION SPLINT

A fixation splint is a nonflexible device attached to a limb to maintain stability. It may be a padded board, a piece of heavy cardboard, or an aluminum splint molded to fit the extremity (Figure 10-15). Whatever the construction, it must be long enough to be secured well above and below the fracture site.

Apply gentle traction while an assistant places the splint (Figure 10-16). Be sure that the splint is

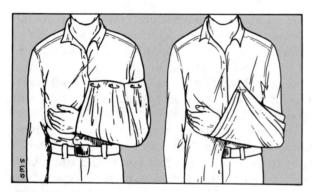

FIGURE 10-13. Improvised forearm sling.

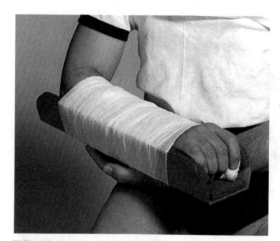

FIGURE 10-15. Cardboard splint of the lower arm.

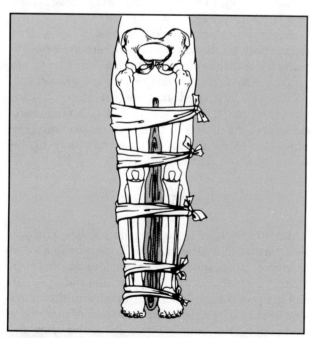

FIGURE 10-14. Improvised self-splint.

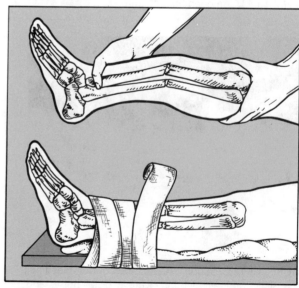

FIGURE 10-16. Applying a fixation splint. Grasp limb above and below the break and apply slight traction.

padded adequately to assure even pressure along the extremity. While your assistant maintains traction, wrap the limb to the splint with self-adhering bandages or cravats, tightly enough to hold the splint firmly to the extremity but not so tight as to cut off circulation. See Figure 10-17 for an example of the REEL splint, a commercial fixation splint.

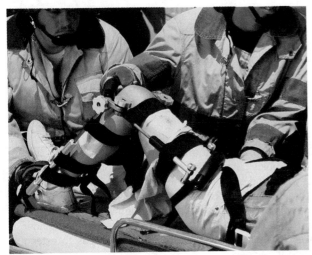

FIGURE 10-17. The REEL splint, which can be adapted to arm or leg splinting.

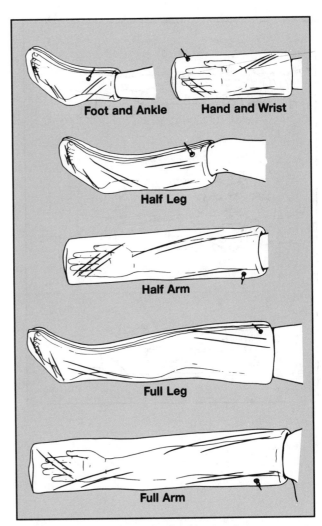

Foot and Ankle   Hand and Wrist

Half Leg

Half Arm

Full Leg

Full Arm

FIGURE 10-18. Examples of inflatable air splints.

INFLATABLE SPLINTS

Inflatable splints can be used to immobilize fractures of the lower leg or forearm (Figure 10-18). When applying inflatable splints, follow these guidelines (Figure 10-19):

1. Remove clothing from the splint area.

2. If the air splint is not equipped with a zipper, gather the splint on your arm so that the bottom edge is just above your wrist.

3. Grasp the victim's hand or foot while your assistant holds traction above the fracture. Slide the air splint over your hand onto the victim's arm or leg. The hand or foot of the injured limb should always be included in the splint. Clothing under the splint should be removed prior to this application.

4. The air splint should be positioned free of wrinkles.

5. While you maintain traction, your assistant inflates the splint by mouth.

6. If the air splint has a zipper, position it over the injured area while your assistant maintains traction above and below the splint. Zip up the splint, and inflate it.

7. In either instance, the splint should be inflated just to the point at which your finger will make a slight dent against the splint.

Air splints must be monitored carefully to be certain that they do not lose pressure or become overinflated. Overinflation is particularly apt to occur when the splint is applied in a cold area and the victim is moved to a warmer area. The air in the splint will then expand. Temperature, as well as surrounding air pressure, can cause detrimental changes.

Another problem is that many air splints completely enclose the hand or foot, making it difficult to check circulation except visually.

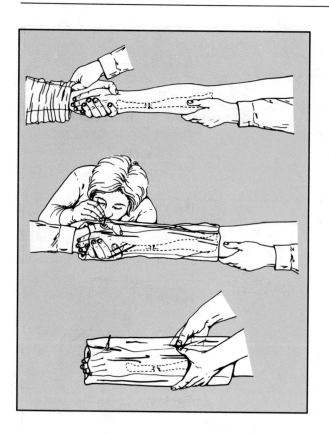

FIGURE 10-19. Grasp the victim's hand or foot while your assistant holds traction above the fracture. Slide the air splint over your hand onto the victim's arm or leg. While you maintain traction, have your assistant inflate the splint by mouth. If the splint has a zipper, apply it to the injured area. Zip up the splint, and inflate it just to the point at which your finger makes a slight dent against it. The splint needs to extend beyond the fingers.

| **10** | **SELF-TEST** | **10** |

Student: _____ Date: _____

Course: _____ Section #: _____

PART I: True/False   If you believe that the statement is true, circle the T. If you believe that the statement is false, circle the F.

T F   1. It usually is impossible to tell the difference between a sprain and a closed fracture without X-ray.

T F   2. For a fractured leg, a simple substitute for a splint is to tape or tie the injured leg to the uninjured one.

T F   3. To test for fracture, you should ask the victim to try to move the injured part or walk on the injured leg.

T F   4. In cases of suspected dislocation, you should correct the deformity before splinting it.

T F   5. If you suspect a fracture of the lower arm you should immobilize the wrist and lower arm, but not the elbow.

T F   6. If a fracture victim is unconscious, you should always assume that he has sustained spinal injury and take appropriate precautions.

T F   7. Permanent nerve damage can result from a splint that is too tight; you should watch carefully for signs of discoloration or swelling, and loosen the splint if necessary.

T F   8. Heat should be applied to a sprained joint for the first twenty-four hours.

T F   9. A sign of strain is immediate and profuse swelling.

T F   10. The First Aider should not attempt to straighten a deformity that involves a joint.

PART II: Multiple Choice   For each question, circle the answer that best reflects an accurate statement.

1. The primary objective in first-aid care for a fracture is to:
   a. set the bone.
   b. immobilize the fracture.
   c. push a protruding bone end back into its original position.
   d. all of the above.

2. To treat a sprain, you should not:
   a. soak the sprained area in hot water to relieve pain.
   b. pack the sprain in ice to reduce swelling.
   c. apply cold packs to the sprain.
   d. soak the sprained area in ice water.

3. In cases of fracture, the purpose of a splint is to:
   a. reduce the chance of shock.
   b. decrease pain.
   c. prevent motion of the injured limb.
   d. prevent further injury.
   e. all of the above.

4. What is a sign or symptom of a strain?
   a. immediate swelling.
   b. inability to move.
   c. sharp pain that lasts for prolonged periods.
   d. a sudden burning sensation.

5. Ligaments connect:
   a. muscle to tendon.
   b. muscle to bone.
   c. bone to bone.
   d. muscle to muscle.

6. An injury in which ligaments are partially torn is called a:
   a. sprain.
   b. strain.
   c. tendonitis.
   d. dislocation.

7. Displacement of a bone end from a joint with associated ligament damage is called:
   a. strain.
   b. sprain.
   c. dislocation.
   d. fracture.

8. The principal symptoms of a dislocation are:
   a. pain and a feeling of pressure over the joint.
   b. loss of motion and deformity.
   c. deformity and loss of pulse.
   d. numbness and pain.

PART III: Matching

1. A fracture is a crack or break in a skeletal bone. In the table below, label the diagrams with the correct description from the left-hand column.

A. Greenstick

B. Transverse

C. Spiral

D. Oblique

E. Comminuted

F. Impacted

_A_   _B_   _C_   _D_   _E_   _F_

2. Muscle, joint, and bone injuries are among the most common types of injuries encountered by First Aiders. There are four major types of muscle, joint, and bone injuries. In the chart below, provide the emergency care for each by choosing the appropriate number for each box.

	DEFINITION	FIRST AID	CHOICES
Strains	Overstraining of muscles and/or tendons, causing muscle bundles and tendons to stretch and possibly rupture.	1	1. Heat if no swelling, plenty of rest.
			2. Control any bleeding and immobilize.
Sprains	Injury to ligaments around joint or joint covering, producing undue stretching or tearing of these tissues.	3	3. Rest, Ice, Compression, Elevation.
Dislocations	Displacement of bone ends that form the joint.	4	4. Don't try to reduce; splint and apply cold. Treat for shock.
Fractures	Crack or break in skeletal bone, either open or closed fractures.	2	

PART IV: What Would You Do If:

You are assisting a young lady by the side of the road. She was horseback riding, became panicked when the horse began running, and fell off, placing her hands out in front of her to break the fall. The right elbow is very painful and grossly deformed.

1. List the steps you would take after you reach the victim.

2. What would you suggest is wrong with the victim, and why?

3. What first aid would you give the victim?

PART V: Practical Skills Check-Off

_____ has satisfactorily passed the following practical skills:
Student's Name

	Date	Partner Check	Inst. Init.
1. Identified major musculoskeletal sites on his/her body.	__/__/__	☐	_____
2. Performed a victim assessment for musculoskeletal injuries.	__/__/__	☐	_____
3. Applied proper emergency care for a strain.	__/__/__	☐	_____
Applied proper emergency care for a sprain.	__/__/__	☐	_____
Applied proper emergency care for a dislocation.	__/__/__	☐	_____
4. Applied proper emergency care for a fracture.	__/__/__	☐	_____

FRACTURES OF THE UPPER AND LOWER EXTREMITIES

Fractures to the upper extremities are very common. When a person falls, he automatically stretches out his hands to break the fall. The hands receive the full weight of the body, which can result in fractures anywhere between the hand and the clavicle.

The bones of the pelvis and lower extremities are very strong because they must bear considerable weight. Therefore, these bones typically are fractured from severe trauma due to heavy blows, falls, and automobile accidents.

When dealing with a fracture victim, first conduct a primary assessment and take the victim's history to identify and provide emergency care for life-threatening problems (fractures are seldom life-threatening) (Figure 11-1).

As in the majority of first-aid cases, phone or otherwise activate the EMS system as soon as possible. If the EMS response time will be just a few minutes, keep the fracture victim quiet, treat for shock, and let the Paramedics and/or EMTs perform the splinting. If, however, the EMS response time will be lengthy, or you are isolated and will be transporting the victim, pursue splinting, then evaluate and monitor distal NEUROVASCULAR function while you transport.

FRACTURES OF THE COLLARBONE (CLAVICLE)

Fractures of the collarbone often occur when a person falls with the hand outstretched or when he sustains a blow to the shoulder. Signs and symptoms of collarbone fractures include:

■ The arm on the injured side is partially or completely immobile.

149

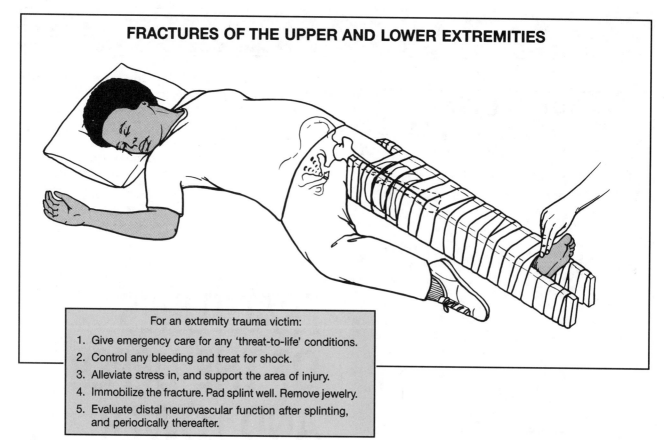

FRACTURES OF THE UPPER AND LOWER EXTREMITIES

For an extremity trauma victim:
1. Give emergency care for any 'threat-to-life' conditions.
2. Control any bleeding and treat for shock.
3. Alleviate stress in, and support the area of injury.
4. Immobilize the fracture. Pad splint well. Remove jewelry.
5. Evaluate distal neurovascular function after splinting, and periodically thereafter.

FIGURE 11-1.

- The shoulder on the injured side is lower and droops forward.
- The victim tends to keep the forearm bent across the chest and supports the arm on the injured side at the elbow with the other hand.
- The victim tilts his head in the direction of the injury with the chin turned in the opposite direction.
- The collarbone may appear crooked or deformed.

EMERGENCY CARE

Emergency care for a fractured collarbone involves the application of a sling and swathe.

To apply a sling and **SWATHE** (Figure 11-2):

1. Place a triangular bandage (about forty by forty by fifty-five inches) over the victim's chest, with the long edge parallel to the uninjured side. (An option is to first place a pillow between the arm and chest.)

2. Place the arm on the injured side in a flexed position on the bandage so that the point of the triangle extends beyond the injured elbow.

3. Fold the lower edge of the triangle up over the bent arm, and tie it to the other end of the bandage at the side of the neck (not over the spine).

4. Bring the point of the bandage forward over the elbow, and pin it securely to the sling front, or twist the point end until it is snug, and tie a single knot to hold it in place.

5. Position the bandage so that the fingers remain slightly exposed. Check them often for signs of restricted circulation.

6. Slide a wide cravat under the small of the victim's back. Raise the cravat to the chest, and tie it securely to the uninjured side.

7. Continue to monitor during transport.

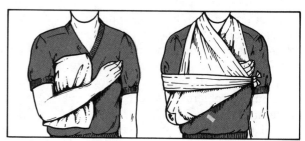

FIGURE 11-2. Immobilizing a fractured collarbone or scapula.

FRACTURES OF THE SCAPULA

Fracture of the **SCAPULA** is not a common injury. When a scapula fracture occurs, it usually is the result of a direct blow. Signs and symptoms are:

▪ Pain and swelling in the injured area.

▪ The victim is unable to swing his arm backward or forward from the shoulder.

EMERGENCY CARE

Emergency care for a fractured scapula is the same as for a fractured collarbone (Figure 11-2):

1. Place the victim's forearm in a triangular bandage sling.
2. Secure the arm to the chest by wrapping a wide cravat bandage around the chest and back, and across the forearm on the injured side. Tie the bandage just below the point of the shoulder.

FRACTURES OF THE HUMERUS

Fractures of the **HUMERUS** (upper one-third of the arm) may be hard to detect because a bone break close to the shoulder causes less pain and disability than a break at the mid-shaft. This type of injury is also difficult to immobilize. A victim may sustain a fracture *anywhere* along the humerus, however, and other fracture sites along the humerus are not difficult to detect. If the mechanism of injury suggests a possible fracture and the victim has pain, treat as a fracture.

EMERGENCY CARE

Emergency care for a fracture of the humerus is as follows (Figure 11-3):

1. Place a pad (i.e., towel) between the arm and the body. Place a padded splint (i.e., newspaper or

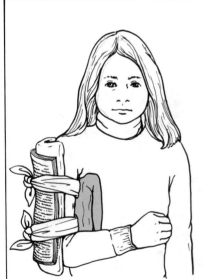
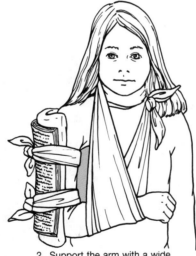
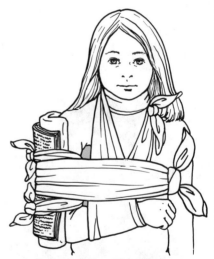

Emergency care for a fracture of the humerus is as follows:

1. Place a pad (i.e., towel) between the arm and the body. Place a padded splint (i.e., newspaper or board) along the outer side of the arm. Tie it to the arm.

2. Support the arm with a wide cravat bandage. The knot should not press against the neck.

3. Use a wide cravat bandage as a swathe to bind the arm to the chest. A broken clavicle (collarbone) can be splinted the same way except the padded splint along the outer side of the arm is not used.
4. Check the distal pulse at the artery. Check motor ability by asking the victim to move the fingers. Check sensory ability by touching a finger and asking which digit was touched.
5. Monitor the fractured extremity frequently.

FIGURE 11-3. Emergency care for a fracture of the humerus.

board) along the outer side of the arm. Tie it to the arm.

2. Support the arm with a wide cravat bandage. The knot should not press against the neck.

3. Use a wide cravat bandage as a swathe to bind the arm to the chest. A broken clavicle (collarbone can be splinted the same way, except that the padded splint along the outer side of the arm is not used.

4. Check the distal pulse at the artery. Check motor ability by asking the victim to move the fingers. Check sensory ability by touching a finger and asking which digit was touched.

5. Monitor the fractured extremity frequently.

FRACTURES OF THE ELBOW

EMERGENCY CARE

The type of emergency care required for a fractured elbow depends upon the position of the elbow at the time of the injury (Figures 11-4–11-6).

1. If the arm is bent at the time of injury:
   - Do not try to straighten the arm.
   - Immobilize the elbow in the position found.
   - Place the forearm in a sling to the distal end of the fifth digit.
   - Bind the arm to the chest.

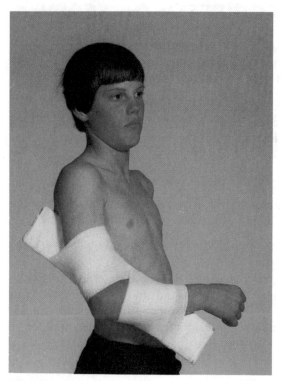

FIGURE 11-5. Immobilizing a fractured elbow with a board splint.

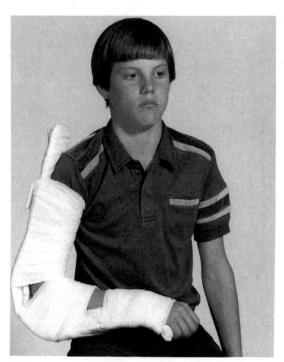

FIGURE 11-4. A ladder splint is formed to the injured limb, well padded, and secured with gauze rolls.

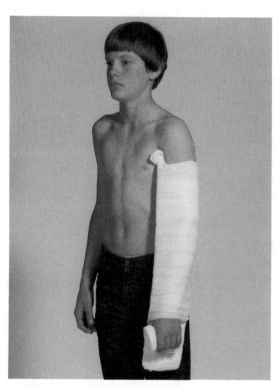

FIGURE 11-6. Splint a dislocated or fractured elbow in the position found.

2. If the elbow is straight at the time of injury:
   - Do not try to bend the arm.
   - Place a pad under the victim's **AXILLA** (armpit).
   - Apply a well-padded splint (or a ladder splint) to the elbow, or center a pillow at the elbow and pin the ends together around the arm.
   - Have the victim lie down, and elevate the injured arm.

FRACTURES OF THE FOREARM AND WRIST

EMERGENCY CARE

For a midforearm fracture (Figures 11-7–11-11):

1. Remove all clothing and jewelry from or near the injury site.
2. Apply gentle in-line pressure; hold until the splint is on.
3. Apply the splint without losing pressure.

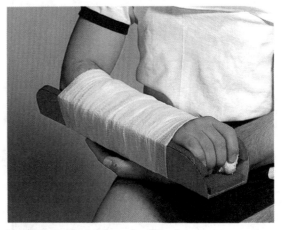

FIGURE 11-7. Cardboard splint of the lower arm.

4. Check distal pulse and sensation.
5. Continue checking the fractured extremity for swelling and circulation en route to the hospital if you transport.

── SPLINTING A FRACTURED FOREARM ──

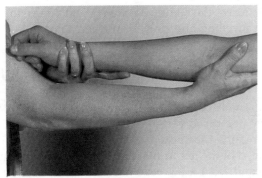

FIGURE 11-8. A fractured, angulated forearm may be straightened by gently pulling in opposite directions on the long axis of the arm.

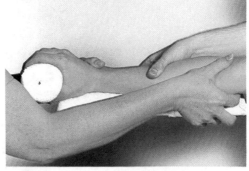

FIGURE 11-9. A well-padded splint that extends beyond both joints is positioned into place. Continue traction.

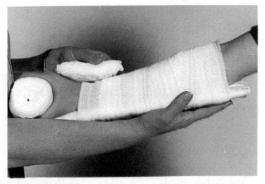

FIGURE 11-10. Splint is securely bandaged into place.

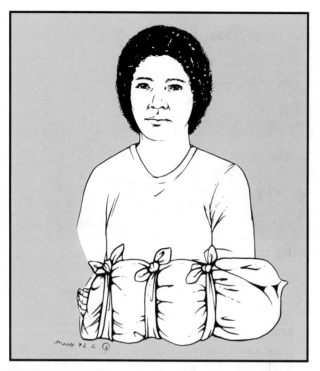

FIGURE 11-11. Pillow splint for fractures of the forearm, wrist, and hand.

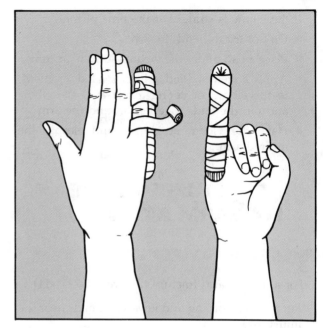

FIGURE 11-12. Fractured finger splinted with a tongue depressor.

FRACTURES OF THE HAND AND FINGERS

EMERGENCY CARE

If the break is a closed fracture of a single finger (Figure 11-12):

1. Place the injured finger in a comfortable position, usually slightly bent.
2. Apply a padded splint to prevent movement. Fractures of the fingers can be splinted with a tongue depressor, a commercial aluminum splint, or even an adjacent finger (but not the thumb)!
3. Elevate the hand.

If the hand has been crushed severely:

1. Do not cleanse the wound.
2. Place a ball of gauze or padded cloth in the victim's hand so that the fingers can curve around the ball (position of function). Cover the entire hand with sterile 4-by-4s.
3. Apply splints.

4. Keep the hand elevated at all times to reduce swelling and prevent further damage.

FRACTURES OF THE PELVIS

The **PELVIC GIRDLE** is formed by the **SACRUM** (lowest five fused vertebrae) and the pelvic bone. It also contains the sockets of the hip joint into which the head of the femur fits. Fractures of the pelvis usually result from a squeeze on the hips or from a direct blow and may puncture the enclosed organs.

Signs and symptoms of a pelvic fracture include:

- Marked pain at the fracture site.
- Severe shock.

EMERGENCY CARE

Every injury causing severe pelvic pain should be cared for like a spinal fracture.

1. Handle the victim as little as possible. Activate the EMS system.
2. Keep the victim quiet, treat for shock, and wait for the ambulance.
3. If you have to deal with the situation yourself, carefully place the victim on a firm, wide, rigid support (e.g., backboard) to stabilize the back.

4. If it is necessary to move the victim, do so without bending the victim's hips or waist.

5. Gently turn the victim to the back in such a way that all parts of the body are turned at the same time. The four-man logroll should be used. Transport the victim on his back.

6. Transport the victim to a physician as soon as possible.

FRACTURES OF THE HIP

A hip fracture is a break in the proximal or upper end of the **FEMUR** (thighbone) or a fracture of the socket (when the bone is forced into it). Hip fractures are common among elderly victims who fall while standing or walking. In this case, the fracture is caused by the twisting force exerted on the femur during the fall.

Other victims, such as those involved in automobile accidents, sustain hip fractures from the force that pushes the thighbone into the socket. The victim usually will lie with the affected leg turned outward, and the leg may appear to be shortened. Blood loss can be severe, and shock is common.

EMERGENCY CARE

To care for hip fractures (Figure 11-13):

1. Immobilize the pelvic girdle in a comfortable position.

2. Place pillows, a folded blanket, or some other soft object between and underneath the legs.

3. With the victim's knees bent, strap the legs together with belts, bandages, or straps.

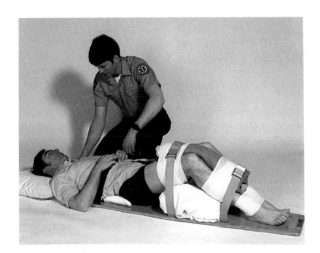

FIGURE 11-13. Immobilizing a fracture or dislocation of the hip or pelvis.

4. Watch the victim for signs and symptoms of shock, and give emergency care accordingly.

5. Transport the victim on a rigid stretcher, such as a backboard.

FRACTURES OF THE SHAFT OF THE FEMUR

A fractured femur usually causes the following (Figure 11-14):

- Marked deformity.
- Pain and swelling.
- Circulation impairment in the foot.
- Possibility of open fracture. Such fractures commonly result from falls and automobile accidents.
- Possible major blood loss; be alert for signs of shock.
- Limb shortening due to muscle contractures.

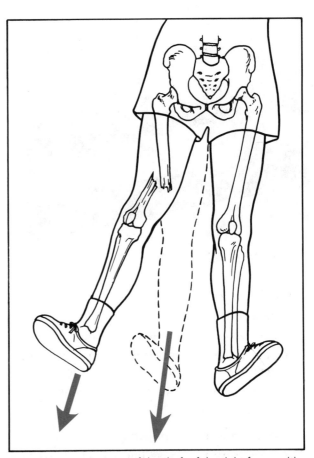

FIGURE 11-14. Fracture of the shaft of the right femur with angulation, shortening, and rotation of the limb below the fracture site. Apply gentle traction parallel to the normal axis of the fractured leg.

EMERGENCY CARE

The care for a fracture of the femur calls for splinting to immobilize the limb and to reduce pain and blood loss. **TRACTION SPLINTS** are used exclusively on femur fractures, usually midshaft fractures. *Use a traction splint only if you have the proper training and equipment.* Application of a traction splint is discussed in the next section of this chapter. You may also use board splints. You will need two, both padded.

1. The outside board should be long enough to reach from the victim's armpit to below his heel. The inner splint should be long enough to reach from the groin to below the heel.

2. Slide the cravat bandages underneath the victim at the ankle, knee, and lower back.

3. Position the padded splints, and add extra padding at the knee and ankle.

4. Tie the cravat bandages snugly around the chest, flank, groin, knee, and ankle (Figure 11-15).

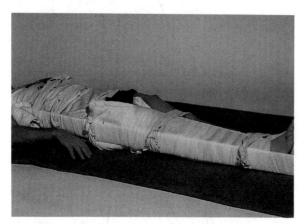

FIGURE 11-15. Immobilizing a high femur fracture with a fixation splint.

5. If transportation is short and immediate:
   - Place a blanket between the victim's legs.
   - Bind the legs together with cravat bandages. Stay well away from the fracture site.
   - Keep the victim warm, and give him emergency care for shock.

6. If an open wound is present:
   - Do not try to cleanse the wound unless it is grossly contaminated. (An open fracture is always contaminated and will require surgical care).

- Cut away any contaminated clothing.
- Cover the wound with a sterile, bulky pad, and control hemorrhage with gentle pressure.
- Secure the dressing and splint.

TRACTION SPLINTS

Fractures of the femur and some fractures below the knee can be treated with the traction splint. *Never use a traction splint if the fracture is within one to two inches of the knee or ankle. Traction splints are not generally used for hip fractures.*

Because the femur is the largest bone in the body, and because the fibula and tibia support each other, it takes a great amount of stress to fracture a lower extremity. Tissue damage frequently occurs — soft tissue may be torn or stretched, and the exploding action of the bone as it breaks sends sharp spicules of bone ends through blood vessels, nerves, and muscles. Severe damage and pain result; muscles contract and go into spasm in response to the pain, leading to further damage.

Soft thigh tissue contains some of the largest blood vessels in the body, and massive hemorrhage may occur when thigh tissue is severed. Because the thigh expands to accommodate the volume of blood, the victim can go into serious shock without losing any blood externally. Open thigh wounds, on the other hand, can result in a rapid loss of blood. Damage to vital motor nerves, also located in the thigh, can cause permanent disability.

A traction splint provides a counterpull, and it alleviates the pain, reduces blood loss, and minimizes further injury. It is not intended to reduce the fracture, but simply to *immobilize the bone ends and prevent further injury.*

Applying a Traction Splint

To apply a traction splint (Figures 11-16–11-23):

1. The first rescuer removes or cuts away clothing to expose the fracture site completely and controls any bleeding. (Make sure that a possible hemorrhaging wound on the back of the thigh does not go unexposed.) Dress and bandage open wounds.

2. The second rescuer checks and records circulation and neurological status distal to the injury, then stabilizes the limb.

3. The second rescuer applies manual traction to the injured leg by grasping the lower part of the heel

— APPLYING A TRACTION SPLINT —

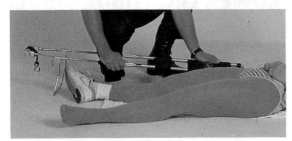

FIGURE 11-16. Expose, dress, and bandage any wound. Adjust splint for length: (1) Unlock splint and fold down heel stand. Slide up the splint until aligned with ankle; (2) Adjust to desired length; tighten sleeves; (3) Position opened leg support straps.

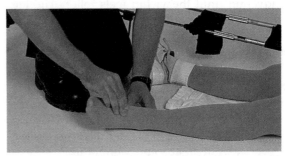

FIGURE 11-17. Palpate the distal pulse to check circulation, then stabilize the limb.

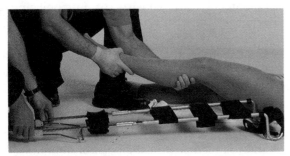

FIGURE 11-18. Move adjusted splint to injured leg and make final adjustments. Brace the fracture with your hand under the fracture site or as close as possible to it.

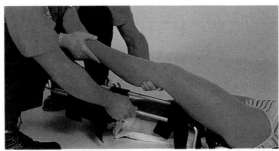

FIGURE 11-19. Rescuer 2 applies manual traction. Rescuer 1 places the splint into proper position.

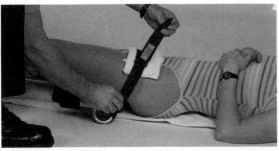

FIGURE 11-20. Rescuer 1 positions splint and attaches padded ischial strap; Rescuer 2 continues traction.

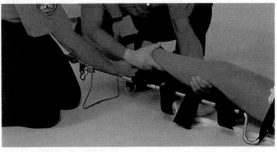

FIGURE 11-21. Rescuer 2 continues with manual traction; Rescuer 1 applies ankle strap. Lower edge of urethane sponge is even with bottom edge of heel. Wrap ankle hitch around foot. Tape, or a cravat, can hold the ankle hitch in place if it slips.

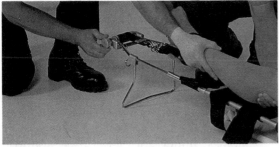

FIGURE 11-22. Rescuer 1 inserts S ring into D rings. Rescuer 2 maintains traction; Rescuer 1 applies mechanical traction until the victim feels relief.

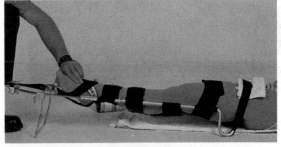

FIGURE 11-23. Leg support straps are fastened in place. Rescuer monitors distal pulse and neurological status. Adjust location of heel stand to victim's comfort.

with one hand and placing the other hand under the slightly bent knee. He then exerts a strong, steady pull until the victim feels relief. The leg should be elevated sufficiently for the splint to be applied properly by the first rescuer. The second rescuer maintains traction of the leg until traction is applied with the splint.

4. The first rescuer simultaneously adjusts the splint for length and makes all other necessary preparations to apply the splint. In doing so, remember that movements of the injured leg must be kept at an absolute minimum.

5. Apply the traction splint.

FRACTURES OF THE PATELLA (KNEECAP)

Fractures of the patella often result from a direct blow or from muscle pull on the cap when control of the knee is lost. Pain and swelling occur, and there may be deformity and/or impaired circulation of the foot.

EMERGENCY CARE

Apply one of the following splints:

1. Pillow or blanket splint (Figure 11-24).

2. A padded splint that extends from the buttocks to below the heel on the back of the leg.

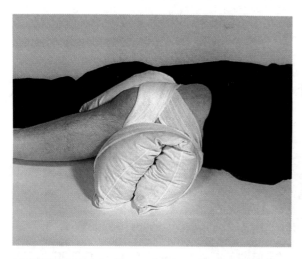

FIGURE 11-24. A pillow splint for a fractured patella or a dislocated knee.

FRACTURES OF THE LOWER LEG (TIBIA, FIBULA)

Open fractures of the lower leg are common because of the thin layers of skin and tissue surrounding these bones. Fractures of the fibula may not be apparent, because this bone does not support any body weight and is splinted naturally by the tibia. Impaired circulation in the foot may occur.

EMERGENCY CARE

Emergency care consists of immobilizing the injury:

1. Gently straighten the leg by applying traction. Grasp the extremity, one hand above and one hand below the fracture site. Provide two to five pounds of gentle counterpressure until the extremity returns to its normal anatomical position. If you meet any resistance in the leg, stop and immobilize it in the position found.

2. Check the distal pulse by palpating the dorsalis pedis artery on the anterior surface of the foot. Check distal movement and sensation by asking the victim to wiggle his toes, and ask if he can feel you touch each toe. If the victim is unconscious, gently palpate the foot for injuries.

3. Gently remove the victim's clothing and shoes so that you can observe the injured extremity for changes and prevent soft-tissue injury from pressure caused by swelling. Cut the seam of the pant leg or skirt, and remove the shoe and sock or hose. Maintain traction during this process.

4. In an emergency, with no other equipment available, place blankets between the victim's legs, and tie the legs together (Figure 11-25). To do this, push cravat bandages under both legs with a stick. Place a folded blanket, two coats, or other material between the victim's legs. Tie the victim's legs together so that the injured leg is immobilized by the uninjured leg.

5. If you have the proper equipment, use two well-padded, long splints at the sides of the legs and feet (Figure 11-26). Use a stick to push cravat bandages under the leg. Place well-padded boards or other suitable objects of proper length along the inner and outer sides of the fractured leg. Tie the splints snugly in place, with the knots pressing against the outside splint.

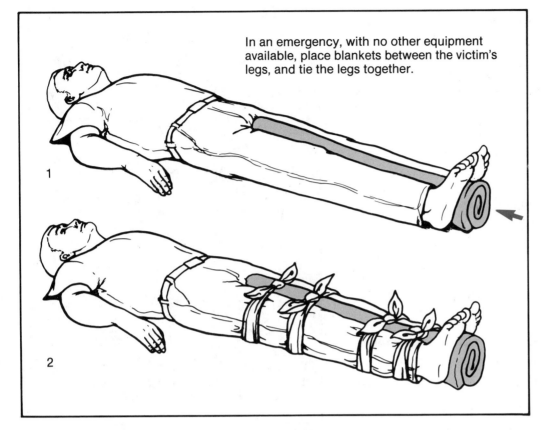

In an emergency, with no other equipment available, place blankets between the victim's legs, and tie the legs together.

FIGURE 11-25.

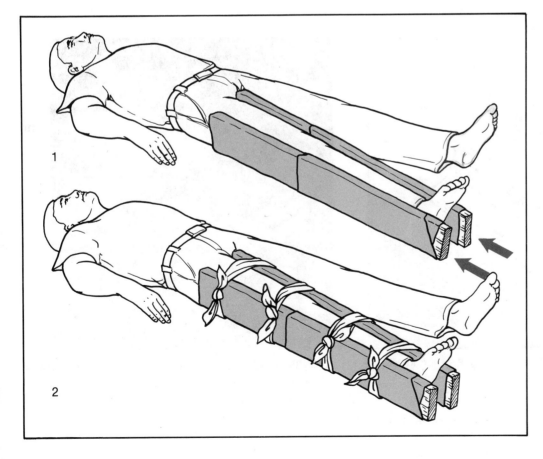

FIGURE 11-26.

FRACTURES OF THE ANKLE AND FOOT

Ankle fractures are most commonly caused by direct blows from heavy, crushing objects, by twisting, and by jumps and falls. Toes are broken frequently by blows or stubbing.

EMERGENCY CARE

Provide the following emergency care:

1. Have the victim lie down.

2. Carefully remove his shoes and socks, unless shoe removal will cause additional injury.

3. Do not try to reduce any deformity.

4. Elevate the limb.

5. Apply a dressing if the victim has an open wound.

6. Use an air splint (Figure 11-27), or wrap a pillow around the ankle and tie it to the ankle with cravat bandages (Figure 11-28). You can also place a splint on the bottom of the foot and secure it with cravat bandages (Figure 11-29).

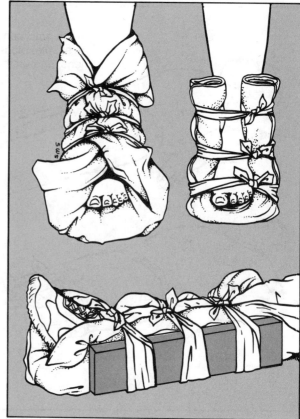

FIGURE 11-28. Immobilizing a fracture of the ankle and foot. Always untie laces if a shoe is left on the foot.

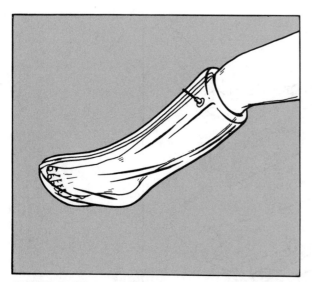

FIGURE 11-27. Immobilizing a fracture of the lower leg, ankle, or foot with a pneumatic splint.

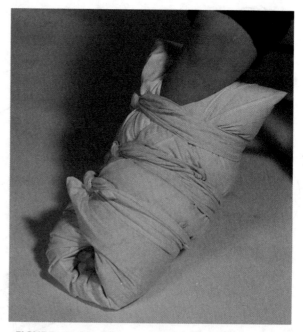

FIGURE 11-29. Pillow splint for a crushed foot or fractured ankle.

| **11** | **SELF-TEST** | **11** |

Student: _____ Date: _____

Course: _____ Section #: _____

PART I: True/False   If you believe that the statement is true, circle the T. If you believe that the statement is false, circle the F.

T   F   1. In an open fracture, the wound is always contaminated.

T   F   2. In cases of ankle and/or foot fracture, you should leave the victim's shoe and stocking on to provide support and lessen the chance of further injury.

T   F   3. A fracture is a crack or splinter in a bone that is not broken.

T   F   4. A closed fracture may become an open fracture through mishandling or motion during transport.

T   F   5. The only accurate diagnosis of closed fracture is made by X-ray, but if you suspect that a fracture is present, you should treat it accordingly, even without X-ray confirmation.

T   F   6. A splint should be placed directly against the skin without padding or dressings for maximum effectiveness.

T   F   7. A splint should not extend beyond the joints above and below the suspected fracture.

T   F   8. A fractured elbow should always be immobilized in the position in which it is found.

PART II: Multiple Choice   For each question, circle the answer that best reflects an accurate statement.

1. To treat an open fracture, do the following:
    a. wash the wound thoroughly with either disinfectant or clear running water.
    b. control bleeding with pressure through a dressing.
    c. if bone is protruding, do not cover the wound.
    d. replace bone fragments before covering the wound with a dressing.

2. To treat an open fracture of the upper arm:
    a. cover the wound with a compression dressing that will control bleeding.
    b. place a pad between the arm and the body.
    c. apply a splint that does not press against the wound.
    d. all of the above.

3. If you suspect a fracture of the upper arm, you should immobilize:
    a. the elbow.
    b. the upper arm.
    c. the shoulder.
    d. all of the above.

4. Emergency care for a fractured collarbone involves:
    a. splinting the entire arm so that all joints are immobile.
    b. putting the arm in a sling and binding the arm to the chest.
    c. tying the straightened arm to the chest and torso.
    d. lying the victim down — a collarbone cannot be splinted, so the victim should not move around.

5. What should a First Aider do to immobilize a fractured elbow when the arm is bent?
    a. bend the arm across the chest, immobilize.
    b. straighten the arm and immobilize.
    c. immobilize in the line of deformity in which it is found.
    d. do not immobilize; transport immediately.

6. Fractures about the hip are best handled by a/an:
    a. blanket splint, with the victim's legs strapped together.
    b. traction splint.
    c. air splint.
    d. sling and swathe.

7. An improvised board splint for the high femur should reach from the _____ to _____.
    a. armpit, below the heel.
    b. waist, knee.
    c. waist, heel.
    d. armpit, below the knee.

8. A First Aider should apply traction with a traction splint until:
    a. the limb is noticeably stretched.
    b. the victim feels relief.
    c. the bone ends realign.
    d. the fracture is reduced.

9. A fractured patella should be splinted with:
    a. a traction splint.
    b. an air splint.
    c. a pillow or blanket splint.
    d. two padded boards.

PART III: Matching

1. **Traction Splints**

The major steps of applying a traction splint, listed below, are out of order. List them in the proper order.

1. Apply manual traction to the injured leg.
2. Apply the traction splint.
3. Expose, dress, and bandage any wound.
4. Check the limb and record circulation and neurological status.
5. Adjust the splint for length.
6. Apply the ankle strap or ankle hitch.
7. Apply mechanical traction.
8. Monitor distal pulse.
9. Fasten the leg support straps in place.

1. _____   6. _____

2. _____   7. _____

3. _____   8. _____

4. _____   9. _____

5. _____

PART IV: What Would You Do If:

At the scene of an automobile accident, you diagnose a young man as having a closed fractured femur about midthigh. He also has a fracture of the pelvis on the opposite side of the leg injury.

1. What first aid would you administer if an ambulance will reach you within ten minutes?

2. How would you splint the fractures if no ambulance can respond and you will have to transport the victim to a medical facility?

PART V: Practical Skills Check-Off

_____ has satisfactorily passed the following practical skills:
Student's Name

	Date	Partner Check	Inst. Init.
1. Splinted a collarbone.	_/_/_	☐	_____
2. Splinted a humerus.	_/_/_	☐	_____
3. Splinted an elbow.	_/_/_	☐	_____
4. Splinted a forearm and wrist.	_/_/_	☐	_____
5. Splinted a hand and fingers.	_/_/_	☐	_____
6. Splinted a pelvis (optional).	_/_/_	☐	_____
7. Splinted a hip.	_/_/_	☐	_____
8. Splinted a femur (fixation).	_/_/_	☐	_____
9. Splinted a femur (traction) (optional).	_/_/_	☐	_____
10. Splinted a patella.	_/_/_	☐	_____
11. Splinted a lower leg (tibia, fibula).	_/_/_	☐	_____
12. Splinted an ankle and foot.	_/_/_	☐	_____

HEAD INJURIES

Head injury is exceeded only by stroke as a cause of major neurological trauma. In one recent year, 114,000 accident deaths occurred in the United States, and head injury was primarily responsible for most of these deaths.

Injuries of the head are some of the most serious and difficult first-aid emergencies to handle. The victim is often confused or unconscious, making assessment difficult. And many injuries of the head are life-threatening: if you handle a head-injured victim improperly, you can cause permanent damage or death.

One of the most beautiful and complex designs in existence, the human **NERVOUS SYSTEM** weighs less than twenty pounds, yet consists of a computer and an electrical distribution system that automatically monitor and control every function of the body. It routinely makes thousands of adjustments every second to control blood pressure and respiration, eliminate infection, protect from injury, and permit nourishment. Simply stated, it makes it possible for us to adapt in every way to our environment.

This complex system is fragile and can be damaged easily. However, the nervous system is well protected against most kinds of injury by bones (the skull and the **SKELETON**) and a series of membranes

and fluids designed to protect and cushion it from injury. Nevertheless, serious injury can occur, and it is important to be able to recognize the common signs and symptoms of head injury.

PHYSIOLOGY OF BRAIN INJURY

The **BRAIN** itself is enclosed in the skull — a rigid, unyielding case. If the brain tissue swells or if intracranial bleeding occurs, the brain at first tries to compensate for the lack of room in which to expand.

When an area of the brain is injured, the blood vessels in the brain dilate so that more blood can flow to the injured area. If that fails, the blood vessels undergo further changes that cause serous fluid to leak into the affected area. As a result, the brain is diluted with water, thus lowering the level of carbon dioxide in the brain tissue.

When such leakage occurs, edema (swelling) results. The volume of the brain increases, leaving less space inside the skull for the blood and **CEREBROSPINAL FLUID**. At first, nothing happens: the brain stops producing cerebrospinal fluid, absorbs existing cerebrospinal fluid more rapidly, and employs several means of decreasing the amount of blood that it receives from the circulatory system.

However, the brain's compensation techniques can go only so far. Soon, intracranial pressure rises, and blood flow throughout the brain becomes inadequate. As a result, the brain cannot function normally, and swelling increases.

VICTIM ASSESSMENT

Do a primary survey to detect any life-threatening problems and correct them. Get an immediate description of key signs and symptoms (Figure 12-1), then watch constantly for changes. Immobilization of a spinal injury can wait, *but there must absolutely be no movement of the victim until you can immobilize him.* The primary assessment should be done in the following order:

AIRWAY

Maintaining an adequate airway is the most vital element in the emergency care of head injury, because the most serious complication is lack of oxygen to the brain. In correcting an airway, never hyperextend the neck (a high percentage of head injury is accompanied by cervical-spine injury); use the modified jaw-thrust maneuver to protect the cervical spine.

CHECK THE HEAD

Using extreme care, check the victim's head (Figures 12-2 and 12-3).

1. Look for depressions, fractures, lacerations deformities, bruising around the eyes, bruising behind the ears, and other obvious problems. See Chapter 2.

2. *Never palpate a wound; never probe a wound to determine its depth; never separate the edges of a wound to explore it; and never remove impaled objects.*

3. Check the victim's pupils. Are they equal? Are they constricted or dilated? Do they react to light?

4. The face should be the same on both sides; if it is not, the victim may have some paralysis.

5. Look to see whether blood and/or cerebrospinal fluid are dripping from the nose, ears, or mouth. If so, do not attempt to stop the flow; dress the dripping area lightly with sterile gauze to absorb the flow, but make sure that you do not create any pressure (Figure 12-4).

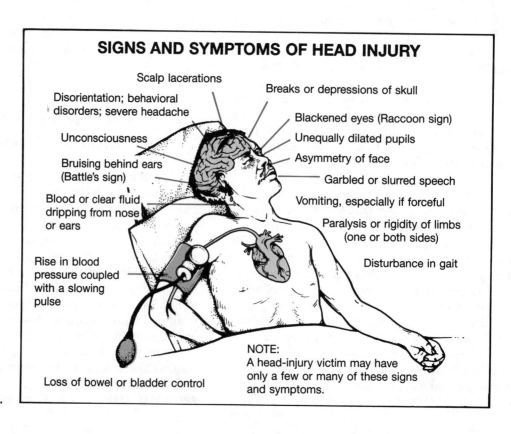

SIGNS AND SYMPTOMS OF HEAD INJURY

Scalp lacerations

Disorientation; behavioral disorders; severe headache

Unconsciousness

Bruising behind ears (Battle's sign)

Blood or clear fluid dripping from nose or ears

Rise in blood pressure coupled with a slowing pulse

Loss of bowel or bladder control

Breaks or depressions of skull

Blackened eyes (Raccoon sign)

Unequally dilated pupils

Asymmetry of face

Garbled or slurred speech

Vomiting, especially if forceful

Paralysis or rigidity of limbs (one or both sides)

Disturbance in gait

NOTE:
A head-injury victim may have only a few or many of these signs and symptoms.

FIGURE 12-1.

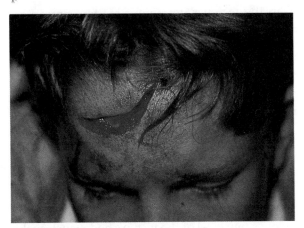

FIGURE 12-2. Always suspect and assess for spinal injury in a head-injured victim.

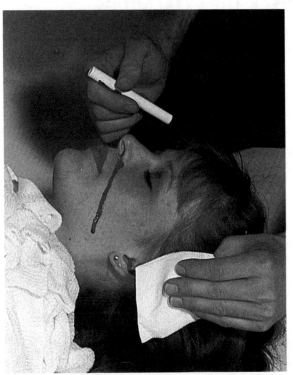

FIGURE 12-4. Blood and/or cerebrospinal fluid may come from the ears and/or nose of a victim of head injury. Turn victim's head to the side to allow drainage, and cover lightly with dressing. Do not block drainage.

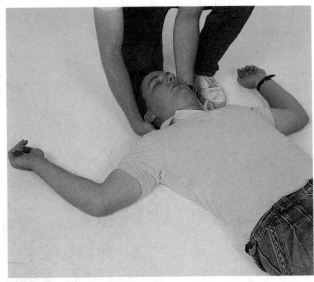

FIGURE 12-3. Carefully check the head for injuries.

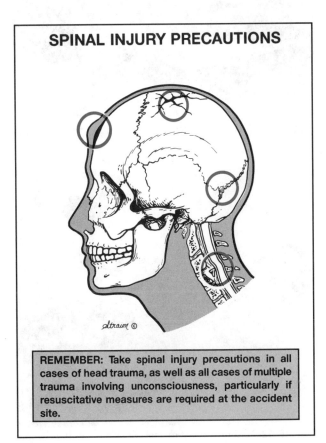

SPINAL INJURY PRECAUTIONS

REMEMBER: Take spinal injury precautions in all cases of head trauma, as well as all cases of multiple trauma involving unconsciousness, particularly if resuscitative measures are required at the accident site.

FIGURE 12-5.

CHECK THE NECK AND SPINE

Maintaining light in-line stabilization:

1. Check the neck and spine for lacerations, bruises, swelling, protrusions, spaces, or other obvious deformities.

2. Use axial head in-line stabilization and a logroll to examine the victim's back. See Chapter 13.

3. Ask the victim about any tenderness, pain, or muscle spasm.

4. *Remember that you will probably not be able to see any deformity even if there is significant spinal injury* (Figure 12-5).

CHECK THE EXTREMITIES

Check the victim's arms and legs for paralysis or loss of sensation. Loss of function or sensation occurs below the point where the spine is injured, but you should check the arms even if the legs seem injured (the injury could be a fracture, not a spinal injury). See Chapter 2.

MOTOR FUNCTION

1. Check the muscle tone of the victim's face by asking him to clench his teeth and grimace at you. Does the face seem symmetrical? If not, the victim may have suffered a stroke.

2. Can he feel your touch on the feet/hands and legs/arms (Figures 12-6 and 12-7)?

3. Can the victim wiggle his toes/fingers and raise the extremities?

4. Can the victim determine if his toes/fingers are being moved up or down?

5. Ask the victim to grasp your index and third fingers of both hands simultaneously; assess the grip strength of his hands. Are they about the same (Figure 12-8)?

6. Ask the victim to push against your palms with both feet, then pull upward with both feet against your palms (Figure 12-9). If you notice an inequality in muscle tone between the victim's left and right sides, ask if it is normal. Unequal muscle tone can signal brain damage or acute spinal-cord injury. Motor function that is absent below some level of the victim's body (such as the nipple line) usually suggests spinal-cord damage. (Checking foot strength should be done very cautiously; it can cause movement that can aggravate spinal injury. If you suspect spinal injury, do not perform this test.) When possible, **this is best left to trained emergency personnel.**

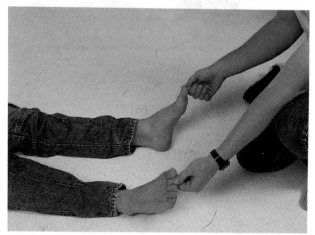

FIGURE 12-6. Can the victim feel touch on the toes and feet?

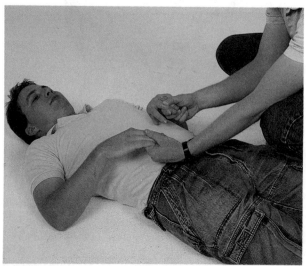

FIGURE 12-7. Can the victim feel touch on the hands and fingers?

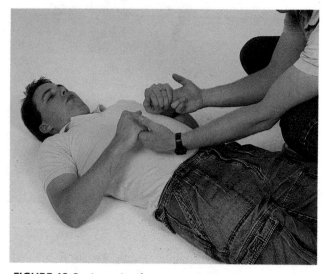

FIGURE 12-8. Assessing for grip strength.

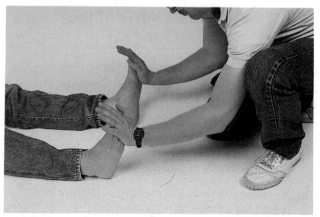

FIGURE 12-9. Assessing for foot strength.

SKULL FRACTURE

Skull fracture is not an uncommon head injury; it can be open or closed. The skull fracture itself does not cause disability and death; rather, it is the *underlying damage* that leads to serious consequences. Skull fracture itself presents no danger if it is not accompanied by brain injury, hematoma, cerebrospinal fluid leakage, or subsequent infection.

There are four basic types of skull fracture (Figure 12-10):

- **Depressed.** An object strikes the skull, leaving an obvious depression or deformity; bone fragments are often driven into the membranes or the brain itself by the force of the impact.

- **Linear.** The most common type of skull fracture (80 percent of all skull fractures are linear), it leaves a thin-line crack in the skull. Linear fractures are the least serious, and most difficult to detect, of all skull fractures.

- **Comminuted.** A comminuted fracture appears at the point of impact, with multiple cracks radiating from the center (it looks like a cracked eggshell).

- **Basal.** A basal skull fracture occurs when there is a break in the bed of the skull; it is often the result of a linear fracture that extends to the floor of the skull. Difficult to detect even by X-ray, a basal skull fracture often causes extensive damage.

SIGNS AND SYMPTOMS OF SKULL FRACTURE

The primary function of the skull is to protect the brain from injury. When the skull is fractured, part of the brain's protective armor is compromised, and serious brain injury can result.

You should suspect skull fracture with any significant trauma to the head. An open skull fracture is visible, but even a closed skull fracture will result in some signs and symptoms. Some are obvious, such as deformity or your ability to see the skull itself through lacerations. Skull fracture can exist without the usual signs, but you should look for the following (Figure 12-11):

- Obvious deformity of the skull.

- Visible damage to the skull, visible through lacerations in the scalp.

- Pain, tenderness, or swelling at the site of injury.

- Clear or pinkish fluid dripping from the nose, the ears, the mouth, or a wound in the head, or bleeding from any or all of these.

TYPES OF SKULL FRACTURE

Penetrating skull fracture

Lacerated brain tissue

Linear

Comminuted

Basal

Depressed

FIGURE 12-10.

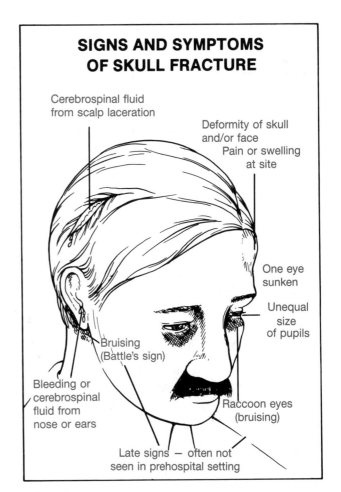

SIGNS AND SYMPTOMS OF SKULL FRACTURE

Cerebrospinal fluid from scalp laceration

Deformity of skull and/or face
Pain or swelling at site

One eye sunken

Unequal size of pupils

Bruising (Battle's sign)

Bleeding or cerebrospinal fluid from nose or ears

Raccoon eyes (bruising)

Late signs — often not seen in prehospital setting

FIGURE 12-11.

- Purplish discoloration or bruising over the mastoid process behind the ear (**BATTLE'S SIGN**).
- Unequal pupil size.
- One eye misplaced in relation to the other eye.
- Purplish discoloration under or around the eyes in the absence of trauma to the eyes (**RACCOON'S SIGN**).

INJURIES TO THE BRAIN

Injuries to the brain can be open or closed. In closed head injuries, the scalp may be lacerated, but the skull not exposed; there will be no opening to the brain. Brain damage, however, can nonetheless be extensive and is often more severe in closed head injuries than in open head injuries. The brain can be damaged whether or not the skull is fractured, since the amount of injury depends mainly on the mechanism of injury and the force involved. In general, however, brain tissue is susceptible to the same kinds of injury as any soft tissue — contusion, laceration, and puncture wounds (Figure 12-12). Abrasion is not common in the brain because of the smooth interior of the skull that encloses it.

CONCUSSION

The most common and least serious brain injury is **CONCUSSION**, a temporary loss of the brain's ability to function that occurs when the brain sustains a blow, regardless of whether other injuries occurred. There is no detectable damage to the brain from a concussion.

A concussion normally causes some disturbance of brain function ranging from momentary confusion to complete loss of consciousness, and it usually causes headache. If the victim loses consciousness, it is usually brief (lasting only a few minutes) and does not recur. Generally, any victim who is unconscious for more than five minutes usually is observed in the hospital for twenty-four hours.

Signs and Symptoms

Depending on where the force is absorbed in the brain, the signs of simple concussion might include the following:

- Momentary confusion.
- Confusion that lasts for several minutes.
- Inability to recall the incident and, sometimes, the period just before and after it (retrograde **AMNESIA**).

- Repeated questioning about what happened.
- Mild to moderate irritability or resistance to treatment.
- Combativeness.
- Verbal abuse.
- Inability to answer questions or obey commands appropriately.
- Persistent vomiting.
- **INCONTINENCE** of urine or feces.
- Restlessness.
- Seizures.

The key distinguishing factor in concussion is that its effects appear immediately or soon after impact, and then they disappear, usually within forty-eight hours; recovery is complete. An injury that causes symptoms that develop several minutes after an incident or symptoms that do not subside over time is not a concussion, but a more serious injury.

CONTUSION

A contusion, or bruising and swelling of the brain tissue, can accompany concussion. It causes bleeding into the surrounding tissues but may or may not cause increased intracranial pressure, even in cases of open head injury. Contusion is usually caused by **COUP-CONTRECOUP** or acceleration-deceleration injury (Figure 12-13). A victim with signs of concussion that do not clear up probably has suffered a contusion.

Signs and Symptoms

Signs and symptoms of contusion include the initial signs and symptoms of concussion, plus one or more of the following:

- Loss of consciousness ranging from hours to months; upon return to consciousness, the victim will not be able to remember the incident or the events immediately preceding and following it.
- Paralysis, ranging from one-sided to total.
- Unequal pupils.
- Forceful or repeated vomiting.
- Alteration of vital signs.

Contusion can lead to swelling of the brain tissue, which can result in permanent disability or death.

HEAD INJURY AND BRAIN TRAUMA

Trauma

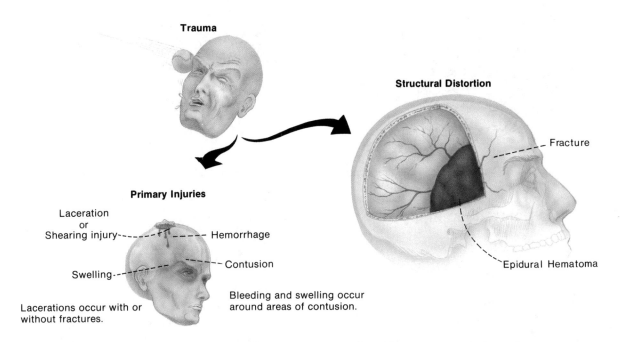

Structural Distortion

Fracture

Epidural Hematoma

Primary Injuries

Laceration
or
Shearing injury

Hemorrhage

Contusion

Swelling

Lacerations occur with or without fractures.

Bleeding and swelling occur around areas of contusion.

Secondary Factors

Contusions with pressure may result in loss of consciousness.

Respiratory and circulatory changes may result from primary brain injury.

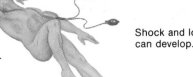

Shock and low blood pressure can develop.

Brain Damage

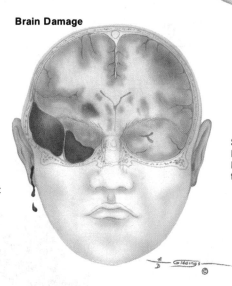

Signs & Symptoms

-Deformity of the skull.
-Drainage of spinal fluid or blood from nose and ears.
-Black eyes.
-Disorientation or confusion.
-Unconsciousness or coma.
-Unequal pupils or pupils that don't respond to light.
-Partial or total paralysis.

Subdural and/or epidural hematomas and brain swelling lead to increased pressure on the brain.

FIGURE 12-12.

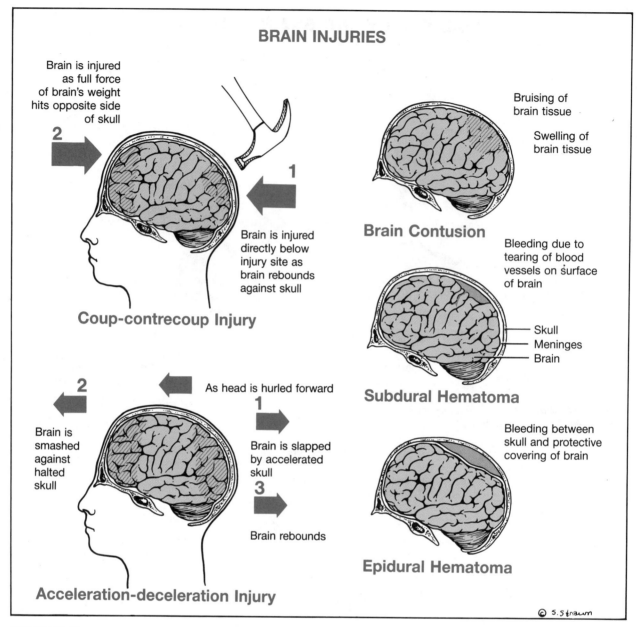

BRAIN INJURIES

Brain is injured as full force of brain's weight hits opposite side of skull

2

1

Brain is injured directly below injury site as brain rebounds against skull

Coup-contrecoup Injury

Bruising of brain tissue

Swelling of brain tissue

Brain Contusion

Bleeding due to tearing of blood vessels on surface of brain

Skull
Meninges
Brain

Subdural Hematoma

2

As head is hurled forward

1

Brain is slapped by accelerated skull

3

Brain rebounds

Brain is smashed against halted skull

Acceleration-deceleration Injury

Bleeding between skull and protective covering of brain

Epidural Hematoma

© S. Strawn

FIGURE 12-13.

LACERATION

Like contusion, a laceration of brain tissue can occur in either an open or closed head injury; often it occurs when an object penetrates the skull and lacerates the brain. It is a permanent injury, almost always results in bleeding, and can cause massive disruption of the nervous system (Figure 12-14).

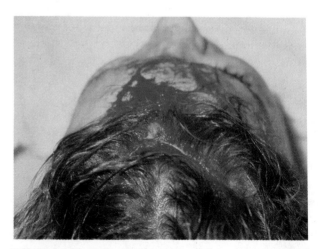

FIGURE 12-14. Open head injury.

PUNCTURE WOUND

A puncture wound of the brain occurs when an object passes through the skull and enters the brain tissue, where it lodges in the brain. It is common in shootings and industrial accidents and often involves bullets, knives, or ice picks. An extreme emergency, it almost always results in long-term damage but is not necessarily fatal. *Never try to remove the object.* If an object is impaled in the head and is visible, immobilize it with soft bulky dressings and dress it with sterile dressings. If an object has penetrated the skull and you cannot see it, cover the wound lightly with sterile dressings. Permit drainage of blood in both cases, and position the victim for shock if bleeding is heavy. *Never apply firm pressure to the head following an injury that might have caused skull fracture.*

OPEN AND CLOSED HEAD INJURY

An open head injury is accompanied by a break in the skull, such as that caused by fracture or an impaled object. It involves direct local damage to the involved tissue, but it also can result in brain damage due to infection, laceration of the brain tissue, or punctures of the brain by objects that invade the cranium after penetrating the skull.

Closed head injury works a little differently. The skull is a nondistensible container with three contents whose individual volumes can vary, but whose total volume cannot: they include the brain tissue, the blood, and the cerebrospinal fluid. As mentioned earlier, the injured brain tries to compensate in a variety of ways by causing fluid levels to decrease. Basal skull fractures are likely to permit the leakage of cerebrospinal fluid; under these circumstances, the cerebrospinal fluid usually is mixed with blood. If so, it can form a characteristic "target sign" when dripped on a sheet or pillowcase. But the rigid skull can hold only so much total volume, and if the brain tissue swells or bleeding occurs, pressure results, causing considerable damage.

SIGNS AND SYMPTOMS OF BRAIN INJURY

Signs and symptoms of brain injury should signal you to a true emergency: brain injury is a serious condition that needs immediate management. In addition to the signs of skull fracture, a victim of brain injury may exhibit any of the following signs or symptoms:

- Loss of consciousness or changes in mental state, ranging from confusion to complete loss of consciousness; deterioration in the level of consciousness almost always indicates hemorrhage and calls for immediate action.
- Paralysis or **FLACCIDITY**, usually on only one side of the body.
- Rigidity of all limbs (present with severe brainstem injury).
- Asymmetry of facial movements, squinting, or drooping.
- Unequal or unresponsive pupils.
- Loss of vision or disturbance of vision in one or both eyes.
- Ringing in the ears or loss of hearing in one or both ears.
- Loss of balance; staggering or stumbling gait.
- Confusion, increasing in severity with time.
- Disorientation regarding persons, place, time, or purpose.
- Memory impairment.
- Nervousness, anxiety, restlessness, or violent behavior.
- Personality changes.
- Rise in body temperature.
- Slow, full heartbeat that gradually becomes rapid and weak (very late sign of serious head injury).
- High blood pressure combined with slow pulse.
- Rapid, labored breathing or disturbances in the pattern of breathing.
- Vomiting (any vomiting in an adult, usually about an hour after injury, or vomiting in a child more than two or three times).
- Obvious signs of injury (such as depression of the skull).
- Tenderness, muscle spasm, or displacement in the neck.
- Garbled speech, repetitive speech, inability to form words, or inability to understand written or spoken language.
- Bowel or bladder incontinence.
- Scalp laceration (a force great enough to lacerate the scalp can be great enough to damage the brain or skull; even with no brain damage, scalp laceration can lead to infection).

EMERGENCY CARE FOR HEAD INJURY

Before beginning any emergency care for head injury assess the victim's level of consciousness; a victim who worsens needs immediate transport to a hospital. Urgent transport is vital. Activate the EMS system immediately.

Whenever you care for a victim of head injury, *always* assume that neck and/or spinal injury also exist. Handle the victim with extreme care, and immobilize the neck and back as early as possible. Keep the victim at rest throughout emergency care.

> **Caution: When possible, head injuries should be cared for by trained emergency medical personnel.**

General emergency care guidelines for head injuries include the following.

1. The top priority is establishing and maintaining an open airway with adequate oxygenation; oxygen deficiency in the brain is the most frequent cause of death following head injury. See Chapter 3.

   - Use the modified jaw-thrust technique to open the airway without further injuring the spine.

   - Remove any foreign bodies from the mouth, and suction blood and mucus.

   - Maintain an open airway and, if necessary, administer artificial ventilation. Take extreme care not to hyperextend the neck.

- Maintain neutral positioning of the head and neck (Figures 12-15 and 12-16) and, if possible, apply a cervical collar (Figures 12-17–12-19) and stabilize the head and neck until the victim can

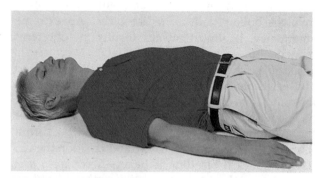

FIGURE 12-15. The victim's head and neck should be in a neutral, in-line position.

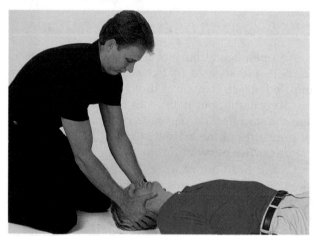

FIGURE 12-16. Maintaining neutral positioning of the head and neck.

EXAMPLES OF CERVICAL COLLARS

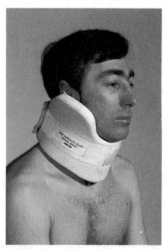

FIGURE 12-17. Hare cervical collar.

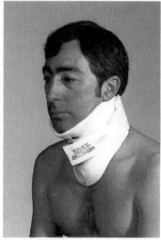

FIGURE 12-18. STIFNECK® cervical collar.

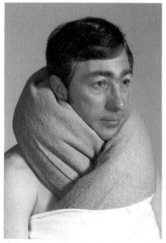

FIGURE 12-19. Improvised cervical collar.

be immobilized fully and fastened to a back-board. See Chapter 13.

■ The victim may vomit, so protect against aspiration; be prepared to roll the secured victim as necessary if vomiting occurs.

2. Closely monitor the victim's breathing; administer artificial ventilation if necessary.

3. Face and scalp wounds may bleed heavily, but they usually are easy to control with direct pressure.

■ Guard against shock from blood loss.

■ Control bleeding from other wounds, but do not attempt to stop the flow of blood or cerebrospinal fluid from the ears or nose. If cerebrospinal fluid is leaking from the nose, ear, or head wound, cover loosely with a completely sterile gauze dressing to avoid introducing contaminants into the central nervous system; the dressing should absorb, but not stop, the flow.

■ For other wounds, use gentle, continuous direct pressure with sterile gauze only as needed to control bleeding.

■ Never exact direct pressure on a head wound that may be accompanied by skull fracture — you could drive fragments of the skull into brain tissue or could seriously increase intracranial pressure.

■ Never apply pressure if you can see brain matter or bone fragments.

■ Apply pressure only at the edges of a fracture over solid, intact bone, to control heavy bleeding.

4. If there is a protruding object:
■ Immobilize it with soft, bulky dressings, and dress the wound with sterile dressings.

■ Never try to remove a penetrating object.

5. If the victim shows signs of shock (high pulse rate, low blood pressure), elevate the foot of the backboard or stretcher — follow local protocol. *Note:* Shock is rarely caused by an isolated head injury — it always signals the possibility of additional injuries. However, it frequently results in brain damage or death. Avoid overheating; look for and care for other internal injuries.

6. At least 10 percent of those who are unconscious following a fall or car accident also have sustained cervical-spine injury. In general, assume that all unconscious trauma victims have sustained spinal-column injury. Maintain neutral positioning of the head and neck (Figure 12-20), and if possible apply a rigid extrication-type **CERVICAL COLLAR** to immobilize the cervical spine.

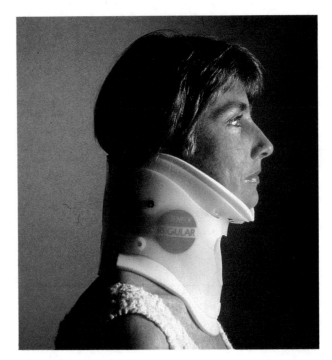

FIGURE 12-20. Proper-sized rigid extrication collar with the chin flush with end of the chin piece.

Make sure that the collar is sized for the victim; it should fit firmly under the chin and snugly against the collarbone. When in doubt about cervical-spine injury, always immobilize the neck. See Chapter 13. **Caution: When possible, head and spinal injuries should be cared for by trained emergency medical personnel. Do not attempt procedures that you have not been trained to do.**

7. Monitor vital signs, watching for changes. Treat as appropriate. If body temperature increases, sponge the victim with cool water or place a cool compress on his forehead.

8. If the victim is conscious, talk to him; if you continue to stimulate him, you may be able to prevent him from losing consciousness.

9. Time is of the essence. Activate the EMS system as soon as possible. If possible, someone should be sent to activate the EMS system while emergency care is being rendered.

■ While waiting for the emergency team to arrive, dress facial and scalp wounds as necessary.

■ Continue to monitor vital signs.

■ Stay alert to the possibility of vomiting, and work quickly to prevent aspiration.

■ Continually monitor the airway and the victim's neurological status.

| **12** | **SELF-TEST** | **12** |

Student: _____   Date: _____

Course: _____   Section #: _____

PART I: True/False   If you believe that the statement is true, circle the T. If you believe that the statement is false, circle the F.

T   F   1. Head injury is the number-one cause of major neurological trauma.

T   F   2. In a head-injured victim, it is best to use the head-tilt/chin-lift maneuver to open the airway.

T   F   3. Forceful (projectile) vomiting may be a sign of a head injury.

T   F   4. Pupillary response is the most important part of the primary assessment for a head-injured victim.

T   F   5. You can usually see some spinal deformity if a spinal injury also is present.

T   F   6. Immobilization of a spinal injury should be done before the primary assessment is completed.

T   F   7. A basal skull fracture is the most common and least serious.

T   F   8. A concussion is the most serious and least common brain injury.

T   F   9. Face and scalp wounds may bleed heavily but usually are easy to control.

T   F   10. At least 10 percent of victims who are unconscious following a fall or car accident have also sustained cervical-spine damage.

PART II: Multiple Choice   For each question, circle the answer that best reflects an accurate statement.

1. If a victim has blood or cerebrospinal fluid draining from the ears but shows no indication of a spinal injury, the first step in emergency care is to:

    a. Stabilize the neck.
    b. stop the flow of blood and cerebrospinal fluid.
    c. complete the body survey.
    d. establish and maintain and open airway.

2. Which of the following methods for maintaining an open airway should be used on an unconscious victim with a head injury?

    a. chin lift only.
    b. head-tilt/chin-lift.
    c. modified jaw thrust.
    d. head-tilt/neck-lift.

3. A subdural hematoma of the brain is:

    a. bleeding due to tearing of a blood vessel on the surface of the brain.
    b. swelling of the brain tissue.
    c. bruising of the brain tissue.
    d. bleeding between the skull and protective covering of the brain.

4. Brain damage is usually far more severe in a/an _____ than in a/an _____.

    a. closed head injury/open head injury.
    b. open head injury/closed head injury.
    c. basal skull fracture/depressed skull fracture.
    d. stroke/comminuted fracture.

5. When a foreign object is impaled in the skull, the First Aider should:

    a. not remove the object, but carefully stabilize it in place.
    b. remove the object and apply a loose sterile dressing.
    c. not remove the object unless it will hinder transportation.
    d. remove the object and pack the wound carefully with sterile pads.

6. Place in order the following steps in the primary assessment of a victim with suspected head and spinal-cord injuries: (1) maintain an open airway; (2) check the neck and spine; (3) check motor function; (4) check the head; (5) check the extremities.

    a. 1, 3, 4, 2, 5.
    b. 1, 2, 3, 4, 5.
    c. 1, 4, 3, 2, 5.
    d. 1, 4, 2, 3, 5.

7. A comminuted skull fracture is one where:

    a. the fracture is not in the area of impact or injury.
    b. the skull is depressed.
    c. scalp laceration and brain laceration are present.
    d. multiple cracks radiate from the center of impact.

8. When the victim has a bleeding, open head wound, the First Aider should:

    a. apply a snug pressure bandage.
    b. apply a loose sterile dressing to aid the clotting process.
    c. apply pressure to the carotid artery.
    d. lightly apply pressure to the wound with sterile dressings.

9. What is the most important guide to gauging the severity of a head injury?

    a. the victim's response to pain stimulus.
    b. level of consciousness.
    c. draining of cerebrospinal fluid.
    d. paralysis of the limbs.

10. What is the most common characteristic of Battle's sign?

    a. unequal dilation of the pupils.
    b. discoloration of the soft tissue under the eyes.
    c. a bruise-like mark behind either ear.
    d. one eye that appears sunken.

11. In a head laceration where the injury causes an opening to the brain, you should:
    a. apply direct pressure to the laceration to stop the bleeding.
    b. lightly cover the laceration but do not pack it to restrict bleeding or fluid flow.
    c. apply direct pressure to the laceration but release it periodically to reduce pressure in the brain.
    d. cover with an occlusive dressing to prevent contamination.

12. The *most* important clue in head injuries is:
    a. how the victim responds to pain stimulus.
    b. the level of consciousness.
    c. how the victim changes.
    d. the victim's ability to move.

13. Amnesia from a concussion is generally:
    a. temporary and normal.
    b. an indication of more serious damage.
    c. concussion.
    d. ordinary for one to two weeks.

14. An epidural hematoma:
    a. is less serious than a subdural hematoma.
    b. is caused by pooling of venous blood.
    c. is caused by blood pooling between the skull and protective covering of the brain.
    d. can be relieved by elevating the head.

15. A concussion is:
    a. trauma to the head.
    b. observable brain damage.
    c. loss of consciousness.
    d. temporary loss of the brain's ability to function.

16. Which of the following is an event in an acceleration-deceleration injury to the brain?
    a. the brain is slapped against the skull as the head is hurled forward.
    b. the brain rebounds against the other side of the skull.
    c. the skull stops suddenly and the brain is smashed against it.
    d. all of these answers.

| PART III: Matching | Match the descriptive terms in the right-hand column with the correct signs and symptoms in the left-hand column. |

Signs and Symptoms

_____ 1. Pulse.

_____ 2. Temperature.

_____ 3. Limbs.

_____ 4. Blood pressure.

_____ 5. Vomiting.

_____ 6. Bowel and bladder.

_____ 7. Facial movements.

_____ 8. Headache.

_____ 9. Pupils.

_____ 10. Battle's sign.

Descriptive Terms That May Indicate Head Injury

A. Especially, if forceful.

B. Inability to control.

C. Asymmetry.

D. Slowing.

E. Slowing and increase.

F. Slow or rapid.

G. Severe.

H. Rigid.

I. Rise.

J. Unequal size.

K. Bluish tinge of skin surrounding ear.

| PART IV: What Would You Do If: |

1. A five-year-old child falls off a high fence, hitting his head on a concrete driveway. He has an open wound on the forehead, he is unconscious, and he has blood-tinged fluid draining from his left ear.

2. You are at a park where a teenage boy has been hit in the head with a baseball. He is in a prone position and has a large swelling on the side of his head. Bystanders say that he has been unconscious, but he is conscious now. He seems confused, restless, and irritable and is vomiting.

| PART V: Practical Skills Check-Off | _____ has satisfactorily passed the following practical skills: |
| | Student's Name |

	Date	Partner Check	Inst. Init.
1. Describe and demonstrate how to assess for possible spinal injury in a head-injured victim.	___/___/___	☐	_____

CHAPTER THIRTEEN

OBJECTIVES

- Describe the common mechanisms of spinal injury.
- Describe and demonstrate how to assess for spinal-cord injury.
- Recognize the signs and symptoms of spinal injury.
- Describe and demonstrate how to give emergency care and immobilize a spine-injured victim.

When possible, it is best to leave the care of suspected spinal injuries to professional rescue personnel. Do not attempt emergency-care procedures unless you have been trained adequately. Always follow local protocol.

INJURIES TO THE SPINE

S PINAL-CORD injuries are some of the most formidable and traumatic injuries to care for: spinal-cord injury affects most other organ systems, and improper handling can kill the victim.

Spinal injury can result from any force that pushes the spine beyond its normal weight-bearing ability or its normal limits of motion. Any trauma severe enough to cause injury to the brain (including a simple fall) can also cause injury to the spine. Especially prone to injury are the **CERVICAL** and **LUMBAR SPINE**. You should always suspect spinal-cord injury if head injury exists. If any vertebrae are crushed or displaced, the cord at that point may be severed, torn, compressed, or stretched, causing permanent damage.

The four top causes of spinal-cord injury, in order, are car accidents, shallow-water swimming/diving accidents, motorcycle accidents, and other injuries and falls. Fifty percent of all spinal-cord accidents result in paralysis from the neck down; the other half produce paralysis from the waist down.

Most victims of spinal injury are males (by a four-to-one ratio when compared to females) between the ages of fifteen and thirty. Approximately 43 percent are related to motor-vehicle accidents, and another 21 percent are attributable to violent crimes. Many sports — including diving/swimming, skiing, sledding, and football — cause accidents that lead to spinal damage.

Some parts of the spine are far more susceptible to injury than others. Half of all spinal injuries occur in the neck, and half of those result in complete paralysis. Fewer injuries involve the **THORACIC VERTEBRAE** or the **SACRAL** and **COCCYGEAL VERTEBRAE**, which have little movement but are designed to bear weight (Figure 13-1).

Spinal injuries affect not only the spine, but often most other organ and bodily functions; improperly assessed and treated, they can result in catastrophic changes in a victim's quality of life. Obviously, proper emergency care is critical.

Do not attempt any of the procedures described in this chapter without adequate training and practice.

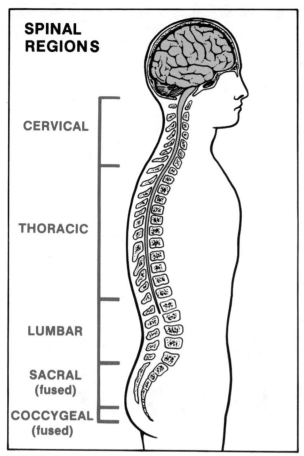

FIGURE 13-1.

mechanism of injury suggests it, even if your assessment does not indicate spinal-cord damage. *Always suspect spinal-cord damage if the victim has extreme discomfort in the neck, if he cannot turn his neck from side to side, or if he suffers numbness in his hands and/or feet (Figure 13-3). Paralysis or pain, pain upon movement, or tenderness anywhere along the spine are reliable indicators of possible spinal-cord injury.*

If the victim is unconscious, assume that he has suffered spinal-cord injury and give emergency care accordingly. If the victim is conscious, perform the following assessment (the victim should be able to pass all tests easily and without pain or restriction (see Chapter 12, Figures 12-6–12-9):

1. Touch the victim's foot and leg; ask him if he feels your touch. Repeat with the other foot and leg.
2. Ask the victim to wiggle his toes.
3. Touch the victim's hand and arm; ask him if he feels your touch. Repeat with the other hand and arm.
4. Ask the victim to wiggle his fingers.
5. Ask the victim to grasp your hand as though he were going to shake your hand; then ask him to squeeze your hand. His grip should be strong and firm and should not cause pain. Have him repeat the procedure with his other hand.

MECHANISMS OF SPINAL INJURY

The basic mechanisms that cause spinal injury include the following (Figure 13-2):

▪ Sudden compression (the weight of the body is driven against the head).
▪ Distraction (sudden "pulling apart" of the spine stretches and tears the cord).
▪ Excessive rotation.
▪ Excessive flexion or extension.
▪ Sudden, forceful lateral bending.

ASSESSMENT OF SPINAL-CORD INJURY

Remember that even if a victim can move or walk around, he may still be injured. Therefore, always treat as if spinal-cord injury is present if the

SIGNS AND SYMPTOMS OF SPINAL INJURY

Remember that a fracture of one spot on the spine usually is associated with a fracture in other areas of the spine. The general signs and symptoms of spinal injury include the following (Figure 13-4):

▪ Pain that accompanies movement; suspect spinal injury if the victim complains of pain when moving an apparently uninjured neck, shoulders, or legs. Pain from spinal injury may be localized, and the victim should be able to indicate exactly where it hurts. *Never ask the victim to move, never allow him to move, and never move him yourself to test pain; base your assessment on any movement that occurred before you arrived on the scene.*

▪ Pain independent of movement. Such pain is generally intermittent instead of constant, and it may occur anywhere along the spine between the top of the head and the tops of the legs. If the lower spinal cord or column is injured, the victim may feel pain in his legs.

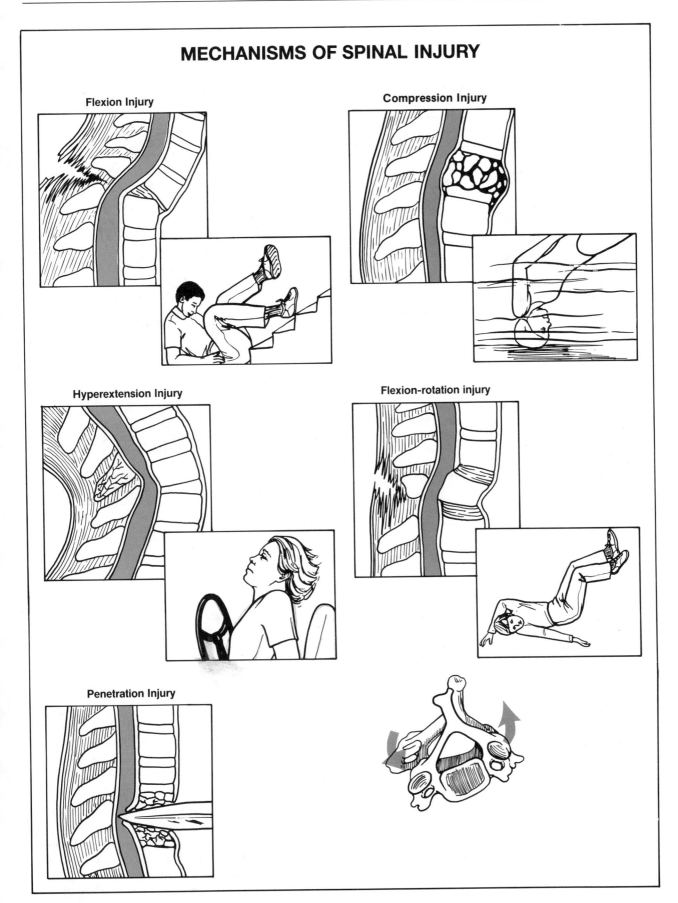

MECHANISMS OF SPINAL INJURY

Flexion Injury

Compression Injury

Hyperextension Injury

Flexion-rotation injury

Penetration Injury

FIGURE 13-2.

CONSIDERATIONS IN CERVICAL SPINE INJURY

NOTE:
Persons with neck injuries may have paralyzed chest muscles and damage to nerves affecting size of blood vessels. Breathing can **then** be accomplished only by the diaphragm. Inadequate breathing and shock may occur.

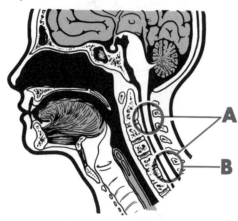

Spine injuries are most common at the cervical level (A). The prime hazard is cord damage (B), which may result from trauma per se or from well-meaning but injudicious management **following** the accident. RULE: In all cases of neck injury, treat the victim as if there **is** a cervical fracture, until proven otherwise.

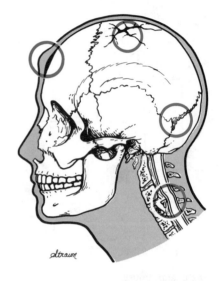

REMEMBER: Take spinal-injury precautions in **all** cases of head trauma, as well as all cases of multiple trauma involving unconsciousness, particularly if resuscitative measures are required at the accident site.

FIGURE 13-3.

■ Lacerations, cuts, punctures, or bruises over or around the spine (these indicate forceful injury). Injuries of the cervical spine may be accompanied by bruises or cuts on the head or face.

■ Obvious deformity of the spine (not a usual sign). *Never have the victim remove his clothing in order to examine his back, since the movement may aggravate any existing injury. The clothing can be cut away.*

■ Loss of response to pain or other stimuli.

■ Numbness, tingling, or weakness in the arms and/or legs.

■ Weakness, loss of sensation, or paralysis below the level of injury. In a conscious victim, paralysis of the extremities is considered the most reliable sign of spinal injury.

■ Loss of function in either the upper or lower extremities.

■ Tenderness during gentle palpation.

■ Impaired breathing, especially breathing that involves little or no chest movement and only slight abdominal movement (an indication that the victim is breathing with the diaphragm alone). The diaphragm may continue to function even though the chest wall muscles are paralyzed.

■ Loss of bowel and/or bladder control.

■ Signs and symptoms of severe shock. Neurogenic shock, while often self-limiting, is severe when the nervous system has been injured and no longer controls the dilation and constriction of the blood vessels. You should suspect spinal injury in a victim with severe shock, even if there are no other signs or symptoms of spinal injury.

SIGNS OF POSSIBLE SPINAL CORD INJURY

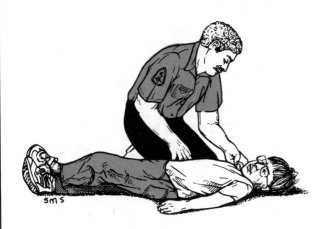

PAIN. The victim may be aware of unprovoked pain in the area of injury.

TENDERNESS. Gently touching the suspected area may result in increased pain.

DEFORMITY. Deformity is rare, although there may be an abnormal bend or bony prominence.

CUTS AND BRUISES. Victims with neck fractures may have cuts and bruises on the head, or face. Victims with injuries in other areas of the spine will have bruises on the shoulders, back, or abdomen.

PARALYSIS. If the victim is unable to move or feels no sensation in some part of his body, he may have a spinal fracture, with cord injury.

PAINFUL MOVEMENT. If the victim tries to move, the pain may increase — never try to move the injured area for the victim.

STEPS FOR CHECKING SIGNS AND SYMPTOMS

CONSCIOUS VICTIMS	UNCONSCIOUS VICTIMS
■ Ask: What happened? Where does it hurt? Can you move your hands and feet? Can you feel me touching your hands (feet)? Can you raise your legs and arms?	■ Assess for breathing.
■ Look: for bruises, cuts, deformities.	■ Look: for cuts, bruises, deformities.
■ Feel: for areas of tenderness, deformity, abnormal sensation.	■ Feel: for deformities, sensation.
	■ Ask others: What happened?
■ The victim's strength can be determined by having him squeeze the rescuer's hand or by checking pressure against the foot (Figure 12-6–12-9 in Chapter 12).	■ Probe the soles of the feet, then the palms of the hands with a sharp object to check for response.

FIGURE 13-4.

EMERGENCY CARE FOR SPINAL INJURY

The general rule for management of spinal injury is to support and immobilize the spine, the head, the torso, and the pelvis. Your goal is to end up with a victim who is immobilized properly on a long **SPINE BOARD** or other rigid support (Figure 13-5). When in doubt, always immobilize a victim you even *suspect* of having spinal injury; it is best to over-treat than to risk further injury.

General guidelines for care are:

1. The first priority is to ensure an adequate air supply by maintaining an open airway and adequate ventilations.

■ Unless the victim complains of pain when you do so, place the head in a neutral position and maintain that position manually until the victim can be fastened to a full-body immobilizer.

■ Administer artificial ventilation as necessary.

■ If the victim complains when you attempt to position the head, do not persist. Immobilize the head as found.

■ If the victim's throat is blocked by his tongue, lift the chin straight up without moving or hyperextending the neck; use the modified jaw-thrust technique.

■ If the victim is still not getting enough air, administer artificial ventilation.

EMERGENCY CARE FOR SUSPECTED SPINAL INJURY

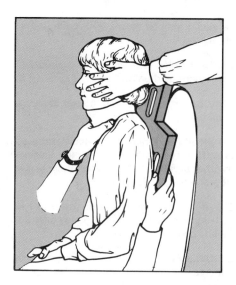

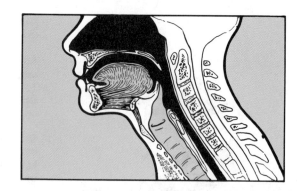

Take every precaution against converting a spinal injury into cord damage. In vehicular accidents, immobilize cervical spine before removing victim (spine board, cervical collar, rolled blanket, etc.). Advise the conscious victim not to move the head. A helmet should be removed unless there is difficulty in removing it. *Follow local protocol.* In such cases, immobilize on spine board with helmet in place.

Is there respiratory difficulty? Remember that the airway has first priority. If resuscitative measures are indicated, support the head, immobilize the neck,and move the victim to a flat surface with help. Check the mouth for obstruction (dentures, tongue, etc.), and ventilate, giving all care to minimize motion of the neck. Control severe bleeding by direct pressure. If necessary, initiate CPR.

Keep in mind that respiratory paralysis may occur with cervical spine injury and that death may occur rapidly if respiratory assistance is delayed. Unless it is necessary to change a victim's position to maintain an open airway or there is some other compelling reason, it is best to splint the neck or back in the original position of deformity.

Be alert for shock and vomiting. If necessary, administer artificial ventilation.

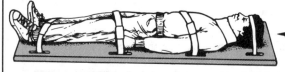

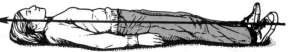

Immobilize victim before moving. As soon as possible, transfer to a firm stretcher or spine board and restrict head movement with tape, sandbags, collar, rolled towels, and/or blankets.

Provide emotional support, and activate the EMS system as soon as possible.

Always support the head in neutral alignment with body. Avoid flexion, extension, lateral movement, rotation, and traction.

FIGURE 13-5.

- Ensure an adequate airway continuously throughout emergency care. Underventilation is the most serious problem in head and spinal injury.

2. Maintain a neutral position of the head and neck (Figure 13-6). If you encounter resistance, stabilize the neck in the position in which you find it.

3. Stabilize the head and neck while another rescuer removes the victim's jewelry, etc. Holding the victim's hair out of the way and keeping the head and neck in normal anatomical position, apply a rigid cervical collar (Figure 13-7) or extrication collar (if available and you are trained to do so). (See Chapter 12, Figures 12-17–12-18, 12-20). This will act as a temporary immobilizer and protect the victim's airway when you have inadequate manpower or multiple victims. Remember that a collar is like most splints: it requires application by two trained rescuers — one to immobilize manually, and the other to apply the hardware.

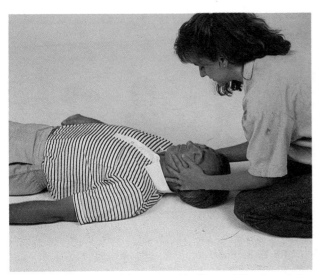

FIGURE 13-6. Maintaining neutral in-line stabilization of the head and neck.

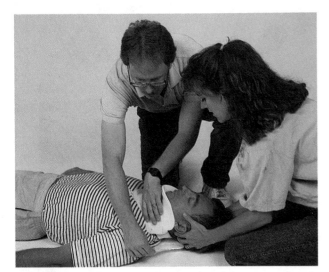

FIGURE 13-7. Support the head and neck in a neutral position while applying a cervical collar.

- Be sure to use a collar of the proper size for the victim. If you do, the victim's head will be in a neutral position, but in order to talk to you he will have to speak with his teeth clenched.

- If you do not have a collar, improvise one with a blanket (see Chapter 12, Figure 12-19). Maintain a neutral position while you are applying the collar, and have another rescuer maintain a neutral position continuously until the victim is secured to a long spine board. Make sure that the collar fits the victim properly: it should fit firmly under the chin and snugly against the collarbone.

4. Check pulse and circulation; perform cardio-pulmonary resuscitation if necessary, but do not move the victim.

   - Control any hemorrhage that is threatening life.

   - Never try to stop the flow of blood from the nose or ears — it could contain cerebrospinal fluid and cause a fatal buildup of pressure.

   - Never apply pressure to a bleeding head wound if you suspect skull fracture; you could push fragments of skull into brain tissue.

5. Secure the victim to a rigid support, preferably a long spine board, as soon as all life-threatening conditions have been stabilized.

   - If you have to turn the victim over to get him on the backboard, logroll him as a unit with his head aligned and without moving his neck (Figures 13-8 and 13-9). Maintain manual stabilization, keeping the body in alignment.

   - To position the victim on the backboard, place the board parallel to the victim. Roll the victim on his side, maintaining neutral position of the head and neck, slide the board under the victim, and return him to a supine position on the board (Figures 13-10–13-12).

6. Strap the victim securely to the backboard; the torso should not be able to move or shift in any direction (Figure 13-13).

   - The victim should be strapped at his shoulders, chest, hips, knees, and ankles with his wrists tied loosely together; make sure that straps do not cause pressure at the sites of other injury.

   - Strap the victim's head down last so that any body movement during strapping will not cause movement in the neck.

   - The strap across the chest should not be so tight that it inhibits movement of the chest muscles and impairs breathing.

   - Use extreme caution during strapping so that you do not rotate the victim when applying and tightening straps.

   - The victim's head should be firmly strapped or taped to the board and surrounded with rolled towels, rolled blankets, or some other pliable objects. If you place light padding under the head, you can help prevent hyperextension of the neck; however, use caution not to flex the neck. Never place padding behind the neck itself. If the victim vomits, your strapping

THREE-RESCUER LOGROLL FOR SPINAL INJURY

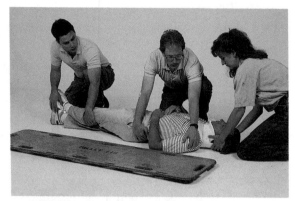

FIGURE 13-8. Maintain support for the head and neck while preparing for logroll.

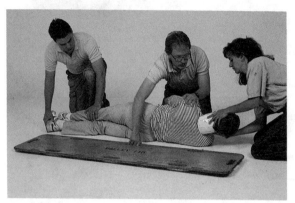

FIGURE 13-9. Roll victim onto side at command of rescuer, maintaining in-line stabilization.

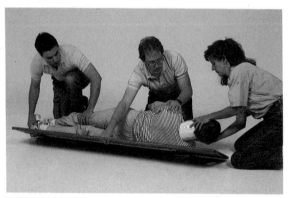

FIGURE 13-10. Examine the back, and move spine board into place.

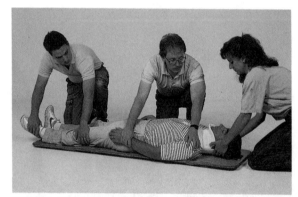

FIGURE 13-11. Lower victim onto spine board at command of rescuer maintaining in-line stabilization, and center victim on the board.

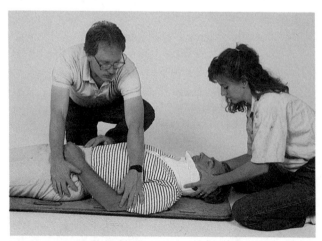

FIGURE 13-12. Maintain in-line stabilization while positioning victim on a long spine board.

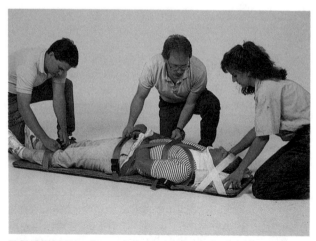

FIGURE 13-13. Strap victim securely to the backboard.

technique should be good enough to enable you to roll the victim onto his left side several times without any change in body position.

■ If the victim is found in a sitting position (Figures 13-14), apply a cervical collar, then immobilize with a short spine board; take care not to put the chin strap or chin cup on the victim (it prevents him from opening his mouth if he needs to vomit).

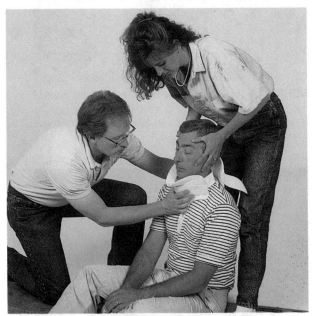

FIGURE 13-14. Maintain in-line stabilization while applying a cervical collar on a victim in a sitting position.

■ **Note:** Anytime a victim vigorously resists the placement of an immobilizer, consider eliminating it, even to the point of not immobilizing that part of the victim's body at all. It may be that in some instances, a victim can harm himself more by struggling against an immobilizer than by lying quietly without one.

7. Treat for shock. Cover the victim to avoid heat loss, but do not allow overheating. Elevate the foot of the long board about twelve inches.

HELMET REMOVAL

The key to finding disorders of any kind is in looking for them in the first place. Thorough assessment is impossible as long as the victim is fully clothed, and that applies especially to protective headgear. The only time when a helmet should not be removed in the field is when the victim complains of pain during removal. *Follow local protocol regarding removing of helmets; it is controversial in some areas, and should only be done if the rescuer has had appropriate training and emergency personnel are not available.*

Always involve at least two rescuers. Never attempt to remove a helmet yourself; wait for help. If the victim requires resuscitation in the meantime, remove the faceguard or shield and perform resuscitation without removing the helmet. As mentioned, if the victim complains of increased pain when you try to remove the helmet, leave the helmet on and immobilize the head.

The steps for removal of a full-face helmet are as follows:

1. If there is a chin strap, unfasten it (Figure 13-15).

2. One rescuer applies manual neutral positioning for the head, while a second rescuer grasps the helmet and pulls both lower margins away from the victim's head (Figure 13-16). This provides added clearance for the victim's ears.

3. The second rescuer slips the helmet off of the victim's head, while the first rescuer continues to maintain neutral positioning (Figure 13-17–13-18).

4. The second rescuer discards the helmet and assumes responsibility for neutral positioning of the head, while the first rescuer obtains and applies a firm cervical collar (extrication type) of the correct size (see Figures 13-6 and 13-7). The victim's spine is then further immobilized by means of a backboard and immobilizer for the head.

HELMET REMOVAL

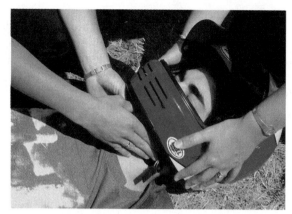

FIGURE 13-15. Maintain manual neutral positioning and unfasten chin strap.

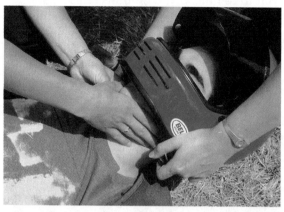

FIGURE 13-16. One rescuer applies manual neutral positioning while the second rescuer grasps the helmet and pulls both lower margins away from the victim's head.

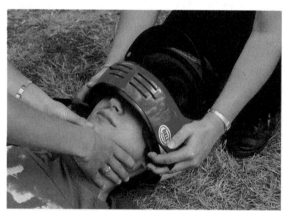

FIGURE 13-17. The second rescuer slips the helmet off of the victim's head, while the other rescuer continues to maintain neutral positioning.

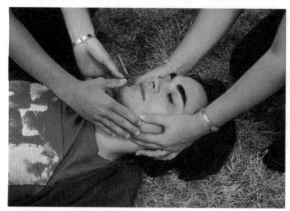

FIGURE 13-18. After the helmet is removed, neutral positioning is maintained in preparation for application of a rigid extrication collar.

Helmet removal can be dangerous and should not be performed by a First Aider unless absolutely necessary and he has had appropriate training. Always follow local protocol.

| 13 | **SELF-TEST** | 13 |

Student: _____ Date: _____

Course: _____ Section #: _____

PART I: True/False   If you believe that the statement is true, circle the T. If you believe that the statement is false, circle the F.

T   F   1. Most victims of spinal injury are males between the ages of twelve and fifteen.

T   F   2. The thoracic spine is the most easily injured region of the spine.

T   F   3. It is not possible for a spine-injured victim to move or walk around.

T   F   4. A fracture on one place of the spine is usually associated with fractures in other areas of the spine.

T   F   5. Spinal-injury precautions should be taken in all cases of head trauma.

T   F   6. The general rule for management of spinal injury is to support and immobilize the spine, the head, the torso, and the pelvis.

T   F   7. Even if the victim complains of pain, place the head in a neutral position.

T   F   8. The airway is the first priority in a spine-injured victim.

T   F   9. Ask the spine-injured victim to remove his shirt so that you can inspect his back.

T   F   10. You should suspect spine injury in a victim of severe shock.

T   F   11. Fifty percent of all spinal-cord injuries result in paralysis from the neck down.

T   F   12. Always immobilize a spine-injured victim, even if they vigorously resist.

T   F   13. With proper precautions one rescuer can safely remove a victim's helmet.

T   F   14. Once a spine-injured victim has been secured to a rigid support elevate the foot end about twelve inches.

T   F   15. Always pad behind the neck of the victim when on a rigid support.

T   F   16. Applying a cervical collar requires two rescuers.

T   F   17. Respiratory paralysis may occur with cervical-spine injury.

T   F   18. Overventilation is a serious problem in head and spinal injury.

T   F   19. Any trauma severe enough to cause injury to the brain can also cause injury to the spine.

T   F   20. Hyperextension of the neck is the best procedure for opening the airway of a spine-injured victim.

PART II: Multiple Choice   For each question, circle the answer that best reflects an accurate statement.

1. The largest number of cervical-spine injuries are due to:
    a. falls.
    b. acts of violence.
    c. motor-vehicle accidents.
    d. sports injuries.

2. Which of the following is *not* a sign of spinal injury?
    a. numbness and tingling in arms and/or legs.
    b. loss of response to pain.
    c. loss of bowel or bladder control.
    d. position of the legs.

3. What is the initial procedure if spinal-cord injury is suspected?
    a. establish a secure airway.
    b. stop hemorrhage.
    c. treat for shock.
    d. move the victim to a more comfortable position.

4. To maintain an airway for a person who you suspect has a spinal injury:
    a. have a trained professional perform a tracheotomy.
    b. use the chin lift or modified jaw-thrust technique.
    c. hyperextend the neck.
    d. use the head-tilt/chin-lift technique.

5. The areas of the spine most susceptible to injury are:
    a. mid-thoracic, upper lumbar.
    b. lower thoracic, coccyx.
    c. lumbar, coccyx.
    d. cervical, lumbar.

6. When should a helmet *not* be removed when there is a suspected head injury?
    a. if the victim complains of increased pain as a result of attempts to remove the helmet.
    b. when the victim is unconscious.
    c. when the victim has a head injury.
    d. all of these answers.

7. A First Aider can check for spinal-cord damage in a conscious victim by:
   a. asking the victim to wiggle his fingers and toes.
   b. asking the victim to speak.
   c. asking the victim to read.
   d. checking the victim's reflexes at the knees or elbows.

8. In most cases, victims with suspected spinal injuries should be transported to a medical center:
   a. as quickly as possible.
   b. after immobilization with a spine board.
   c. in any comfortable position.
   d. after vital signs have been stabilized.

9. Most spinal-cord injury victims are:
   a. elderly men.
   b. young men.
   c. teenagers.
   d. young women.

10. Which of the following statements about emergency care of spinal injuries is *not* true?
    a. open airway with modified jaw-thrust technique.
    b. help the victim move into a comfortable position.
    c. advise the conscious victim not to move his head.
    d. in-line support should be applied to the head.

11. Paralysis of the lower extremities may indicate spinal-cord damage in the:
    a. neck.
    b. upper back.
    c. entire length below the neck.
    d. lower back.

PART III: What Would You Do If:

1. You are going to a small outdoor swimming pool, where a teenage boy has dived into the pool and hit his head on the bottom. When you arrive, you find that his friends have removed him from the pool. He is unconscious and in a supine position.

2. You are at the scene of an automobile accident and find a woman who was thrown out of one of the vehicles. She is in a sitting position, has a large forehead laceration, and is complaining of neck pain.

PART IV: Practical Skills Check-Off

_____ has satisfactorily passed the following practical skills:
Student's Name

	Date	Partner Check	Inst. Init.
1. Demonstrate how to assess for suspected spinal injury.	__/__/__	☐	_____
2. Demonstrate how to maintain neutral in-line stabilization of the head and neck.	__/__/__	☐	_____
3. Demonstrate how to apply a cervical collar.	__/__/__	☐	_____
4. Demonstrate how to immobilize a suspected spine-injured victim.	__/__/__	☐	_____

CHAPTER FOURTEEN

OBJECTIVES

■ Describe and demonstrate how to give emergency care for a foreign object in the eye.

■ Describe and demonstrate how to give appropriate emergency care for common eye injuries involving the orbits, eyelids, globe, impaled objects and eviscerated eyeball.

■ Describe the basic rules for emergency eye care.

INJURIES TO THE EYE

Few true **OCULAR** (eye) emergencies occur, but when they do, they tend to be very urgent. It is important that you be well enough informed to suspect them in the appropriate settings (Figure 14-1).

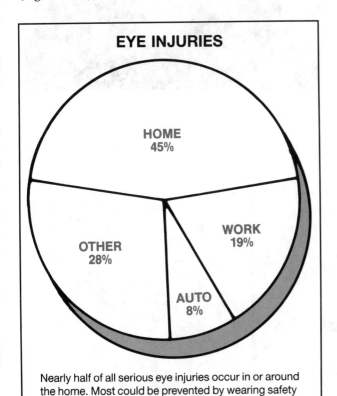

EYE INJURIES

HOME
45%

OTHER
28%

WORK
19%

AUTO
8%

Nearly half of all serious eye injuries occur in or around the home. Most could be prevented by wearing safety glasses while doing chores.

Source: Katherine A. Randall, *Sightsaving.*

FIGURE 14-1.

FOREIGN OBJECTS IN THE EYE

Foreign objects, such as particles of dirt, sand, cinders, coal dust, or fine pieces of metal, frequently are blown or driven into the eye and lodge there. They not only cause discomfort, but if not removed may cause **INFLAMMATION** or possible infection, and/or may scratch the **CORNEA**. Fortunately, through an increased flow of tears, nature dislodges many of these substances before any harm is done. In no case should the eye be rubbed, since rubbing may cause scratching of the delicate eye tissues or force a foreign particle with sharp edges into the tissues, making removal difficult. It is always much safer for the First Aider to transport the person to a physician or activate the EMS system than to attempt to remove foreign particles from the eye.

However, if removal of a foreign particle is necessary, the procedure is as follows:

1. Flush the eye with clean water, if available, holding the eyelids apart (Figure 14-2). *Follow local protocol* — some EMS systems do not recommend flushing the eye except in cases of chemical burns.

2. Often, a foreign object lodged under the upper eyelid can be removed by drawing the upper lid down over the lower lid; as the upper lid returns to its normal position, the undersurfaces will be drawn over the lashes of the lower lid and the foreign body removed by the wiping action of the eyelashes.

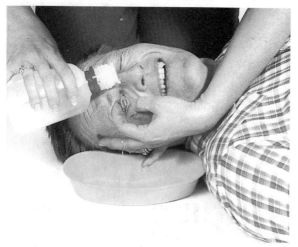

FIGURE 14-2. Flushing foreign particle out of the eye.

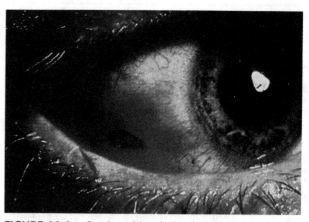

FIGURE 14-4. Foreign object lodged in the eye.

3. A foreign object in the eye also may be removed by grasping the eyelashes of the upper lid and turning the lid over a cotton swab or similar object (Figure 14-3). The particle may then be carefully removed from the eyelid with the corner of a piece of sterile gauze.

4. Particles lodged under the lower lid may be removed by pulling down the lower lid, exposing the inner surface (Figure 14-3). The corner of a piece of sterile gauze can be used to remove the foreign object.

Should a foreign object become lodged in the eyeball, (Figure 14-4), do not attempt to disturb it, as it may be forced deeper into the eye and result in further damage. Place a bandage compress over *both eyes* (Figure 14-5).

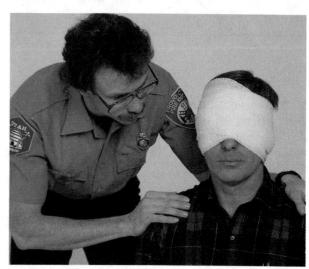

FIGURE 14-5. If a foreign object becomes lodged in an eye, bandage both eyes to minimize motion.

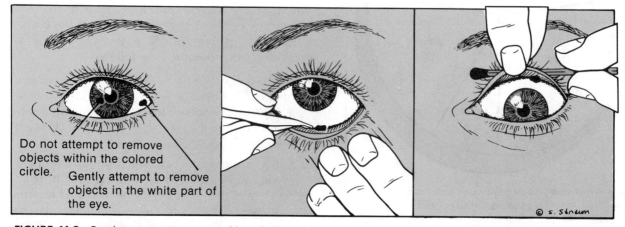

Do not attempt to remove objects within the colored circle. Gently attempt to remove objects in the white part of the eye.

FIGURE 14-3. Gently attempt to remove objects in the white part of the eye. Using two fingers, gently pull down the lower eyelid while the victim looks up. Carefully pull up the upper eyelid as the victim looks down. A matchstick or cotton swab can help you to grip the lid as shown.

Gentleness is essential in handling eye injuries. If difficulty is experienced in removing a foreign object from the eye, transport the victim to the hospital at once.

INJURY TO THE ORBITS

Trauma to the face may result in the fracture of one or several of the bones of the skull that form the **ORBITS** (eye sockets). A victim with an **ORBITAL FRACTURE** may complain of double vision and, due to nerve damage, may manifest loss of sensation above the eyebrow or over the cheek. In some cases, massive nasal discharge may occur; in others, markedly decreased vision (Figure 14-6).

Fractures of the lower part of the socket are the most common and can cause paralysis of upward gaze (the victim's eyes will not be able to follow your finger upward). Hence, it is important to check all possible eye movements in the victim sustaining possible facial fractures.

Orbital fractures require hospitalization and possible surgery.

1. Activate the EMS system, and keep the victim in a sitting position.
2. If no associated injury to the **GLOBE** (eyeball) is apparent, ice packs may be used over the injured area to reduce swelling.

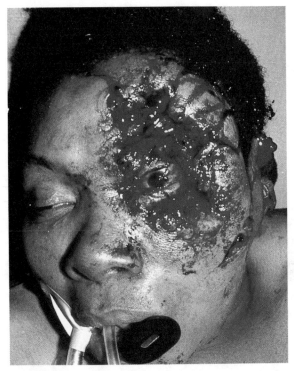

FIGURE 14-6.   Eye orbit injury.

3. However, if globe injury is suspected, or if you are in doubt, avoid using ice packs and keep the victim in a supine position.

LID INJURIES

Lid injuries include ecchymosis (black eyes), burns, and lacerations (Figure 14-7). In general, little can be done for these injuries in the field beyond gentle patching. First aid consists of controlling bleeding and protecting the injured tissue and underlying structures as you would any soft-tissue injury.

1. Eyelid bleeding can be profuse but usually can be controlled with light pressure. Only a light dressing should be used, and *no* pressure should be used if the eyeball itself is injured.
2. Cover the uninjured eye with a bandage to decrease movement of the injured eye.
3. If the eyelids do not cover the eyeball, use a light, moist dressing to prevent drying.

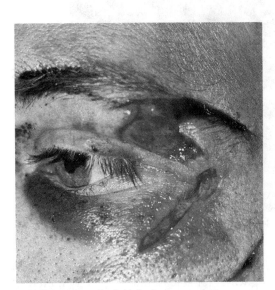

FIGURE 14-7.   Eyelid injury.

INJURIES TO THE GLOBE

Injuries to the globe include bruising, lacerations, foreign objects, and abrasions and generally are best treated in the emergency department, where specialized equipment is available. Patches lightly applied to *both* eyes and keeping the victim in a supine position are all that are necessary in the field. Cold compresses may give some pain relief. The exceptions are chemical burns, especially **ALKALINE** burns, which rapidly lead to total blindness. In any victim suffering chemical burns to the eye, try to determine the cause of the burn and, if possible, send the substance with the victim to the emergency room. The victim should be kept flat on his back.

CHEMICAL BURNS OF THE EYE

Quite common, chemical burns of the eye (Figure 14-8) constitute the most urgent emergency related to eye injuries; the first ten minutes following injury are crucial to the final outcome. In all chemical burns of the eye, begin immediate, continuous **IRRIGATION** with water; it need not be sterile, but should be clean.

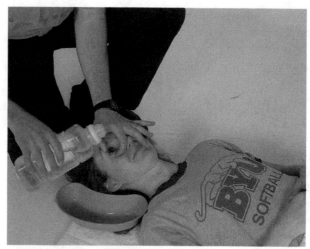

FIGURE 14-9. Chemical burns of the eye should be continuously irrigated for fifteen to thirty minutes.

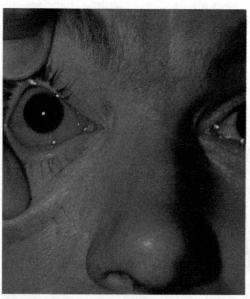

FIGURE 14-8. Chemical burn of the eye.

1. Continuously irrigate the affected eye with running water for at least fifteen to thirty minutes, beginning as soon as you encounter the victim (Figure 14-9).

2. Contact lenses must be removed or flushed out; if not, they will trap chemicals between the contact lens and the cornea. *Follow local protocol.*

3. Remove any solid particles from the surface of the eye with a moistened cotton swab.

4. It may be easiest to place the victim on his side, with a basin or towels under his head, and to direct clean water into the eye while gently holding the eyelid open.

5. You may have to force the lids open, since the victim may be unable to do so because of pain.

6. Irrigation should be continued until medical help is obtained.

7. Do not use any irrigants other than clean water.

8. Never irrigate the eye with any chemical antidote, including dilute vinegar, sodium bicarbonate, or alcohol.

9. If only one eye is affected, irrigate away from the unaffected eye.

10. Activate the EMS system.

IMPALED OBJECTS IN THE EYE

Objects impaled or embedded in the eye (Figure 14-10) should be removed only by a physician. Penetrating objects must be protected from accidental movement or removal until the victim receives medical attention.

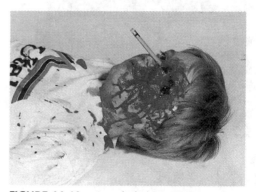

FIGURE 14-10. Impaled object in eye.

Impaled objects in the eye should be treated with great urgency, especially if a metallic object is involved; it can rust rapidly, leaving a permanent rust ring.

To give emergency care for impaled objects in the eye:

1. Manipulate the eye as little as possible during emergency care.

2. Tell the victim that both eyes must be bandaged to protect the injured eye.

3. Stabilize the head with sandbags or large pads, and always activate the EMS system, keeping the victim on his back.

4. Encircle the eye with a gauze dressing or other suitable material, such as soft, sterile cloth; do not apply pressure.

5. Position a metal shield, a crushed cup, or a cone over the embedded object. The object should not touch the top or sides of the cup (Figure 14-11).

6. Hold the cup and dressing in place with a bandage compress or roller bandage that covers both eyes. It is important to bandage both eyes to prevent movement of the injured eye (Figure 14-12).

7. Give the victim nothing by mouth in case he needs general anesthesia when he reaches the hospital.

8. Never leave the victim alone, as he might panic with both eyes covered. Keep the victim in hand contact so that he will always know someone is there.

9. If the victim is unconscious, close his uninjured eye before bandaging to prevent drying of tissues, which can cause additional eye injury. Closing the eye allows normal tears to keep the eye moist.

EVISCERATED EYEBALL

During a serious injury, the eyeball may be knocked out of the socket (extruded or avulsed) (Figure 14-13). Do not attempt to replace the eyeball into the socket.

1. Cover the eye with a moist covering and a protective cup without applying pressure to the eye.

2. Apply a bandage compress or roller bandage that covers both eyes.

3. The victim should be kept in a face-up position with the head immobilized.

4. Activate the EMS system.

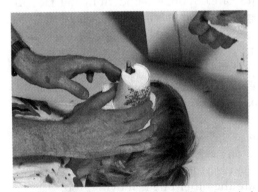

FIGURE 14-11. Dress and stabilize impaled object.

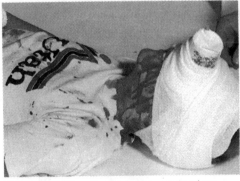

FIGURE 14-12. Bandage the cup in place.

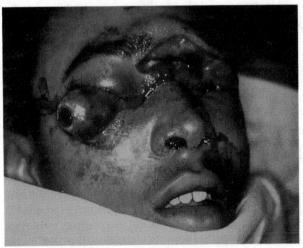

FIGURE 14-13. Extruded eyeball.

OTHER EYE INJURIES

In virtually all other medical emergencies involving the eye, you need only patch the affected eye and either transport the victim to the hospital or activate the EMS system. *Follow local protocol.* While many of these represent critical emergencies, there is little that you can accomplish besides safeguarding the eye from further irritation. Such situations include:

- Eye infections — these are manifested by redness and discharge of pus.

- Acute **GLAUCOMA** — the victim complains of eyeache, headache, nausea, and of seeing halos around lights. His eye is red, his pupil does not react to light, and his cornea is hazy. His eyeball is much harder — more swollen — than the "normal," soft-feeling eye. Glaucoma is an emergency that leads to blindness.

- **RETINAL DETACHMENT** — the victim complains of a curtain blocking his field of vision, together with light flashes or dark spots in front of his eyes. In this situation, *gentle care* is crucial. The victim should lie flat on his back while waiting for emergency personnel.

- **BLACK EYE** — any blow forceful enough to cause hemorrhage to the skin surrounding the eye may also damage the eye itself. It is difficult to determine whether the eyeball has been injured. One way is to ask the victim details about his eyesight. Vision is blurred in the ordinary black eye. However, if the opposing eye is covered and sight in the black eye is impaired, the eyeball probably has been damaged. Double vision with both eyes open also indicates eyeball damage. Activate the EMS system immediately.

- Cornea abrasion — depending on the severity of the scrape, the victim may require transport to an emergency room, usually to obtain medication for pain relief. Bandage both eyes; continue to calmly reassure the victim.

- **LIGHT BURNS** — welding flash, **SNOWBLINDNESS**. **ULTRAVIOLET LIGHT BURNS** of the cornea can be frighteningly painful, and they usually do not cause pain or signs and symptoms until three to six hours after exposure. Symptoms will disappear in two to five days. The victim should remain in a dark room and avoid additional exposure. The pain may be decreased by covering both eyes with a moist dressing and having the victim lie flat. The victim should be seen by a physician.

- **HEAT BURNS** — the eyelids may be the only area burned in a heat burn. Do not attempt to open the eyelids if they are burned. The eye should be covered loosely with a sterile, moist dressing, and the EMS system should be activated or the victim transported to a physician.

BASIC RULES FOR EMERGENCY EYE CARE

Remember these basic rules when giving emergency eye care:

- Do not irrigate the injured eye. *The obvious exception is a chemical or detergent injury to the eye.* If the injury does not involve chemicals, you will only end up scratching the eye surface. If the eye has been perforated, damage incurred in washing it will be irreversible.

- Do not put salves or medicine into the injured eye. They will probably do more harm than good. The physician is the only one equipped to administer medication.

- Do not remove blood or blood clots from the eye. Blood contains antiseptics that will help the injured eye. Bleeding from an eye injury is usually not severe enough to require **TRANSFUSION** or immediate care. Sponge blood from the face to help keep the victim comfortable. Leave the eye alone.

- Do not try to force the eyelid open unless you have to wash out chemicals.

- Have the victim lie down and keep quiet. Never let a victim with an eye injury walk without help, especially up or down stairs.

- Limit use of the *uninjured* eye; it usually is best to patch it along with the injured eye. Eyes move together, and if the victim is using one eye, chances are the other one is moving, too.

- Do not allow the victim to eat. In case general anesthesia is required at the hospital, food in the stomach will complicate the procedure.

- Never panic. It will upset the victim and cause you to lose valuable calmness needed in effective care.

- An eye emergency should always be seen by a physician.

| **14** | **SELF-TEST** | **14** |

Student: _____ Date: _____

Course: _____ Section #: _____

PART I: True/False   If you believe that the statement is true, circle the T. If you believe that the statement is false, circle the F.

T   F   1. Most eye injuries occur in the work-place setting.

(T) F   2. Both eyes should be bandaged if a foreign object is lodged in just one eye.

T   (F) 3. It is always best to gently try and remove an object lodged in the eyeball.

(T) F   4. Eyelid bleeding usually can be controlled with light pressure.

T   F   5. Moist dressings should never be used on the eye.

T   (F) 6. A chemical burn of the eye should be flushed (irrigated) for at least five minutes.

T   F   7. Never force the eyelids open in an attempt to irrigate a chemical burn.

T   (F) 8. Milk is a good irrigator for chemical burns of the eye.

T   F   9. The medical term for a retinal detachment is ecchymosis.

(T) F   10. It is best to irrigate all eye injuries with clean water.

(T) F   11. If a foreign object becomes lodged in an eye, bandage both eyes to minimize motion.

T   F   12. Fractures of the upper part of the eye socket are most common.

(T) F   13. Never use cold compresses on injuries to the globe.

(T) F   14. If the eyelids do not cover the eyeball in a lid injury, use a light, moist dressing to prevent drying.

T   (F) 15. Do not attempt to remove contact lenses, particularly in a chemical burn.

T   F   16. Even though only one eye is affected in a chemical burn always irrigate both eyes.

T   F   17. In retinal detachment the victim usually complains of seeing halos around lights.

T   F   18. Corneal abrasions can be serious but little pain is involved.

T   F   19. Do not attempt to open eyelids if they are burned.

(T) F   20. Do not remove blood or blood clots from the eye.

PART II: Multiple Choice   For each question, circle the answer that best reflects an accurate statement.

1. The first priority in treating a chemical burn to the eye is to:
   a. immediately begin irrigating the eye with clean water.
   b. immediately begin irrigating the eye with a chemical antidote.
   c. immediately instruct the victim to close the eye and transport him to a medical center.
   d. apply a cold compress to the affected eye.

2. If a pencil or other sharp object becomes impaled in the eye: (1) stabilize the head; (2) position a cup over the pencil and hold in place with roller bandage; (3) cover both eyes with a bandage; (4) position the victim on the unaffected side.
   a. 1, 2, and 3.
   b. 1, 2, 3, and 4.
   c. 1, 3, and 4.
   d. 1 and 2.

3. When a victim has a foreign object imbedded in the globe of the eye:
   a. remove the object and then dress and bandage the eye.
   b. place a loose dressing over the object.
   c. prepare a thick dressing and secure a protective cone over the impaled object, leaving the uninjured eye unbandaged.
   d. prepare a thick dressing and secure a protective cone over the object, bandaging the uninjured eye also.

4. If an eyeball is knocked out of the socket:
   a. do not attempt to put the eye back in the socket.
   b. cover the extruded eyeball with a thick dressing moistened with clean water.
   c. cover both the injured and uninjured eyes with a thick dressing.
   d. gently and carefully replace the eyeball in the socket and cover with a dressing.

5. To remove a piece of dust from the eye, the first effort should be to:

   a. turn the upper lid over a cotton swab and remove the object with sterile gauze.
   b. pull down the lower lid and use sterile gauze to wipe away the foreign object.
   c. flush the eye with clean water.
   d. draw the upper lid down over the lower lid.

6. Eyelid injuries should be:

   a. irrigated with cool water.
   b. covered with a compress and roller bandages.
   c. treated with antibiotic salve.
   d. covered with a light dressing.

7. In all chemical burns of the eye:

   a. irrigate with water and vinegar solution.
   b. have the victim blink repeatedly and wash the eyes.
   c. irrigate continuously for fifteen to thirty minutes.
   d. irrigate the eyes with sodium bicarbonate.

8. If removal of a foreign object from the eye becomes necessary, the first maneuver is to:

   a. flush the eye with clean water if local protocol permits.
   b. pull the lower lid down and use a piece of gauze to remove the foreign body.
   c. turn the upper lid over a cotton swab or similar object.
   d. draw the upper lid down over the lower lid.

9. Acute glaucoma is characterized by:

   a. light flashes.
   b. corneal burns.
   c. a harder and more swollen than normal eyeball.
   d. pus discharge.

10. Which of the following is a basic rule of giving emergency eye care?

    a. flush the injured eye with water in case of heat burns.
    b. do not force the eyelid open (unless you have to wash out chemicals).
    c. administer eye drops to soothe eye injuries.
    d. gently sponge blood from the injured eye.

11. Eyelid injuries should be:

    a. irrigated with cool water.
    b. covered with a compress and roller bandages.
    c. treated with antibiotic salve.
    d. covered with a light dressing.

PART III: Matching: Match the emergency-care procedures in the right-hand column with the correct injury in the left-hand column.

Injury	Emergency Care
_____1. Foreign bodies in the eye.	A. Position a cup or cone over the injured eye and bandage.
_____2. Injury to the orbits.	B. Check all possible eye movements.
_____3. Lid injuries.	C. Cover eyes with a sterile, moist dressing.
_____4. Injuries to the globe.	D. Cover the eyes with a light dressing (moist if necessary).
_____5. Chemical burns.	E. Flush the eyes with clean water.
_____6. Impaled objects in the eye.	F. Keep victim lying on his back.
_____7. Retinal detachment.	G. Continuously irrigate the affected eye for fifteen to thirty minutes.
_____8. Heat burns.	H. Patches applied lightly to the eyes and cold compresses may give pain relief.

PART IV: What Would You Do If:

1. You are at a construction site where a carpenter was cutting some lumber with a power rip saw. A fragment of wood flew into his eye and was lodged in the eyeball.

2. A young child knocks an open can of gasoline from a high shelf in her family's garage, and some of the spilled gasoline gets in one of her eyes.

3. You witness a fight and find a victim lying on his back with a small pocket knife blade impaled in his left eye.

PART IV: Practical Skills Check-Off _____ has satisfactorily passed the following practical skills:
Student's Name

	Date	Partner Check	Inst. Init.
1. Demonstrate how to remove a foreign particle from the eye.	__/__/__	☐	_____
2. Demonstrate how to irrigate (flush) a chemical burn to the eye.	__/__/__	☐	_____
3. Demonstrate how to stabilize an impaled object in the eye.	__/__/__	☐	_____

CHAPTER FIFTEEN

OBJECTIVES

■ Recognize how facial and throat injuries can lead to airway obstruction and spinal injury.

■ Describe and demonstrate how to provide emergency care for various types of face and throat injuries.

■ Describe and demonstrate how to care for avulsed teeth.

■ Describe and demonstrate how to care for facial fractures.

INJURIES TO THE FACE AND THROAT

INJURIES TO THE FACE

The specialized structures of the face, prone to injury because of their location, can be permanently and irreversibly damaged. While some injuries to the face are minor, many face and throat injuries are life-threatening because they compromise the upper airway, impairing the victim's ability to breathe. In addition, many injuries of the face and throat stem from impacts strong enough to cause cervical-spine damage or skull fracture (Figure 15-1 and 15-2).

EMERGENCY CARE

Care for injuries to the face the same way as for other soft-tissue injuries, with these distinctions:

1. Check the airway — foreign bodies, the tongue, fractures, swelling, and bleeding can all compromise the airway following facial injury.

2. Completely immobilize the neck to prevent aggravation of possible cervical-spine injuries, which can accompany facial injuries.

3. Control bleeding with pressure; apply extremely gentle pressure if you suspect that bones beneath the wound may have been fractured or shattered (especially if the brain may be damaged by bone fragments).

4. Turn the victim prone or on one side with his face down to facilitate drainage of blood. If you suspect spinal injury, immobilize the victim before turning him, or logroll and immobilize him on his side. See Chapter 13.

5. Use dressings and pressure bandages for wounds of the face.

6. Apply ice to reduce swelling and bleeding.

7. If nerves, tendons, or blood vessels have been exposed, cover them with a moist, sterile bandage.

8. Injuries to the mouth that involve bleeding are especially serious, because blood running down the throat can choke the victim or cause him to vomit.

   ■ Tilt the victim's head, and lift his chin to maintain the airway. Use modified jaw thrust if spinal injury is suspected.

   ■ Allow drainage as necessary to remove blood or foreign material.

9. Check for avulsed teeth, and salvage them if you can.

10. Monitor carefully for facial **EDEMA** (swelling) that could compromise breathing.

    ■ If the victim shows signs of respiratory distress (such as noisy breathing, cool skin, or cyanosis), position him in a semi-sitting position with his knees raised.

    ■ Tilt his head forward to promote drainage.

━ INJURIES TO THE FACE ━

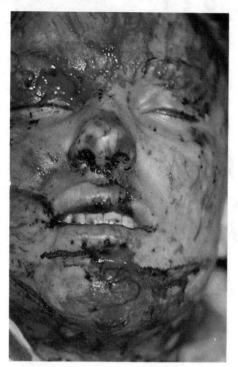

FIGURE 15-1.

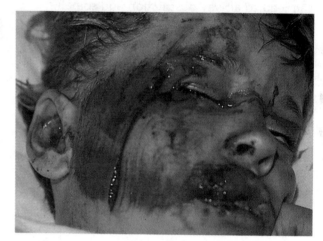

FIGURE 15-2

11. Remove any object impaled in the cheek (see Chapter 8). This is the only situation in which an impaled object should be removed (the other possible exception to the general rule is an object that is impaled in the airway, obstructing breathing).

   ■ The inside of the cheek should be felt gently to determine whether the impaled object has penetrated all the way through. If this is the case, carefully pull it out from the same side through which it entered. (If removal proves difficult, leave the impaled object in place.)

   ■ When the object has been removed, pack the inside of the cheek between the teeth and the cheek with sterile gauze, and place a pressure dressing and bandage over the outside of the wound.

   ■ If bleeding is profuse, position the victim so that blood will drain out of his mouth rather than into his throat.

12. Remember that facial trauma can be very upsetting to the victim and brings with it fears of disfigurement. Treat the victim with understanding and reassurance.

TRAUMA TO THE MOUTH AND JAW

In victims with trauma to the mouth and jaw, it is *essential*, when possible, to immobilize the head and neck with a backboard and cervical collar to protect against aggravation of cervical-spine and spinal injuries, which commonly accompany this kind of trauma.

Victims who sustain significant trauma to the face may also have fractures of the jaw and damage to or loss of teeth (Figures 15-3–15-6).

EMERGENCY CARE

Emergency care is aimed at the following:

1. Establish an airway.

   ■ Inspect the mouth for small fragments of teeth or dentures on which the victim might choke, and remove them.

── COMMON INJURIES OF THE MOUTH, JAW, AND CHIN ──

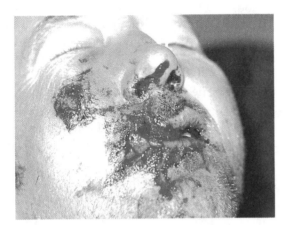

FIGURE 15-3

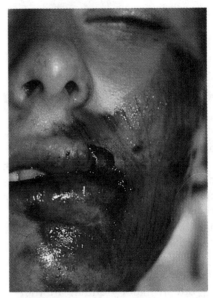

FIGURE 15-4

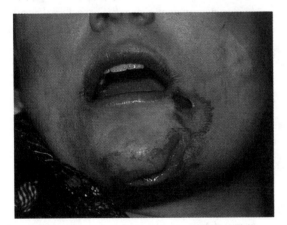

FIGURE 15-5

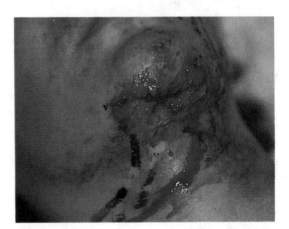

FIGURE 15-6

- Position the victim to allow drainage of any blood from the mouth and throat. The face, richly supplied with blood, may bleed freely and profusely.

2. Examine the mouth for broken or missing teeth.
   - If a tooth has been lost, try to find it!
   - If you find a missing tooth, rinse it with cold water; gently pick off any remaining debris (*never* scrub the tooth); put the tooth in a cup containing milk, or saliva; and send it with the victim.
   - Never handle the tooth by the root; there may still be ligament fibers attached that could enable successful reimplantation.

- If you cannot find teeth that have been knocked out, assume that the victim has swallowed or aspirated them until proven otherwise.

- Control bleeding from the socket with a gauze pad. Never use disinfectant or other cleansers to clean the tooth, and do not allow the tooth to dry.

- If an avulsed tooth is reimplanted within thirty minutes, there is about a 90 percent success rate. However, if a tooth has been out of the socket 150 minutes, the success rate drops to 20 percent.

3. Send any dentures or pieces of dentures with the victim.

FRACTURES OF THE FACE AND LOWER JAW

MAXILLOFACIAL fractures may be simple — such as undisplaced nasal fractures — or extensive, involving severe lacerations, bony fractures, and nerve damage (Figure 15-7). Victims with this type of injury will require assistance and transport to a hospital emergency room.

The first priority in caring for a victim with a facial fracture is establishing and maintaining the airway. The airway can be compromised by blood, edema, or structural defects. Facial fractures are rarely life-threatening, but in major trauma, another part of the body may sustain a serious injury. Consider and assess the entire victim:

1. Before considering any care, assess the victim for possible cervical, thoracic, and lumbar spine fracture or injury.

2. Check for tearing or rupture of the eyeball — common in victims who wear contact lenses and who have suffered facial trauma.

3. Check for facial burns — they indicate smoke and heat inhalation.

4. Check for **LONG BONE** fractures in extremities. Splint them before caring for facial fracture.

5. Check for rib fractures. Take measures to prevent possible hemothorax or pneumothorax. See Chapter 16.

6. Check for injury to the abdomen. See Chapter 17.

THE FACE

Signs and symptoms of facial fractures include:

■ Distortion of facial features.

■ Numbness or pain.

■ Severe bruising and swelling.

■ Bleeding from nose and mouth.

■ Limited jaw motion.

■ Teeth do not meet normally.

■ Double vision when bone around the eye is fractured.

■ Irregularities in the facial bones that can be felt before swelling occurs.

Emergency Care

Especially in blunt injuries and severe facial wounds, emergency-care objectives are to control hemorrhage and clear the airway.

1. Clear the airway. With both conscious and unconscious victims, if no neck injury exists, support the head with your hand, pull the jaw or jaw fragments upward, and hold the tongue down and forward. Remove dentures and foreign debris from the mouth.

2. Check for neck and spinal injuries.

3. After immobilizing for neck or spinal injuries, position the victim to allow for drainage.

4. Place bandages carefully to allow for vomiting and blood drainage.

■ Nose fractures — if the fracture is an open fracture, apply a sterile compress and bandage as for a nose wound, making sure that the bandage is not too tight.

■ Upper jaw or cheekbone fractures — if an open wound is present, treat it as a facial wound; if there is no open wound, a dressing is not necessary.

THE LOWER JAW

Signs and symptoms of lower-jaw fractures are (Figure 15-8):

■ Victim's mouth is usually open.

■ Saliva mixed with blood may flow from the corners of the mouth.

■ Talking is painful and difficult.

■ Teeth are often missing, loosened, or uneven.

■ Even if teeth are not missing, the victim will complain that teeth do not "fit together right."

■ There may be pain in the areas around the ears.

Emergency Care

Emergency care for a fractured lower jaw requires:

1. Clearing and maintaining an open airway.

2. Caring for open wounds.

3. Carefully immobilizing the lower jaw with cervical collar or cravats. Monitor for vomiting. *Follow local protocol.*

FACIAL FRACTURES

Facial fractures often result from impact injuries to the face. The main danger of facial fractures is airway problems. Bone fragments and blood may obstruct the airway. Common signs of a fractured jaw may include irregularity of bite, loss of teeth, bleeding in the mouth, deformity and/or loose bone segments, increased salivation, and the inability to swallow or talk.

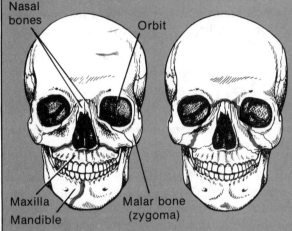

Nasal bones
Orbit
Maxilla
Mandible
Malar bone (zygoma)

Maxilla and Mandible Fracture

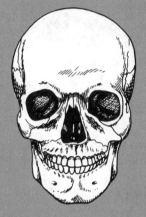

Maxilla-nasal-orbital Fracture

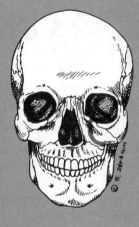

Nasal-orbital Fracture

Malar (cheek) Fracture

EMERGENCY CARE

Emergency care is the same as for soft-tissue injuries with special attention to clearing the airway of any obstructing materials, teeth, blood, etc.
- Maintain open airway, allowing for drainage if necessary.
- If necessary, assist ventilation. Control bleeding with as little pressure as is necessary so as not to displace fractures. The use of the temporal and facial pressure points may be necessary.
- Dress and bandage open wounds.
- Continually monitor airway.
- If necessary, immobilize mandible (lower jaw). However, if there is considerable bleeding in the mouth, it is best to not immobilize because it may compromise the airway.
- Keep victim quiet, and be very gentle so fracture areas will not displace or do further damage to other tissues.
- The victim who is not bleeding should be put in a semi-reclining position unless spinal injuries are suspected. Victims with bleeding facial injuries should be positioned on their sides with head turned down for draining.
- Always suspect and assess for spinal injuries, and take necessary immobilization precautions.
- Assess for other possible injuries.
- Activate the EMS system.

FIGURE 15-7.

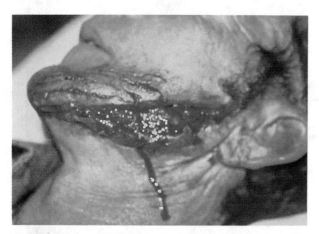

FIGURE 15-8. Soft-tissue injuries and fracture of the lower jaw.

INJURIES OF THE NOSE

Soft-tissue injuries of the nose should be cared for similar to other soft-tissue injuries, with special care being taken to maintain an open airway and position the victim so that blood does not drain into the throat (Figures 15-9 and 15-10).

NOSEBLEEDS

Nosebleeds are a relatively common reason for emergency calls. For complete information on managing nosebleed emergencies, see Chapter 5 on control of bleeding.

FOREIGN OBJECTS IN THE NOSE

Foreign objects in the nose are usually a problem among small children. The best emergency care is to reassure and calm the child and parent, then transport the victim to a hospital.

Tissue damage and impaction can result from probing and inadequate attempts at removal. Special lighting and instruments available at the hospital minimize the risk of removal.

NASAL FRACTURES

A broken nose can usually be identified by swelling and deformity. To treat, apply ice compresses to reduce swelling, and transport the victim to a physician.

INJURIES OF THE EAR

Cuts and lacerations of the ear occur frequently; occasionally, a section of the ear may be severed (Figures 15-11 and 15-12). Treat as for other soft-tissue injuries. Save any avulsed parts and send with the victim to the hospital. When dressing an injured ear, it is recommended that you place part of the dressing between the ear and the side of the head.

FOREIGN OBJECTS IN THE EAR

Foreign objects in the **EXTERNAL EAR** are a common problem among children. Some children have an irresistible compulsion to stuff their ears with small objects, such as beans and peanuts. *Leave the ear alone*, and transport the victim to the hospital, where good lighting and appropriate equipment are available.

— INJURIES OF THE NOSE —

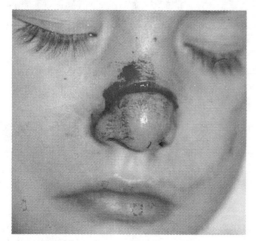

FIGURE 15-9.

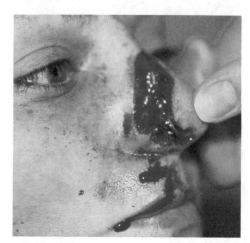

FIGURE 15-10.

INJURIES OF THE EAR

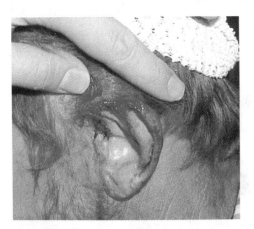

FIGURE 15-11.

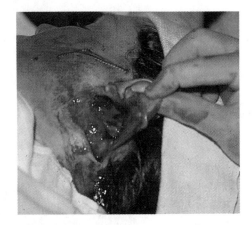

FIGURE 15-12.

INJURIES OF THE THROAT

The throat can be injured by any crushing blow. Common causes include hanging (attempted suicide), impact with a steering wheel, or running or riding into a stretched wire or clothesline. The throat may also be lacerated, which may result in bleeding from a major artery or vein and air bubbles entering the blood vessels (Figures 15-13 and 15-14).

Maintaining an airway is extremely important in throat injuries, because blood clots when exposed to air can threaten the airway (Figure 15-15).

1. Position the victim to allow for drainage.

2. If breathing is impaired, reassure the victim and, if necessary, administer artificial ventilation.

3. If tolerated by the victim and his airway status, keep the victim lying down to lessen the chance of air entering the blood vessels.

4. Control bleeding with slight to moderate pressure and bulky dressings. Be cautious when applying pressure — too much pressure will occlude carotid flow to the brain.

5. Position the victim on the left side with his feet elevated if bleeding is significant.

6. Apply an occlusive dressing.

7. Treat for shock.

8. When caring for bleeding wounds, never probe open wounds or use circumferential bandages that can interfere with blood flow on the uninjured side of the neck and also impair respiration.

9. Activate the EMS system.

INJURIES OF THE THROAT

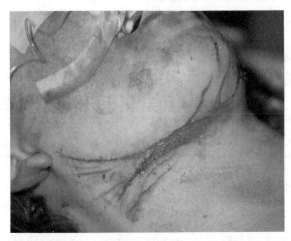

FIGURE 15-13.

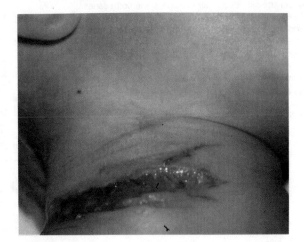

FIGURE 15-14.

COMMON NECK AND THROAT INJURIES

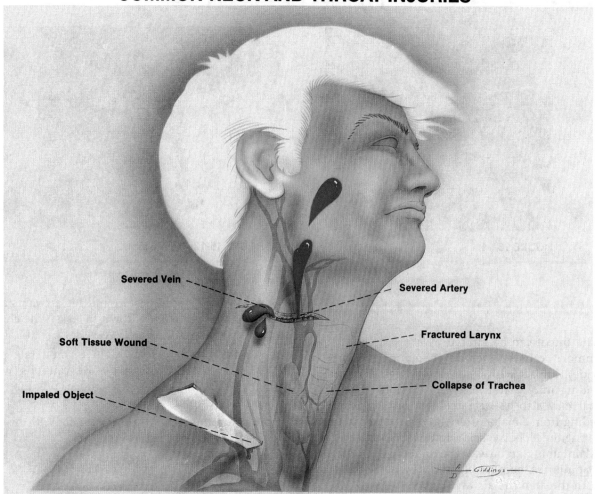

Severed Vein

Severed Artery

Soft Tissue Wound

Fractured Larynx

Collapse of Trachea

Impaled Object

BLUNT OR CRUSHING TRAUMA

- Loss of voice.
- Severe airway obstruction even though the mouth and nose are clean and no foreign body is present.
- Deformity, contusions, or depressions in the neck.
- Swelling in the neck and sometimes face and chest. When the swollen areas are touched there are crackling sensations under the skin due to air leakage in the soft tissues.
- If one of the above signs is present, it is an extreme emergency, and the victim needs to be transported to a medical facility immediately.
- Calm and reassure the victim, encouraging him to breathe slowly.
- Administer artificial ventilation as needed.
- Be alert for possible cervical-spine injuries, and take appropriate immobilization measures.
- Activate the EMS system immediately.

OPEN INJURIES

- Serious open wounds of the neck can cause profuse bleeding.
- If an **artery** has been severed and there is bright red spurting blood, apply direct pressure with a sterile (if possible) bulky dressing. If blood soaks through the dressing, do not remove it — just add another dressing on the first one. Maintain firm pressure with your hand until you arrive at the hospital. CAUTION: Pressure dressing around the neck can compromise the airway.
- Do not apply pressure over the airway or on both sides of the neck at the same time.
- If necessary, apply pressure to the carotid pressure point. Do not apply pressure on both carotid arteries at the same time. If there is an impaled object, stabilize in place with bulky dressings. Do not remove.
- Keep victim supine with legs slightly elevated, and activate the EMS system immediately.
- If a large **vein** (profuse, steady flow of dark red to maroon-colored blood) is severed, attempt to control bleeding using direct pressure with a bulky dressing. If bleeding is controlled, cover with an occlusive dressing.
- If bleeding is not immediately controlled, apply pressure above and below the point of bleeding. It is imperative that air not be allowed to be sucked into the vein (air embolism) and be carried into the circulatory system. This can be rapidly fatal. This is more likely to occur if the victim is sitting or standing.
- Cover wound with an occlusive dressing or plastic wrap, and tape all edges snugly to form an airtight seal over the severed vein.
- Position the victim on his side.
- Activate the EMS system. Administer artificial ventilation as needed.
- Monitor airway.

FIGURE 15-15.

| **15** | **SELF-TEST** | **15** |

Student: _____ Date: _____

Course: _____ Section #: _____

PART I: True/False   If you believe that the statement is true, circle the T. If you believe that the statement is false, circle the F.

T   F   1. Victims of trauma to the mouth and face should usually have their head and neck immobilized.

T   F   2. If you find a missing tooth, scrub it thoroughly and pack it in ice.

T   F   3. A tooth should only be handled by the root.

T   F   4. Do not clean a knocked-out tooth with a disinfectant, and do not allow it to dry.

T   F   5. Before considering any emergency care, examine the victim for possible spinal injury.

T   F   6. Place bandages carefully to allow for vomiting and blood drainage.

T   F   7. In injuries to the nose, be sure that the victim is positioned to allow for blood to drain into the throat rather than into the mouth.

T   F   8. The best emergency care for foreign objects in the nose and ear is to calm, reassure, and transport to a physician.

T   F   9. Never apply ice or cold packs to a suspected nasal fracture.

T   F   10. When dressing an injured ear, do not place part of the dressing between the ear and the side of the head.

T   F   11. Keep victims with throat injuries in a sitting position.

T   F   12. Never probe open wounds of the throat, and do not use circumferential bandages.

T   F   13. Once bleeding has been controlled from a large severed neck vein, cover the wound with an occlusive dressing.

T   F   14. If an artery in the neck has been severed, apply pressure to both carotid arteries at the same time.

T   F   15. Do not apply any pressure to a facial wound for control of bleeding if you suspect that the bones beneath the wound may be fractured.

T   F   16. If a facial injury victim shows signs of respiratory distress, position him in a semi-sitting position with his knees raised.

T   F   17. If an avulsed tooth is reimplanted within two hours, there is a ninety percent success rate.

T   F   18. With facial fractures, it is always best to immobilize the mandible.

T   F   19. The first priority in caring for a victim with a facial fracture is immobilization.

T   F   20. Victims with facial fractures that are not bleeding should be put in a semi-reclining position unless spinal injures are suspected.

PART II: Multiple Choice   For each question, circle the answer that best reflects an accurate statement.

1. Which of the following is *not* a recommended practice in treating a victim with trauma to the face?
   a. keep victims who are not bleeding in a semi-reclining position.
   b. immobilize the head and neck using a backboard and extrication collar.
   c. examine the mouth for broken or missing teeth, and transport any teeth or denture material with the victim to the hospital.
   d. use heavy direct pressure to control bleeding of facial injuries.

2. When caring for victims with injuries to the soft tissues in the mouth:
   a. place cotton balls into tooth sockets to control bleeding.
   b. wrap any dislodged teeth in dry sterile gauze.
   c. check for and remove any dislodged teeth, crowns, or bridges.
   d. all of these answers.

3. Bleeding from the socket of a dislodged tooth when the victim is conscious may be controlled by:
   a. applying pressure to the socket with the tip of the index finger.
   b. rinsing the mouth with ice water.
   c. inserting firmly packed cotton balls into the socket.
   d. having the victim bite down on a pad of sterile gauze placed over the socket.

4. A whole tooth can sometimes be replanted. The key to successful replanting is to keep the dislodged tooth:
   a. in an airtight bag.
   b. moist.
   c. warm.
   d. covered with baking soda.

5. If any blood vessels, nerves, or muscles are exposed as a result of a facial wound:

   a. apply an ice pack.
   b. cover them with a moist dressing.
   c. apply a sterile dressing and cover it with an airtight seal.
   d. none of these answers.

6. When a victim sustains a possible facial fracture:

   a. keep the victim lying down with the head and neck immobilized.
   b. check all possible eye movements.
   c. use ice packs over the area.
   d. flush the area with clean water.

7. The first means to be used for controlling bleeding of facial injuries is:

   a. elevation.
   b. flushing the wound.
   c. gentle, direct pressure.
   d. use of pressure points.

8. The most important aim of emergency care of jaw fractures is to:

   a. find teeth that have been knocked out.
   b. apply wraps to keep the lower jaw stable.
   c. ensure an airway.
   d. pack the area in ice to help control swelling.

9. A tooth can be replanted if:

   a. it is kept moist.
   b. the bone structure of the mouth is not damaged.
   c. a dentist is seen up to forty-eight hours after the tooth has been lost.
   d. the dentin of the tooth is intact.

10. Which of the following is *not* a sign or symptom of blunt or crushing trauma to the neck?

    a. crackling sensations under the skin from air leakage in soft tissues.
    b. deformity and/or contusions of the neck.
    c. loss of voice.
    d. severe external bleeding.

11. What is the best position for a victim with a bleeding throat injury?

    a. lying on left side with head down.
    b. lying on his stomach.
    c. sitting up.
    d. lying on his back.

12. Which of the following is *not* true about a cheek wound?

    a. you should not try to remove any foreign object impaled in the cheek.
    b. a gauze pad or dressing should be placed inside the mouth and held in place.
    c. you should check for bleeding into the mouth or throat that might obstruct the airway.
    d. all of these statements are true.

13. If a blood vessel in the neck is lacerated:

    a. place the victim in a sitting position to decrease the chance of an air embolism.
    b. apply pressure to the carotid artery in both sides of the neck.
    c. apply pressure above and below the point of bleeding.
    d. all of these answers.

14. A victim with a bleeding throat injury should be placed in what position?

    a. on the stomach with the head slightly elevated.
    b. lying on the left side with the head down.
    c. sitting up with the head up.
    d. on the back with the head down.

PART III: What Would You Do If:

1. You are at the scene of a motorcycle accident. The victim was not wearing a helmet and has abrasions and lacerations around the mouth and lower jaw.

2. A construction worker is hit with some falling lighting fixtures. He has one partially avulsed ear and a deep nose laceration.

PART IV: Practical Skills Check-Off

_____ has satisfactorily passed the following practical skills:
Student's Name

	Date	Partner Check	Inst. Init.
1. Demonstrate and explain how to care for an avulsed tooth.	___/___/___	☐	_____
2. Demonstrate how to immobilize the mandible (lower jaw).	___/___/___	☐	_____
3. Demonstrate how to care for an open wound of the neck.	___/___/___	☐	_____

INJURIES TO THE CHEST

CHEST INJURIES

All chest injuries should be considered life-threatening until proven otherwise, and you should always assume cardiac damage until it is ruled out. There are two general categories of chest injury: closed and open. In closed (blunt) chest injuries, the skin remains unbroken; it can be caused by a wide range of accidents, and commonly occurs from the blunt trauma of being struck by a falling object, being buried in a cave-in, or being thrown against a steering wheel in an automobile accident. Although the skin may not sustain any lacerations, serious underlying damage can occur, especially lacerations to the heart and lungs when deceleration forces them against the ribs.

In an open (penetrating) chest injury, the skin is broken, usually by a bullet or knife or by the end of a broken rib protruding through the skin. Although the skin is broken, the same injuries may be present as if the injury were closed (lacerations to the heart and lungs). In addition, the entry of air into the **THORAX** can interfere with breathing.

The main types of chest injury include:

■ Blunt trauma (a forceful blow to the chest).

■ Penetrating injury (a sharp object penetrates the chest wall).

■ Compression injury (the chest cavity compresses rapidly, usually as the result of an automobile accident).

Blunt trauma, potentially deadly, includes complications such as bruising of heart and/or lung tissue, **FLAIL CHEST**, pneumothorax, hemothorax, collapsed lungs, and injury to the aorta and other major vessels (Figure 16-1). If you suspect any of these, activate the EMS system immediately.

GENERAL SIGNS AND SYMPTOMS OF CHEST INJURY

Whether the injury is open or closed, certain signs and symptoms will occur in major chest trauma, many of them simultaneously. The major signs and symptoms of chest trauma include (Figure 16-2):

■ Cyanosis (bluish coloring of the fingernails, fingertips, lips, or skin).

■ **DYSPNEA** (shortness of breath or difficulty in breathing).

■ Tracheal deviation.

EMERGENCY CARE OF CHEST INJURIES

HEMOTHORAX

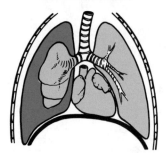

Blood leaks into the chest cavity from lacerated vessels or the lung itself and the lung collapses.

PNEUMOTHORAX

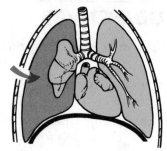

Air enters the chest cavity through a sucking wound or leaks from a lacerated lung. The lung cannot expand.

SPONTANEOUS PNEUMOTHORAX

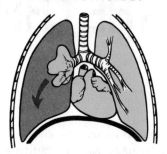

Air leaks into the chest from a weak area in the lung surface and the lung collapses. (Not necessarily related to trauma.)

TENSION PNEUMOTHORAX

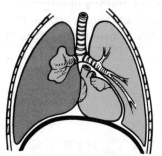

Air continuously leaks out the lung. It collapses, pressure rises, and the collapsed lung is forced against the heart and other lung.

EMERGENCY CARE

- Remove clothing to assess for open wounds; always check for an exit wound on back.
- Maintain an open airway and assist with ventilation as needed.
- Seal any open sucking wounds with an airtight dressing (plastic wrap, aluminum foil, Vaseline, gauze, etc.). Tape all edges snugly. *Follow local protocol.* If necessary, seal the wound with your hands until proper dressing can be prepared.
- Be alert for tension pneumothorax. If it develops, unseal the dressing for a few seconds to release pressure, then reseal.
- Do not remove impaled objects; stabilize with bulky dressings and bandage in place.
- Care for other bleeding and wounds with direct pressure and appropriate dressings, bandaged in place.
- Treat for shock.
- Continually monitor vital signs.
- Calm and reassure victim.
- Be alert for vomiting, coughing of blood and secretions from the mouth. Prevent aspiration and be ready to position for drainage.
- Put the victim in semi-reclining position or lying on his injured side if breathing is easier and/or you suspect internal bleeding.
- Activate the EMS system immediately.

FIGURE 16-1.

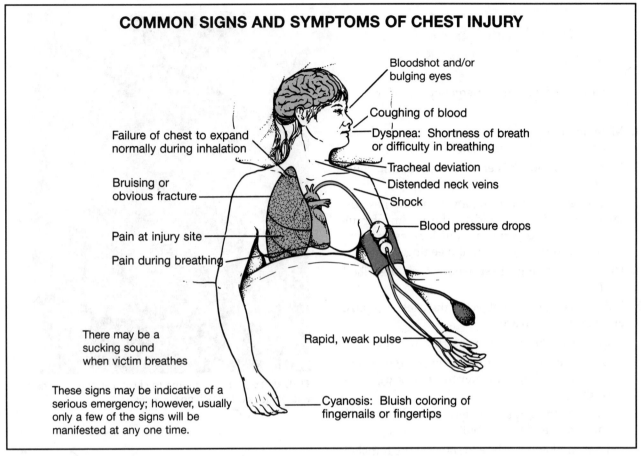

FIGURE 16-2.

- Pain during breathing.
- Distended neck veins.
- Pain at the injury site or pain near an injury that is made worse by breathing.
- Coughing up of blood (**HEMOPTYSIS**), usually bright red and frothy.
- Failure of chest (one or both sides) to expand normally during inhalation.
- Shock.
- Rapid, weak pulse, also indicating shock.
- Bruising or obvious fracture.

Two of the most important signs are the respiratory rate and any change in the normal breathing pattern. Depending on the physical fitness of the victim, he breathes normally (in an uninjured state) from twelve to twenty times each minute without strain, pain, or difficulty. If a victim breathes more than twenty-four times per minute, experiences pain when he breathes, or finds it difficult to take a deep breath, he probably has sustained a chest injury.

Broken ribs, bruising of the lungs, or severe lung disease can cause pain in the chest that is aggravated by breathing. Shortness of breath may be caused by failure of the chest to expand normally, fully, or properly; by obstruction of the airway; by compression of a lung (due to blood or air within the chest cavity); by loss of nervous control over breathing; or by lung disease (such as chronic obstructive pulmonary disease).

The failure of the chest wall to expand properly may result from direct injury to the chest wall, injury to the nerves that control the chest-wall muscles, or injury to the part of the brain that controls respirations.

Lacerations of lung tissue allows blood to seep into the lungs; the victim tries to clear it out by coughing. A victim coughing up blood may have lacerated tissue of the lungs or the bronchial tubes.

EMERGENCY CARE PRINCIPLES FOR CHEST INJURIES

Provide the following emergency care for chest injuries:

1. Maintain an open airway; your first priority is to ensure adequate ventilation.

2. If necessary, administer mouth-to-mouth ventilation.

3. Control external bleeding; a victim who has sustained chest injury could be the victim of multiple injuries, so perform a quick assessment to detect *any* source of external bleeding.

4. Dress penetrating chest wounds as described later.

5. If there is an impaled object in the chest, stabilize and bandage in place.

   ▪ Cut away clothing to expose the wound.

   ▪ Dress the wound around the impaled object to control bleeding and prevent a sucking chest wound.

   ▪ Stabilize the impaled object with rolls of self-adhering bandages or bulky dressings.

   ▪ Tape bandages in place to stabilize the impaled object.

6. Activate the EMS system immediately.

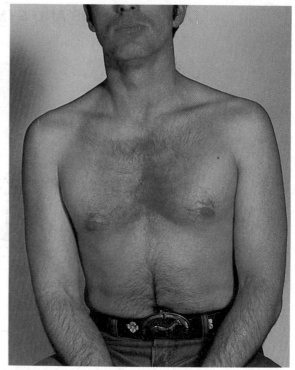

FIGURE 16-3. Blunt trauma to chest, causing flail chest and paradoxical breathing.

FLAIL CHEST

Flail chest results when the chest wall becomes unstable due to fractures of the sternum (breastbone), the cartilage connecting the ribs to the sternum, and/or the ribs. It can affect the front, back, or sides of the rib cage. It most often occurs when two or more adjacent ribs are broken, each in two or more places; the segment of chest wall between them becomes free-floating. The free-floating segment is referred to as the "flail area," and the motion of that area is opposite the motion of the rest of the chest (Figures 16-3 and 16-4). When the victim inhales, the area collapses or does not expand; when he exhales, it protrudes while the rest of the chest wall contracts. This produces an unstable chest-wall segment which markedly interferes with ventilation (**PARADOXICAL BREATHING**) (Figure 16-5).

Flail chest can be a life-threatening injury because it usually involves bruising of the lung tissues beneath the flail area and can lead to inadequate

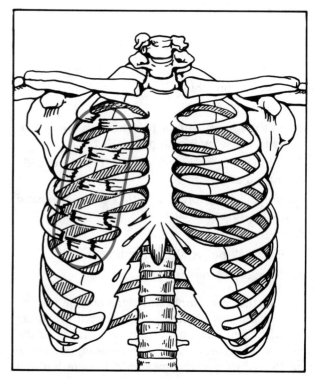

FIGURE 16-4. Flail chest occurs when blunt trauma causes fracture of two or more ribs, in more than one place.

FLAIL CHEST: PARADOXICAL BREATHING

EXPIRATION

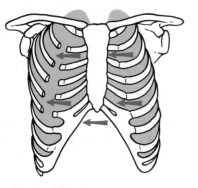

Injured chest wall moves out
Uninjured chest wall moves in

INSPIRATION

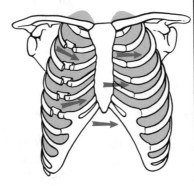

Injured chest wall collapses in
Uninjured chest wall moves out

EMERGENCY CARE

- Have victim lie on back.
- Remove clothing from chest area.
- Tape a small pillow or thick, heavy dressing over the injury site.
- Maintain open airway and assist ventilations as needed.
- Treat for shock.
- Regularly monitor vital signs.
- If you suspect internal bleeding, or if the victim has increased pain and discomfort in semi-sitting position, have victim lie on the injured side.
- Activate the EMS system immediately.

FIGURE 16-5.

oxygenation of the heart. The fractured bone ends may also puncture a lung. Flail chest may involve serious intrathoracic bleeding from the **COSTAL** arteries and veins, which can lead to shock. The victim must be stabilized and transported as rapidly as possible to a medical facility.

Signs and symptoms of flail chest include:

- Paradoxical breathing, almost always accompanied by severe pain.
- Swelling over the injured area.
- Signs of shock.
- Increasing airway resistance.
- Victim's attempt to splint his chest wall with his hands and arms.

To check for flail chest, have the victim lie on his back. Place your hands gently on the victim's chest and check for symmetry of the sides as he breathes. Bare his chest and stand at his feet, watching for a seesaw motion of his chest while he breathes. It can be extremely difficult to detect flail chest in an obese or muscular person. Remember, flail chest can be excruciating — the victim may not want to relinquish guarding of his chest.

EMERGENCY CARE

To care for flail chest:

1. Maintain an open airway and administer artificial ventilation if necessary.

2. Use *gentle* palpation to locate the edges of the flail section.

3. Stabilize the flail site with a pad of dressings or a pillow; the stabilizing object must weigh less than five pounds (Figure 16-6). Secure it with wide cravats, straps, or tape to increase victim comfort.

4. Position the victim with the flail segment against an external support in a semi-sitting position or lying on the injured side if a sitting position causes discomfort.

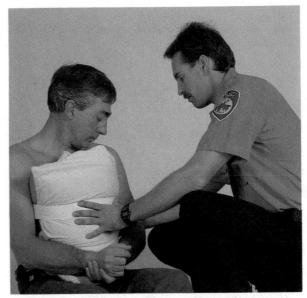

FIGURE 16-6. Stabilize flail chest by applying a pillow or bulky dressing and transport in a semi-sitting position.

5. Monitor vital signs closely; give care for shock.

6. Activate the EMS system immediately. If you suspect internal bleeding, position the victim in a semi-sitting position if he experiences too much pain lying on his injured side.

COMPRESSION INJURIES AND TRAUMATIC ASPHYXIA

A life-threatening emergency, severe and sudden compression of a victim's chest (such as when a person is thrown against a steering wheel) causes a rapid increase in intrathoracic pressure and results in a group of symptoms. Most serious, the sternum exerts sudden and severe pressure on the heart.

Traumatic **ASPHYXIA** occurs from a sudden compression of the chest wall; when it occurs, the blood is forced the wrong way out of the heart (from the right side of the heart rather than the left side) and back into the veins, particularly those of the head and shoulders. Signs and symptoms of traumatic asphyxia include:

- Severe shock.
- Distended neck veins.
- Bloodshot, protruding eyes.
- Cyanotic tongue and lips.
- Hemoptysis (coughing up blood) or vomiting blood.
- Swollen, cyanotic appearance of the head, neck, and shoulders.

Rib fractures and flail chest may also be caused by the sudden impact.

EMERGENCY CARE

To care for compression injuries and traumatic asphyxia:

1. Maintain an open airway.

2. Administer artificial ventilation as needed.

3. Control any bleeding that results from the trauma.

4. Monitor the victim closely and watch for complications. Put the victim in a semi-reclining position or on his injured side if breathing is easier and/or you suspect internal bleeding.

5. Activate the EMS system.

BROKEN RIBS

While broken ribs themselves are not life-threatening, they can cause injuries that *are*. While rib fracture is uncommon in children, direct blows or blunt trauma to the chest often result in fractured ribs in adults. The ribs most often fractured are the fifth through the tenth (those in the middle of the rib cage). The upper ribs are difficult to fracture because they are protected by the bony shoulder girdle, and the lower ribs are not attached to the sternum and can withstand greater impact. Pneumothorax, hemothorax (see Figure 16-1), **SUBCUTANEOUS EMPHYSEMA**, and lacerated intercostal vessels are common potential complications of rib fracture.

The most common symptom of rib fracture is pain at the fracture site (Figure 16-7). It usually hurts the victim to move, cough, or breathe deeply. The victim probably will take shallow breaths and will likely want to hold his hand over the area, since immobilization often offers some pain relief (Figure 16-8). Other signs and symptoms, which may or may not be present, include:

- Grating sound upon palpation.
- Chest deformity.

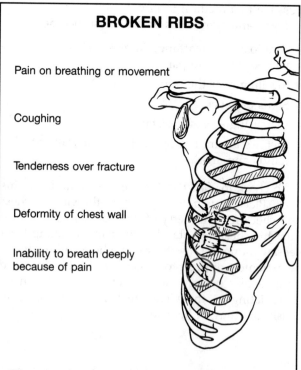

BROKEN RIBS

Pain on breathing or movement

Coughing

Tenderness over fracture

Deformity of chest wall

Inability to breath deeply because of pain

If lung has been punctured, the victim may cough up frothy blood and feel a crackling sensation under the fingertips as you feel the area of the fracture (subcutaneous emphysema).

FIGURE 16-7.

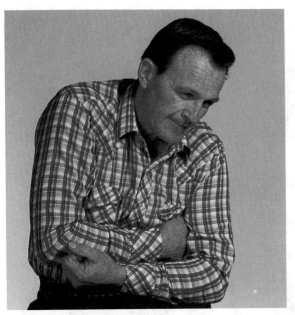

FIGURE 16-8. Typical "guarded" position of victim with rib fractures.

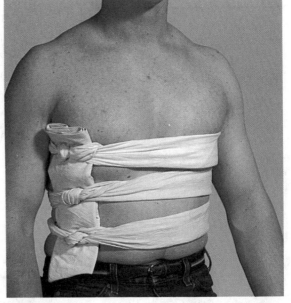

FIGURE 16-9. Immobilizing fractured ribs with cravats or roller bandage and pad.

- Shallow, uncoordinated breathing.
- Crackling sensation near the fracture site.
- Bruising or lacerations at the suspected fracture site.

EMERGENCY CARE

If only one rib has been fractured and no danger exists of heart or lung laceration, you should usually not bind the chest. However, since X-ray examination is necessary for diagnosis, you should always assume that multiple ribs have been broken and immobilize liberally.

The greatest priority in emergency care is to make sure that the victim can breathe adequately by splinting the chest as needed. Give the victim a pillow or blanket to hold against the fractured ribs for support. If the victim is unconscious or cannot splint his own ribs, treat as follows:

1. Apply three cravat bandages or one elastic bandage around the chest to support the ribs. Center the first bandage immediately below the site of the pain. Place the second bandage above the site of the pain. Place the third bandage around the lower half of the victim's chest to restrict movements and relieve pain (Figure 16-9).

2. Have the victim exhale.

3. Tie the two bandages over a pad on the uninjured side before allowing the victim to inhale. This will reduce the movement of the ribs caused by breathing.

4. Make sure that the bandages are snug but that they do not interfere with breathing.

5. As an alternative, use a sling and swathe, utilizing the victim's arm as a splint and support. Placing the forearm of the injured side across the chest, use a cravat to hold it in place as a swathe (Figures 16-10–16-12). Placing a pad between the arm and chest can help reduce pain. However, a sling and swathe can be used without a pad.

6. *Do not* tape the ribs or use continuous strapping; such bandaging can cause complications.

7. Place the victim in a semi-prone position, injured side down.

8. Activate the EMS system, and assist ventilations if needed.

9. *Do not* wrap the victim's chest if the ribs are depressed or if frothy blood is coming from the victim's mouth — both indicate a punctured lung. If there is an open wound on the chest, cover it immediately with an occlusive dressing.

HEMOTHORAX

Like pneumothorax, hemothorax fills up the chest cavity with blood (rather than air) and creates

APPLYING A SLING AND SWATHE

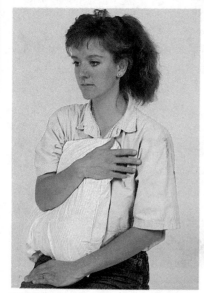

FIGURE 16-10. Place a pad between the arm and chest.

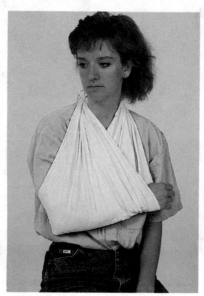

FIGURE 16-11. Supporting with a sling.

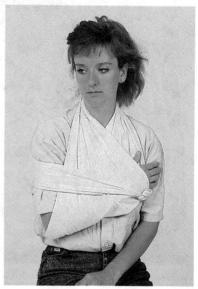

FIGURE 16-12. Immobilizing the arm and sling with a swathe.

pressure on the heart and lungs. The lungs cannot expand, and the same process occurs as with pneumothorax. In addition, severe bleeding can cause shock (see Figures 16-1 and 16-13).

Hemothorax occurs as a result of blunt or penetrating trauma to the chest caused by either open or closed chest wounds. It often accompanies pneumothorax. The blood usually originates from lacerated blood vessels in the chest wall or chest cavity; in rare cases, it results from a lacerated lung. The severity of the hemothorax depends on the amount of blood lost into the chest cavity.

If the hemothorax is small, it may be asymptomatic. Otherwise, the signs and symptoms of hemothorax are similar to those of pneumothorax; the following may or may not be present:

- Shock (due to blood loss).
- Rapid heartbeat.
- Rapid, shallow breathing.
- Absent breath sounds on the injured side.
- Tightness of the chest.
- Weak, thready pulse.
- Bruising over the injured area.
- Confusion and anxiety.

- Hemoptysis (coughing up blood) or blood flecks on the victim's lips.
- Frothy or bloody sputum.

EMERGENCY CARE

To care for a victim of hemothorax:

1. *Do not waste time — activate the EMS system immediately.* Keep the victim in a semi-reclining position unless shock is suspected.
2. Administer artificial ventilation if necessary.
3. Control bleeding from any external wounds with a pressure dressing.
4. Treat for shock.

TENSION PNEUMOTHORAX

TENSION PNEUMOTHORAX is one of the most life-threatening chest injuries. In tension pneumothorax, air continuously leaks out of the lung and becomes trapped in the pleural space. Once the process of compression within the chest cavity due

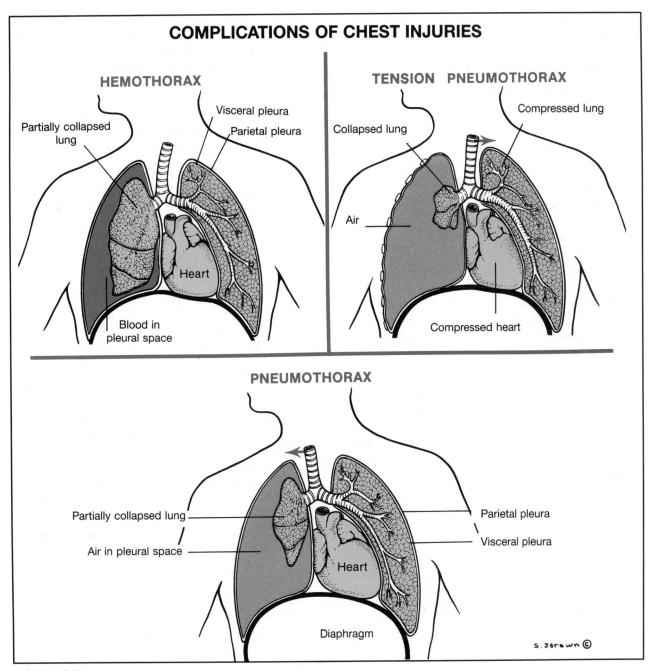

FIGURE 16-13.

to the presence of air begins, it worsens progressively with each breath until the lung on the affected side is reduced to the size of a small ball (sometimes only a few inches in diameter). Even after the lung can be compressed no more, air continues to leak into the pleural space and the pressure continues to rise, pressing the collapsed lung against the heart and the lung on the opposite side (see Figure 16-1 and 16-13). The remaining lung then starts to collapse

The extreme pressure in the chest cavity prevents blood from returning to the heart through the veins, and the blood is no longer pumped out. Death can occur rapidly, sometimes within minutes.

Signs and symptoms of tension pneumothorax include:

■ Obvious and increasing difficulty in breathing.

■ Bulging of neck veins with tracheal deviation.

- Bulging of the chest wall above the collarbone and between the ribs.
- Reduced breathing sounds on one side of the chest and eventually on both sides.
- Tracheal deviation to the uninjured side.
- Falling blood pressure and narrowing pulse pressure.
- Rapid, weak pulse.
- Uneven chest movements during breathing.
- Cyanosis.
- Extreme anxiety.

EMERGENCY CARE

Tension pneumothorax is one of the few emergencies in which seconds strictly count. Emergency care is aimed at activating the EMS system immediately and at relieving the increasing pressure in the pleural cavity. To care for tension pneumothorax, do the following:

1. Activate the EMS system immediately.
2. If you have bandaged a sucking chest wound, try releasing the dressing for a few seconds; if there is a tension pneumothorax, air will rush out of the wound. Release the dressing during expiration of air, and reapply it during inspiration; leave one corner untaped to allow for release of pressure.
3. Administer artificial ventilation as necessary.
4. Treat for shock.

PNEUMOTHORAX

Pneumothorax occurs when air from a wound site enters the chest cavity but not the lung. The pressure of the air in the chest cavity presses against the lung, separating it from the chest wall and causing it to collapse (see Figures 16-1 and 16-13). The volume of the lung is reduced, resulting in respiratory arrest.

Air can enter the chest cavity in one of two ways: either from a sucking wound that allows air to enter from the outside (open pneumothorax), or from air that leaks out of a lung due to laceration. Once the lung is ruptured, it does not expand properly with breathing, and within minutes the victim suffers from a lack of oxygen.

In some cases, called **SPONTANEOUS PNEUMOTHORAX**, the lung does not collapse because of injury, but because a congenitally weak area on the

surface of the lung ruptures (see Figure 16-1). The weakened lung loses its ability to expand, and the victim experiences sharp chest pain and mild to severe respiratory distress. Spontaneous pneumothorax is common among smokers or emphysema victims, especially if they are emaciated.

Suspect pneumothorax if a victim suffers a sudden shortness of breath without an obvious cause. Other signs and symptoms include:

- Sudden, sharp chest pain.
- Failure of the lung to expand with inhalation, causing decreased or absent breath sounds on the affected side.

EMERGENCY CARE

Emergency care for pneumothorax includes the following:

1. Clear and maintain an open airway.
2. Administer artificial ventilation as needed.
3. Cover any open chest wounds. If necessary, use your hand; preferably, apply an occlusive dressing to cover the wound (the dressing should be at least two inches wider than the wound on all sides). Tape the dressing to the chest, leaving one corner untaped to allow release of pressure.
4. Monitor the victim closely; a pneumothorax can become a tension pneumothorax if pressure builds. If tension pneumothorax develops, briefly remove the occlusive dressing.
5. Activate the EMS system as soon as possible.

SUCKING CHEST WOUNDS (OPEN PNEUMOTHORAX)

In open chest wounds, air from the environment sometimes enters the chest cavity when the chest is expanded during the victim's normal breathing. It moves through the wound as the victim inhales; when the victim exhales, air is forced back out of the wound. Each time the victim breathes, a moist sucking or bubbling is produced as the air passes in and out of the wound. In addition, there will be decreased breath sounds (Figure 16-14).

Pneumothorax results when air enters the chest cavity but does not enter the lung from the wound site. The pressure of the air in the chest cavity presses against the lung, causing it to collapse.

Air can enter the chest cavity in two ways: (1) from a sucking wound that allows air to enter from outside; or (2) from air that leaks out of the opposite lung due to laceration. Once the lung is compressed, it does not expand properly with breathing, and within minutes the victim suffers from a lack of oxygen.

EMERGENCY CARE

To care for open pneumothorax:

1. Apply an airtight dressing (occlusive) over the sucking wound *immediately* to prevent serious respiratory problems (Figure 16-15). Household plastic wrap is not strong enough — use a nonporous material like aluminum foil or Vaseline gauze held in place with a pressure dressing. Your goal should be to create an airtight seal over the wound and prevent air from passing through the wound. The dressing must be large enough so that it is not sucked into the wound; there should be at least two inches of overlap on all sides.

2. Tape the dressing to the chest, leaving one corner untaped to prevent a buildup of pressure (Figure 16-16). *Follow local protocol.*

SUCKING CHEST WOUND

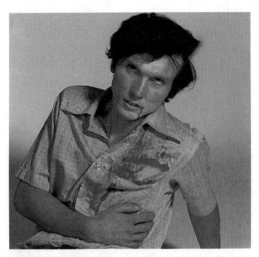

FIGURE 16-14. Sucking chest wound and possible pneumothorax.

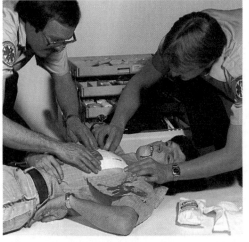

FIGURE 16-15. Position occlusive covering, which should contact the chest wall directly.

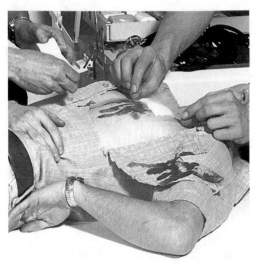

FIGURE 16-16. Tape dressing and occlusive covering in place.

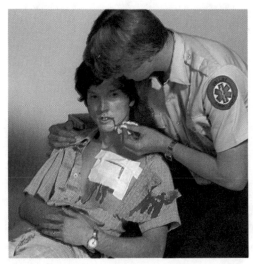

FIGURE 16-17. Position victim to ease breathing.

3. Administer artificial ventilation as necessary.

4. Activate the EMS system keeping the victim either sitting up or in some other position of comfort that is least painful and allows for the least labored breathing (Figure 16-17).

PENETRATING INJURY

The most common penetrating chest injury is from a stab or gunshot wound. In addition to the possibility of lacerating the great vessels in the chest, penetrating injury can result in massive bleeding, sucking chest wounds (open pneumothorax), pneumothorax, hemothorax, an impaled object in the chest, or laceration of the heart and lungs. It can be a fatal injury.

EMERGENCY CARE

Surgical intervention is required. First aid in the field is as follows:

1. Open and maintain an airway.

2. Administer artificial ventilation as necessary.

3. Place the victim in a shock position, on his back with his feet elevated ten to twelve inches, unless other injuries contraindicate this position.

4. Activate the EMS system immediately, monitoring the victim closely while waiting for emergency personnel.

For more information on penetrating injuries, see Chapter 8.

| **16** | **SELF-TEST** | **16** |

Student: _____ Date: _____

Course: _____ Section #: _____

PART I: True/False   If you believe that the statement is true, circle the T. If you believe that the statement is false, circle the F.

T   F   1. Traumatic asphyxia occurs from a sudden compression of the chest wall.

T   F   2. Flail chest most often occurs when two or more adjacent ribs are broken in two or more places.

T   F   3. In paradoxical breathing, the injured chest wall moves in and the uninjured chest wall moves out.

T   F   4. Paradoxical breathing is rarely accompanied by pain.

T   F   5. Stabilize a flail chest with pads or a pillow.

T   F   6. Position a flail chest victim so that the flail segment is not against any external support.

T   F   7. A rib-fracture victim usually will take shallow breaths.

T   F   8. The greatest priority in the treatment of rib fractures is to make sure that the victim can breathe adequately.

T   F   9. Do not tape the ribs or use continuous strapping.

T   F   10. A rib-fracture victim should be placed in a supine position.

T   T   11. If a victim with a rib fracture has frothy blood coming from his mouth, the bandages should be applied more tightly.

PART II: Multiple Choice   For each question, circle the answer that best reflects an accurate statement.

1. In what position should you place a victim with broken ribs?
    a. semi-sitting.
    b. upright.
    c. semi-prone, injured side down.
    d. flat on the back.

2. Where should cravat bandages be applied to an uncomplicated rib fracture?
    a. have the victim inhale and tie bandages on the injured side.
    b. have the victim exhale and tie bandages on the injured side.
    c. have the victim inhale and tie bandages on the uninjured side.
    d. have the victim exhale and tie bandages on the uninjured side.

3. Which of the following is *not* a sign or symptom of a chest injury?
    a. coughing blood.
    b. shock.
    c. strong, bounding pulse.
    d. distended neck veins.

4. The condition where blood leaks into the chest cavity from lacerated vessels or from the lung, causing the lung to compress, is called:
    a. pneumothorax.
    b. flail chest.
    c. traumatic asphyxia.
    d. hemothorax.

5. A flail chest may be the result of:
    a. a perforated lung.
    b. fractures of the sternum, cartilage, or ribs.
    c. a puncture wound to the chest.
    d. a cervical-spine injury.

6. Paradoxical breathing occurs when:
    a. compression injuries cause gasping breaths interspersed with extremely shallow breathing.
    b. lack of oxygen from a compressed lung.
    c. air remains in the chest cavity outside the lungs.
    d. the motion of the injured chest area is opposite the motion of the remainder of the chest.

7. If tension pneumothorax is suspected in a victim with a bandaged sucking chest wound:
    a. add further dressing to halt the loss of air.
    b. try releasing the dressing for a few seconds to see if the pressure is relieved.
    c. remove all dressings completely.
    d. delay transport until further assessment is completed.

8. What characteristic do pneumothorax, tension pneumothorax, and hemothorax have in common?
    a. pressure buildup in the chest cavity, causing the lung(s) to compress.
    b. air entering the chest cavity.
    c. blood in the chest cavity.
    d. all of these answers.

9. If the victim has suffered a stab wound to the chest:
    a. remove the penetrating object if possible.
    b. listen for "sucking" chest wounds.
    c. apply direct pressure to the penetrating object to control bleeding.
    d. concentrate on cleansing the wound.

10. Two general categories of chest wounds are:
    a. open and closed.
    b. simple and compound.
    c. fracture and puncture.
    d. lung-related and heart-related.

11. The chest wall will fail to expand if:
    a. there is direct injury to the chest wall.
    b. there is an injury to the nerves that control the chest wall muscles.
    c. there is an injury to the part of the brain that controls breathing.
    d. all of the above.

12. The most serious threat posed by injuries to the chest and rib cage is possible damage to the _____ in the chest cavity.
    a. stomach and intestinal organs.
    b. intercostal muscles.
    c. cartilage.
    d. heart and lungs.

13. To stabilize flail chest:
    a. apply an airtight dressing over the flail area.
    b. place a pillow over the flail area and secure with tape.
    c. put sandbags on either side of the victim's chest and bandage in place.
    d. maintain the victim in a semi-reclining position.

14. Traumatic asphyxia is caused by:
    a. blunt trauma.
    b. pneumothorax.
    c. severe compression of the chest.
    d. heart contusions.

15. Pneumothorax occurs when:
    a. air enters the chest cavity but does not enter the lung from a wound site.
    b. the descending aorta is lacerated.
    c. blood fills up the chest cavity.
    d. three or more ribs break and the chest wall that lies over the break area collapses.

16. The primary consideration in treating a sucking chest wound is:
    a. stopping the air leak.
    b. controlling the bleeding.
    c. treating for shock.
    d. preventing infection.

17. Which area of the ribs is most often fractured?
    a. middle.
    b. lower.
    c. upper.
    d. floating.

18. Which of the following is *not* an appropriate material to use for treatment of a sucking chest wound?
    a. plastic wrap.
    b. aluminum foil.
    c. Vaseline, gauze pads.
    d. single-layer gauze.

PART III: Matching:

_____1. Air leaks into the chest from a weak area in the lung surface.

_____2. Blood leaks into the chest cavity.

_____3. Air continuously leaks out of the lung and the lung collapses.

_____4. Air enters the chest cavity through a sucking wound.

_____5. Sudden compression of chest wall.

A. Traumatic asphyxia.

B. Hemothorax.

C. Spontaneous pneumothorax.

D. Tension pneumothorax.

E. Pneumothorax.

PART IV: What Would You Do If:

1. A middle-aged man sustains a hard blow to the chest in a family football game. It hurts the victim to move, cough, or breathe deeply. He holds his hand over a painful area on the left side of his chest, and there is some chest deformity and a grating sound upon palpation.

2. A victim has been stabbed in the chest with a large kitchen knife. When you arrive, the knife has been removed. When the victim breathes, there is a bubbling produced at the wound site.

PART IV: Practical Skills Check-Off

_____ has satisfactorily passed the following practical skills:
Student's Name

	Date	Partner Check	Inst. Init.
1. Demonstrate how to position a chest-injury victim (semi-sitting or on injured side.	__/__/__	☐	_____
2. Demonstrate how to stabilize a flail chest.	__/__/__	☐	_____
3. Demonstrate how to immobilize for fractured ribs.	__/__/__	☐	_____
4. Demonstrate how to care for a sucking chest wound.	__/__/__	☐	_____

INJURIES TO THE ABDOMEN AND GENITALIA

A wide range of accidents, from motor vehicle accidents to shootings or blunt trauma, affect the organs of the abdomen. And because the **ABDOMINAL CAVITY** contains not only vital organs but a rich supply of blood vessels, major abdominal injuries are life-threatening and demand prompt and proper first aid.

Injuries to the **GENITALIA**, while embarrassing and frightening, are seldom life-threatening. However, you have an important duty to protect the victim from public embarrassment and to provide emotional support.

THE ABDOMINAL CAVITY

The abdominal cavity contains the major organs of the **GASTROINTESTINAL TRACT**, and in a woman it also contains the internal sex organs — the **OVARIES, FALLOPIAN TUBES,** and **UTERUS**. The abdominal cavity is separated from the thoracic cavity by the diaphragm.

The abdominal cavity is well protected above by the thorax, below by the heavy ring of pelvic bones, and at the sides and in back by thick tough muscles, the lower ribs, and the spinal column. It is protected in front by flat muscular layers, which for greater strength run in different directions in the abdominal wall.

ABDOMINAL INJURIES

Victims involved in fights, falls, or automobile accidents should always be suspected of having sustained injury to the abdominal area. Injuries might range from severe hemorrhage, resulting in shock, to a rupture of the diaphragm, which forces abdominal organs into the chest cavity (Figure 17-1). Almost all injuries to the abdominal area require surgical repair.

Blunt trauma is serious, because it can involve any of the vascular organs surrounding and adjacent to the abdomen. Injuries to the **LIVER, KIDNEYS, PANCREAS, SPLEEN,** and **GALLBLADDER** may cause severe hemorrhaging that can result in death.

OPEN WOUNDS

A wound in which the skin is broken and the abdominal cavity is penetrated is extremely dangerous because of possible damage to internal organs. The **STOMACH** or **INTESTINE** may be perforated, internal bleeding may occur, and infection may develop.

It is sometimes difficult to determine whether internal organs have been injured; in the presence of open abdominal wounds, assume that organ damage has occurred. Generally, signs and symptoms include:

■ Severe abdominal tenderness.

INJURIES TO THE CHEST, ABDOMEN AND PELVIC CAVITY

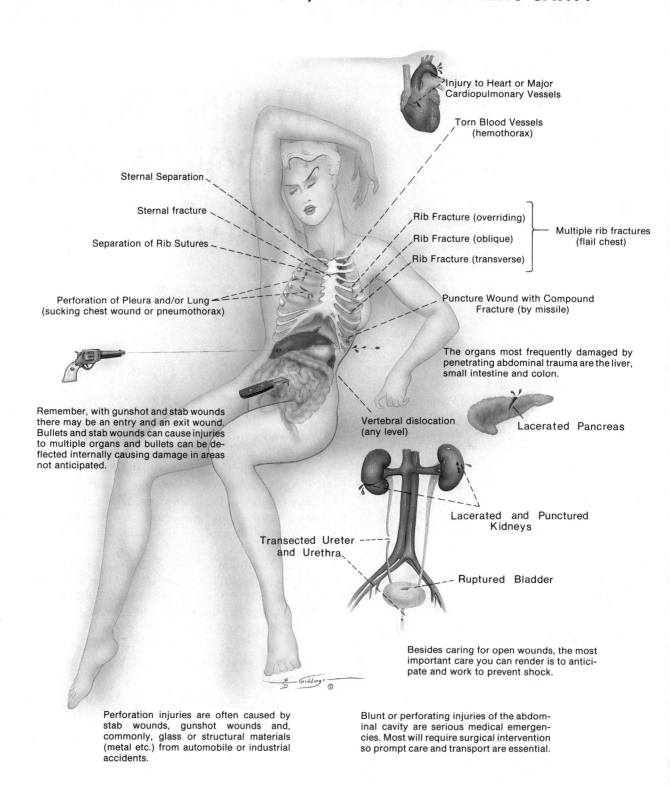

Injury to Heart or Major Cardiopulmonary Vessels

Torn Blood Vessels (hemothorax)

Sternal Separation

Sternal fracture

Separation of Rib Sutures

Rib Fracture (overriding)

Rib Fracture (oblique)

Rib Fracture (transverse)

Multiple rib fractures (flail chest)

Perforation of Pleura and/or Lung (sucking chest wound or pneumothorax)

Puncture Wound with Compound Fracture (by missile)

The organs most frequently damaged by penetrating abdominal trauma are the liver, small intestine and colon.

Remember, with gunshot and stab wounds there may be an entry and an exit wound. Bullets and stab wounds can cause injuries to multiple organs and bullets can be deflected internally causing damage in areas not anticipated.

Vertebral dislocation (any level)

Lacerated Pancreas

Lacerated and Punctured Kidneys

Transected Ureter and Urethra

Ruptured Bladder

Besides caring for open wounds, the most important care you can render is to anticipate and work to prevent shock.

Perforation injuries are often caused by stab wounds, gunshot wounds and, commonly, glass or structural materials (metal etc.) from automobile or industrial accidents.

Blunt or perforating injuries of the abdominal cavity are serious medical emergencies. Most will require surgical intervention so prompt care and transport are essential.

FIGURE 17-1.

- Abdominal muscle rigidity.
- Abdominal distention.
- Intense pain.
- Severe shock.
- Nausea and/or vomiting.
- Abdominal muscle spasm.

CLOSED WOUNDS (INTERNAL INJURIES)

In closed abdominal wounds, the abdomen has been damaged by a severe blow or crushing injury, but the skin remains unbroken. Such wounds may be extremely dangerous, because serious injury to the internal organs, internal hemorrhage, and shock may occur. See also Chapter 25.

GENERAL SIGNS AND SYMPTOMS OF ABDOMINAL INJURIES

Victims with abdominal injuries may exhibit any of the following (Figure 17-2):

- The abdomen may be distended.
- The abdomen may be rigid and tender with pain felt in an area other than the site of injury.
- The victim may have pain that begins as mild discomfort and then progresses to an intolerable pain.
- The victim may protect his abdomen.
- The victim prefers to lie still with legs drawn up in the **FETAL POSITION** (Figure 17-3).
- Pain may radiate to either shoulder.
- There may be abdominal cramping.
- There may be rapid, shallow breathing.
- The pulse may be rapid.
- Open wounds and penetrations may be evident.
- The victim may be nauseated and may vomit.
- Organs may protrude through open wounds (**EVISCERATION**) (Figure 17-4).
- Fractures may be evident.
- There may be obvious lacerations and puncture wounds in the abdomen.
- The victim may be in shock.
- The victim may be vomiting blood.

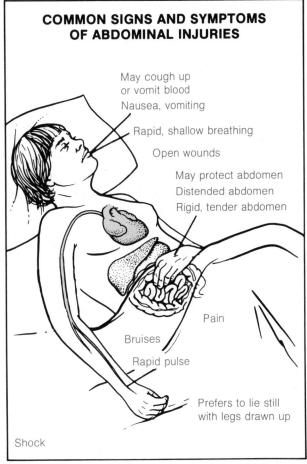

COMMON SIGNS AND SYMPTOMS OF ABDOMINAL INJURIES

May cough up or vomit blood
Nausea, vomiting
Rapid, shallow breathing
Open wounds
May protect abdomen
Distended abdomen
Rigid, tender abdomen
Pain
Bruises
Rapid pulse
Prefers to lie still with legs drawn up
Shock

FIGURE 17-2.

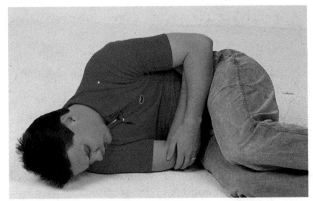

FIGURE 17-3. Victims with abdominal injuries often lie with their legs drawn up in the fetal position.

- Back pain may be present if the kidneys have been injured.
- The victim may be very weak or very thirsty.

GENERAL EMERGENCY CARE FOR ABDOMINAL INJURIES

As with all injured victims, top priorities are airway, breathing, and circulation. Additionally, provide the following emergency care for abdominal injuries:

1. Remove clothing from the abdominal area to allow for adequate assessment.

2. Suspect shock, and work diligently to prevent it. Keep the victim warm, but do not overheat.

3. Control bleeding and dress all open wounds with a dry, sterile dressing.

4. If organs are protruding, do not touch them and do *not* attempt to replace them within the abdominal cavity. Cover them with a sterile dressing and keep the dressing moistened with clean water. Apply an occlusive dressing to retain moisture and protect from contaminants.

5. The victim is usually most comfortable lying on his back with his knees flexed; elevate his feet if possible.

6. Be alert for vomiting. Maintain an open airway by positioning the victim for adequate drainage.

7. Constantly monitor vital signs and abdominal condition.

8. Do not remove penetrating or impaled objects. Dress the wounds around the impaled object to control bleeding, stabilize the impaled object with bulky dressings, and bandage in place to prevent movement.

9. Immobilize the victim if you suspect pelvic fracture.

10. Do not give the victim anything by mouth.

11. Activate the EMS system as quickly as possible.

ABDOMINAL EVISCERATIONS

An evisceration bandage is used when an abdominal laceration wound has resulted in a protrusion of the abdominal contents. In such cases (Figures 17-4–17-8):

1. Suspect shock and work to prevent it.

2. Constantly monitor vital signs.

3. Do *not* touch protruding organs.

4. Do *not* try to replace organs within the abdomen.

5. Cover the organs with a clean, moist, sterile dressing. Use sterile gauze compresses if available, and moisten them with clean water. *Never* use absorbent cotton or any material that clings

when wet, such as paper towels or toilet tissue. *Note:* Some areas are using a dry occlusive dressing, while others recommend moistening the dressing with water. Follow local protocol.

6. Cover the dressing with clean aluminum foil to retain moisture and warmth.

7. Gently wrap the dressing in place with a bandage or clean sheet.

8. Place the victim in a supine position with knees flexed and supported.

9. Activate the EMS system immediately.

RUPTURE OR HERNIAS

The most common form of rupture or **HERNIA** is a protrusion of a portion of an internal organ through the wall of the abdomen. Most ruptures occur in or just above the groin, but they may occur at other places over the abdomen. Ruptures result from a combination of weakness of the tissues and muscular strain.

The signs and symptoms of a rupture are as follows:

- Sharp, stinging pain.
- Feeling of something giving way at the site of the rupture.
- Swelling.
- Possible nausea and vomiting.

To care for a hernia (Figure 17-9):

1. Lie the victim on his back with the knees well drawn up.

2. Place a blanket or similar padding under the knees.

3. Never attempt to force the protrusion back into the cavity.

4. Cover the victim with a blanket.

5. Activate the EMS system.

6. Treat the victim for shock if it is present.

GENITOURINARY SYSTEM INJURIES

MALE GENITALIA

While injuries to the external male genitalia — lacerations, avulsions, abrasions, penetrations, and contusions — are excruciatingly painful, they are not necessarily life-threatening. However, the

ABDOMINAL EVISCERATION

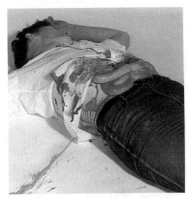

FIGURE 17-4. Abdominal eviscera-tion — an open wound resulting in protrusion of intestines.

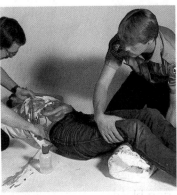

FIGURE 17-5. Cut away clothing from wound and support knees in a flexed position.

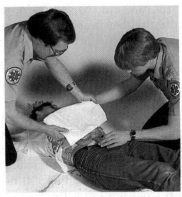

FIGURE 17-6. Place dressing over wound. **Do not attempt to replace intestines within abdomen.**

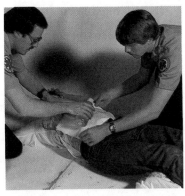

FIGURE 17-7. Moisten dressing with clean water. It is best to pre-moisten before application. Note: in some areas, dry dressings are recom-mended. Follow local protocol.

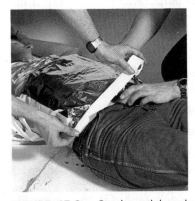

FIGURE 17-8. Gently and loosely tape the dressing in place, then apply an occlusive material such as aluminum foil or plastic wrap. Tape loosely over dressing to keep dress-ing moist.

amount of pain involved and the nature of the injury can cause great concern to the victim. Act in a calm, professional way, and protect the victim from onlookers.

Penis

The skin of the **PENIS** can be torn or avulsed, par-ticularly in an uncircumcised victim, and most com-monly in an industrial accident. To give emergency care:

1. Wrap the penis in a soft, sterile dressing mois-tened with sterile saline solution.

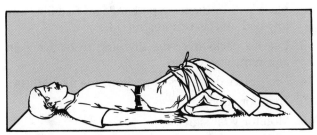

FIGURE 17-9. Emergency care for a rupture or hernia.

2. Apply an ice bag to the penis to relieve pain and reduce swelling.

3. If you can find the torn skin, wrap it in sterile gauze that has been moistened with clean water; send it with the victim to the hospital.

4. Never remove penetrating objects; stabilize them with bulky dressings prior to transport.

5. Always preserve avulsed parts.

6. In some cases, the penis itself may be partially or completely amputated, and blood loss may be significant. Apply direct pressure with a sterile pressure dressing to the remaining stump of the penis to control blood loss. If necessary, apply a tourniquet until direct pressure can bring bleeding under control. Activate the EMS system as quickly as possible.

7. If you can find the amputated penis, wrap it in a sterile dressing moistened with clean water, place it in a plastic bag and send it to the hospital with the victim.

Tears of the **FORESKIN** or laceration of the skin just underneath the ridge can result in heavy bleeding. To give emergency care:

1. Use pressure to control the bleeding.

2. Apply ice to reduce swelling and relieve pain.

3. Activate the EMS system.

Sometimes the penis gets caught in the zipper of pants, an injury that usually occurs among children. To care for this emergency:

1. If only one or two teeth of the zipper are involved, try to gently unzip the pants and free the penis. It may be easiest to cut off the zipper fastener and gently separate the teeth.

2. If the victim is unusually upset or if a long section of skin is caught, cut the zipper out of the pants to make the victim more comfortable.

3. Apply ice to reduce swelling and relieve pain.

4. Transport the victim to a physician.

Urethra

Lacerations of the **URETHRA**, while uncommon, can result from **STRADDLE INJURIES**, forceful blunt trauma to the abdomen, and penetrating objects. Signs and symptoms of urethral laceration include:

- Blood in the urine.

- Bleeding from the urethral opening.

- Urge to void or difficulty in voiding.

- Distended bladder.

To care for this emergency:

1. If there is bleeding from the urethral opening, apply direct pressure with a dry, sterile dressing to control bleeding.

2. Do not remove penetrating objects; stabilize them with bulky dressings.

3. Transport, instructing the victim not to urinate during transport, or activate the EMS system.

Scrotum and Testicles

A direct blow to the **SCROTUM** can cause the **TESTES** to rupture, or can result in a pooling of blood around them, causing tremendous pain and a feeling of pressure.

To care for this emergency:

1. Apply ice to the entire crotch area to reduce swelling, bleeding, and pain.

2. Activate the EMS system.

3. If scrotal skin becomes avulsed, try to find it. Wrap it in moist, sterile gauze, and send it with the victim to the hospital.

4. Dress the scrotum itself in a sterile dressing moistened with clean water, and control bleeding with pressure.

FEMALE GENITALIA

Injuries to the external female genitalia are rare but can follow straddle injuries or sexual assault. Because the area is richly supplied with blood vessels and nerves, the injury can cause blinding pain and considerable bleeding; however, it is not usually life-threatening. To care for this emergency:

1. Control bleeding with local pressure, using moist compresses.

2. Dress the wounds, and keep the dressing in place with a diaper-type bandage. Stabilize any impaled objects or foreign bodies.

3. Use ice packs over the dressing to relieve pain and reduce swelling.

4. *Never* place dressings or packs inside the **VAGINA**.

5. Treat for shock.

6. Monitor vital signs.

7. Activate the EMS system as soon as possible.

| **17** | **SELF-TEST** | **17** |

Student: _____ Date: _____

Course: _____ Section #: _____

PART I: True/False   If you believe that the statement is true, circle the T. If you believe that the statement is false, circle the F.

T   F   1. Blunt or perforating injuries of the abdominal cavity are serious medical emergencies.

T   F   2. The organs most frequently damaged by penetrating abdominal trauma are the liver, small intestine, and colon.

T   F   3. Victims with abdominal pain may have pain that radiates to either shoulder.

T   F   4. Common signs and symptoms of abdominal injuries include slow, shallow breathing, and rapid pulse.

T   F   5. If organs are protruding from the abdomen, gently try to replace them in the abdominal cavity.

T   F   6. A victim with abdominal injury is usually most comfortable in a prone position.

T   F   7. Do not remove penetrating or impaled objects from the abdomen.

T   F   8. The most common hernia is a protrusion of a portion of an internal organ through the wall of the abdomen.

T   F   9. Most hernias occur in or just below the groin.

T   F   10. A dull, pulsating pain is the most common symptom of a hernia.

T   F   11. To treat a victim with a hernia, lie him on his back with the knees drawn up.

T   F   12. Penetrating objects of the penis should be removed.

T   F   13. Bleeding from an injury to the penis or female genitalia should always be controlled at the femoral pressure point.

T   F   14. Injuries to the male and female genital area can be treated with ice to reduce swelling and relieve pain.

T   F   15. Bleeding from the female genital area should be treated by placing dressings or packs inside the vagina.

PART II: Multiple Choice   For each question, circle the answer that best reflects an accurate statement.

1. What symptom would a victim with abdominal injuries exhibit?
   a. deep, labored breathing.
   b. dangerously slow pulse.
   c. pain radiating into the legs.
   d. prefers to lie still with legs drawn up.

2. Which of the following is *not* appropriate care for abdominal injuries?
   a. carefully remove impaled objects.
   b. do not give the victim anything by mouth.
   c. work to prevent shock.
   d. have the victim lie on his back with legs flexed.

3. Emergency care for a rupture or hernia includes:
   a. never attempt to force the protrusion back into the cavity.
   b. lie the victim on his back with legs straight.
   c. administer aspirin with small quantities of water.
   d. place a cold compress on the area.

4. Eviscerated organs should be:
   a. replaced within the abdomen.
   b. covered with a dry dressing only.
   c. covered with a moist sterile and occlusive dressing.
   d. rinsed thoroughly with copious amounts of water and replaced within the abdomen.

5. When the penis is partially or completely amputated, first:
   a. pack the area in ice.
   b. elevate the area.
   c. apply direct pressure.
   d. apply a tourniquet to the remaining stump to control blood loss.

6. Which of the following is *not* a sign or symptom of rupture or hernia?
   a. swelling.
   b. nausea and vomiting.
   c. feeling of something giving way.
   d. dull ache.

7. Which of the following is *not* a correct means of treating injuries to the female genitalia?
   a. apply local pressure.
   b. dress wounds.
   c. hold dressings in place with a diaper-like bandage.
   d. place dressings inside the vagina.

8. Which of the following is *not* a recommended guideline in caring for injuries to the male genitalia?
   a. preserve any avulsed parts.
   b. use pressure to control bleeding.
   c. quickly remove any penetrating object to relieve pain.
   d. wrap the injury in a moist, sterile dressing.

9. The proper emergency care of testicular rupture is to:
   a. apply a tourniquet to the scrotum.
   b. use pressure to control bleeding.
   c. apply a pressure dressing and bandage.
   d. apply ice packs to the area.

10. Lacerations of the urethra or ureters:
   a. are common.
   b. are usually caused by penetrating injuries to the abdomen.
   c. are usually not indicated by blood in the urine.
   d. seldom require medical care.

11. Injuries to the external male genitalia:
    a. are usually life-threatening medical emergencies.
    b. are usually very painful and embarrassing to the victim.
    c. usually cause little concern to the victim.
    d. all of the above.

12. The most common form of rupture or hernia occurs when:
    a. a portion of an internal organ protrudes through the abdominal wall.
    b. a portion of a thoracic organ protrudes through the thoracic wall.
    c. veins or arteries become weak and bulge or rupture.
    d. any of the above.

13. Do all of the following for abdominal injuries, except:
    a. gently replace protruding organs within the abdominal cavity.
    b. suspect shock and work to prevent it.
    c. control bleeding and dress all open wounds.
    d. be alert for vomiting and protect the airway.

PART III: What Would You Do If:

1. You are at the scene of a construction site where a worker has fallen on some reinforcing rods. He is lying on his back and has an obvious abdominal evisceration.

2. You are at a home where a victim has been lifting and moving heavy boxes. He complains of nausea and sharp, stinging pain just above the groin. There is swelling and protrusion in the area of pain.

PART IV: Practical Skills Check-Off

_____ has satisfactorily passed the following practical skills:
Student's Name

	Date	Partner Check	Inst. Init.
1. Demonstrate how to care for an abdominal evisceration.	__/__/__	☐	_____
2. Demonstrate how to care for a hernia victim.	__/__/__	☐	_____

CHAPTER EIGHTEEN

OBJECTIVES

- ■ Understand the incidence and seriousness of poisoning and various ways in which poisons can enter the body.

- ■ Identify the common signs and symptoms of ingested, inhaled, and absorbed poisons.

- ■ Describe the appropriate emergency care for specific types of poisoning.

POISONING EMERGENCIES

Each year in the United States, thousands of people die from suicidal or accidental poisonings. Poisoning is now the fifth most common cause of accidental death in the United States and ranks first among children (Figure 18-1). Each year, it is estimated that 3 percent of all children in the United States require treatment for poisoning.

In addition to the fatalities, approximately one million cases of nonfatal poisonings occur because

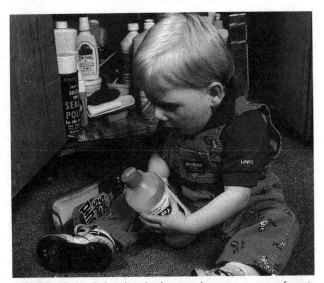

FIGURE 18-1. Poisoning is the number-one cause of accidental death among children.

of exposure to substances such as industrial chemicals, cleaning agents, plant and insect sprays, and medications — in fact, two-thirds of all poisonings, in all age groups involve drugs. As a result, trained First Aiders are very likely to encounter poisoning emergencies, especially involving children.

A poison is any substance — liquid, solid, or gas — that impairs health or causes death by its chemical action when it is introduced in relatively small amounts into the body or onto the skin surface. Some substances that are otherwise harmless become deadly if used incorrectly. It is critical that you learn to recognize signs and symptoms of poisoning and that you become able to administer effective emergency care.

Poisons may enter the body in the following ways:

- ■ **INGESTION**, or through the mouth (medication, household cleaners, agricultural products, and chemicals).

- ■ Inhalation in the form of noxious dusts, gases, fumes, or mists (**CARBON MONOXIDE**, **CHLORINE**, **AMMONIA**, insect sprays, chemical gases).

- ■ Injection into the body tissues or bloodstream by hypodermic needles or as bites of **RABID** animals, poisonous snakes, or poisonous insects (snakebite, spider bite, insect sting). See Chapter 20.

- ■ **ABSORPTION** through the skin (as with mercury or certain other poisonous liquids) or contact with the skin (as with poisonous plants and certain fungi).

INGESTED POISONS

In the United States alone, eight to ten million poisonings each year occur in the form of ingestion; thousands of those victims die. The most common agents involved are **SALICYLATES** (aspirin), **ACETAMINOPHEN**, alcohol, detergents/soaps, and petroleum distillates.

Ingested poisons usually remain in the stomach only a short time; the stomach absorbs substances only minimally. Rather, absorption takes place after the poison has passed into the small intestine. Thus, much of the management of poisoning is aimed at trying to rid the body of the poison before it gains access to the intestinal tract.

The chief causes of poisoning by ingestion are:

- Overdose of medicine (intentional or accidental).
- Medicines, household cleaners, and chemicals within reach of children.
- Combining drugs and alcohol.
- Storing poisons in food or drink containers.
- Carelessness.

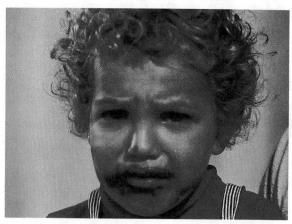

FIGURE 18-2. Skin discoloration — possible poisoning.

- Unconsciousness or varying levels of unconsciousness.
- Convulsions or seizures.

SIGNS AND SYMPTOMS

The signs and symptoms of poisoning by ingestion are variable, depending on the substances involved. The most common signs and symptoms are (Figures 18-2 and 18-3):

- Dilated or constricted pupils.
- Nausea, retching, vomiting, and diarrhea.
- Severe abdominal pain, tenderness, distension, and cramps.
- Slowed or abnormal respiration and circulation.
- Excessive salivation or foaming at the mouth.
- Excessive sweating.
- Excessive tear formation.
- Burns or stains around the mouth, pain in the mouth or throat, pain upon swallowing (corrosive poisons may corrode, burn, or destroy the tissues of the mouth, throat, and stomach).
- Unusual breath or body odors.
- Signs of shock.
- Characteristic chemical odors on the breath (such as that left by turpentine).

POISON CENTERS

For every case of ingested poisoning, call the nearest poison center (a regional one, if possible) for advice. Officials at the center can help you decide which first-aid measures are a priority and can help you formulate an effective plan. The poison center can also provide information on any available antidote that may be appropriate.

Calls to poison centers are toll-free, and most are staffed twenty-four hours per day by experienced professionals. Each center also is connected to a network of consultants nationwide who can answer questions about almost any toxin. Information on the poison center's computer is updated every ninety days to provide the latest information on treatment options and antidotes. Centers also provide followup telephone calls, monitoring the victim's progress and making treatment suggestions until the victim is either hospitalized or asymptomatic.

Contacting the poison center in case of ingested poisoning is safer and more reliable than following manufacturer's label cautions, especially since label information may be incomplete, too generic, or too outdated to be effective. However, initial victim assessment and emergency care should not be delayed to accommodate a call to the poison center.

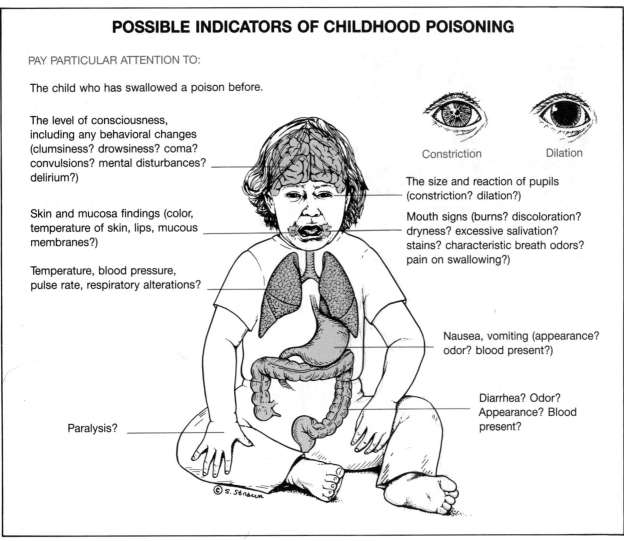

POSSIBLE INDICATORS OF CHILDHOOD POISONING

PAY PARTICULAR ATTENTION TO:

The child who has swallowed a poison before.

The level of consciousness, including any behavioral changes (clumsiness? drowsiness? coma? convulsions? mental disturbances? delirium?)

Skin and mucosa findings (color, temperature of skin, lips, mucous membranes?)

Temperature, blood pressure, pulse rate, respiratory alterations?

Paralysis?

Constriction   Dilation

The size and reaction of pupils (constriction? dilation?)

Mouth signs (burns? discoloration? dryness? excessive salivation? stains? characteristic breath odors? pain on swallowing?)

Nausea, vomiting (appearance? odor? blood present?)

Diarrhea? Odor? Appearance? Blood present?

© S. Schaun

FIGURE 18-3.

EMERGENCY CARE FOR INGESTED POISONS

The priorities in caring for this type of emergency are airway, breathing, and circulation. Follow these guidelines:

1. **Maintain the airway.** This cannot be overemphasized! The sleepy or **COMATOSE** victim is in constant danger of aspiration — maintaining the airway is one of your primary responsibilities.

2. **Keep the airway clear with proper positioning.** Secretions may be profuse following the ingestion of certain poisons, so be prepared to place the victim on his side with his head tilted down to allow for proper drainage.

3. **Induce vomiting.** If the victim has ingested poison within the past thirty to sixty minutes, the general rule is to induce vomiting to empty the stomach. *Follow local protocol.* There are some important exceptions for which you should *never* induce vomiting; they are itemized under number 4 in this list. The method of choice of inducing vomiting is to use **SYRUP OF IPECAC** (See Figure 18-4). However, there is some controversy about First Aiders using ipecac — follow local protocol. To induce vomiting:

   ■ Have the victim drink water; an adult needs eight ounces, a child four ounces.

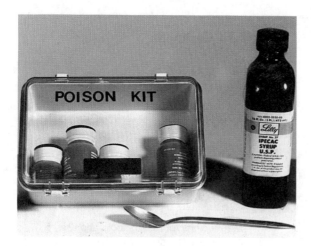

FIGURE 18-4. Emergency care kit for poisoning includes syrup of ipecac and activated charcoal.

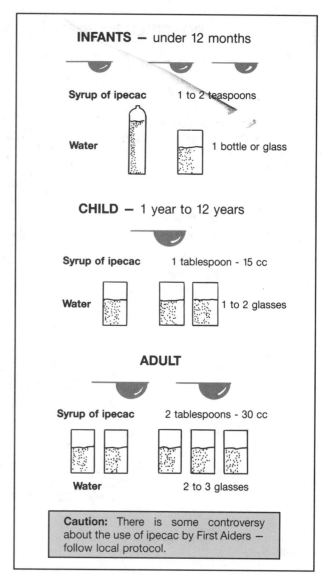

FIGURE 18-5. How to induce vomiting.

- Administer syrup of ipecac. *Make sure that you are using syrup of ipecac, NOT ipecac fluid extract, which is fourteen times more potent — and it can be fatal at the listed doses.* Syrup of ipecac doses are: adult, two tablespoons (thirty cubic centimeters); children one year and older, one tablespoon (fifteen cubic centimeters); infants under twelve months, one to two teaspoons (five to ten cubic centimeters). Follow an infant's dose with one bottle of water, a child's with one to two glasses of water, and an adult's with two to three glasses of water (Figure 18-5). When possible, it is recommended that children under twelve months be "ipecaced" in a health-care facility — follow local protocol.

- Have the victim sit and lean forward to prevent vomitus from being aspirated into the lungs. Place an infant or small child on his stomach with his head lower than the rest of his body, his face pointed downward.

- Do not delay transport or activation of the EMS system while waiting for the victim to vomit. Syrup of ipecac may take up to twenty minutes to work; vomiting almost always occurs after one dose if you allow enough time for it to work. While a second dose is seldom necessary, you can repeat your initial dosage *once* if the victim does not vomit after twenty minutes.

- If the victim does not vomit after the second dose, you must transport him to a hospital immediately.

- When the victim stops vomiting from the ipecac, give him **ACTIVATED CHARCOAL** — a

specially treated, steam-cleaned charcoal that can absorb many times its weight in contaminants. Mix at least two tablespoons of dry charcoal in a glass of tap water to make a slurry. (Many poison antidote kits contain a premixed charcoal slurry that should *not* be mixed with water.) Give the mixture to children in an opaque container, since they may be reluctant to drink it. *Never give activated charcoal before or together with syrup of ipecac, because the charcoal will inactivate the ipecac and render it ineffective. Many feel that activated charcoal should not be used in a first-aid setting — follow local protocol.*

- Give the victim nothing by mouth for one hour following vomiting.

▪ Never allow the victim to fall asleep in a supine position after vomiting; vomiting could recur, and the victim could aspirate.

4. As mentioned, *there are times when you should NOT induce vomiting* — follow local protocol. As a general rule, you should never induce vomiting in the following cases (Figure 18-6):

▪ The victim is younger than six months of age.

▪ The victim is stuporous or comatose; the vomitus may be aspirated into the lungs, causing pneumonia.

▪ The victim has no gag reflex.

▪ The victim is having or has had seizures.

▪ The victim shows signs or symptoms of acute myocardial infarction.

▪ The victim has ingested corrosives (strong acids or alkalis). These include many household cleaners that can damage the esophagus and lining of the mouth as they are ejected.

▪ The victim has ingested petroleum distillates or products (such as kerosene, gasoline, lighter fluid, or furniture polish). You may be instructed to induce vomiting anyway if the victim has ingested excessive amounts or if he has swallowed an extremely toxic product, such as a pesticide or one containing heavy metals. Check with your local poison center.

▪ The victim has ingested a convulsant, such as **STRYCHNINE** (often found in mouse poisons); vomiting may induce convulsions.

▪ The victim is in the last trimester of pregnancy.

▪ When in doubt, call for advice, follow local protocol, and follow the recommendations of the poison center.

▪ If the victim has swallowed acid, alkali, or petroleum distillates and is in complete control of his airway, administer one to two glasses of milk or water to help wash out and coat the esophagus and dilute the poison.

5. If a child has handled or been poisoned by a corrosive substance, always wash his hands and fingers thoroughly to prevent any damage to his eyes if he rubs them. If in doubt, flush his eyes with water.

6. Be prepared to manage shock, coma, seizures, and cardiac arrest as detailed in other chapters of this book. Mouth-to-mouth resuscitation may be dangerous if the victim still has poison on his lips, tongue, or the skin surrounding his mouth. Use a handkerchief or a pocket face mask.

7. Do not use milk or carbonated beverages with syrup of ipecac.

8. Do not give mustard or salt to induce vomiting.

9. If syrup of ipecac is not available, *as a last resort* you can induce vomiting by using the end of a napkin- or handkerchief-padded spoon to tickle the back of the throat and stimulate the gag reflex. Vomiting may be more effectively induced if you first give the victim several glasses of warm water. If the victim is a child, administer a cup of water and place him face down across your knees before tickling his throat.

10. Activate the EMS system immediately.

WHEN NOT TO INDUCE VOMITING IN A POISONING EMERGENCY

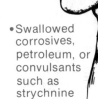

- Having heart attack
- Having seizure
- Unconscious or stuporous
- Swallowed corrosives, petroleum, or convulsants such as strychnine

> When in doubt always call for advice and follow recommendation of a physician and/or local poison center.

FIGURE 18-6.

INHALED POISONS

About 1,400 people die each year in the United States as a result of inhaling poisonous vapors and fumes, some of which are present without any sign. Most toxic inhalation occurs as a result of fire. It is critical that care be immediate, because the body absorbs inhaled poisons rapidly.

Common sources of inhaled poison include:

- Carbon monoxide.
- Carbon dioxide from industrial sites, sewers, and wells.
- Chlorine gas (common around swimming pools).
- Fumes from liquid chemicals and sprays.
- Chemical warfare agents (such as tear gas, nerve gas, and vomit gas).
- Ammonia.
- Sulphur dioxide (used in the home and commercially to make ice).
- Anesthetic gases (ether, nitrous oxide, chloroform).
- Solvents used in dry cleaning, degreasing agents, or fire extinguishers.
- Industrial gases.
- Incomplete combustion of natural gas.
- Hydrogen sulfide (sewer gas).

SIGNS AND SYMPTOMS OF INHALED POISONING

The general signs and symptoms of inhaled poisoning include the following:

- Severe headache.
- Nausea and/or vomiting.
- Cough, stridor, wheezing, or rales.
- Shortness of breath.
- Chest pain or tightness.
- Facial burns.
- Signs of respiratory tract burns, including singed nasal hairs, soot in sputum, or soot in throat.
- Burning or tearing eyes.
- Burning sensation in the throat or chest.
- Cyanosis.
- Confusion.
- Dizziness.
- Varying levels of consciousness.

CARBON MONOXIDE POISONING

The most common gas that causes poisoning is carbon monoxide — present in paint remover, aerosols, coal, charcoal briquettes, tobacco, gasoline, insulating materials, building materials, exhaust fumes of internal combustion engines (such as cars), lanterns, sewer gas, charcoal grills, and gas that is manufactured for cooking and heating. More than 2,500 people die each year from carbon-monoxide poisoning.

Carbon monoxide is completely nonirritating, tasteless, colorless, and odorless. It is formed by the incomplete combustion of gasoline, coal, kerosene, plastic, wood, and natural gas. The primary sources of carbon monoxide are home-heating devices and exhaust fumes from automobiles.

The initial symptoms of poisoning include headache, weakness, agitation, confusion, and slight dizziness. As the poisoning progresses, the victim suffers dim vision, spots before the eyes, sensitivity of the eyes to light, temporary blindness or hearing loss, and eventually, convulsions, coma, and death. If the victim is not removed from the source quickly, he will become unconscious and will have trouble breathing. It takes only a few minutes to die from carbon monoxide poisoning. Death is so certain, in fact, that more than half of all suicides in the United States each year are committed with automobile exhaust, which is 7 percent carbon monoxide.

The signs and symptoms of acute carbon-monoxide poisoning are the same in adults and children and depend on the percentage of carbon monoxide in the blood. They may range from subtle central-nervous-system effects to coma and death. The range of signs and symptoms includes the following (Figure 18-7):

- Throbbing headache (low levels of carbon monoxide).
- Nausea (low levels).
- Shortness of breath (low levels).
- Irritability, confusion, loss of judgment (higher levels).
- Increased heart and breathing rate (higher levels).
- Dizziness (higher levels).
- Yawning (higher levels).
- Faintness (higher levels).
- Lethargy and stupor (higher levels).
- Seizures (higher levels).
- Heart arrhythmias, chest pain (higher levels).
- Skin color normal at first, becoming pale, then becoming cyanotic as poisoning progresses. In late stages at very high levels, mucous membranes and skin become bright cherry-red in color, sometimes blistering. Cherry-red lips are not commonly seen and occur at higher levels.
- Temporary loss of vision (higher levels).

Approximately 10 to 30 percent of all carbon monoxide poisoning victims have a delay in the onset of symptoms that may be several weeks. If

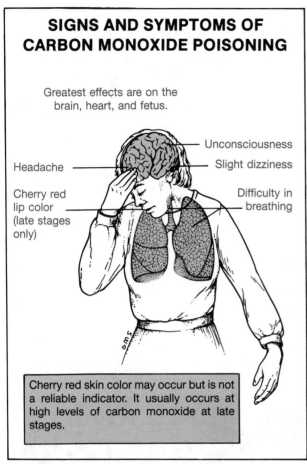

SIGNS AND SYMPTOMS OF CARBON MONOXIDE POISONING

Greatest effects are on the brain, heart, and fetus.

Headache

Cherry red lip color (late stages only)

Unconsciousness

Slight dizziness

Difficulty in breathing

Cherry red skin color may occur but is not a reliable indicator. It usually occurs at high levels of carbon monoxide at late stages.

FIGURE 18-7.

such a delay occurs, the symptoms are usually irreversible. Signs and symptoms of delayed poisoning include:

- Flu-like illness (look for a persistent flu-like illness without fever or upper respiratory infection).
- Irritability.
- Memory loss.
- Inability to concentrate.
- Inability to think abstractly.
- Personality changes.
- Uncontrolled crying.

EMERGENCY CARE FOR INHALED POISONS

- *Protect yourself first!* Safeguarding your own health, get the victim into fresh air immediately, removing him from the source of the poison. If the victim is in a closed garage or room, call a rescue squad or the fire department. Remember — the presence of carbon monoxide is difficult to

detect. Do not delay unnecessarily in an area that may be contaminated. If there are no contraindicating injuries, have the victim lie down with his head elevated.

2. Loosen all tight-fitting clothing, especially around the neck and over the chest.

3. If the victim is not breathing, start artificial ventilation immediately, and continue until the victim is breathing on his own. Do not interrupt the artificial ventilation for any reason. If necessary, administer CPR.

4. Treat the victim for shock and keep him completely inactive and quiet.

5. Transport the victim to a physician or activate the EMS system immediately, even if he seems to have recovered (awakening or seeming alertness can be false signs of recovery).

6. Contact the poison center for further instructions.

ABSORBED POISONS

Absorbed poisons — those that enter through the skin — generally cause burns, lesions, and inflammation. Corrosives or other chemicals that are splashed into the eyes cause extreme burning pain, excessive tearing, and the inability to open the eye.

EMERGENCY CARE FOR ABSORBED POISONS

Whenever a victim has corrosives or chemicals on the skin or in the eyes, contact the regional poison center immediately. Guidelines for treating chemical burns of the eyes are found in Chapter 14. General emergency care for absorbed poisons is as follows:

1. Protecting your own hands with gloves, carefully remove all contaminated clothing. Take extreme care not to spread the contamination as you are removing the victim's clothing.

2. Blot dry any liquid toxins on the victim's skin.

3. Brush any solid toxins from the victim's skin, taking extreme care not to abrade the skin and not to spread the contamination.

4. Irrigate the victim's skin copiously with running water when possible (a shower or garden hose is ideal). Make sure that you protect bystanders and the victim from further contamination. Do two separate washings.

5. Carefully check "hidden" areas, such as the nailbeds, skin creases, areas between the fingers and toes, and any hair.

6. Transport the victim to a physician or activate the EMS system.

POISONOUS PLANTS

INGESTION OF A POISONOUS PLANT

A number of common backyard and household plants are poisonous if they are eaten. The United States Public Health Service estimates that 12,000 children eat potentially poisonous plants every year. And the plants involved are not exotic — they include morning glory, rhubarb leaves, buttercup, daisy, daffodil, lily of the valley, narcissus, tulip, azalea, English ivy, mistletoe berries, iris, hyacinth, laurel, philodendron, rhododendron, wisteria, delphinium, and certain parts of the tomato, potato, and petunia plants.

Signs and symptoms of plant ingestion depend, of course, on the plant that was ingested; each one has individual toxins. The most common signs and symptoms include:

- Intense burning of the tongue and mouth.
- Nausea and vomiting.
- Diarrhea.
- Watering of the mouth, nose, and eyes.
- Seizures.
- Excessive sweating.
- Weakness.
- Paralysis.
- Stomach pain.
- Dilated pupils.
- Fever.
- Hallucinations.
- Abdominal cramps.
- Respiratory depression.

Emergency Care for Ingestion of Poisonous Plants

Emergency care for ingestion of poisonous plants consists of the following:

1. Induce vomiting with syrup of ipecac. Follow the guidelines listed under ingested poisons.
2. Administer activated charcoal after all vomiting has stopped.
3. Provide basic supportive care; apply cold compresses to the mouth to ease pain and itching.
4. Activate the EMS system immediately.

SKIN CONTACT WITH A POISONOUS PLANT

Poison ivy (Figure 18-8) thrives in sun and in light shade. It usually grows in the form of a trailing vine that sends out numerous kinky brown footlets that are slightly thickened at the tips. It can also grow in the form of a bush and can attain heights of ten feet or more. Poison sumac (Figure 18-9) is a tall shrub or slender tree, usually growing along swamps and ponds in wooded areas. Poison oak (Figure 18-10) resembles poison ivy, with one important difference: the poison oak leaves have rounded, lobed leaflets instead of leaflets that are jagged or entire. Poison oak is found mostly in the Southeast and West. Other plants that can cause mild to severe **DERMATITIS** include stinging nettle, crown of thorns, buttercup, mayapple, marsh marigold, candelabra cactus, brown-eyed Susan, shasta daisy, and chrysanthemum.

Signs and symptoms of contact with a poisonous plant generally include the following:

- Blisters at the site of contact (it generally takes two to seven days for the rash to form, but severe

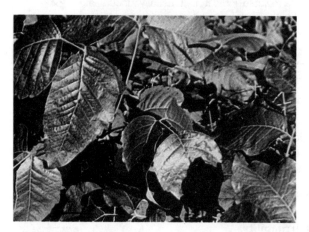

FIGURE 18-8. Poison ivy.

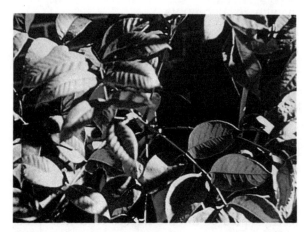

FIGURE 18-9. Poison sumac.

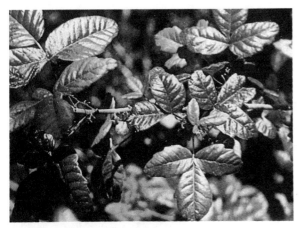

FIGURE 18-10. Poison oak.

contact can cause a rash within twelve hours) (Figure 18-11).

- Itching and burning.
- Swelling.
- Pain if the reaction is severe.
- Other areas of contact can cause **CONJUNCTIVITIS**, asthma, and other allergic reactions.

If the rash is scratched, secondary infections can occur. The rash usually disappears in one to two weeks in cases of mild exposure, and up to three weeks when exposure is more severe.

Toxin on the hands may spread the rash to other parts of the body, but the clear fluid that weeps from the rash will not spread the rash or infect new sites.

Emergency Care for Skin Contact with a Poisonous Plant

The following emergency care is recommended:

1. Remove any clothing that may have plant oils on it. Be careful not to spread contamination as you

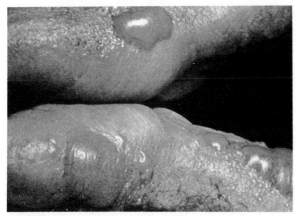

FIGURE 18-11. Blisters from poisonous plant contact.

remove the victim's clothing, and protect your own skin from exposure.

2. Wash the exposed skin thoroughly as soon as possible after contact to limit the spread of plant oils. Speed counts! Wash within five minutes, if possible. Do not use soap — it causes plant oils to spread. Ideally, you should pour rubbing alcohol (follow local protocol) over the area and rinse it with cool water. Then flood the exposed skin with cool water and pat — do not rub — dry. Make sure to scrub under the fingernails to remove any plant oils there.

3. Apply cold compresses to help reduce swelling and irritation.

4. Apply soothing lotions to help reduce swelling and irritation; use calamine or calamine/antihistamine, but steer away from others, since they can worsen the allergic reaction.

5. Keep the area clean and dry, and instruct the victim not to scratch the rash.

6. If a severe exposure does not respond to the above-outlined emergency care, have the victim see a physician.

FOOD POISONING

Food poisoning occurs when food that contains bacteria or the toxins that bacteria produce is eaten. Illness can be caused either by the bacteria itself or by the toxins produced by the bacteria.

STAPHYLOCOCCUS

The most common food-borne illness, **STAPHYLOCOCCUS** poisoning, is caused by bacterial toxins and causes inflammation and irritation of the stomach and intestinal linings. One to five hours after eating the affected food, the victim will experience sudden and violent nausea and vomiting, abdominal cramps, and diarrhea. There is no fever. In severe cases, shock may develop. Recovery is rapid, sometimes within three hours and rarely beyond twenty-four hours.

Staphylococcus poisoning usually is caused by food that is prepared ahead of time and kept warm in warming trays or a warm oven.

Emergency care consists of controlling vomiting and diarrhea to prevent dehydration, and giving care for shock. Do not give the victim anything to eat or drink until his vomiting and diarrhea have stopped. Extremely young or old victims may need to be hospitalized to control dehydration.

CLOSTRIDIUM PERFRINGENS

CLOSTRIDIUM PERFRINGENS food poisoning results when food is prepared in large quantities and is allowed to sit at room temperature (or in an ineffective steamer). The infection may also result if food is not refrigerated at a low enough temperature (the bacteria thrive in environments anywhere from 40°F. to 140°F.).

Nausea, abdominal cramps, and diarrhea are common symptoms; vomiting is rare. Onset of symptoms occurs usually after six to twenty-four hours; the illness rarely lasts longer than twenty-four hours. To treat, control dehydration.

SALMONELLA

Symptoms of **SALMONELLA** poisoning usually appear twelve to twenty-four hours (and sometimes up to seventy-two hours) following ingestion of a contaminated food. Salmonella poisoning is caused by a living bacteria. The victim suffers diarrhea, fever, nausea, vomiting, and abdominal cramps with occasional chills. Weakness and dehydration may result. Salmonella poisoning can be prevented through proper cooking and cleanliness of the cooking area and cooking utensils (see Figure 18-12).

Emergency care consists of controlling vomiting and diarrhea to prevent dehydration. Antibiotic therapy may be needed for victims under one year of age or the elderly. These victims should be seen by a physician.

BOTULISM

Early recognition of **BOTULISM** and fast care are necessary to save a victim's life. Botulism, which is uncommon, can be deadly. Botulism blocks transmission of impulses from the nerves to the muscles; it causes severe weakness, paralysis, and death. The toxin, unfortunately, is tasteless, so a victim can eat spoiled food without knowing it.

Detection of botulism is difficult because it resembles so many other problems. Symptoms usually do not appear for approximately twenty-four hours after eating; if the victim lives, they linger for weeks. While the diagnosis of botulism may require sophisticated testing, suspect botulism in any victim who develops a dry, sore mouth and throat and difficulty focusing the eyes (or blurred or double vision) after a period of fatigue. Other signs and symptoms include problems speaking and swallowing, weakness or paralysis, limited eye movement, dilated pupils, paralysis of the breathing muscles,

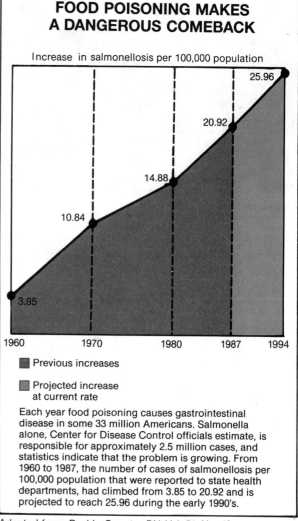

FOOD POISONING MAKES A DANGEROUS COMEBACK

Increase in salmonellosis per 100,000 population

25.96
20.92
14.88
10.84
3.85

1960   1970   1980   1987   1994

■ Previous increases

■ Projected increase at current rate

Each year food poisoning causes gastrointestinal disease in some 33 million Americans. Salmonella alone, Center for Disease Control officials estimate, is responsible for approximately 2.5 million cases, and statistics indicate that the problem is growing. From 1960 to 1987, the number of cases of salmonellosis per 100,000 population that were reported to state health departments, had climbed from 3.85 to 20.92 and is projected to reach 25.96 during the early 1990's.

Adapted from: Paul L. Cerrato, *RN*, Vol. 51, No. 10.
FIGURE 18-12.

decreased tendon reflexes, and impaired speech. Any pain that is experienced is generally from a headache in the front part of the head. Breathing difficulty may develop.

The major sources of botulism poisoning occur when food is improperly stored after it is cooked: home-canned foods have been culprits, but 42 percent of all reported cases have occurred from foods served in restaurants.

A physician must administer antitoxins; because they carry risks, they can be administered only in a hospital. Induce vomiting to rid the victim of any remaining spoiled food. If breathing muscles are paralyzed, open the airway and administer artificial ventilation. Activate the EMS system *immediately*.

| 18 | SELF-TEST | 18 |

Student: _____   Date: _____

Course: _____   Section #: _____

PART I: True/False   If you believe that the statement is true, circle the T. If you believe that the statement is false, circle the F.

(T) F   1. Ingestion of poisonous plants is a common poisoning emergency in children.

(T) F   2. A victim of an inhaled poison should be given syrup of ipecac.

T F   3. Cherry-red lips are a common early sign of carbon-monoxide poisoning.

T F   4. Approximately 10 to 30 percent of all carbon-monoxide poisoning victims have a delay of up to several weeks of onset of symptoms.

T F   5. A throbbing headache is a symptom of low-level carbon-monoxide poisoning.

T F   6. Activated charcoal should be given together with syrup of ipecac for ingested poisoning emergencies.

T F   7. In a poisoning emergency where syrup of ipecac is used, transport should be delayed until the victim vomits.

T F   8. A victim of poisoning should be kept in a semi-sitting position.

T F   9. Initial symptoms of carbon-monoxide poisoning include headache, weakness, agitation, confusion, and dizziness.

PART II: Multiple Choice   For each question, circle the answer that best reflects an accurate statement.

1. Poisoning is now the _____fifth_____ most common cause of death in the United States.
    a. first.
    b. third.
    c. fifth.
    d. second.

2. Which of the following is *not* a way that poisons may enter the body?
    a. absorption.
    b. emesis.
    c. inhalation.
    d. injection.

3. In *all but one* of the following victims, the First Aider should *not* induce vomiting:
    a. a victim who has ingested petroleum products.
    b. a victim in early pregnancy.
    c. a stuporous victim.
    d. a victim with seizures.

4. The usual dose of syrup of ipecac for a child over one year of age is:
    a. 15 milliliters (1 tablespoon) with 1 to 2 glasses of water.
    b. 30 milliliters (2 tablespoons) with 2 to 3 glasses of water.
    c. 15 milliliters (1 tablespoon) with one half glass of water.
    d. 30 milliliters (2 tablespoons) with 1 to 2 glasses of water.

5. The common signs and symptoms of poisoning by ingestion are:
    a. nausea, vomiting, diarrhea.
    b. severe abdominal pain or cramps.
    c. excessive salivation or sweating.
    d. all of these answers.

6. If the victim has ingested poison, vomiting should *never* be induced when:
    a. the victim has severe abdominal pain and cramps.
    b. the victim is stuporous or unconscious.
    c. diarrhea is present.
    d. respiration and circulation are slowed.

7. Syrup of ipecac is an effective means of inducing vomiting. What is the proper dose for eliminating poisons in an adult?
    a. one teaspoon.
    b. one tablespoon.
    c. two tablespoons.
    d. three tablespoons.

8. To induce vomiting, syrup of ipecac should be followed by:
    a. rigorous exercise.
    b. large doses of activated charcoal.
    c. two to three glasses of water.
    d. nothing, syrup of ipecac works by itself.

9. It is critical that care be given immediately to the person who has inhaled poison because:
    a. inhaled poisons are more toxic than ingested poisons.
    b. the body absorbs inhaled poisons rapidly.
    c. inhaled poisons remain in the system longer than ingested poisons.
    d. the victim may experience convulsions that make treatment difficult.

10. What is a characteristic symptom of carbon-monoxide poisoning?
    a. headache.
    b. cool, pale skin.
    c. complaints of a strange taste in the mouth.
    d. stains around the mouth.

11. What is the initial emergency-care procedure for inhalation poisonings?
    a. remove the victim to fresh air.
    b. begin mouth-to-mouth resuscitation.
    c. treat the victim for shock.
    d. seek medical care immediately.

12. What signs and symptoms do poison ivy, poison oak, and poison sumac have in common?
    a. a red rash that does not itch.
    b. nausea and vomiting.
    c. initial redness of the affected area followed by bumps and blisters.
    d. all of these answers.

13. The First Aider's primary responsibility in the emergency care of poisoning is to:
    a. maintain the airway and prevent aspiration of vomitus.
    b. determine what substance caused the poisoning.
    c. assess the level of consciousness.
    d. assess respirations.

14. Symptoms of salmonella poisoning usually appear:
    a. two to three days after ingestion of contaminated food.
    b. gradually, becoming worse within six to eight hours.
    c. suddenly, within one to two hours of eating contaminated food.
    d. within twelve to twenty-four hours after ingestion of contaminated food.

15. The difference in appearance between poison ivy and poison oak is:
    a. poison oak has round leaves while poison ivy has jagged leaves.
    b. poison ivy has greenish-white berries, while poison oak has red berries.
    c. poison ivy leaves are dull, while poison oak leaves are shiny.
    d. all of these answers.

16. Emergency care for the victim who has ingested a strong alkali or acid should include:
    a. neutralization of the acid or alkali with activated charcoal.
    b. dilution with water and immediate transportation.
    c. inducement of vomiting with syrup of ipecac.
    d. all of these answers.

17. After vomiting has ceased, give a victim:
    a. activated charcoal.
    b. lemon juice in a glass of water.
    c. raw egg to coat the stomach.
    d. more ipecac and water.

18. A late stage symptom often indicating carbon monoxide poisoning results when the lips turn:
    a. cyanotic blue.
    b. cyanotic gray.
    c. cherry red.
    d. pale marble white.

19. The most common form of food poisoning results from contamination of the food by:
    a. staphylococcus.
    b. salmonella.
    c. streptococcus.
    d. clostridium.

20. Which of the following is *not* true of staphylococcus-caused food poisoning?
    a. the symptoms usually appear one to five hours after eating.
    b. recovery usually occurs in three to five days.
    c. victims should not eat or drink until diarrhea stops.
    d. the victim may experience diarrhea, abdominal cramping, nausea, and/or vomiting.

21. If a victim experiences double vision and impaired speech after eating canned peaches, the First Aider should suspect:
    a. salmonella poisoning.
    b. botulism.
    c. staph poisoning.
    d. perfringens poisoning.

PART III: Matching: For each poisoning situation listed at the left, indicate when vomiting should or should not be induced.

Poisoning Situation	Emergency Care
_____1. The stuporous or comatose victim.	A. Induce vomiting.
_____2. The last trimester pregnant victim.	B. Do not induce vomiting.
_____3. The victim with possible acute myocardial infarction.	
_____4. The victim has no gag reflex.	
_____5. The victim who has ingested corrosives (strong acids or alkalis).	
_____6. The victim with seizures.	
_____7. The victim who has ingested petroleum products (kerosene, gasoline, lighter fluid, furniture polish).	
_____8. The victim who has ingested a convulsant, iodides, silver nitrate (styptic pencil), or strychnine.	

PART IV: What Would You Do If:

1. A neighbor child (approximately two years old) drank some insecticide being stored in a soda-pop bottle. The boy has severe abdominal pain and is vomiting. His respiration is slowing, and he is starting to show signs of shock.

2. A teenage boy is found in his garage with the car motor running and the doors closed. When you arrive, he has been removed from the garage. He is unconscious, has a rapid heart and breathing rate, and is cyanotic.

PART V: Practical Skills Check-Off _____ has satisfactorily passed the following practical skills:
Student's Name

	Date	Partner Check	Inst. Init.
1. Describe and demonstrate how to induce vomiting and administer activated charcoal.	___/___/___	☐	_____

CHAPTER NINETEEN

OBJECTIVES

■ Know the general terminology relating to drug/alcohol dependency.

■ Explain how to determine if an emergency is drug/alcohol related and the factors that may make it life-threatening.

■ Review the various drug groups, including alcohol, and identify the signs and symptoms associated with their use.

■ Describe the general guidelines for managing a drug/alcohol emergency, including the talk-down technique.

■ Describe emergency care and special precautions for dealing with the PCP user.

DRUG AND ALCOHOL EMERGENCIES

D rugs and alcohol are misused and abused by a variety of individuals. **ALCOHOLISM** strikes all classes and almost every age group; in the United States alone, there are ten million alcoholics. Alcohol is directly involved in approximately 30,000 deaths and 500,000 injuries each year as a result of automobile accidents, and it is a factor in half of all arrests for criminal activity. Because of its deleterious effects on the liver, pancreas, central nervous system, and other body organs, alcohol reduces the average life span of an alcoholic by ten to twelve years (Figures 19-1–19-9).

It is important to become familiar with the various categories of commonly abused drugs, learn their effects on the body, recognize signs and symptoms of **OVERDOSE** and **WITHDRAWAL**, and know the principles of emergency care.

Background information concerning each drug group is provided in Table 19-1 to help you understand the seriousness and complexity of drug and alcohol emergencies. It is not expected that you will remember everything about each of the drug groups. The information that is most important for you to remember concerns emergency care for drug and alcohol abuse and overdose.

GENERAL TERMINOLOGY

DRUG ABUSE is defined as the self-administration of drugs (or of a single drug) in a manner that is not in accord with approved medical or social patterns. **COMPULSIVE DRUG USE** refers to the situation in which an individual becomes preoccupied with the use and procurement of the drug. Compulsive drug use usually leads to **ADDICTION** characterized by physical and/or psychological dependence.

PHYSICAL DEPENDENCE is defined by the appearance of an observable **ABSTINENCE SYNDROME** or withdrawal following the abrupt discontinuation of a drug that has been used regularly. Physical dependence signs and symptoms are different for different drug classes (such as **NARCOTICS, DEPRESSANTS**, or **STIMULANTS**), but physical dependence can always be identified by the presence of abstinence syndromes.

A physically dependent person will usually have one set of signs and symptoms due to drug use and an opposite set when the drug is withheld. **OPIATES**, for example, reduce gastrointestinal activity. When a person who is physically dependent on opiates is denied the drug, he suffers the opposite effect of increased gastrointestinal activity.

ALCOHOL AND DRUG ABUSE DISORDERS

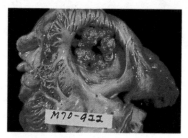

FIGURE 19-1. Fungal damaged heart from drug injection.

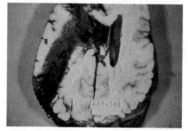

FIGURE 19-2. Bullet wound to brain, alcohol-related.

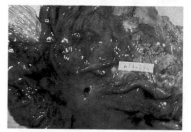

FIGURE 19-3. Chronic gastric ulcer from alcohol use.

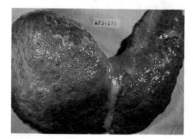

FIGURE 19-4. Alcoholic cirrhosis of liver.

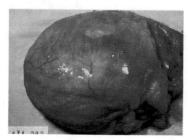

FIGURE 19-5. Enlarged, weak heart, alcohol-induced.

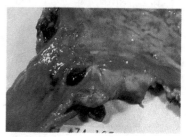

FIGURE 19-6. Ruptured vein in esophagus, causing severe internal bleeding. Alcohol-induced.

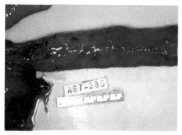

FIGURE 19-7. Dilated esophageal veins from chronic alcohol use.

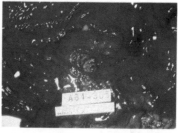

FIGURE 19-8. Internal bleeding from an ulcer caused by chronic alcohol use.

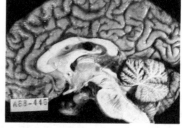

FIGURE 19-9. Brain damage (cerebellum) from chronic alcohol use.

Physical dependence is not a "normal" physiological condition. It represents adaptation by the bodily systems to the presence of the drug. When a person becomes physically dependent, then, the absence of the drug has a significant physiological impact.

PSYCHOLOGICAL DEPENDENCE refers to a condition in which the individual experiences a strong *need* to use the drug repeatedly, even in the absence of physical dependence. The state of psychological dependence is sometimes called **HABITUATION**.

While most drug therapy has traditionally centered on treating physical dependence, psychological dependence is often more compelling and critical. Some drugs produce no physical dependence at all but produce intense psychological dependence.

One of the difficulties with psychological dependence is that the person is "rewarded" for taking the drug. He becomes motivated, feels good, and thinks that he is capable of doing marvelous things. In many cases, the drug is used to escape feelings of depression.

TABLE 19-1	**EMERGENCY CONSEQUENCES OF COMMONLY ABUSED DRUGS**	
DRUG CLUSTER	**MOST COMMON DRUG OF ABUSE**	**CONSEQUENCE OF ABUSE**
STIMULANTS AND APPETITE SUPRESSANTS	AMPHETAMINES Caffeine Cocaine Ephedrine Methylphenidate Nicotine Over-the-Counter Preparations	Moderate dosages cause increased alertness, mood elevation, excitation, euphoria, increased pulse rate and blood pressure, insomnia, loss of appetite. "Recreational" use of cocaine, even in small doses, can cause severe cardiac toxicity, including angina pectoris, arrhythmias, and myocardial infarcts. Overdoses can cause agitation, violence, paranoia, increase in body temperature, hallucinations, convulsions, possible death. Cocaine overdose causes excitement, euphoria, rapid respiration, elevated blood pressure, cyanosis, paralysis, loss of reflexes, and can lead to circulatory failure and death. Although the degree of physical addiction is not known, sudden withdrawal can cause apathy, long periods of sleep, irritability, depression, disorientation.
CANNABIS PRODUCTS	Hashish Marijuana THC (Tetrahydrocannabinol)	Moderate dosages cause euphoria, relaxed inhibitions, increased appetite, dry mouth, disoriented behavior. Overdoses can cause fatigue, tremors, paranoia, possible psychosis. Although the degree of physical addiction is not known, sudden withdrawal can cause insomnia, hyperactivity, and decreased appetite is occasionally reported.
DEPRESSANTS — NARCOTICS AND OPIATES	Codeine Heroin Methadone Morphine Opium (90% of opiate-dependent abusers will have a mixed overdose)	Moderate dosages cause euphoria, drowsiness, lethargy, respiratory depression, constricted pupils, constipation, nausea. Overdoses can cause slow and shallow breathing, clammy skin, convulsions, coma, possible death. Sudden withdrawal results in watery eyes, runny nose, yawning, restlessness, rapid pulse, elevated blood pressure, diarrhea, loss of appetite, irritability, tremors, panic, chills and sweating, cramps, nausea, needle tracks.
DEPRESSANTS — SEDATIVES AND TRANQUILIZERS	Alcohol Antihistamines Barbiturates Chloralhydrate, Other Non-Barbiturate, Nonbenzodiazepine, Sedatives, Over-the-Counter Preparations, Diazepam and Other Benzodiazepines, Other Major Tranquilizers, Other Minor Tranquilizers	Moderate dosages can result in slurred speech, drowsiness, impaired thinking, incoordination, disorientation, drunken behavior without odor of alcohol. Overdose can result in CNS depression, shallow respiration, cold and clammy skin, dilated pupils, weak and rapid pulse, coma, respiratory/circulatory failure, possible death. Aggressive and suicidal behavior may also occur. Sudden withdrawal results in anxiety, insomnia, tremors, delirium, convulsions, possible death.
PSYCHEDELIC DRUGS (Hallucinogens)	DET (N, N-Diethyltryptamine) DMT (N, N-Dimethytryptamine) LSD (Lysergic Acid Diethylamide) Mescaline MDA (3, 4 Methylenedioxyamphetamine) PCP (PHENCYCLIDINE) STP (DOM-2, 5-Dimethoxy, 4-Methylamphetamine)	Moderate dosages can result in motor disturbances, anxiety, paranoia, delusions of persecution, illusions and hallucinations, poor perception of time and distance. Overdose can result in longer, more intense "trip" episodes, psychosis or exacerbation of a pre-existing psychiatric problem, and possible death. Flashbacks can occur months or years after the original dose. PCP may also cause paralysis, violence, rage, status epilepticus.
INHALANTS	Medical Anesthetics Gasoline and Kerosene Glues and Organic Cements Lighter Fluid Lacquer and Varnish Thinners Aerosol Propellants	Moderate dosages cause excitement, euphoria, feelings of drunkenness, giddiness, loss of inhibitions, aggressiveness, delusions, depression, drowsiness, headache, nausea. Overdoses can cause loss of memory, delirium, glazed eyes, slurred speech, drowsiness, hallucinations, confusion, unsteady gait, and erratic heart beat and pulse are possible. Sudden withdrawal results in insomnia, decreased appetite, depression, irritability, headache. Death can result from suffocation or from a phenomenon called SSD ("sudden sniffing death"), which is still poorly understood but which might follow myocardial infarction.

TOLERANCE refers to a situation in which, after repeated exposures to a given drug, achieving the desired effect requires larger doses. The magnitude of tolerance can be measured by comparing the results obtained from the initial dose of the drug with those obtained from subsequent doses.

In many instances, tolerance works within a drug class, i.e., tolerance to one **BARBITURATE** produces a tolerance to all barbiturates. In addition, tolerance may develop in response to only some actions of a particular drug. Tolerance to the different effects of a drug does not necessarily develop at the same rate or with the same degree.

The extent of tolerance and the rate of its development depend on the individual, the drug, the dose, the frequency of dose, and the method of administration. Most tolerance results from frequent and continuous exposure to the drug. An increase in dosage will again produce the desired results. With some drugs, however, the user reaches a plateau, and the desired effect cannot be obtained with *any* dosage. Remember — with **STREET DRUGS**, there is no quality assurance. A "dime bag" that produces moderate euphoria today could be a lethal dose tomorrow!

Addiction involves physical and psychological dependence, tolerance, and compulsive drug use. It is characterized by overwhelming involvement in the use of a drug.

HOW TO DETERMINE IF AN EMERGENCY IS DRUG/ALCOHOL RELATED

Because abuse of drugs and alcohol produces signs that mimic a number of systemic disorders or diseases, it is often difficult to assess a condition as a drug or alcohol emergency. This is especially true if a victim is unconscious. See Table 19-1.

If you suspect that an unconscious victim might be experiencing a drug or alcohol emergency, do the following:

- Inspect the area immediately around the victim for evidence of drug or alcohol use — empty or partially filled pill bottles, syringes, empty liquor bottles, and so on.
- Check the victim's mouth for signs of partially dissolved pills or tablets that may still be in his mouth. (If present, remove.)
- Smell the victim's breath for traces of alcohol. (Be sure that you do not confuse a musky, fruity, or acetone odor for alcohol — all three can be indicative of diabetic coma.)

- Remember — many serious diseases (such as diabetes and epilepsy) resemble drug overdose or abuse. Do not make the mistake of assuming that ingested drugs are the only reason a person may be stuporous or have slurred speech. *Never jump to conclusions.*

HOW TO DETERMINE IF AN ALCOHOL/DRUG EMERGENCY IS LIFE-THREATENING

If you suspect drug or alcohol ingestion at a dangerous level, observe the victim briefly for these six signs and symptoms that indicate a life-threatening emergency (Figure 19-10):

- **Unconsciousness.** The victim cannot be awakened, or, if you can awaken him, he lapses back into unconsciousness almost immediately. He appears to be in a deep sleep or coma.
- **Breathing difficulties.** The victim's breathing may have stopped, may be weak and shallow, or may be weak and strong in cycles. The victim's exhalations may be raspy, rattling, or noisy. The victim's skin may be cyanotic, indicating that he is not receiving enough oxygenated blood.
- **Fever.** Any temperature above 100°F. (38°C.) may indicate a dangerous situation when drugs and/or alcohol are involved.
- **Abnormal pulse rate or irregular pulse.** Normal range for pulse rate is between 60 and 100 beats per minute for an adult; any pulse that is below or above that acceptable range may indicate danger, as does a pulse that is irregular (not rhythmical).
- **Vomiting while not fully conscious.** A person who is stuporous, semiconscious, and who vomits runs a high risk of aspirating the vomitus, creating serious breathing difficulties.
- **Convulsions.** An impending convulsion may be indicated by twitching of the face, trunk, arms, or legs; muscle rigidity; or muscle spasm. A victim who is experiencing a series of violent jerking movements and spasms is having a convulsion.

OBSERVATION AND ASSESSMENT

The most important information to be gathered from the victim concerns the level of consciousness

DRUG AND ALCOHOL EMERGENCY INDICATORS

If any of the following six danger signs are present, no matter what caused the crisis, the victim's life may be threatened and there is an immediate need for emergency care and medical assistance.

1
Unconsciousness:
The victim cannot be awakened from what appears to be a deep sleep or coma. If awakened for a short period of time, he almost immediately relapses into unconsciousness.

3
Raised temperature:
As a guide it may be stated that any temperature above 100°F. or 38°C. falls into this category.

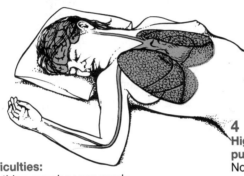

4
High or low pulse rate, or an irregular pulse:
Normal range for pulse rate is between 60 and 100 beats per minute for an adult; any pulse that is below or above that acceptable range indicates danger, as does a pulse that is irregular (not rhythmical).

2
Respiratory difficulties:
The victim's breathing may be very weak, strong and weak in cycles, or may stop altogether. Inhalation or expiration may be noisy. If the victim's skin is bluish (cyanotic), he is almost certainly not receiving enough oxygen, but the absence of cyanosis does not necessarily mean that respiratory difficulties are not severe.

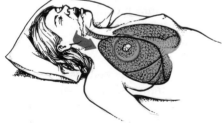

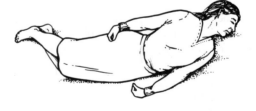

5
Vomiting while semi-conscious or unconscious:
If the victim vomits while semi-conscious or unconscious, the prime danger consists of the possibility that he may breathe vomitus back into his lungs, causing further respiratory difficulties.

6
Convulsions or seizures:
Muscle rigidity, spasm, or twitching of face, trunk muscles, or extremities may indicate an impending convulsion with a series of violent muscle spasms and jerking movements.

FIGURE 19-10.

and vital signs. The severity of the intoxication can be determined by observing the following:

- Whether the victim is awake and will answer questions.

- Whether the victim withdraws from painful stimuli.

- Whether respirations are adequate.

- Whether the circulatory system is functioning properly (blood pressure, pulse, skin color).

Typically most victims will fall into one of three categories:

1. Awake, claiming to have ingested a medicine — the victim answers questions and is alert and aware.

2. Semicomatose — the victim will respond appropriately to verbal or noxious stimuli but fall asleep when the stimulus is removed.

3. Comatose — the victim cannot be aroused to consciousness by verbal or noxious stimuli.

ALCOHOL EMERGENCIES

The alcoholic syndrome usually consists of problem drinking, during which alcohol is used frequently to relieve tensions or other emotional difficulties, and the stage of true addiction, in which abstinence from drinking causes major withdrawal symptoms.

Alcoholism occurs in all social strata. The alcoholic differs from the true social drinker in that he usually begins drinking early in the day, is more prone to drink alone or secretly, and may periodically go on prolonged binges characterized by loss of memory ("blackout periods"). Abstinence from alcohol is likely to produce withdrawal symptoms, such as tremulousness, anxiety, or **DELIRIUM TREMENS (DTs)**. As the alcoholic becomes more dependent upon drinking, his performance at work and relationships with friends and family are likely to deteriorate. Absences from work, emotional disturbances, and automobile accidents become more frequent (Figure 19-11).

ACUTE INTOXICATION

Acute intoxication depends on the amount of alcohol consumed. The signs include drowsiness, disordered speech and gait, and behavior that is violent, destructive, or erratic. But beware — *this picture may be mimicked precisely by the diabetic victim in*

INSULIN SHOCK. Therefore, be suspicious and when in doubt give sugar. If the victim is not diabetic, no harm will be done; many nondiabetic alcoholics have significant **HYPOGLYCEMIA** anyway. Also be alert to the possibility that the victim may have taken a combination of alcohol and sedative drugs.

Give the alcoholic in a coma the same emergency care as you would give any other comatose victim. Give attention to the airway, and monitor the victim carefully.

WITHDRAWAL SYNDROME

Withdrawal syndrome comprises a wide spectrum of signs and symptoms ranging from acute anxiety and tremulousness to DTs. The most common signs and symptoms include:

- Insomnia.
- Muscular weakness.
- Fever.
- Seizures.
- Disorientation, confusion, and thought-process disorders.
- Hallucinations.
- Anorexia.
- Nausea and vomiting.

Early withdrawal almost always begins within one to two days after the last drink; it is very frightening to the victim but is rarely life-threatening. DTs — a severe, life-threatening condition with a mortality rate of approximately 15 percent — can occur between one and fourteen days after the victim's last drink, most commonly within two to five days. A single episode of DTs lasts between one and three days; multiple episodes can last as long as one month.

DTs are characterized by severe confusion, loss of memory, tremors, restlessness, extremely high fever, dilated pupils, profuse sweating, insomnia, nausea, diarrhea, and almost always hallucinations, mostly of a frightening nature (snakes, spiders, or rats, for example). DTs should be suspected in any victim with delirium of unknown cause; reassurance is all that is necessary from the First Aider.

Seizures are very common in alcoholic withdrawal, but not in DTs. The seizures tend to occur early in the withdrawal period, usually during the first twenty-four hours of abstinence; 90 percent of all alcohol-induced seizures occur within seven to forty-eight hours after the victim's last drink. One-third of all who have seizures in early withdrawal will progress to DTs if left untreated or if treated inadequately.

ALCOHOL EMERGENCIES

CAUTION　　These signs can mean illnesses or injuries other than alcohol abuse (e.g., epilepsy, diabetes, head injury).

It is therefore especially important that the person with apparent alcohol on his breath (which can smell like the acetone breath of a diabetic) not be immediately dismissed as a drunk.
He should be carefully checked for other illnesses/injuries.

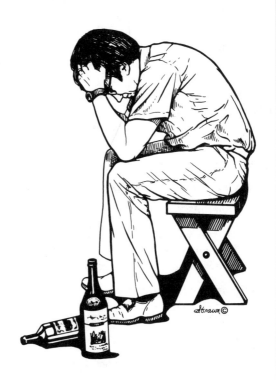

SIGNS
The signs of alcohol intoxication are familiar to all:
- Odor of alcohol on breath
- Swaying/unsteadiness
- Slurred speech
- Nausea/vomiting
- Flushed face

EFFECTS
Alcohol affects a person's judgement, vision, reaction time and coordination. In very large quantities, it can cause death by paralyzing the respiratory center of the brain.

DEPRESSANT
Alcohol is a depressant, not a stimulant. Many people think it is a stimulant since its first effect is to reduce tension and give a mild feeling of euphoria or exhilaration.

ALCOHOL COMBINES WITH OTHER DEPRESSANTS
When alcohol is taken in combination with analgesics, tranquilizers, antihistamines, barbiturates, etc., the depressant effects will be added together and, in some instances, the resultant effect will be greater than the expected combined effects of the two drugs.

MANAGEMENT

The intoxicated victim should be given the same attention given to victims with other illnesses/injuries.

The intoxicated victim needs constant watching to be sure that he doesn't aspirate vomitus and that he maintains respirations.

WITHDRAWAL PROBLEMS

An alcoholic who suddenly stops drinking can suffer from severe withdrawal problems. Sudden withdrawal will often result in DT's (delerium tremens).

Signs include:
1. Shaking hands
2. Restlessness
3. Confusion
4. Hallucinations
5. Sometimes maniacal behavior

The victim must be protected from hurting himself.

FIGURE 19-11.

GENERAL GUIDELINES FOR MANAGING A DRUG/ALCOHOL CRISIS

The conscious victim with a drug- or alcohol-related emergency is often experiencing severe emotional stress. In such instances, the most important tools are the verbal and nonverbal communication skills of the First Aider. The goal is to establish and maintain rapport, create trust, and build a short-term working relationship that will lower anxiety, produce a clearer understanding of the problem at hand, and identify the resources necessary to cope with it.

The following guidelines may be helpful in reducing emotional overreaction by helping the victim make sense out of what is happening to him:

1. Provide a reality base.

   ■ Identify yourself and your position.

   ■ Use the victim's name.

   ■ Based on the victim's response, introduce as much familiarity as possible, e.g., persons, objects, newspapers, TV programs.

   ■ Be calm and self-assured.

2. Provide appropriate nonverbal support.

   ■ Maintain eye contact.

   ■ Maintain a relaxed body posture. Be quiet, calm, and gentle.

   ■ Touch the victim if it seems appropriate.

3. Encourage communication.

   ■ Communicate directly with the victim, not through others.

   ■ Ask clear, simple questions.

   ■ Ask questions slowly, one at a time.

   ■ Try not to ask questions that require a simple "yes" or "no."

   ■ Tolerate repetition; do not become impatient.

4. Foster confidence.

   ■ Be nonjudgmental. Do not accuse the victim.

   ■ Help the victim gain confidence in you.

   ■ Listen carefully.

   ■ Respond to feelings; let the victim know that you understand his feelings.

   ■ Identify and reinforce progress.

DEALING WITH HYPERVENTILATION VICTIMS

Hyperventilation is common in drug-abusing victims. It can be a manifestation of acute anxiety, but it also may indicate **METABOLIC ACIDOSIS**, severe pain, drug withdrawal, or aspirin poisoning.

Hyperventilation in a drug emergency should be cared for as a medical disorder and *not* as anxiety hyperventilation. *Do not* have the victim breathe into a paper bag.

Often it is difficult to provide a quiet, reassuring environment in an emergency setting. The hyperventilating victim should be removed from the crisis situation as soon as possible and should not be left alone. Listen (in a nonjudgmental way) to the problems of the victim, and respond to the victim's questions regarding his condition in a calm, confident manner.

GENERAL PROCEDURES FOR OVERDOSE

The general goals in handling an overdose victim are to protect the victim and yourself, to calm the victim without harming him, and to prevent physical injury, aspiration, and **HYPERTHERMIA**. An overdose of almost any drug will cause poisoning and should be cared for at once. Emergency care is limited for a person suffering from drug poisoning, but the following procedures can be done. Your two primary goals should be to monitor the victim's vital signs and to provide basic life support. The following guidelines apply to all drug and alcohol emergencies:

■ Do not panic. Treat the victim calmly. Squelch your impulses to throw cold water on the victim or to move him around. Of course, you should move a victim if he is inhaling a harmful substance or if he is in immediate danger.

■ If the victim is conscious, try to get him to sit or lie down.

■ Quickly assess the situation. Because symptoms of drug abuse resemble those of other diseases, it is important that you obtain as much information as possible. If the victim is conscious, ask him what he has taken. If the victim is unconscious, ask friends or family members who may know what has happened. However, do not spend a lot of time finding out what has happened at this stage; there may be life-threatening symptoms that need to be handled directly. You can always come back for further assessment once the victim is under control.

- Establish and maintain a clear airway. Remove anything from the mouth or throat that might pose a breathing hazard, including false teeth, blood, mucus, or vomitus.

- Administer artificial ventilation if needed.

- Turn the victm's head to the side and downward toward the ground in case of vomiting.

- Monitor the victim's vital signs frequently. Various drugs can cause changes in respiration, heart rate, blood pressure, and the central nervous system. In case of respiratory or cardiac complications, care for the life-threatening situations immediately.

- Watch overdose victims carefully; they can be conscious one minute and lapse into unconsciousness the next.

- Try to maintain proper body temperature.

- Take measures to correct or prevent shock.

- If the victim is conscious, induce vomiting, particularly if the drug has been ingested within the last thirty minutes. *Follow local protocol.* This course of action depends, however, on where the crisis occurred and the drug taken. If the victim can be taken to a hospital within minutes, induced vomiting is unnecessary. On the other hand, in an isolated setting where medical care is not promptly available, induced vomiting is useful. Of course, if the drug has been taken intravenously or by inhalation (sniffing), induced vomiting will not help. Nor should vomiting be induced in stuporous victims who may become comatose within minutes because the danger of aspiration of vomitus is too great. For directions on induced vomiting, see Chapter 18.

- If the victim is conscious, reassure him of his well-being, and explain who you are and that you are trying to help him (Figure 19-12).

- Speak firmly to the victim. Be understanding and assuring. Have an accepting, nonjudgmental attitude toward the victim; *never* ridicule or criticize him.

- Perform a brief physical assessment to eliminate possibilities of complications or other injuries.

- Activate the EMS system as soon as possible.

- If there is time prior to the emergency personnel arriving, search the area around the victim for tablets, capsules, pill bottles or boxes (especially empty ones), syringes, other drug paraphernalia, ampules, prescriptions, hospital attendance cards, or physician's notes that might help you identify what drug the victim has taken. Have any such evidence transported to the hospital along with the victim.

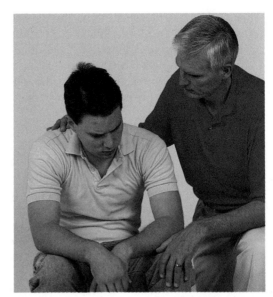

FIGURE 19-12. Reassure the victim. Explain who you are and that you're trying to help.

- Reduce stimuli as much as possible; lower the lights if you can, and let the victim rest in a calm, quiet atmosphere.

- If the victim is agitated, move him to a quiet place where he can be observed and where he will have little interaction with others. It is critical that you calm the victim who seems to be agitated or paranoid. Carefully explain each step of care.

- Encourage deep breathing exercises to help the victim stay calm.

- If the victim becomes increasingly excited and approaches or reaches a delirious phase, be firm but friendly in dealing with him. Some victims will be in an excited phase when the emergency team arrives. This is a common problem with overdoses of amphetamines, antidepressants, and some over-the-counter medications. If necessary, make proper efforts to restrain the victim to protect him from himself, and try to obtain help. Call police if necessary.

- *Do not* jump to conclusions — do not make decisions based solely on the victim's personal appearance, the fact that you detect an alcoholic odor, or the victim's companions.

- *Do not* accuse or criticize the victim.

- *Do not* leave intoxicated victims alone; make sure that they are attended and observed at all times.

THE TALK-DOWN TECHNIQUE

The dangers associated with the hallucinogens and with marijuana are primarily psychological in nature. These may be evident as intense anxiety or panic states (**BAD TRIPS**), depressive or paranoid reactions, mood changes, disorientation, and an inability to distinguish between reality and fantasy. Some prolonged psychotic reactions to psychedelic drugs have been reported, particularly with persons already psychologically disturbed.

The talk-down technique has been established as the preferred method for handling bad trips. This technique involves nonmoralizing, comforting, personal support from an experienced individual. It is aided by limiting external stimulation, such as intense light or loud sounds, and having the person lie down and relax.

Never use the talk-down technique for victims who have used PCP, because it may further aggravate them.

The goal of talking-down is to reduce the victim's anxiety, panic, depression, or confusion. Follow these steps:

1. Make the victim feel welcome. Remain relaxed and sympathetic. Because a victim can become suddenly hostile, have a companion with you. Be calm, but be authoritative.

2. Reassure the victim that his strange mental condition is a result of ingestion of the drug and that he *will* return to normal. Help him realize that he is not mentally ill.

3. Identify yourself clearly. Tell the victim who you are and what you are doing to help him. Be careful not to invade the victim's "personal space" until you have established rapport with him; try to stay approximately eight to ten feet away until you sense that the victim has some trust in you. Never touch the victim until he gives you permission *unless* he suddenly poses a threat to your safety or to his own safety.

4. Help the victim verbalize what is happening to him. Review for the victim what is going on in his trip; ask him questions.

5. Reiterate simple and concrete statements. Repeat and confirm what the victim says so that he knows you are listening to him. Orient the victim to time and place: be absolutely clear in letting the victim know where he is, what is happening to him, and who is with him. Help him identify surrounding objects that will probably be familiar to him, a process that helps with his self-identification. Listen for clues that will let you know whether the victim is anxious; if he is, discuss those anxieties with him. Help him work through them. Help him conquer guilt feelings.

6. Forewarn the victim about what will happen to him as the drug begins to wear off. He will probably be confused one minute and experience mental clarity the next. Again, help him understand that this is due to the drug, not to mental illness.

7. Activate the EMS system as soon as possible.

PHENCYCLIDINE (PCP)

One of the most dangerous hallucinogens — and one that deserves separate treatment — is phencyclidine (PCP). Nothing has so bewildered and amazed researchers as PCP — a drug that is cheap, easy to make, and easy to take and that is related to horrible psychological effects (some of which can last for years).

Physical signs and symptoms of moderate PCP intoxication include extreme agitation, involuntary horizontal and vertical movement of the eyes, unresponsiveness to pain, severe muscular rigidity, production of excessive bronchial and oral secretions (leading to choking in some cases), and hypertension. Signs and symptoms during moderate intoxication tend to come in spurts — a victim may seem to have no reaction and may suddenly flare into frantic activity (physical and mental). Three of the most severe reactions stemming from high doses of PCP are psychological ones; schizophrenia, paranoia, and memory loss — in some cases permanent.

The PCP victim may be combative and require restraint. Your first priority is to protect yourself; if you are injured, you will not be able to help the victim! It is critical that you provide reassurance that will not frighten or further upset the victim. Most victims will be confused and upset; adverse emergency-care efforts can increase psychological harm. Keep the victim in a quiet, nonstimulating environment. *Talking-down — a method recommended for other victims of hallucinogenic drugs — should not be used with PCP victims, since it will probably aggravate them further.*

Since PCP acts as an anesthetic, the victim will probably be unaware of any injuries sustained. Check quickly to determine whether there are any injuries that need attention. If there are, administer emergency care before continuing with psychological care. Restrain a victim who attempts to harm others. Keep the lights in the room as dim as you can (they will need to be bright enough, however, to monitor signs and otherwise care for the victim). Do whatever you can to minimize the confusion. Most PCP victims will require minimal care, but vital signs will still need to be monitored regularly. Therefore, you should activate the EMS system as quickly as possible while you work to calm him.

| **19** | **SELF-TEST** | **19** |

Student: _____ Date: _____

Course: _____ Section #: _____

PART I: True/False   If you believe that the statement is true, circle the T. If you believe that the statement is false, circle the F.

T   F   1. Stimulant overdose often causes slow and shallow breathing.

T   F   2. Inhalant overdose causes symptoms very much like stimulant overdose.

T   F   3. The most important information about a drug overdose is what kind of drug was used.

T   F   4. Seizures are rare in alcoholic withdrawal.

T   F   5. The most severe reactions from PCP use include paranoia and memory loss.

T   F   6. Vomiting should be induced if the drug overdose has happened anytime in the last three hours.

T   F   7. Hyperventilating drug-emergency victims should be encouraged to breathe into a paper bag.

T   F   8. DTs that occur one to two days after the last drink are rarely life-threatening.

PART II: Multiple Choice   For each question, circle the answer that best reflects an accurate statement.

1. Typically, most emergency drug/alcohol victims fall into *all but one* of the following consciousness categories:
    a. semicomatose.
    b. awake.
    c. comatose.
    d. hyperactive.

2. A common emergency among drug-abusing victims is:
    a. hyperventilation.
    b. cardiac arrhythmias.
    c. convulsions.
    d. tremors.

3. Hyperventilation in a drug emergency should be treated by:
    a. removing the victim from the crisis situation as soon as possible.
    b. quieting the victim and leaving him alone to calm down.
    c. encouraging the victim to place his head lower than his knees.
    d. having the victim breathe into a paper bag.

4. The most important information to be gathered from an emergency drug/alcohol victim concerns:
    a. the type of drug taken.
    b. whether a lethal dose of the drug has been taken.
    c. level of consciousness and vital signs.
    d. whether a victim is armed.

5. A pulse rate _____ should be considered a life-threatening drug emergency in an adult:
    a. below 60 or above 100.
    b. below 60 or above 130.
    c. below 60 or above 120.
    d. below 80 or above 100.

6. Which of the following is the most serious danger from overdose of a depressant drug?
    a. decrease in body temperature.
    b. allergic reaction.
    c. loss of inhibition.
    d. respiratory depression.

7. Which of the following is *not* a recommended procedure in dealing with a drug-overdose victim?
    a. induce vomiting if the victim is conscious and the drug was ingested within the last thirty minutes.
    b. be alert for allergic reactions.
    c. splash cold water on the victim who is semi-comatose.
    d. be firm in dealing with the victim.

8. Which of the following is *not* a major indicator of a drug or alcohol emergency?
    a. slurred speech.
    b. high, low, or irregular pulse.
    c. temperature above 100 degrees F. or 38 degrees C.
    d. convulsions or seizures.

9. Which of the following may indicate that an alcohol/drug emergency is life-threatening?
    a. pancreatitis.
    b. impaired coordination.
    c. vomiting while not fully conscious.
    d. disturbance of vision.

10. Which of the following is *not* a guideline for dealing with an overdose victim?
    a. if the victim is conscious, induce vomiting.
    b. throw a little cold water on a victim who appears semi-conscious.
    c. be alert for allergic reactions.
    d. be firm but friendly in dealing with the victim.

11. What is the preferred method for handling an individual experiencing a "bad trip?"
    a. throw cold water on the victim.
    b. the "talk-down" technique.
    c. get the victim to walk around.
    d. put the victim in an isolated room where he cannot hurt himself.

12. Which of the following is part of the "talk-down" technique for communicating with a drug/alcohol emergency victim:
    a. forewarn the victim about what will happen when the drug starts to wear off.
    b. restrain a violent victim if necessary.
    c. allow the victim some time alone if he feels that he needs it.
    d. encourage the victim to rest and sleep.

13. The signs of acute intoxication may be mimicked by a _____ victim.
    a. comatose.
    b. diabetic (insulin shock).
    c. convulsive.
    d. violent.

14. When you encounter an alcohol-abuse victim, which of the following signs indicates that medical attention is needed immediately?

    a. grand mal seizures.
    b. high blood pressure.
    c. hypoglycemia.
    d. increased breathing rate.

15. Which of the following is *not* a guideline for managing a drug/alcohol crisis?

    a. encourage the victim to communicate.
    b. provide appropriate nonverbal support for the victim.
    c. provide a reality base for the victim.
    d. let the victim make decisions on what he needs to do.

16. Delirium tremens occurs as a result of:

    a. alcohol overdose.
    b. alcohol taken with tranquilizers.
    c. high alcohol concentrations ingested very quickly.
    d. alcohol withdrawal.

17. Which of the following is *not* a symptom of delirium tremens due to alcohol withdrawal?

    a. confusion.
    b. hallucinations.
    c. shaking hands.
    d. deep, comatose sleep.

18. Which of the following is the most serious danger from overdose of a depressant drug?

    a. decreased in body temperature.
    b. allergic reaction.
    c. loss of inhibition.
    d. respiratory depression.

19. Phencyclidine, better known as angel dust or PCP, is:

    a. a very dangerous hallucinogen, and extremely unpredictable.
    b. physically addicting.
    c. a central nervous system depressant.
    d. a drug that has a wide margin of safety.

20. Which of the following is *not* a stimulant?

    a. amphetamines.
    b. caffeine.
    c. valium.
    d. cocaine.

21. Heroin is a:

    a. hallucinogen.
    b. narcotic.
    c. barbiturate.
    d. stimulant.

22. Serious potential danger from inhalants includes:

    a. altered heart rhythm.
    b. allergic reaction that produces hay fever symptoms.
    c. hallucinations and delusions.
    d. psychic dependence.

PART III: Matching: Choose the definition on the right that best matches the term on the left.

Terms	Definitions
_____1. Drug abuse	A. Condition in which the victim experiences a strong need to experience the drug repeatedly.
_____2. Compulsive drug use	B. leads to addiction characterized by physical or psychological dependence.
_____3. Physical dependence	C. Refers to the situation in which, after repeated exposures to a given drug, achieving the desired effect requires larger doses.
_____4. Psychological dependence	D. Involves physical and psychological dependence, tolerance, and compulsive drug use.
_____5. Habituation	E. The self-administration of drugs (or of a single drug) in a manner that is not in accord with approved medical or social patterns.
_____6. Tolerance	F. Sometimes called psychological dependence.
_____7. Addiction	G. Appearance of an observable abstinence syndrome following the abrupt discontinuation of a drug that has been used regularly.

PART IV: What Would You Do If:

1. You are at an apartment where you find a young man who has apparently overdosed on drugs. He is unconscious and has a raised temperature, irregular pulse, and weak respiration.

2. You find an older man unconscious in an alley. He has an alcohol odor, respiratory depression, and signs of shock.

PART V: Practical Skills Check-Off   _____ has satisfactorily passed the following practical skills:
                                          Student's Name

	Date	Partner Check	Inst. Init.
1. Describe and demonstrate the general crisis-intervention guidelines for dealing with a drug/alcohol emergency.	___/___/___	☐	_____

BITES AND STINGS

Insect bites and stings are common, and most are considered minor. It is only when the insect is poisonous or when the victim has an allergic reaction and runs the risk of developing **ANAPHYLACTIC SHOCK** that the situation becomes an emergency. Even under those conditions, prompt emergency care can save lives and prevent permanent tissue damage.

SNAKEBITE

About 45,000 people every year are bitten by snakes in the United States; of those, 7,000 involve poisonous snakes, and of those treated, only about fifteen die. More than half of the poisonous snakebites involve children, and most occur between April and October.

About 20 of the 120 species of snakes in the United States are poisonous; they include rattlesnakes, coral snakes, water moccasins, and copperheads (Figures 20-1–20-4). There are poisonous snakes in every state except Alaska, Hawaii, and Maine. Of the poisonous bites in the United States,

55 percent are from rattlesnakes, 34 percent from copperheads, 10 percent from water moccasins, and 1 percent from coral snakes. Seventy percent of the fatalities are from rattlesnake bites, and between 95 and 98 percent of the bites occur on extremities (Figures 20-5 and 20-6).

Nonpoisonous snakebites are not considered serious and are generally treated as minor wounds; only poisonous snakebites are considered medical emergencies. Symptoms generally occur immediately, but only about one-third of all bites manifest symptoms. When no symptoms occur, probably no venom was injected into the victim. In 50 percent of coral snake bites, no venom is injected because the coral snake has to "chew" the skin for envenomation to occur. In as many as 25 percent of all venomous pit-viper bites, no venom is injected, possibly because the fangs may be injured, the venom sacs may be empty at the time of the bite, or the snake may not use the fangs when it strikes.

Signs that indicate a poisonous snakebite include:

■ The bite consists of one or two distinct puncture wounds (Figure 20-6). Nonpoisonous snakes usually leave a series of small, shallow puncture

COMMON POISONOUS SNAKES

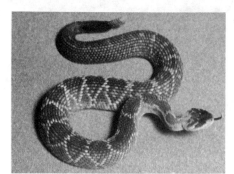

FIGURE 20-1. Rattlesnake.

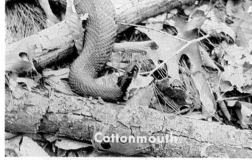

FIGURE 20-2. Cottonmouth.

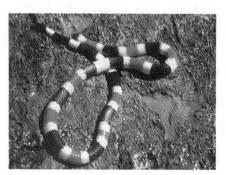

FIGURE 20-3. Coral snake.

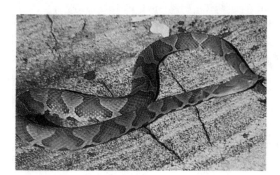

FIGURE 20-4. Copperhead.

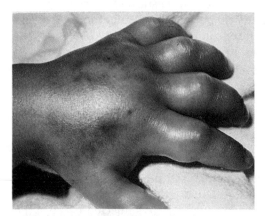

FIGURE 20-5. Snakebite to the hand.

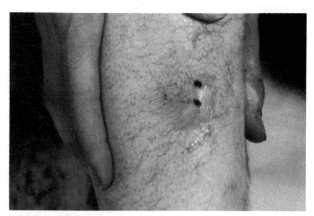

FIGURE 20-6. Rattlesnake bite.

wounds because they have teeth instead of fangs. (The exception is the coral snake, which leaves a semicircular marking from its teeth.) Because some poisonous snakes also have teeth, fang *and* teeth marks may be apparent. The presence of teeth marks does not rule out a poisonous bite,

but the presence of fang marks *always* confirms poison (Figure 20-7).

■ The victim experiences severe pain and burning almost immediately, but always within four hours of the incident.

POISONOUS SNAKEBITES

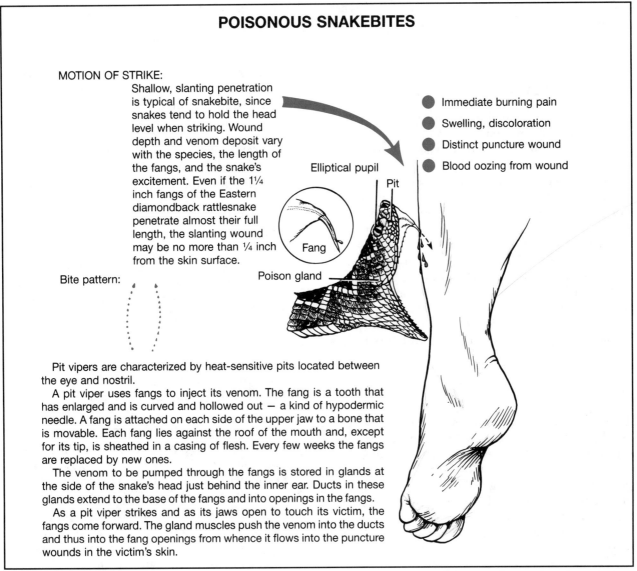

MOTION OF STRIKE:

Shallow, slanting penetration is typical of snakebite, since snakes tend to hold the head level when striking. Wound depth and venom deposit vary with the species, the length of the fangs, and the snake's excitement. Even if the 1¼ inch fangs of the Eastern diamondback rattlesnake penetrate almost their full length, the slanting wound may be no more than ¼ inch from the skin surface.

Bite pattern:

Elliptical pupil

Pit

Fang

Poison gland

- Immediate burning pain
- Swelling, discoloration
- Distinct puncture wound
- Blood oozing from wound

Pit vipers are characterized by heat-sensitive pits located between the eye and nostril.

A pit viper uses fangs to inject its venom. The fang is a tooth that has enlarged and is curved and hollowed out — a kind of hypodermic needle. A fang is attached on each side of the upper jaw to a bone that is movable. Each fang lies against the roof of the mouth and, except for its tip, is sheathed in a casing of flesh. Every few weeks the fangs are replaced by new ones.

The venom to be pumped through the fangs is stored in glands at the side of the snake's head just behind the inner ear. Ducts in these glands extend to the base of the fangs and into openings in the fangs.

As a pit viper strikes and as its jaws open to touch its victim, the fangs come forward. The gland muscles push the venom into the ducts and thus into the fang openings from whence it flows into the puncture wounds in the victim's skin.

FIGURE 20-7.

The wound begins to swell and discolor usually immediately, but always within four hours. Most poisonous snakes have the following characteristics:

- Large fangs; nonpoisonous snakes have small teeth. The two fangs of a poisonous snake are hollow and work like a hypodermic needle. (The exception is the coral snake, a poisonous snake that does not have fangs.)

- Elliptical pupils (vertical slits, much like those of a cat); nonvenomous snakes have round pupils.

- Presence of a pit. Venomous snakes (often called pit vipers) have a telltale pit between the eye and the mouth. The pit, a heat-sensing organ, makes it possible for the snake to strike a warm-blooded victim accurately, even if the snake cannot see the victim.

- A variety of differently shaped blotches on backgrounds of pink, yellow olive, tan, gray or brown skin.

- A triangular head that is larger than the neck, such as in the diamondback rattlesnake.

There is one exception to all of this: the coral snake, a highly poisonous snake that resembles a number of nonpoisonous snakes, does not have fangs and has round pupils. Because its mouth is so small and its teeth are short, most coral snakes inflict bites on the toes and fingers. Coral snakes are small and are ringed with red, yellow, and black; the red and yellow touch each other.

EMERGENCY CARE

The care for a snakebite depends on whether the victim was bitten by a pit viper (rattlesnake, copperhead, or cottonmouth) or coral snake. Remember to protect yourself against snakebite. If you can safely kill and transport the snake with the victim, do so. It will allow the physician to identify the snake. Try not to crush the head, since the head often has identifying features. Snakes can often be found within a twenty-foot radius of the area in which the bite occurred. *Caution:* Pit vipers can retain the striking reflex for about an hour after death.

The priorities of emergency care for snakebite are to limit the spread of the venom and to transport the victim without delay. Chances for recovery are great if the victim receives care within two hours of the bite.

Pit Viper

The severity of a pit viper bite is gauged by how rapidly symptoms develop, which depends on how much poison was injected. As a general rule, you can safely assume that the victim has not been poisoned if the burning pain characteristic of pit-viper bite does not develop within one hour of the time the victim was bitten.

Signs and symptoms of pit-viper bite include the following:

- Immediate and severe burning pain and swelling around the fang marks, usually within five minutes. The entire extremity generally swells within eight to thirty-six hours.
- Purplish discoloration around the bite, usually developing within two to three hours.
- Numbness and possible blistering around the bite, generally within several hours.
- Nausea and vomiting.
- Rapid heartbeat, low blood pressure, weakness, and fainting.
- Numbness and tingling of the tongue and mouth.
- Excessive sweating.
- Fever and chills.
- Muscular twitching.
- Convulsions.
- Dimmed vision.
- Headache.

Consider the bite to be severe if the victim develops signs or symptoms of shock, paralysis, blurred vision, or convulsions, or if he becomes unconscious.

Priorities in a pit viper are to maintain basic life support — airway, breathing, and circulation. Follow these guidelines:

1. Move the victim away from the snake to prevent repeated bites.

2. Have the victim lie down, and keep him calm and quiet. Maintain direct eye contact, and speak in a soothing, reassuring voice. Remember that many snakebite victims will be hysterical — snakebite can cause tremendous psychological trauma. Continually reassure the victim as you give him emergency care. Activity increases circulation, and circulation increases the absorption of venom.

3. Keep the bitten extremity lower than the heart, and immobilize it in a functional position. Remove any rings, bracelets, or other jewelry that could impede circulation if swelling occurs.

4. Wipe the wound area with alcohol, soap and water, hydrogen peroxide, or other mild antiseptic. *Follow local protocol.* Take special care not to scrub or tear the tissues; cleanse the area very carefully, since envenomation makes the tissues extremely fragile. Irrigate the entire wound area with clean water.

5. Find the fang marks. Wrap a flat band that is at least three-fourths of a inch wide around the extremity two to four inches above the fang marks, between the bite site and the heart. Follow local protocol. The band should be tight enough to stop the flow of blood through the veins but not through the arteries. You should be able to slip two fingers between the victim's skin and the constricting band (Figure 20-8). *Make sure that you adjust the constricting band as swelling occurs so that it does not become too tight. Never* place constricting bands on either side of a joint, around a joint, or around the head, neck, or trunk.

6. Apply suction to the wound directly over the fang marks. *Follow local protocol.* An extractor from a snakebite kit is ideal (Figure 20-9). The suction must be strong and be applied within the first five minutes to be effective. After thirty minutes, the venom is diffused and cannot be removed by suction.

7. The most effective recommendation for snakebite care is to transport the victim to a medical facility for antivenin therapy.

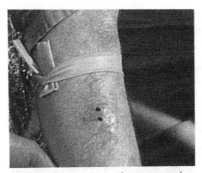

FIGURE 20-8. For poisonous snake-bite (pit vipers), apply a constricting band above the bite. The band should be tight enough to slow surface circulation, but should not interfere with arterial blood flow. It should be loose enough so that the fingers can be inserted under the band.

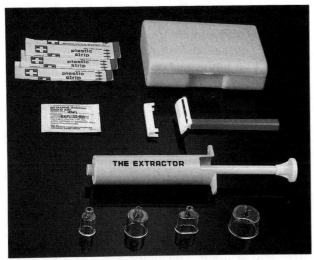

FIGURE 20-9. An extractor kit for suctioning venom. In some EMS areas, commercial snakebite kits are recommended. However, emergency care for snakebite is controversial in some areas. *Follow local protocol.*

8. Use basic-life-support procedures as appropriate, and treat the victim for shock. Monitor vital signs, keeping the victim warm and lying down. Give the victim nothing by mouth.

9. Arrange to transport the victim to the hospital as soon as possible, or activate the EMS system even if he shows no signs of envenomation. Be prepared to perform CPR. If the victim is more than a one hour walking distance of a car, it is probably best to send someone for help, *follow local protocol.*

10. *Never* apply ice to the bite area; ice can cause frostbite and tissue sloughing.

Coral Snake

Coral snakes are the most poisonous of all. Fortunately, they account for only 1 to 2 percent of all snakebites in the United States. Instead of having fangs like the pit vipers, the coral snake has several pairs of short, grooved, fanglike teeth in its upper jaw. Thus, it chews its victims instead of striking with a clean blow. The venom from a coral snake is absorbed rapidly into the bloodstream and is disseminated quickly throughout the body.

Signs and symptoms of a coral snake bite are completely different than those of a pit viper. Rather than leaving two distinct fang marks, the coral snake leaves one or more tiny scratch marks in the area of the bite. While a pit-viper bite causes immediate burning pain, little pain or swelling occurs with a coral snake bite, and the victim's tissue usually does not turn black and blue. Usually, in fact, there is *no* pain or swelling at the bite site.

Coral-snake venom has its effects on the central nervous system. One to eight hours after the bite, the victim will experience blurred vision, drooping eyelids, slurred speech, increased salivation and sweating, and drowsiness. As time passes, the victim may develop nausea and vomiting, shock, difficulty in breathing, paralysis, convulsions, and coma. Depending on the size and age of the victim, total central-nervous-system shutdown can occur in as few as ten minutes.

Emergency care for a coral snake bite is similar to that for a pit-viper bite, with a few important additions:

1. Remove the victim's rings, bracelets, or any other jewelry that could impede circulation if swelling occurs.

2. Flush the bite area with warm, soapy water to wash away any remaining poison; use at least several quarts of water.

3. If the bite is on an extremity, apply a constricting band above the bite, following the same restrictions as for pit viper bites. Follow local protocol regarding constricting bands.

4. Apply a coolant bag to the bite (follow local protocol). Never pack the bite area in ice, since you may cause frostbite.

5. Immobilize the extremity, treat the victim for shock, and give nothing by mouth.

6. *Never incise or suction a coral snake bite.*

7. *Transport the victim to a medical facility as quickly as possible, or activate the EMS system.*

INSECT BITES

GENERAL EMERGENCY CARE

In most cases of insect bite, emergency care consists of:

1. Washing the wound thoroughly with soap and water.
2. Covering the wound with a loose dressing to discourage the victim from scratching it.
3. Applying cold compresses to the wound to reduce swelling and ease itching. *Never* pack ice directly on the skin.

Itching should subside within a few hours. If itching persists beyond two days, or if signs of infection develop, seek medical help.

Any victim who develops signs and symptoms of an allergic reaction following an insect bite should be seen by a physician. The signs and symptoms of allergic reaction include:

▪ Burning pain and itching at the bite site.
▪ Itching on the palms of the hands and soles of the feet.
▪ Itching on the neck and the groin.
▪ General body swelling.
▪ A nettle-like rash over the entire body.
▪ Breathing difficulties.

Anaphylactic shock, a life-threatening medical emergency, may follow insect bite. If any of the following signs or symptoms develop, activate the EMS system immediately and perform basic life support (see the anaphylactic shock section of Chapter 6):

▪ Faintness, weakness.
▪ Nausea.
▪ Shock.
▪ Unconsciousness.

SPECIAL CARE FOR SPECIFIC BITES

Black Widow Spider

The black widow spider is characterized by a shiny black body, thin legs, and a crimson red marking on its abdomen, usually in the shape of an hourglass or two triangles (Figure 20-10). Do not be confused by appearances, however — of the five species in the United States, only three are black, and not all have the characteristic red marking.

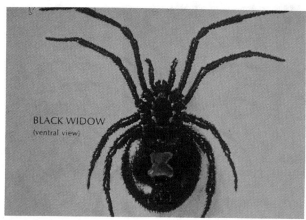

FIGURE 20-10. Black widow spider.

Black widow bites are the leading cause of death from spider bites in the United States. The venom — fourteen times more toxic than rattlesnake venom — causes little local reaction but results in pain and spasm in the large muscle groups within thirty minutes to three hours. Severe bites cause respiratory failure, coma, and death.

Those at highest risk for developing severe bites are children under the age of sixteen, the elderly over the age of sixty, people with chronic illness, and anyone with hypertension.

The most common sign of a black widow bite is high blood pressure. The most recognizable symptoms are flushing, sweating, and grimacing of the face within ten minutes to two hours. Other signs and symptoms include:

▪ A pinprick sensation at the bite site, becoming a dull ache within thirty to forty minutes.
▪ Pain and spasms in the shoulders, back, chest, and abdominal muscles within thirty minutes to three hours.
▪ Rigid, boardlike abdomen.
▪ Restlessness and anxiety.
▪ Fever.
▪ Rash.
▪ Headache.
▪ Vomiting or nausea.

The symptoms of black widow bite generally last from twenty-four to forty-eight hours; the weakness and headache, however, may linger for months.

Emergency care is generally not effective in the long-term treatment of black widow bite. The general goal of emergency care is general wound care and sending the victim to a physician. Follow these guidelines:

1. Administer care for shock.
2. Apply a cold compress to the bite area; do *not* apply ice.
3. Activate the EMS system or transport the victim to the hospital as quickly as possible.
4. Black widow antivenins are risky and are generally used only for high-risk victims. Nevertheless, try to find the spider if you can so that physicians can make a positive identification. They will be able to identify the spider, even if it is crushed, and will not have to guess about treatment regimes.

Brown Recluse Spider

The brown recluse spider is generally brown but can range in color from yellow to dark chocolate brown (Figure 20-11). The characteristic marking is a brown, violin-shaped marking on the upper back. The bite of the brown recluse spider is a serious medical condition: the bite is nonhealing and requires surgical skin grafting to repair (Figure 20-12).

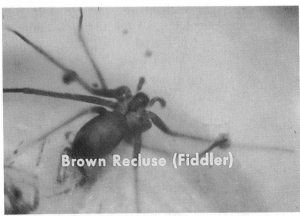

FIGURE 20-11. Brown recluse spider.

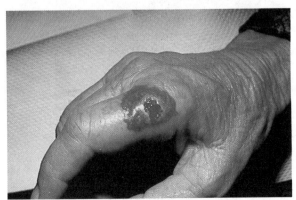

FIGURE 20-12. Brown recluse bite.

Unfortunately, most victims are unaware that they have been bitten, since the bite is often painless at first. Several hours after the bite occurs, the following signs and symptoms result:

▪ Within a few hours, the bite is a bluish area with a white periphery, gradually becoming surrounded with a red halo (a "bulls-eye" pattern).
▪ Within twenty-four hours, the victim develops:
  — Fever (usually of 103°F.).
  — Joint pain.
  — Nausea and vomiting.
  — Chills.
▪ Within seven to ten days, the bite becomes a large ulcer.

Emergency care consists of the following:

1. Administer care for shock.
2. Administer mouth-to-mouth ventilation if needed.
3. Transport the victim to a hospital or activate the EMS system as soon as possible.
4. Again, it is very important that you positively identify the spider so that surgical incision can be done as soon as possible. If you can, send the spider to the hospital with the victim.

Scorpion

Of the three species of scorpion in the United States that sting and inject poisonous venom, only one is generally fatal (Figure 20-13). The severity of the sting depends on the amount of venom injected; scorpion stings can be fatal. Ninety percent of all scorpion stings occur on the hands.

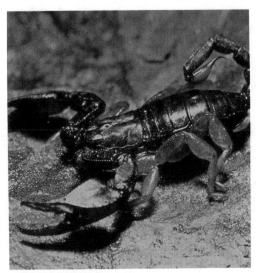

FIGURE 20-13. Scorpion.

Signs and symptoms of scorpion stings include:

- Sharp pain at the sting site.
- Swelling at the sting site, which spreads gradually.
- Discoloration at the sting site.
- Nausea and vomiting.
- Restlessness.
- Drooling.
- Poor coordination.
- Incontinence.
- Seizures.

Emergency care of scorpion stings consists of the following:

1. Apply a flat, constricting band two inches above the sting if it is on an extremity. The band should be tight enough to stop venous, but not arterial, flow; you should be able to slip two fingers between the band and the victim's skin.

2. Apply a cold compress to the sting site to slow the spread of the venom and to reduce swelling. Never use ice.

3. Transport the victim to a physician or activate the EMS system immediately.

Fire Ants

Fire ants bite down into the skin, then sting downwardly as they pivot; the result is a characteristic circular pattern of bites. Fire ant bites produce extremely painful vesicles that are filled with fluid (Figure 20-14). At first the fluid is clear; later it becomes cloudy. The bite causes a sharp, stinging pain followed by swelling.

To care for fire ant bites, watch for any allergic reactions, and transport the victim to a physician.

Ticks

Ticks (Figure 20-15) can cause a serious problem because they can carry tick fever, Rocky Mountain spotted fever, Lyme disease, and other bacterial diseases. In addition, a prolonged attachment of a female tick can cause progressive paralysis that mimics polio; 10 percent of all victims die as a result.

Ticks are visible after they have attached themselves to the skin. However, since they often choose warm, moist areas, you should carefully inspect the victim's scalp, other hairy areas, the armpits, the groin, and skin creases. *Never* pluck an embedded tick head out of the skin — you may force infected blood into the victim.

To remove a tick, follow these guidelines:*

1. Remove a tick as soon as you discover it. The longer the tick remains attached to the skin, the more likely it is that an infection will result.

2. Use tweezers when removing a tick, or cover your fingers with a tissue; if you touch the tick, you may contaminate yourself. However, if you do not have tweezers and cannot cover your fingertips, pull the tick off right away rather than waiting and looking around for an appropriate implement.

3. To remove a tick, grasp it as close as possible to the point where it is attached to the skin. Pull firmly and steadily until the tick is dislodged, then flush it down the toilet. Do not twist or jerk

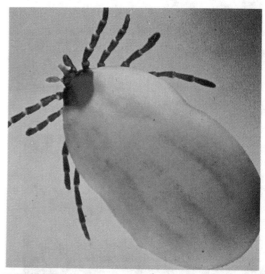

FIGURE 20-15. Engorged tick.

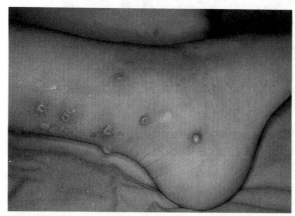

FIGURE 20-14. Fire ant bites.

*Reproduced with permission from *Patient Care*, June 15, 1988, Copyright © 1988, *Patient Care*, Oradell, NJ.

the tick, since this may result in incomplete removal. Avoid squashing an engorged tick during removal: infected blood may spurt into your eyes, mouth, or a cut on the surface of your skin.

4. Once the tick is removed, wash your hands and the bite area thoroughly with soap and water, and apply an antiseptic to the area to prevent a bacterial infection.

5. Remember to have the victim mark the date on his calendar. It documents the exact time of exposure and will serve as a reminder if he needs to seek medical care.

6. If the victim develops fever with chills, headache, or muscle aches after being exposed to a tick, immediate treatment from a physician should be sought.

One of the most serious complications of tick infestation is Rocky Mountain spotted fever, which can occur in victims who are unaware that they have a tick. Signs and symptoms generally develop within seven to ten days of tick infestation and include nausea and vomiting, abdominal pain, headache, generalized weakness, flaccid paralysis, and respiratory failure.

You should also be aware of Lyme disease, which often goes undetected. Its symptoms mimic those of gout, arthritis, fatigue, or multiple sclerosis. It occurs most frequently in New York, New Jersey, Pennsylvania, Connecticut, Massachusetts, Rhode Island, Wisconsin, and Minnesota.

INSECT STINGS

The normal reaction to an insect sting is a sharp, stinging pain followed immediately by an itchy, swollen, painful wheal. Swelling may persist for several days but usually subsides within twenty-four hours. Redness, tenderness, and swelling at or around the sting site — even if severe — in the absence of other symptoms is considered to be a local reaction. Local reactions are rarely serious or life-threatening and can be treated successfully with cold compresses.

But allergic reactions are another story: approximately fifty people die each year in the United States as a result of insect stings. Thousands of people are allergic to the sting of bees, wasps, and hornets, and for those people, stings may cause death — on the average, within ten minutes of the sting, but almost always within the first hour.

The stinging insects that most commonly cause allergic reactions are a group of the hymenoptera —

the insects with membranous wings. These consist of the honeybee, the wasp, the hornet, and the yellow jacket (Figure 20-16). Stings from wasps and bees are more common than all other insect bites combined.

In determining care for a victim, it is important to identify what kind of insect inflicted the sting. Clues in habitat and stinging habit can help in identification. Honeybees leave the stinger and venom sac behind, embedded in the skin; hornets and wasps do not. Hornets prefer trees and shrubs, and yellow jackets stay close to the ground — both hornets and yellow jackets build their nests near the ground. Wasps love attics and build their nests high off the ground in sheltered places, usually under eaves. Honeybees cluster around flowers and flowering shrubs, including the flowering clover in lawns.

SIGNS AND SYMPTOMS OF ANAPHYLAXIS

Signs and symptoms of anaphylaxis include the following (see also the anaphylactic shock section of Chapter 6):

- Faintness.
- Dizziness.
- Generalized itching.
- Hives.
- Flushing.
- Generalized swelling, including the eyelids, lips, and tongue.
- Upper airway obstruction.
- Difficulty swallowing.
- Shortness of breath, wheezing, or stridor.
- Labored breathing.
- Abdominal cramps.
- Confusion.
- Loss of consciousness.
- Convulsions.

In some victims, anaphylactic symptoms may be delayed for as long as two weeks. In those cases, signs and symptoms include:

- Rash.
- Fever.
- Joint pain.
- Neurological problems.
- Secondary infections.

WASPS, BEES, AND FIRE ANTS

The following members of this group commonly attack humans, causing local pain, redness, swelling, and subsequent itching. Always consider the possibility of anaphylaxis.

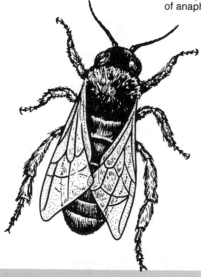

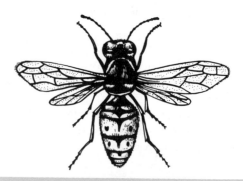

YELLOW JACKET: A principal insect causing sting reactions in the Northeast and Midwest. Yellow jackets tend to dominate in late summer and fall. Nests are located in the ground. Often seen in picnic areas, garbage cans, and food stands because they're carnivores, yellow jackets are ill-tempered and aggressive and can deliver multiple stings at one time. They will often sting without being provoked.

HONEYBEE: Found throughout the United States at anytime of year, except in colder temperatures when they remain in their hives. In the Northeast and Midwest, they are major insects causing sting reactions. Hives are usually found in hollowed out areas such as dead tree trunks. Honeybees principally ingest nectar of plants, so they are often seen in the vicinity of flowers. The honeybee with its barbed stinger will self-eviscerate after a sting, leaving the venom sac and stinger in place.

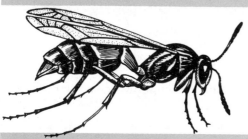

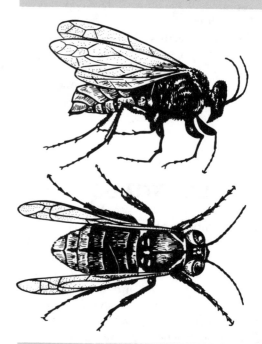

WASPS: The most likely insect to cause sting reactions in the Southeast and Southwest. Wasps tend to nest in small numbers under the eaves of houses and buildings. These are carnivores that are found in picnic areas, garbage cans, and food stands. Can deliver multiple stings at one time.

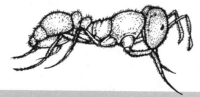

YELLOW HORNET AND WHITE-FACED OR BALD-FACED HORNET: Seen mainly in the spring and early summer. Nests usually found in branches and bushes above ground. These are carnivores that are seen in picnic areas, garbage cans, and food stands. Can deliver multiple stings at one time.

FIRE ANT: The imported fire ant is bright red and lives in loose dirt mounds. It is found throughout the southern states as far west as New Mexico. Fire ants may cause serious illness and/or anaphylaxis. The ant attaches itself to the skin by its strong jaws and swivels its tail-position stinger about, inflicting repeated stings.

Adapted with permission from: John W. Georgitis, "Insect Stings — Responding to the Gamut of Allergic Reactions," *Modern Medicine*

FIGURE 20-16.

EMERGENCY CARE FOR INSECT STINGS

Emergency care consists of the following (Figure 20-17):

1. Lower the affected part below the heart.

2. Apply a constricting band above the sting site if the sting was inflicted on an extremity. The constricting band should be tight enough to restrict the flow of blood through the veins but not through the arteries. Test for tightness by making sure that you can wedge your finger between the band and the skin. Loosen the band once every five to ten minutes to allow the venom to slowly enter the circulatory system. *Do not remove the constricting band until symptoms have been brought under control. Constricting bands are controversial in some EMS areas. Follow local protocol.*

3. If the sting was inflicted by a honeybee and the stinger is still in the skin, remove the stinger by gently scraping against it with your fingernail, with the edge of a knife, or with a credit card (Figure 20-18). Be careful not to *squeeze* the stinger. The venom sac will still be attached, and you will inject additional venom into the area. Make sure that you remove the venom sac — it can continue to secrete venom even though the stinger is detached from the insect.

4. Apply a commercial cold pack or ice bags to the site to relieve pain and swelling.

5. If respirations are not adequate, give mouth-to-mouth ventilation.

6. Keep the victim warm. Have him lie down, and elevate his legs and lower his head if he shows signs and symptoms of (or danger of lapsing into) shock.

7. Activate the EMS system immediately.

8. Make sure that the victim will be under strict observation for the first twenty-four hours to eliminate the possibility of later breathing problems or hemorrhage. Tell family members to take the victim to the hospital immediately if any suspicious signs and symptoms develop.

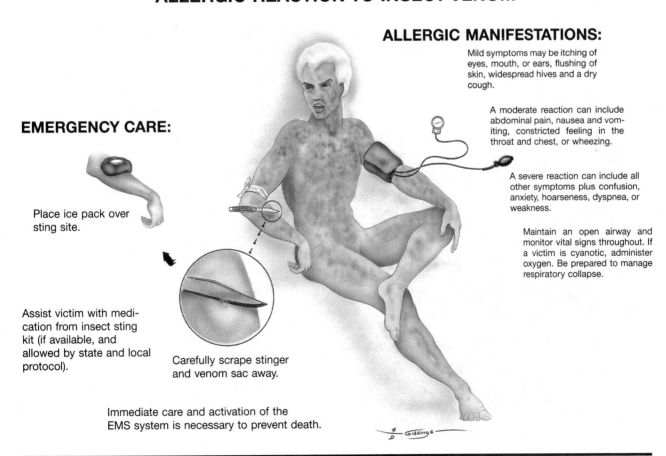

ALLERGIC REACTION TO INSECT VENOM

ALLERGIC MANIFESTATIONS:

Mild symptoms may be itching of eyes, mouth, or ears, flushing of skin, widespread hives and a dry cough.

A moderate reaction can include abdominal pain, nausea and vomiting, constricted feeling in the throat and chest, or wheezing.

A severe reaction can include all other symptoms plus confusion, anxiety, hoarseness, dyspnea, or weakness.

Maintain an open airway and monitor vital signs throughout. If a victim is cyanotic, administer oxygen. Be prepared to manage respiratory collapse.

EMERGENCY CARE:

Place ice pack over sting site.

Assist victim with medication from insect sting kit (if available, and allowed by state and local protocol).

Carefully scrape stinger and venom sac away.

Immediate care and activation of the EMS system is necessary to prevent death.

FIGURE 20-17.

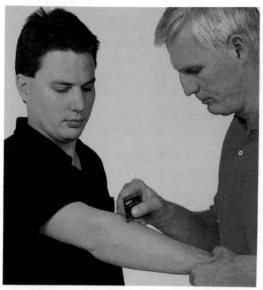

FIGURE 20-18. Scraping a honey-bee stinger away with the edge of a credit card.

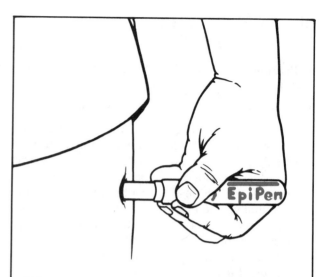

This pressure-activated device delivers a set dose of epinephrine for temporary emergency treatment of anaphylaxis quickly and with minimal pain. This device, or another type of epinephrine delivery system, is included in any of several emergency treatment kits available by prescription.

FIGURE 20-20.

9. If you know that the victim is allergic to stings, do not wait for the signs and symptoms to occur — delay can be fatal. If the victim has a history of severe allergic reactions and has an insect sting kit, assist him in administering the contents of the kit (Figures 20-19 and 20-20). *Follow local protocol.* Activate the EMS system immediately.

MARINE LIFE POISONING

Four-fifths of all organisms on the earth live in the ocean, which covers 71 percent of the earth's surface. Venomous organisms are naturally part of that vast life form; while they usually live in temperate or tropical waters, they can be found in virtually all waters (Figures 20-21–20-32). Most are not aggressive; in fact, most marine-life poisoning occurs when a victim swims into or steps on an animal.

There are differences between the stings and bites of aquatic organisms and those of land organisms. First, the venom of aquatic organisms may produce more extensive tissue damage. Such injuries should be treated as soft-tissue injuries. Second, venoms of aquatic organisms are destroyed by heat; therefore, heat, rather than ice, should be applied to such stings and bites.

EMERGENCY CARE

Care for large bites (such as those from a shark) like any other major trauma:

1. Control bleeding.
2. Treat for shock.
3. Give basic life support.
4. Activate the EMS system.

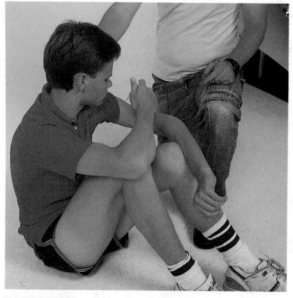

FIGURE 20-19. Assist the victim who has a history of allergic reactions to insect stings and carries a sting kit.

COMMON SOURCES OF MARINE LIFE STINGS AND WOUNDS

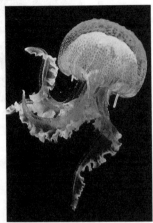

FIGURE 20-21. Jellyfish.

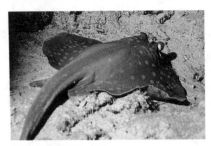

FIGURE 20-22. Stingray.

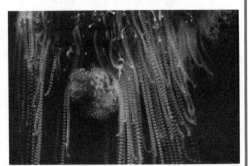

FIGURE 20-23. Tentacles of Portuguese Man-of-War.

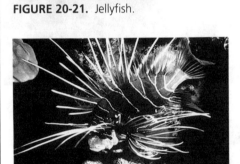

FIGURE 20-24. Lionfish.

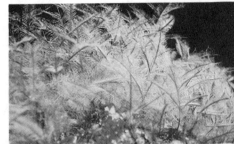

FIGURE 20-25. Feather hydroid.

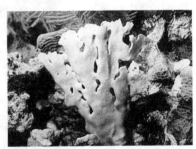

FIGURE 20-27. Fire coral.

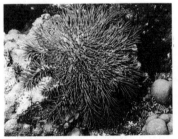

FIGURE 20-28. Crown-of-Thorns Starfish.

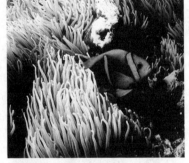

FIGURE 20-26. Sea anemone and clownfish.

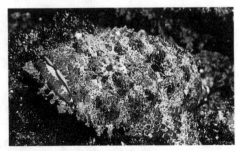

FIGURE 20-30. Scorpion fish.

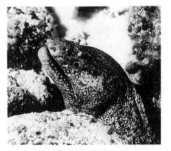

FIGURE 20-31. Moray eel.

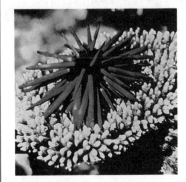

FIGURE 20-29. Sea urchin.

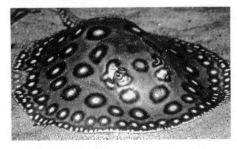

FIGURE 20-32. Stingray

In cases of poisonous injuries, victims may have a wide variety of symptoms, ranging from a minor injury to death. General care for injuries inflicted by most sea animals consists of the following:

1. Apply a constricting band above the sting or bite. Check for a pulse in the limb to ensure that the constricting band is not too tight. It should be tight enough to restrict the flow of blood through the veins but not through the arteries.

2. Remove any material that sticks to the sting site on the surface of the flesh.

3. Irrigate the wound thoroughly with water.

4. If the skin is unbroken, wash the wound with a mild agent such as Alcoholic Zephiran, strong soap solution, or ammonia. *Never scrub the area.* Make sure that washings from the irrigation and the oxidizing agent flow away from the body. *Follow local protocol.*

5. Remove stingers and barbs the same way in which you remove bee stingers. Be careful not to squeeze more venom into the wound. If the stinger is barbed perpendicular to the wound and you are unable to remove it without excessive force, support the stinger or barb, bandage it in place, and wait for surgical removal.

6. Apply heat and maintain the injured area at a temperature of 110° to 114°F. for thirty minutes or while waiting for emergency personnel. Apply heat for another thirty minutes if symptoms recur. In some areas it is being recommended that you pack the affected area with ice or cold packs to reduce swelling. *Follow local protocol. If cold is used, do not chill to the point of frostbite.*

7. Transport the victim immediately to a hospital or activate the EMS system. Position the victim so that gravity does not force return of the venom.

To treat tentacle stings, such as those inflicted by jellyfish, corals, hydras, and anemones, follow these guidelines (Figure 20-33):

1. Remove the victim from the water.

2. Pour rubbing alcohol on the affected area to denature the toxin.

3. Sprinkle the affected area with meat tenderizer to destroy the toxins.

4. Sprinkle the affected area with talcum powder.

5. Transport the victim to a hospital or activate the EMS system.

To treat puncture wounds, such as those inflicted by stingray spines and spiny fish, follow these guidelines (Figure 20-34):

1. Remove the victim from the water.

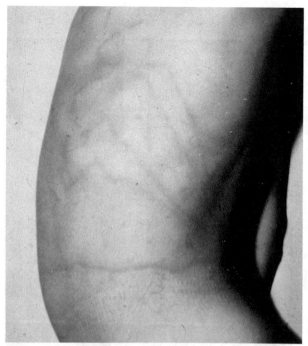

FIGURE 20-33. Jellyfish sting.

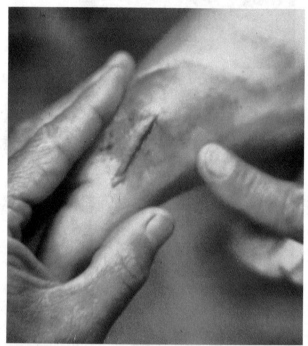

FIGURE 20-34. Stingray sting.

2. Immobilize the injured part.

3. Soak the affected area in hot water for at least thirty minutes, changing the water frequently to maintain its temperature.

4. Transport the victim to a hospital while soaking the injured part, or activate the EMS system.

| 20 | **SELF-TEST** | 20 |

Student: _____   Date: _____

Course: _____   Section #: _____

PART I: True/False   If you believe that the statement is true, circle the T. If you believe that the statement is false, circle the F.

T (F)   1. More than 200 people die each year from poisonous snakebites.

(T) F   2. Most poisonous snakebites in the United States are from rattlesnakes.

T (F)   3. Most fatalities from snakebites are from copperheads.

(T) F   4. Chances of recovery from a poisonous snakebite are great if the victim receives care within two hours of the bite.

(T) F   5. Some of the most common signs and symptoms of a pit viper bite, usually within five minutes, are immediate and severe burning pain and swelling around the fang marks.

T (F)   6. Ice should be applied to a pit viper bite.

T (F)   7. Coral snake bites leave the same distinct fang marks as a pit viper bite.

T (F)   8. A constricting band should not be used with scorpion stings.

T F   9. Approximately fifty people die each year in the United States because of insect stings.

T F   10. Venoms of most aquatic organisms are destroyed by heat.

T F   11. Tentacle stings from a jellyfish should be cleansed with alcohol.

T F   12. Puncture wounds from stingray spines should be soaked in hot water.

PART II: Multiple Choice   For each question, circle the answer that best reflects an accurate statement.

1. Most poisonous snakes have:
   a. multicolored rings around the body.
   b. elliptical pupils.
   c. small teeth.
   d. flat heads.

2. The constricting band applied for a snakebite wound should:
   a. not limit the flow of either arterial or venous blood.
   b. limit the flow of arterial blood but not venous blood.
   c. limit the flow of venous blood but not arterial blood.
   d. limit the flow of both arterial and venous blood.

3. Venoms of aquatic organisms:
   a. may cause severe vomiting.
   b. can cause anaphylactic shock.
   c. are destroyed by heat.
   d. are activated by cold.

4. Which of the following statements about venoms of aquatic organisms is *not* true?
   a. the First Aider should immediately pack wounds from marine organisms in ice.
   b. bites and stings from aquatic organisms should be treated as soft-tissue injuries.
   c. aquatic organism venoms may produce more extensive tissue damage than land organism venoms.
   d. aquatic organism venoms are usually destroyed by heat.

5. Care of the victim who has been bitten by a snake with fangs includes: (1) have the victim lie down, remain quiet, and position the bitten extremity slightly lower than the heart; (2) cleanse the wound area with water and soap or hydrogen peroxide; (3) wrap a constrictive band around the bitten extremity above the fang marks, restricting venous, but not arterial, blood flow; (4) apply suction to the wound.
   a. 1, 2, and 3.
   b. 1, 2, and 4.
   c. 1, 2, 3, and 4.
   d. 2, 3, and 4.

6. Which of the following is *not* a symptom of a coral snake bite?
   a. blurred vision.
   b. paralysis.
   c. black-and-blue skin tissue, accompanied by considerable pain and swelling.
   d. drowsiness and slurred speech.

7. Coral snakes inject poison through:
   a. long fangs in the forward part of the upper jaw.
   b. long fangs in both the upper jaw and the lower jaw.
   c. a chewing motion.
   d. long fangs in the forward part of the lower jaw.

8. Unless contraindicated by local protocol, a First Aider should treat a coral snake bite by:
   a. application of a constricting band and an ice bag.
   b. application of a constricting band only.
   c. incision and suction of the wound area.
   d. application of rubbing alcohol and an ice pack to the wound.

9. The emergency care for black widow and brown recluse bites always has one of the following in common:

   a. administering mouth-to-mouth ventilations.
   b. application of an ice pack.
   c. application of a constricting band.
   d. try to identify the spider.

10. Which of the following should you do as part of the emergency care for a victim of allergic reaction to a sting on the extremity?

    a. apply warm compresses to increase circulation.
    b. elevate the extremity to reduce swelling.
    c. apply a tourniquet above the sting.
    d. apply a constricting band above the sting.

11. The first step in providing emergency care for a honeybee sting is to:

    a. grasp the sac or stinger with a pair of tweezers and gently pull it out.
    b. apply wet mud to the sting area; let it dry.
    c. apply baking soda to the affected area.
    d. remove the stinger by scraping it gently with your fingernail or the edge of a knife.

12. If a sting has been inflicted by a honeybee and the stinger is still in the victim's skin, the First Aider should: (1) never squeeze the area where the sting has occurred; (2) remove the stinger by scraping with a fingernail or knife edge; (3) keep the victim lying down with his legs elevated slightly; (4) apply moist heat to the area of the sting.

    a. 2, 3, and 4.
    b. 1, 2, 3, and 4.
    c. 1, 3, and 4.
    d. 1, 2, and 3.

13. Which of the following is *not* a recommended practice in caring for marine-life poisoning?

    a. vigorously scrub the area.
    b. apply a constricting band between the wound and the heat.
    c. carefully remove stingers or barbs with a knife blade or fingernail.
    d. irrigate the wound with water.

14. Which of the following is *not* a sign or symptom of a poisonous snakebite?

    a. severe pain and burning.
    b. swelling of the wound.
    c. discoloration of the wound.
    d. series of small, shallow puncture wounds.

15. Characteristics of the majority of poisonous snakes include:

    a. irregularly shaped blotches on the skin.
    b. fangs.
    c. elliptical pupils.
    d. all of these answers.

PART III: Matching: Match the type of snake with the characteristics in the left column.

Characteristics	Type of Snake
_____1. Series of small, shallow puncture wounds.	A. Poisonous.
_____2. Wound begins to swell and discolor.	B. Nonpoisonous.
_____3. Differently shaped blotches on background of pink, yellow, olive, tan, gray, or brown skin.	
_____4. Elliptical pupils (vertical slits, much like those of a cat).	
_____5. Large fangs that are hollow.	
_____6. Pain and burning almost immediately.	
_____7. Pit between the eye and mouth.	

PART IV: What Would You Do If:

1. You are in the foothills just outside your community, about twenty minutes from town. You find a teenage boy in shorts who has been bitten by a snake on the lower left leg. There are two distinct puncture wounds. The boy is experiencing severe pain and burning. He is nauseated and sweating and feels weak; his heartbeat is rapid.

2. A young woman is stung by a bee, she is dizzy, has shortness of breath, difficulty swallowing, and generalized itching and swelling.

PART V: Practical Skills Check-Off   _____ has satisfactorily passed the following practical skills:
Student's Name

	Date	Partner Check	Inst. Init.
1. Describe and demonstrate how to give emergency care for a poisonous snakebite (rattlesnake and coral).	__/__/__	☐	_____
2. Describe and demonstrate how to give emergency care for a honeybee sting.	__/__/__	☐	_____

CHAPTER TWENTY-ONE

HEART ATTACK AND OTHER CARDIAC EMERGENCIES

OBJECTIVES

■ Understand coronary artery disease and related risk factors.

■ Describe the cause, signs and symptoms, and emergency care for angina, congestive heart failure, and myocardial infarction.

Heart attacks and associated heart disease are the number-one killer in the United States today. Almost half a million Americans die each year of cardiovascular disease before they can reach a hospital, and almost 29 million more Americans suffer from some form of cardiovascular disease. The most common problem is **CORONARY ARTERY DISEASE**, which usually leads to angina pectoris and may eventually lead to acute myocardial infarction (heart attack) if left untreated.

Because of the critical nature of heart-disease emergencies, every adult with chest pain should be cared for as a heart-attack victim until proven otherwise.

CORONARY ARTERY DISEASE

As the name implies, coronary artery disease affects the arteries that supply the heart with blood by injuring the inner lining of the arterial walls. The two types of coronary artery disease are **ARTERIOSCLEROSIS** and **ATHEROSCLEROSIS**, which is a form of arteriosclerosis, and victims commonly have both kinds.

Atherosclerosis results when fatty substances and other debris are deposited on the inner lining of the arterial wall (Figure 21-1). As a result, the opening of the artery is narrowed, reducing the flow of blood through the affected artery. Another form of arteriosclerosis occurs when calcium is deposited in the walls of the arteries, resulting in loss of arterial elasticity and an increase in blood pressure. Arteriosclerosis generally affects other arteries in

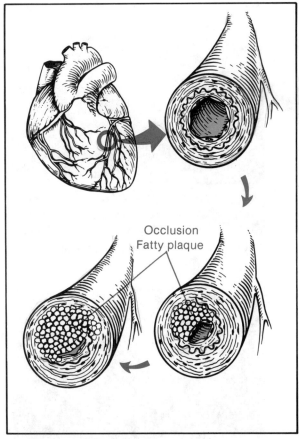

FIGURE 21-1. Fatty deposit buildup in arteries. The deterioration of a normal artery is seen as atherosclerosis develops and begins depositing fatty substances and roughening the channel lining until a clot forms and plugs the artery to deprive the heart muscle of vital blood, which results in heart attack.

Occlusion
Fatty plaque

addition to the coronary arteries, and may lead to hypertension, kidney disease, or stroke.

In coronary artery disease, the opening of the coronary artery is narrowed, restricting the amount of blood that can reach and nourish the heart muscle. Roughened surfaces on the artery cause buildup of additional debris, further narrowing the artery. At some point, the victim may experience angina pectoris (chest pain) or a heart attack because the coronary artery eventually becomes blocked. (Figures 21-2–21-5).

CARDIAC RISK FACTORS

Researchers have identified a number of cardiac risk factors that predispose an individual to coronary artery disease and eventual heart attack. The major risk factors include (Figure 21-6):

- Heredity (a family tendency toward heart disease).
- Sex (males are affected more than females).
- Age (signs and symptoms generally develop after the age of forty).
- Race.
- High serum cholesterol (may be related to eating foods that are high in saturated fats).
- Smoking.
- Sedentary lifestyle.
- Poorly handled stress.

Obviously, the first four factors cannot be controlled; however, with awareness and determination, an individual can change the last four factors and decrease his risk of developing coronary artery disease.

CARDIOVASCULAR DISEASE

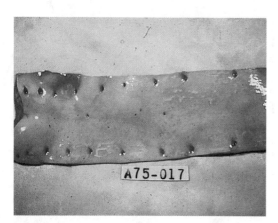

FIGURE 21-2. Inside surface, normal artery.

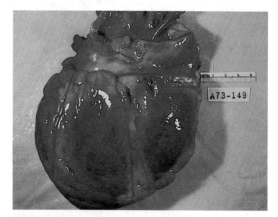

FIGURE 21-3. Myocardial infarction.

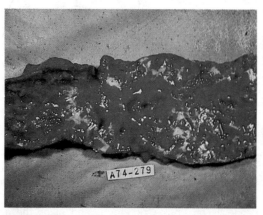

FIGURE 21-4. Inside surface, severe atherosclerosis.

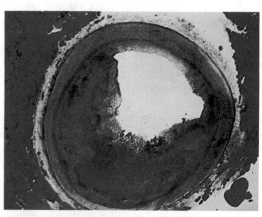

FIGURE 21-5. Artery cross-section, atherosclerosis.

ANGINA PECTORIS

Angina pectoris is actually a set of signs and symptoms that can occur in a victim with serious coronary artery disease. Because of the disease, the coronary arteries are narrowed, and only a limited supply of oxygen-rich blood can be delivered to the heart. Like any muscle, the heart relies on a constant supply of oxygen to function. When the demand for oxygenated blood is greater than the diseased arteries can provide, the person experiences angina pectoris, a brief feeling of pain or discomfort that signals the heart's need for oxygen.

Angina pectoris does not always manifest itself as pain — it may be a feeling of tightness, gripping, heaviness, squeezing, burning, or a dull constriction. The pain is usually on the left side of the chest but may radiate to the jaw, neck, shoulder, arm, or hand (usually on the left side). The pain is sometimes accompanied by nausea, vomiting, and shortness of breath.

Most often angina pectoris occurs because the victim has increased the heart's demand for oxygen by an increased workload, usually by physical activity or emotional excitement, and most often in cold weather. The heart rate may increase as a result of physical activity beyond the victim's limit, emotional stress, or being outdoors in extreme weather (hot, cold, or windy). When the heart's workload is increased, it needs greater amounts of blood — which the diseased arteries are unable to deliver. When there is not enough blood to meet the metabolic needs of the cardiac cells, angina pectoris results. Less commonly, angina may occur without exertion.

Approximately 80 percent of all angina victims are men in their fifties or sixties; angina is reversible

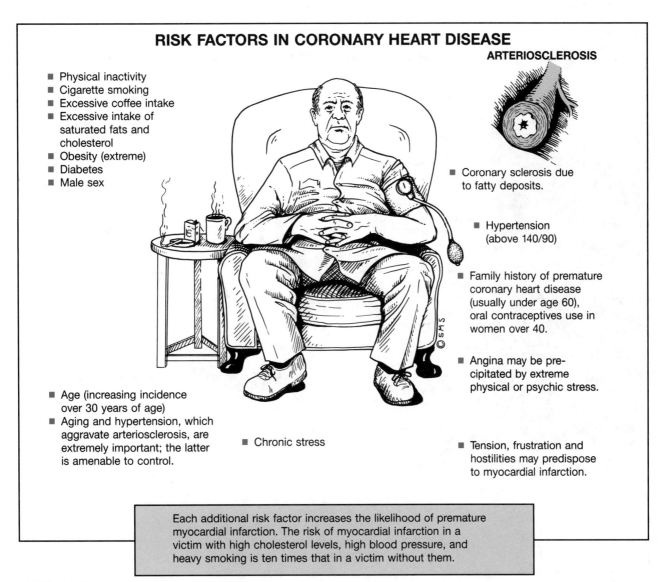

RISK FACTORS IN CORONARY HEART DISEASE

ARTERIOSCLEROSIS

- Physical inactivity
- Cigarette smoking
- Excessive coffee intake
- Excessive intake of saturated fats and cholesterol
- Obesity (extreme)
- Diabetes
- Male sex

- Coronary sclerosis due to fatty deposits.

- Hypertension (above 140/90)

- Family history of premature coronary heart disease (usually under age 60), oral contraceptives use in women over 40.

- Age (increasing incidence over 30 years of age)
- Aging and hypertension, which aggravate arteriosclerosis, are extremely important; the latter is amenable to control.

- Chronic stress

- Angina may be precipitated by extreme physical or psychic stress.

- Tension, frustration and hostilities may predispose to myocardial infarction.

Each additional risk factor increases the likelihood of premature myocardial infarction. The risk of myocardial infarction in a victim with high cholesterol levels, high blood pressure, and heavy smoking is ten times that in a victim without them.

FIGURE 21-6.

and produces no permanent damage to the heart. Pain is generally relieved by rest, usually within a few minutes after the victim stops the activity, calms down, moves indoors, or takes nitroglycerin as prescribed by a physician.

RISK FACTORS

Common risk factors for angina pectoris are:

- The presence of coronary artery disease.
- A history of cardiac problems.
- Cigarette smoking.
- Poor dietary habits.
- A hostile **TYPE A PERSONALITY.**
- **HYPERTENSION.**

Keep in mind, however, that these risk factors may be absent.

SIGNS AND SYMPTOMS

The most common complaint of angina is chest pain that may range from a mild ache to a severe crushing pain. It appears suddenly but usually is associated with physical exertion. Other common signs and symptoms include (Figure 21-7):

- Dyspnea (shortness of breath).
- Profuse perspiration.
- Lightheadedness.
- Palpitations.
- Nausea and/or vomiting.
- Pale, cool, and moist skin.

Remember — it is impossible for a First Aider to differentiate between the pain of angina pectoris and the pain of heart attack. While angina is a transient episode that leaves the heart undamaged, it *is*

DISTINGUISHING ANGINA PECTORIS FROM MYOCARDIAL INFARCTION

	ANGINA PECTORIS	MYOCARDIAL INFARCTION
Location of Pain	Substernal or across chest	Same
Radiation of Pain	Neck, jaw or arms	Same
Nature of Pain	Dull or heavy discomfort with a pressure or squeezing sensation	Same, but maybe more intense
Duration	Usually lasts 3 to 8 minutes rarely longer	Usually lasts longer than 30 minutes
Other Symptoms	Usually none	Perspiration, weakness, nausea, pale gray color
Precipitating Factors	Extremes in weather, exertion, stress, meals	Often none
Factors Giving Relief	Stopping physical activity, reducing stress, nitroglycerin	Nitroglycerin may give incomplete, or no relief

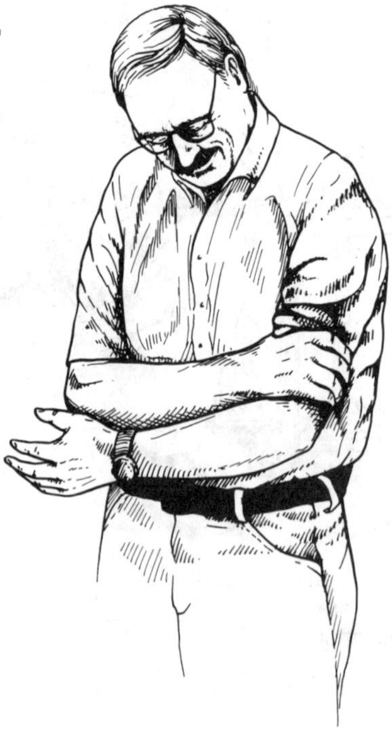

If in doubt as to which condition the victim has, always treat as if it is an acute myocardial infarction.

FIGURE 21-7.

an indication of coronary artery disease and needs to be treated by a physician; left untreated, it may eventually cause heart attack.

See "General Emergency Care for Cardiac Victims" later in this chapter for treating angina.

CONGESTIVE HEART FAILURE

CONGESTIVE HEART FAILURE results when the heart's pumping output does not meet the needs of bodily tissues; i.e., perfusion is inadequate. While there are a number of causes, the most common include myocardial infarction, hypertension, chronic obstructive pulmonary disease, coronary artery disease, and heart valve damage.

SIGNS AND SYMPTOMS

The most dramatic sign of congestive heart failure is **PULMONARY EDEMA**, resulting in severe dyspnea. The victim may also experience the following (Figure 21-8):

- Wheezing.
- Rapid heart rate.
- Increased respiratory rate.
- Paleness or cyanosis.
- Difficulty breathing while lying flat.
- Normal to high blood pressure.
- Feet and lower-extremity edema (swelling).
- Anxiety.
- Mild to severe confusion.
- A desire to sit upright.
- Abdominal distension.
- Distended neck veins.

Remember — while these signs and symptoms are the most common, the victim may have any combination of them, and some victims may have only one or two. Congestive heart failure with respiratory difficulty is life-threatening and requires immediate care.

EMERGENCY CARE

In any victim experiencing severe dyspnea, care for it as follows:

1. Sit the victim upright, legs dangling over the side; this position encourages the flow of fluid out of the lungs and into the extremities.
2. Activate the EMS system immediately.

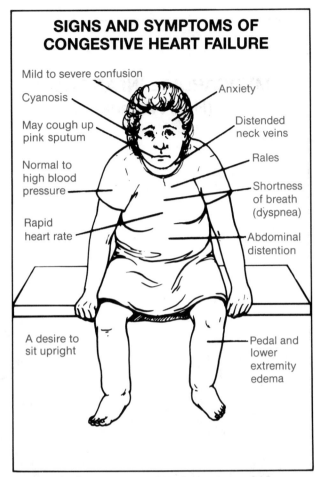

SIGNS AND SYMPTOMS OF CONGESTIVE HEART FAILURE

Mild to severe confusion
Cyanosis
May cough up pink sputum
Normal to high blood pressure
Rapid heart rate
A desire to sit upright
Anxiety
Distended neck veins
Rales
Shortness of breath (dyspnea)
Abdominal distention
Pedal and lower extremity edema

FIGURE 21-8.

MYOCARDIAL INFARCTION

Called a "heart attack" by the lay person, myocardial infarction means death of the myocardium (heart muscle). When blood supply to part of the heart is significantly reduced or stopped completely, the affected part dies. (Figure 21-9).

Myocardial infarction causes four serious consequences:

- **Sudden death.** Nearly half a million people die each year in this country from myocardial infarction before they ever reach a hospital. Most of them die within two hours of first experiencing signs and symptoms of myocardial infarction.
- **Cardiogenic shock.** If 40 percent or more of the left ventricle is damaged after a myocardial infarction, severe impairment of the heart's pumping action results, leading to inadequate circulation of blood. The mortality rate from cardiogenic shock is 80 percent.

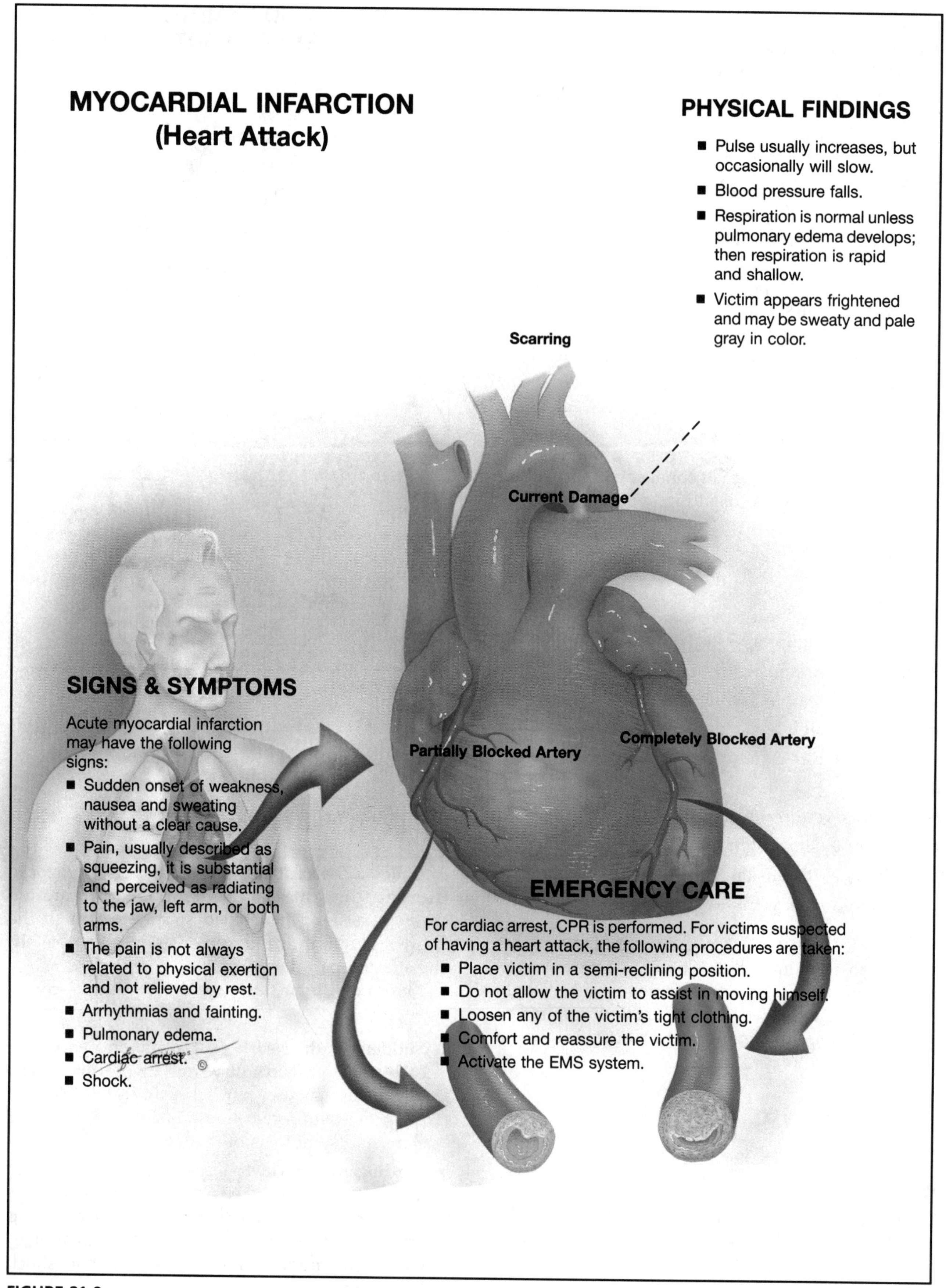

MYOCARDIAL INFARCTION
(Heart Attack)

PHYSICAL FINDINGS

- Pulse usually increases, but occasionally will slow.
- Blood pressure falls.
- Respiration is normal unless pulmonary edema develops; then respiration is rapid and shallow.
- Victim appears frightened and may be sweaty and pale gray in color.

Scarring

Current Damage

SIGNS & SYMPTOMS

Acute myocardial infarction may have the following signs:

- Sudden onset of weakness, nausea and sweating without a clear cause.
- Pain, usually described as squeezing, it is substantial and perceived as radiating to the jaw, left arm, or both arms.
- The pain is not always related to physical exertion and not relieved by rest.
- Arrhythmias and fainting.
- Pulmonary edema.
- Cardiac arrest.
- Shock.

Partially Blocked Artery

Completely Blocked Artery

EMERGENCY CARE

For cardiac arrest, CPR is performed. For victims suspected of having a heart attack, the following procedures are taken:

- Place victim in a semi-reclining position.
- Do not allow the victim to assist in moving himself.
- Loosen any of the victim's tight clothing.
- Comfort and reassure the victim.
- Activate the EMS system.

FIGURE 21-9.

■ **Congestive heart failure**. Congestive heart failure may develop between three and seven days after a myocardial infarction. It often manifests itself as pulmonary edema due to inadequate pumping of the heart.

■ **Cardiac dysrhythmias**. Cardiac dysrhythmias are abnormal heart rhythms that occur following a myocardial infarction, generally caused by an **IRRITABLE HEART** or by injury to the electrical conduction system of the heart.

SIGNS AND SYMPTOMS

The major symptom of a myocardial infarction is chest pain that may range from mild discomfort to a severe crushing pain (Figure 21-10) — *but it should be noted that 25 percent of all myocardial infarction victims have no chest pain at all* (usually the elderly or diabetics). Myocardial infarctions without pain are called silent myocardial infarctions. The pain from myocardial infarction lasts for longer than thirty minutes, and the classical location is substernal radiating to the neck, jaw, left shoulder, and left arm. Remember, however, that chest pain associated with myocardial infarction can be experienced in a great number of ways (Figure 21-11). *Any adult with chest pain should be suspected of myocardial infarction until proven otherwise.*

Other common signs and symptoms of myocardial infarction include the following:

■ Dyspnea.

■ Profuse sweating.

■ Cool, pale, moist skin.

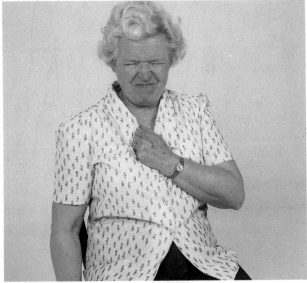

FIGURE 21-10. The major symptom of a myocardial infarction is chest pain.

■ Possible cyanosis.

■ Nausea and/or vomiting.

■ Weakness.

■ Lightheadedness.

■ Anxiety.

■ Feeling of impending doom.

■ Pulse exceeding 100 beats per minute.

■ A pulse less than 60 beats per minute can also be an alarming sign.

■ Fainting.

EMERGENCY CARE

For all possible cases of myocardial infarction, provide the following care:

1. Assess for airway, breathing, and circulation. Assist as necessary.

2. Do not let the victim move on his own; restrict all unnecessary movement, and provide comfort and reassurance to calm the victim.

3. Place the victim in the position of greatest comfort and ease of breathing. A sitting or semi-reclined position is preferred by most victims.

4. Monitor vital signs continuously.

5. Administer artificial ventilation and CPR as necessary.

6. Activate the EMS system immediately.

GENERAL EMERGENCY CARE FOR CARDIAC VICTIMS

A victim with a heart-disease emergency can be given the following general care:

1. Have the victim cease all movement.

2. Place the victim in a semi-reclining or sitting position, or position of comfort.

3. If the problem is a suspected angina attack, ask the victim if he has nitroglycerine. If the victim has tablets and has not already taken them, place one tablet underneath the tongue. This is not allowed in many areas — *follow local protocol.*

4. Make sure that the airway is open and administer artificial ventilation if necessary.

5. Loosen constricting clothing.

6. Maintain body temperature as close to normal as possible.

7. Comfort and reassure the victim.

8. Administer CPR if cardiac arrest occurs.

9. Activate the EMS system immediately.

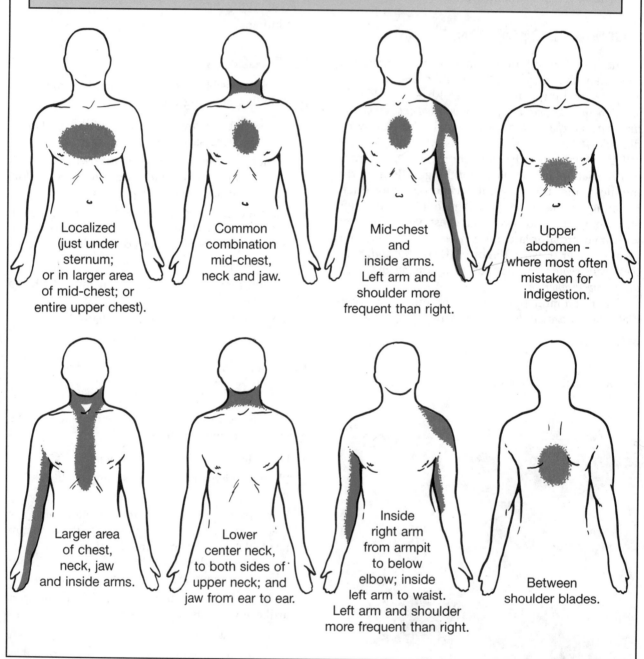

EARLY SIGNALS OF A HEART ATTACK

PAIN, in one form or another, usually accompanies a heart attack and ranges from a mild ache to unbearable severity. When severe, pain is often felt as constricting, like a vise on the chest. Pain also often includes the burning and bloating sensations that usually accompany indigestion. Pain may be continuous and then might subside, but don't ignore it if it does. Pain could occur in any one or combination of locations shown below.

Localized (just under sternum; or in larger area of mid-chest; or entire upper chest).

Common combination mid-chest, neck and jaw.

Mid-chest and inside arms. Left arm and shoulder more frequent than right.

Upper abdomen - where most often mistaken for indigestion.

Larger area of chest, neck, jaw and inside arms.

Lower center neck, to both sides of upper neck; and jaw from ear to ear.

Inside right arm from armpit to below elbow; inside left arm to waist. Left arm and shoulder more frequent than right.

Between shoulder blades.

FIGURE 21-11.

| 21 | **SELF-TEST** | 21 |

Student: _____ Date: _____

Course: _____ Section #: _____

PART I: True/False   If you believe that the statement is true, circle the T. If you believe that the statement is false, circle the F.

T F   1. Atherosclerosis results when fatty substances and other debris are deposited on the inner lining of the arterial wall.

T F   2. Angina does not always manifest itself as pain.

T F   3. Angina pain is usually relieved by rest.

T F   4. Angina pain is usually on the left side.

T F   5. It is quite easy to differentiate between the pain of angina pectoris and the pain of myocardial infarction.

T F   6. Emergency care for a victim with congestive heart failure includes putting the victim in an upright sitting position.

T F   7. A myocardial infarction may cause cardiogenic shock, which has a mortality rate of 80 percent.

T F   8. About 25 percent of all myocardial infarction victims have no chest pain.

T F   9. The pain of myocardial infarction lasts for longer than thirty minutes and is usually substernal, radiating to the neck, jaw, left shoulder, and left arm.

T F 10. Victims of heart-disease emergencies should be put in a prone position.

T F 11. Approximately 80 percent of all angina victims are men in their fifties or sixties.

T F 12. It is usually easy for a First Aider to differentiate between pain of angina and the pain of a heart attack.

T F 13. Congestive heart failure with respiratory difficulty is life-threatening and requires immediate care.

T F 14. Nearly half a million people die each year in this country from myocardial infarction.

T F 15. The major symptom of myocardial infarction is cyanosis.

PART II: Multiple Choice   For each question, circle the answer that best reflects an accurate statement.

1. Which of the following is *not* a type of pain associated with myocardial infarction?
   a. chest, neck, jaw, and inside arms.
   b. mid-chest and inside arms.
   c. lower center neck to upper neck (both sides).
   d. inside right arm from elbow to wrist.

2. In most cases, the pain from myocardial infarction is:
   a. located beneath the breastbone and feels like someone is squeezing the chest.
   b. very sharp, especially during inhalation.
   c. in the upper abdomen and feels like indigestion.
   d. between the shoulder blades in the back.

3. The signs and symptoms of myocardial infarction include all of the following *except*:
   a. pale skin color.
   b. shortness of breath.
   c. decreased pulse rate.
   d. feeling of impending doom.

4. Most acute heart attacks are caused by blockage of the _____ arteries.
   a. cephalic.   c. coronal.
   b. coronary.   d. carotid.

5. The buildup of fatty deposits in arteries is called:
   a. atherosclerosis.
   b. angina pectoris.
   c. coronary thrombosis.
   d. cholesterol.

6. Congestive heart failure:
   a. is the result of congenital heart damage.
   b. may happen within a week of a heart attack due to the heart's inability to pump blood effectively.
   c. usually accompanies a stroke.
   d. is frequently the result of pneumonia.

7. Angina pectoris:
   a. is often accompanied by weakness and nausea.
   b. is a term that describes any kind of chest pain.
   c. usually lasts longer than thirty minutes.
   d. is pain in the heart caused by insufficient oxygen.

8. You are asked to assist a forty-seven-year-old employee who had a sudden onset of severe chest pain that travelled down his left shoulder to his hand. When you arrive, he is short of breath, frightened, and restless. What should you suspect?
   a. stroke.
   b. angina pectoris.
   c. chronic heart failure.
   d. heart attack.

9. Another heart condition, often mistaken for indigestion, is brought on by emotional stress, strenuous exercise, or agitation and is characterized by pain in the chest or arm. This condition is known as:
   a. chronic heart failure.
   b. heart attack.
   c. stroke.
   d. angina pectoris.

10. You would most likely expect which of the following heart conditions to develop over several months?

    a. acute myocardial infarction.
    b. heart attack.
    c. cardiogenic shock.
    d. congestive heart failure.

11. Which of the following is *not* an emergency-care measure for a cardiac victim?

    a. loosen constrictive clothing.
    b. place the victim in a semireclining position.
    c. have the victim cease all movement.
    d. do not help victim administer his medication until a physician has seen him.

12. The term "dyspnea" refers to:

    a. shortness of breath while lying down.
    b. profuse sweating.
    c. lack of oxygen.
    d. shortness of breath.

13. Which of the following is *not* a recommended practice in caring for a conscious, suspected heart-attack victim?

    a. always have the victim transported to a hospital.
    b. comfort and reassure the victim.
    c. loosen any tight-fitting clothing.
    d. keep the victim moving, if possible.

14. Which of the following is true regarding angina pectoris and myocardial infarction?

    a. nitroglycerine often relieves angina pectoris and myocardial infarction.
    b. the pain usually lasts only three to eight minutes in angina pectoris and myocardial infarction.
    c. the pain for both conditions is in the same general area, but it is more intense with angina pectoris.
    d. extremes in weather, physical exertion, or stress usually precipitate a myocardial infarction, but angina pectoris often occurs without warning.

15. Emergency care for a victim with congestive heart failure:

    a. includes watching for signs of angina pectoris.
    b. is exactly the same as that for myocardial infarction.
    c. includes immediate CPR.
    d. sit victim upright with legs dangling over the side.

16. America's number-one killer is:

    a. stroke.
    b. heart attack and heart disease.
    c. accidents.
    d. cancer.

17. Which of the following are risk factors in heart disease: (1) lack of physical exercise; (2) heavy cigarette smoking; (3) dietary indiscretion; (4) hypotension; (5) chronic unhappiness.

    a. 1, 2, and 3.
    b. 1, 2, 3, and 5.
    c. 1, 2, 3, and 4.
    d. 1, 2, 3, 4, and 5.

18. Which of the following statements about the pain experienced as a result of myocardial infarction is *not* true?

    a. the pain is usually centered underneath the breastbone.
    b. the victim often has a squeezing sensation.
    c. the right arm is usually more involved than the left arm.
    d. the pain may be centered in the upper abdomen where it is often mistaken for indigestion.

19. A victim with swelling in the extremities and frothy, pink sputum would be manifesting symptoms of:

    a. angina pectoris.
    b. cardiac arrest.
    c. congestive heart failure.
    d. none of the above.

20. Which of the following statements regarding angina pectoris is true?

    a. nitroglycerine should not be given to an angina pectoris victim.
    b. angina pectoris often results in damage to heart tissues and is sometimes fatal.
    c. administering oxygen can worsen angina pectoris.
    d. angina pectoris is temporary pain that can be brought on by emotional stress.

PART III: What Would You Do If:

1. An older person has been working in his garden and complains of a squeezing, burning, heavy sensation on the left side of his chest. He is nauseous and lightheaded, and has cool, moist skin.

2. You are called at the home of a middle-aged woman who is experiencing severe dyspnea and a rapid heart rate. She has lower-extremity edema and distended neck veins, and seems confused.

PART IV: Practical Skills Check-Off

_____ has satisfactorily passed the following practical skills:
                    Student's Name

	Date	Partner Check	Inst. Init.

1. Describe and demonstrate how to give emergency care for a victim of a myocardial infarction.

___/___/___   ☐   _____

OBJECTIVES

- Understand the types of circulation disturbance in the brain that can cause a stroke.
- Recognize the common signs and symptoms of stroke.
- Describe and demonstrate the appropriate emergency care for stroke.

CHAPTER TWENTY-TWO

STROKE

Stroke is defined as any disease process that impairs circulation to the brain. The third most common cause of death in this country, stroke affects approximately half a million Americans each year. More than half of those die, and many others suffer permanent neurological damage.

Stroke, also known as cerebrovascular accident (CVA), occurs when the blood flow to the brain is interrupted long enough to cause damage, resulting in the sudden onset of brain dysfunction. The characteristics of stroke, which range from the unnoticed to those causing coma, depend on the extent of the stroke, the site of the stroke, and the amount of brain damage that results.

The outcome of stroke — regardless of its cause — depends on the age of the victim, the location and function of the brain cells that were damaged, the extent of the damage, and how rapidly other areas of brain tissue are able to take over the work of the damaged cells (brain cells do not regenerate). Without treatment, recurrence among survivors of stroke is common; with appropriate treatment, recurrence is not common.

According to the American Heart Association Council on Stroke, the most likely candidate for stroke has high blood pressure and a history of brief intermittent stroke episodes called **TRANSIENT ISCHEMIC ATTACKS (TIAs)**. Other predisposing factors in general include diabetes and hardening of the arteries in the heart, neck, and legs. The stroke victim often smokes heavily and has high levels of cholesterol or other fats in the blood. Rarely, stroke may be caused by a migraine headache.

GENERAL CAUSES OF STROKE

The four general causes of interference of the blood supply to the brain are:

- **THROMBUS**.
- **EMBOLUS**.
- Hemorrhage.
- Compression (Figure 22-1).

THROMBUS

The most common cause of stroke occurs when a cerebral artery is blocked by a clot (thrombus) that forms inside the brain; 75 to 85 percent of all strokes are caused by a thrombus. **CEREBRAL THROMBOSIS** usually occurs in those over the age of fifty, and the incidence generally increases with age. The major cause is atherosclerosis. Approximately 60 percent of victims have hypertension, 25 percent have diabetes, and half also have some type of vascular disease.

Up to 75 percent of all thrombus strokes are preceded by one or more transient ischemic attacks, brief "spells" similar to strokes that result when the blockage is incomplete or lasts only a few minutes. In the case of a TIA, the brain cells are injured but they do not die. TIAs often occur in a series over a period of many days, usually getting worse with time. While most TIAs are warning of a possible future stroke, they *can* occasionally occur without being followed by a stroke. They result in no permanent brain damage.

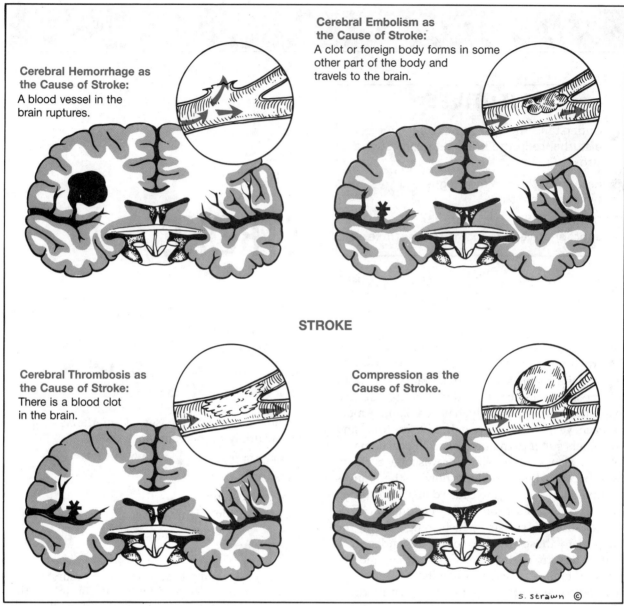

FIGURE 22-1. Causes of stroke.

The symptoms of a TIA last for less than twenty-four hours and usually for less than one hour. All are temporary, leaving no permanent effects; often, only one symptom may be present. The most common symptoms of TIAs include:

- Blindness in one eye.
- Headache.
- Dizziness.
- Lightheadedness.
- Fainting.
- Difficulty in performing familiar acts.

- Temporary paralysis of the face.
- Temporary paralysis of one side of the body.
- Difficulty pronouncing and/or understanding words.
- Inability to recognize familiar objects.

TIAs do *not* cause nausea or vomiting, and often headache is not present. A thrombotic stroke usually occurs gradually in steps and becomes worse over time as the blockage slowly increases. When TIAs are present, they tend to worsen progressively as more brain tissue becomes involved.

EMBOLUS

A stroke may also result when a clot develops elsewhere in the body, travels through the bloodstream, and becomes lodged in one of the cerebral arteries — a condition called cerebral embolism. While embolism strokes are probably much less common than thrombus strokes, they occur much more rapidly; of all strokes, they have the most rapid onset. They often occur in young or middle-aged adults.

Emboli are most often found in people who have existing heart disease that results in uncontrolled and ineffective beating of the heart.

HEMORRHAGE

In 15 to 25 percent of all strokes, the stroke occurs when a diseased blood vessel in the brain bursts, flooding the surrounding brain tissue with blood (Figures 22-2 and 22-3). Hemorrhage is the most dramatic form of stroke, and 80 percent of its victims

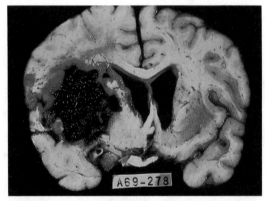

FIGURE 22-2. Cerebrovascular accident (stroke) from cerebral hemorrhage.

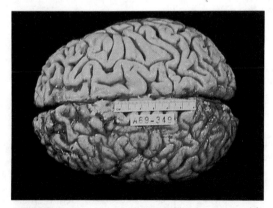

FIGURE 22-3. Stroke-damaged brain — one side.

die. Onset is abrupt, and it rapidly and progressively worsens as more brain tissue becomes involved; however, it does *not* occur in steplike stages, as does thrombotic stroke. While headache is not as common with thrombotic or embolism strokes, up to half of all hemorrhage stroke victims experience severe headache; vomiting is common. Hypertension is also found in more than half of all stroke victims.

Cerebral hemorrhage is most likely to occur when the victim suffers from a combination of hypertension and atherosclerosis. While other forms of stroke usually occur in victims over forty years of age, cerebral hemorrhage can affect victims of any age. However, the incidence does increase progressively over the age of fifty.

COMPRESSION

A small percentage of strokes occur when extreme pressure is applied to a cerebral artery, cutting off blood supply to the adjacent brain tissue and nerves. This pressure — or compression — can be caused by a brain tumor, by displaced cerebral tissue following hemorrhage elsewhere in the brain or following head trauma, or by a clot that forms outside the artery as a result of blood leakage elsewhere in the brain. Compression can also result if a cerebral artery goes into spasm; however, spasms are usually so brief that resulting damage is rarely permanent.

SIGNS AND SYMPTOMS OF STROKE

The signs and symptoms of stroke depend on the location, size, and severity of the stroke. Most signs come on suddenly and are focal in nature. The worst strokes are signalled by rapid and progressive signs and symptoms that are accompanied by the development of new signs and symptoms. Remember that other medical problems — such as epilepsy — can mimic stroke.

The precise signs and symptoms that accompany a stroke depend on the cause. A stroke caused by clotting (thrombus) results in lessening of bodily functions without accompanying pain or seizures; onset is gradual and progresses in a steplike way. A stroke caused by cerebral hemorrhage produces sudden, excruciating headache followed by a rapid loss of consciousness, along with neck rigidity and coma. A stroke caused by an embolus is marked by possible sudden convulsions, paralysis, and abrupt loss of consciousness. A severe headache may occur explosively, although it is possible that no headache at all may occur.

The general signs and symptoms of stroke occur suddenly and may include the following (Figure 22-4):

- An alteration of the level of consciousness:
    - Unexplained dizziness, confusion, or unsteadiness.
    - A change in personality.
    - A change in the level of mental ability, including concentration ability.
    - Decreased consciousness, ranging from dizziness to coma.
    - Convulsions.

- Effects on motor function:
    - Weakness of the arms, legs, or face.
    - Numbness or paralysis of the face, arms, or legs, often on only one side.
    - One-sided weakness or numbness that gradually evolves to general weakness or numbness.
    - Paralysis or weakness on one or both sides of the body; unilateral weakness or paralysis is most common.
    - Mouth drawn to one side of the face or drooping on one side; paralysis of facial muscles, resulting in loss of facial expression and drooping eyelid.

- Effects on sensory function and changes in vision:
    - Loss of vision or temporary dimness of vision, particularly in one eye.
    - Double vision.

- Altered communication abilities:
    - Inability to speak or trouble in speaking or understanding speech.
    - Stuttering.

- Other symptoms:
    - Headache accompanied by a stiff neck (caused by hemorrhage).
    - A sudden, severe headache or a change in the pattern of headaches normally experienced by the victim.
    - Flushed or pale face.
    - Respiratory distress.
    - Pupils unequal in size or reaction, or constricted.
    - Loss of bowel or bladder control.
    - Nausea and/or vomiting.

If the stroke occurs on the left side of the brain, the damage is noticeable on the right side of the body; if the stroke occurs on the right side of the brain, the damage is evident on the left side of the body.

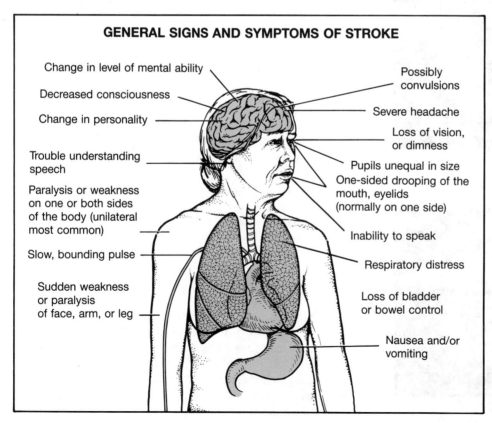

GENERAL SIGNS AND SYMPTOMS OF STROKE

Change in level of mental ability

Decreased consciousness

Change in personality

Trouble understanding speech

Paralysis or weakness on one or both sides of the body (unilateral most common)

Slow, bounding pulse

Sudden weakness or paralysis of face, arm, or leg

Possibly convulsions

Severe headache

Loss of vision, or dimness

Pupils unequal in size
One-sided drooping of the mouth, eyelids (normally on one side)

Inability to speak

Respiratory distress

Loss of bladder or bowel control

Nausea and/or vomiting

FIGURE 22-4. Note: Even though a variety of signs/symptoms may appear in a stroke victim, one may be sufficient reason to begin emergency care.

It is important to note the victim's state of consciousness. Only massive strokes or those involving the brain stem render the victim completely unconscious. These, of course, are the most serious and require the most extensive care. The most critical stroke victim is the one who loses consciousness completely and becomes flaccid (limp) on the involved side; these signs indicate major brain injury.

EMERGENCY CARE

The following steps should be initiated:

1. Handle the victim calmly and carefully; be particularly gentle with paralyzed parts. Maintain a considerate, optimistic, and hopeful attitude. Remember that the victim can hear you, even if he is not able to communicate back, so be careful about what you say in his presence. Say nothing that will increase his anxiety, because anxiety can aggravate the stroke considerably.

2. Position the victim on his back with his head and shoulders slightly raised (about twenty to thirty degrees) to relieve intracranial pressure. Keep the head in a neutral, forward-facing position to maintain arterial and venous flow to and from the head. Use a simple head tilt to keep the tongue from falling back and blocking the throat.

3. Assess the victim's airway and respiration.
   - Clear the airway of any foreign matter, food, or vomitus with a gauze-wrapped finger.
   - Remove all dentures and dental bridges.
   - Administer artificial ventilation and CPR if necessary.
   - If you believe that the victim may choke on vomitus or mucus, turn his head to the side to facilitate drainage.

4. If the victim develops further difficulty in breathing or becomes unconscious, turn him on his side, preferably with the paralyzed side down and well cushioned. If the unconscious victim begins to vomit, turn him on his side, clear his airway, and allow drainage.

5. If the victim's eyelid is affected, gently close the lid and loosely tape it closed to prevent it from drying out.

6. Keep the victim warm, but do not overheat; excessive heat speeds brain damage.

7. Keep the victim absolutely quiet; shield him from curious onlookers.

8. Never give the victim anything to eat or drink; paralysis of the pharynx is common. Never use any kind of stimulant, such as smelling salts.

9. Activate the EMS system as soon as possible.

| **22** | **SELF-TEST** | **22** |

Student: _____ Date: _____

Course: _____ Section #: _____

PART I: True/False   If you believe that the statement is true, circle the T. If you believe that the statement is false, circle the F.

T   F   1.   Strokes are most often caused by severe migraine headaches.

T   F   2.   The most common cause of stroke is a cerebral hemorrhage.

T   F   3.   The major cause of cerebral thrombosis is atherosclerosis.

T   F   4.   Up to 75 percent of all thrombus strokes are preceded by one or more TIAs.

T   F   5.   TIAs are a warning of a possible future stroke.

T   F   6.   TIAs often cause nausea, vomiting, and headaches.

T   F   7.   Emboli are most often found in people who have existing heart disease.

T   F   8.   Over 50 percent of all strokes occur when a blood vessel in the brain bursts.

T   F   9.   Up to half of all hemorrhage-stroke victims experience severe headache.

T   F   10. A small percentage of strokes occur when extreme pressure is applied to a cerebral artery.

T   F   11. The general signs and symptoms of stroke occur suddenly and often include dizziness, confusion, and a change in personality.

T   F   12. The most critical stroke victim is the one who loses consciousness completely and becomes flaccid on the involved side.

T   F   13. Even though a stroke victim may be unresponsive, he may be able to hear and understand what you are saying.

T   F   14. Position a stroke victim in a semi-sitting position.

T   F   15. Strokes that involve coma and neck rigidity are usually caused by cerebral hemorrhage.

T   F   16. Conscious stroke victims should be allowed to take fluids orally.

T   F   17. Stroke is defined as any disease process that impairs circulation to the brain.

T   F   18. Embolism strokes have the least rapid onset.

T   F   19. A stroke caused by an embolus is marked by possible sudden convulsions, paralysis and abrupt loss of consciousness.

T   F   20. Keep the stroke victim as warm as possible — even to the point of overheating.

PART II: Multiple Choice   For each question, circle the answer that best reflects an accurate statement.

1. A stroke usually occurs:

    a. as a result of angina pectoris.
    b. when blood flowing to the brain is cut off.
    c. when blood flowing to the heart is cut off.
    d. as a result of myocardial infarction.

2. Which of the following is *not* a cause of stroke?

    a. cerebral embolism.
    b. cerebral thrombosis.
    c. cerebral hypotension.
    d. cerebral hemorrhage.

3. Which of the following terms describes a blood clot that originates in the brain?

    a. cerebral embolism.
    b. cerebral compression.
    c. cerebral hemorrhage.
    d. cerebral thrombosis.

4. Which of the following are general signs and symptoms of stroke? (1) change in level of mental ability; (2) change in personality; (3) trouble speaking or understanding speech; (4) paralysis or weakness on one or both sides of the body; (5) convulsions; (6) unequal pupils; (7) drooping facial features; (8) loss of bladder or bowel control.

    a. 1, 2, 3, 4, 5, 6, 7, and 8.
    b. 1, 3, 4, 7, and 8.
    c. 3, 4, 5, 6, and 7.
    d. 2, 3, 4, 6, and 7.

5. Which of the following are recommended procedures in the emergency care of a stroke victim? (1) handle the victim calmly; (2) position the victim on his back with head and shoulders slightly raised; (3) remove all dentures, bridges, or false teeth; (4) keep the victim as warm as possible; (5) if the victim is conscious, give small sips of water; (6) administer smelling salts.

    a. 1, 2, 3, and 5.
    b. 1, 2, 3, 4, 5, and 6.
    c. 1, 2, and 3.
    d. 1, 2, 3, and 4.

6. The condition of an unconscious stroke victim can be made worse by:

   a. excessive heat.
   b. inadequate protection of paralyzed limbs.
   c. comments by the First Aider or bystanders on the severity of the victim's condition.
   d. all of these answers.

7. When the blood supply to part of the brain is cut off, impairing the function of cells in that part of the brain, the victim is said to have suffered a(n):

   a. stroke.
   b. epileptic seizure.
   c. angina pectoris attack.
   d. coma.

8. Which of the following is *not* a cause of blood-supply interference in the brain?

   a. compression.
   b. clotting.
   c. convulsions.
   d. hemorrhage.

9. What are the signs and symptoms of stroke?

   a. paralysis, unequal pupils.
   b. slow bounding pulse and paralysis on one side of the body.
   c. inability to speak, unequal pupils.
   d. all of the above.

10. Before an actual stroke, a person may suffer:

    a. convulsions.
    b. complete speech loss.
    c. TIAs.
    d. loss of bladder control.

11. The most critical stroke victim is the:

    a. one who loses consciousness completely and becomes flaccid on the involved side.
    b. one who becomes rigid and completely paralyzed on the involved side.
    c. one who has severe headache and unequal pupils.
    d. one who has loss of vision and inability to speak.

12. What is the emergency care for a stroke victim?

    a. give the victim sips of water.
    b. keep the victim lying down and elevate his feet.
    c. begin CPR.
    d. keep the victim quiet and reassure him.

PART III: What Would You Do If:

1. You are at the home of an elderly person who is complaining of confusion and dizziness. She has weakness in her arms and legs and is having trouble seeing and speaking. She is nauseated and is having some respiratory distress.

2. The same person has paralysis on her left side — including her arm, leg, and face.

PART IV: Practical Skills Check-Off _____ has satisfactorily passed the following practical skills:
Student's Name

	Date	Partner Check	Inst. Init.
1. Describe and demonstrate how to give emergency care to a stroke victim.	__/__/__	☐	_____

CHAPTER TWENTY

OBJECTIVES

- Identify the common causes of dyspnea, including chronic obstructive pulmonary disease (emphysema, bronchitis, and asthma), pneumonia, and hyperventilation.

- Recognize the signs and symptoms that may accompany the various types of emergencies that cause dyspnea.

- Describe and demonstrate how to administer emergency care for each of the causes of dyspnea.

288 • MEDICAL EMERGENCIE
get medical help ea
life with proper r
program. E
Emphysema
more commo
city dwellers
most impo
smoking
is of m
are al

RESPIRATORY EMERGENCIES

DYSPNEA
(SHORTNESS OF BREATH)

Dyspnea, one of the most common medical complaints, is defined as a sensation of shortness of breath — a feeling of air hunger accompanied by labored breathing. Two major sets of circumstances generally accompany dyspnea: in one, air cannot pass easily into the lungs; in the other, air cannot pass easily out of the lungs. Most commonly, there is resistance in either the airway (from obstruction or an inflamed, swollen epiglottis) or in expansion of the lungs.

Dyspnea is not a disease in itself but is a symptom of a number of diseases. Breathing will generally be rapid and shallow, but victims may feel short of breath whether they are breathing rapidly or slowly. Remember that shortness of breath is normal following exercise, fatigue, coughing, or the production of excess sputum. In these cases, the condition is not considered true dyspnea.

Dyspnea can be a gradual process, or it may occur suddenly. Common causes include heart and/or lung diseases or injury.

Take the following steps in giving emergency care:

1. Maintain an open airway. Dyspnea may be caused by aspiration of a foreign body;

immediately check for aspiration, and clear the airway if necessary.

2. Treat for shock.

3. Activate the EMS system.

CHRONIC OBSTRUCTIVE PULMONARY DISEASE (COPD)

The most common obstructive airway diseases are emphysema, chronic bronchitis, and asthma. The most reversible is asthma, while the most irreversible is emphysema; chronic bronchitis falls somewhere in between. The incidence of chronic obstructive pulmonary disease is high: up to 20 percent of the adult population in the United States suffers from some form of it. Of those, 90 percent have emphysema, chronic bronchitis, or both; most have a combination of the two.

EMPHYSEMA AND CHRONIC BRONCHITIS

Emphysema is a progressive disease that cannot be reversed, and as it advances, the victim experiences increasing dyspnea. With chronic bronchitis, on the other hand, the damage cannot be reversed, but the disease process *can* be stopped; victims who

rly can lead a fairly normal
...edication and a good exercise

...and chronic bronchitis are much
... in men than in women and among
... than among rural populations. The
...rtant known factor in COPD is cigarette
...urban air pollution also plays a role, but it
...uch lesser significance. Most COPD victims
...o prone to allergies and a variety of infections

(Figure 23-1). The typical victim is found leaning forward in an attempt to breathe (Figure 23-2). He may be gasping for air, have distended neck veins, and be cyanotic.

Emphysema

Emphysema is characterized by distension of the air spaces (groups of alveoli) beyond the bronchioles, with destructive changes in their walls.

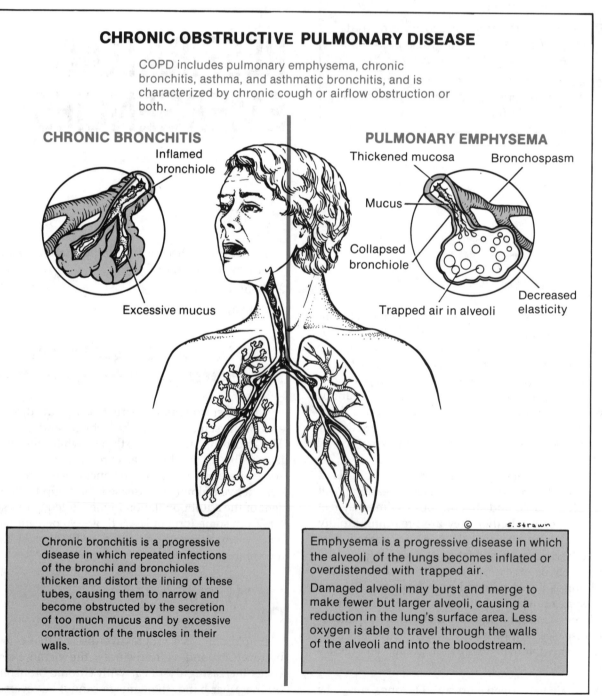

CHRONIC OBSTRUCTIVE PULMONARY DISEASE

COPD includes pulmonary emphysema, chronic bronchitis, asthma, and asthmatic bronchitis, and is characterized by chronic cough or airflow obstruction or both.

CHRONIC BRONCHITIS
Inflamed bronchiole

Excessive mucus

PULMONARY EMPHYSEMA
Thickened mucosa   Bronchospasm

Mucus

Collapsed bronchiole

Trapped air in alveoli   Decreased elasticity

© S. Strawn

Chronic bronchitis is a progressive disease in which repeated infections of the bronchi and bronchioles thicken and distort the lining of these tubes, causing them to narrow and become obstructed by the secretion of too much mucus and by excessive contraction of the muscles in their walls.

Emphysema is a progressive disease in which the alveoli of the lungs becomes inflated or overdistended with trapped air.

Damaged alveoli may burst and merge to make fewer but larger alveoli, causing a reduction in the lung's surface area. Less oxygen is able to travel through the walls of the alveoli and into the bloodstream.

FIGURE 23-1.

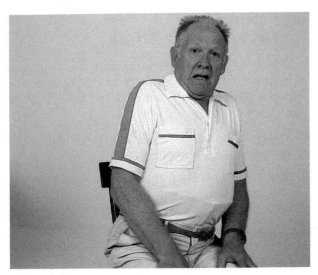

FIGURE 23-2. Victims of emphysema and chronic bronchitis often lean forward in an attempt to breathe.

Basically, the alveoli lose their elasticity, become distended with trapped air, and stop functioning. Air is trapped in the alveoli, causing the small walls to eventually break down. As a result, the total number of alveoli decreases, making it more difficult for the victim to breathe.

The victim with emphysema is often thin, with evidence of weight loss. He generally gives a history of increasing dyspnea on exertion, with progressive limitation of his activity. Coughing may not be a prominent problem; if he does cough, usually only small amounts of mucus are produced. Exhalation is prolonged and difficult, and the victim's lungs remain expanded even after exhalation, causing the chest to appear barrel-shaped. Persons with emphysema are not usually cyanotic, and for this reason they are sometimes referred to as "pink puffers." Respirations are rapid, and the few breath sounds are very distant and difficult to hear. The victim may appear short of breath and may purse his lips during exhalation. As the disease progresses, the victim experiences increasing dyspnea upon exertion.

Chronic Bronchitis

Chronic bronchitis is characterized by inflammation, edema, and excessive mucus production in the bronchial tree. The victim uses his neck and chest muscles to assist his breathing. By definition, chronic bronchitis features a productive cough that has persisted for at least three months out of the year over the past two consecutive years.

The typical victim with chronic bronchitis has almost invariably been a heavy cigarette smoker with many respiratory infections. The bronchitis gets worse with exercise. This victim is usually somewhat short and overweight, with a bluish complexion — features that have given rise to the term "blue bloater" to describe the victim. The victim often has a tendency toward associated heart disease and right heart failure, which causes the cyanosis. The disease also causes peripheral edema and distended neck veins, and most victims experience associated congestive heart failure.

The chronic bronchitic is often coughing, and wheezes can be heard in the chest. High-pitched wheezing occurs during both inhalation and exhalation as the victim struggles to get air in and out of the lungs; low-pitched snoring sounds occur during both inhalation and exhalation as air flows through the narrowed and secretion-choked passageways of the bronchial tree.

Remember that the "pink puffer" and the "blue bloater" represent two extremes of a whole spectrum of problems. Most victims fall somewhere in between the two extremes, manifesting signs and symptoms of both.

Emergency Care

The number-one goal of COPD emergency care is to enhance oxygenation; without it, the victim may die. The major threat to life in COPD is a lack of oxygen. To care for the COPD victim, do the following:

1. Establish an airway.
2. The victim will probably be most comfortable in a sitting or semi-sitting position.
3. If the victim is unconscious, administer artificial ventilation if necessary.
4. Monitor the victim's respiratory rate and depth, and assist ventilations if respiration becomes depressed. *Watch the victim closely for changes in rate and depth.*
5. Maintain the victim's body temperature.
6. Encourage the victim to cough up his secretions.
7. Loosen any restrictive clothing as you comfort and reassure the victim.
8. Activate the EMS system as soon as possible.

ASTHMA

Bronchial asthma is characterized by an increased sensitivity of the trachea, bronchi, and bronchioles to various stimuli, with widespread reversible narrowing of the airways (bronchospasm). There are generally two different degrees of asthma: acute or chronic asthma, with periodic attacks and symptomatic periods between attacks; and status asthmaticus, with a prolonged and life-threatening attack.

There are also generally two different kinds of asthma. Extrinsic asthma, or "allergic" asthma, is usually a reaction to dust, pollen, or other irritants in the atmosphere; it is often seasonal, occurs most often in children, and often clears up after adolescence. Intrinsic, or "nonallergic," asthma is most common in adults and is not due to allergic reaction, but often to infection. It is not seasonal, and is often chronic. Most often, it is caused by emotion, inhaled fumes, viral infections, aspirin, cold air, or some other irritant.

Asthma afflicts approximately 3 percent of the general population, or about 10 million Americans; about 6,000 die from asthma each year. It is most common among children and middle-aged women. Often, the disease is present in more than one member of the same family, and it tends to run in families.

The acute asthmatic attack varies in duration, intensity, and frequency. It reflects airway obstruction due to:

- Bronchospasm (generalized spasm of the bronchi).
- Swelling of the mucous membranes in the bronchial walls.
- Plugging of the bronchi by thick mucus secretions.

The typical acute attack, usually accompanied by a recent respiratory infection, may feature the following signs and symptoms:

- Victim sits upright, often leaning forward, fighting to breathe.
- Spasmodic, unproductive cough (the cough may actually be productive, but because of bronchospasm, the sputum or mucus stays trapped in the bronchial tree, making the cough appear to be unproductive).
- Whistling, high-pitched wheezing, usually audible during exhalation; may also be present on inhalation.
- Very little movement of air during breathing.
- Hyperinflated chest with air trapped in the lungs because of increased obstruction during exhalation.
- Rapid, shallow respirations.
- Rapid pulse (usually exceeding 120 beats per minute).
- Fatigue.

Emergency Care for Acute Asthma Attack

The three goals of emergency care for asthma are to improve oxygenation, relieve bronchospasm, and improve the victim's ventilation. Follow these guidelines:

1. Establish an airway and assist ventilations if necessary.
2. Stay calm, and keep the victim as calm as possible; stress and emotional intensity worsen the asthma. Keep the victim in a position of comfort.
3. If you do not anticipate aspiration, give the victim as much fluid by mouth as he will tolerate; fluids help loosen secretions. *Follow local protocol.*
4. Activate the EMS system.

STATUS ASTHMATICUS

Status asthmaticus is a severe, prolonged asthmatic attack that represents a *dire medical emergency.* Signs and symptoms of status asthmaticus may include the following (Figure 23-3):

- Severe inflation of the chest.
- Extremely labored breathing, with the victim fighting to move air and using accessory muscles of respiration.
- Inaudible breath sounds and wheezes due to negligible movement of air.
- Exhaustion.
- Dehydration.

Do not be fooled by a victim who seems to be suffering from status asthmaticus but who then seems to begin to recover. *He could still be in grave danger.*

To care for status asthmaticus, follow the same general guidelines as with acute asthma, but increase your urgency in establishing care and activating the EMS system. Be sure to maintain a calm, reassuring attitude.

PNEUMONIA

Pneumonia is the medical term used to describe a group of illnesses that are characterized by lung inflammation and fluid- or pus-filled alveoli, leading to inadequately oxygenated blood. Pneumonia is most frequently caused by a bacterial or viral infection, but it can also be caused by inhaled irritants (such as chemicals or smoke) or aspirated materials (such as vomitus).

STATUS ASTHMATICUS

Status asthmaticus is a severe, prolonged asthmatic attack. The acute asthmatic attack involves airway obstruction due to bronchospasm, swelling of mucous membranes in the bronchial walls, and plugging of bronchi by thick mucous secretions. Allergic reactions, respiratory infection, or emotional stress may bring on an attack.

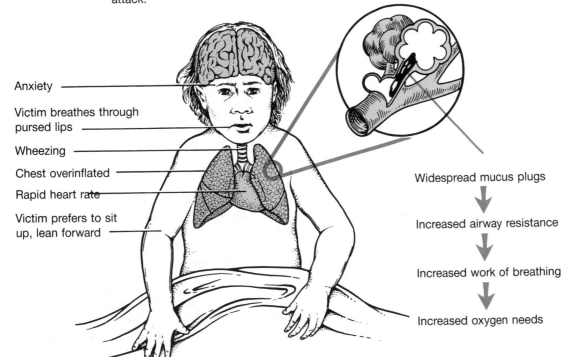

Anxiety

Victim breathes through pursed lips

Wheezing

Chest overinflated

Rapid heart rate

Victim prefers to sit up, lean forward

Widespread mucus plugs

↓

Increased airway resistance

↓

Increased work of breathing

↓

Increased oxygen needs

Note: Even in persons known to have asthma, always consider upper airway obstruction, pulmonary embolism, anaphylaxis, bronchial foreign body (unilateral wheezing), and congestive heart failure ("cardiac asthma").

EMERGENCY CARE

First consideration is the immediate management of shock.

Ventilation: Take appropriate measures to insure breathing. Clear the airway, assist respiration.

Position: Put victim in semi-sitting position or position that helps victim breathe easiest.

Transport: Activate the EMS system immediately while continually monitoring vital signs.

FIGURE 23-3.

SIGNS AND SYMPTOMS

Look for the following signs and symptoms:

- Lung inflammation and obstruction:
  - Chest pain, usually made worse when breathing.
  - Dyspnea.
  - Rapid respiration.
  - Respiratory distress.
  - Productive cough with purulent sputum or mucus.
- Systemic response to infection:
  - Fever (usually exceeding 101 degrees F.).
  - Chills.
  - Hot, dry skin.

EMERGENCY CARE

1. Position the victim so that he is comfortable and can breathe with the least amount of distress; most victims will prefer to sit upright or in a semi-sitting position.
2. Maintain an open airway.
3. Administer plenty of fluids if there are no contraindications; fluids loosen mucus and help prevent dehydration that follows prolonged hyperventilation.
4. Transport the victim to a physician.

HYPERVENTILATION

Hyperventilation syndrome is a collection of signs and symptoms that occur when a victim "over-breathes" or breathes too rapidly. Hyperventilation syndrome is characterized by rapid, deep, or abnormal breathing. The causes of hyperventilation syndrome are varied but usually involve psychological stress. It typically occurs in young, anxious victims, most of whom are unaware that they are breathing abnormally. Hyperventilation may also have a medical origin, such as aspirin overdose. Not everyone who is breathing rapidly or deeply is hyperventilating.

SIGNS AND SYMPTOMS

Whatever the cause, overbreathing can lower the arterial carbon dioxide to an abnormal level, causing the following signs and symptoms:

- Marked anxiety, escalating to panic.

- Dyspnea.
- Dizziness or lightheadedness.
- Blurring of vision.
- Dryness or bitterness of the mouth.
- Numbness and/or tingling of the hands and feet or the area around the mouth.
- Tightness or a "lump" in the throat.
- Pounding of the heart with stabbing pains in the chest.
- A feeling of great tiredness or weakness.
- A feeling of being in a dream.
- A feeling of impending doom.
- Fainting.
- Deep, sighing, rapid respirations with rapid pulse.

EMERGENCY CARE

Prior to beginning emergency care, rule out any organic causes for rapid breathing, such as diabetic coma, trauma, or asthma. If you are certain that none of these life-threatening conditions exist, follow these guidelines:

1. Remain calm and reassuring; listen carefully, show understanding consideration, and try to help the victim calm down.
2. Try to talk the victim into slowing the respiratory rate.
3. Explain to the victim what happened.
4. Transport the victim to an emergency room, or activate the EMS system.

DIZZY, LIGHTHEADED? DON'T BREATHE INTO A BAG

If you feel dizzy, lightheaded, and anxious, you could be having an anxiety attack. But it could also be a heart attack, breathing difficulty, or another health problem. And if you're advised to breathe into a paper bag — a popular remedy for anxiety-related "hyperventilation" (breathing so fast that the carbon dioxide level in your blood falls too low) — *don't do it*, this report warns. Tests on normal healthy people showed that bag rebreathing rarely restores blood gas balance, but often causes dangerous stress to the heart and respiratory system. Because paper bag rebreathing isn't the harmless therapy people had thought, this report says it shouldn't be used without close medical supervision.

(M. Callaham, Annals of Emergency Medicine 18:622, June 1989) As reported in Medical Abstracts Newsletter Volume 9, Number 7.

| 23 | **SELF-TEST** | 23 |

Student: _____ Date: _____

Course: _____ Section #: _____

PART I: True/False   If you believe that the statement is true, circle the T. If you believe that the statement is false, circle the F.

T   F   1. Dyspnea is not a disease itself but is a symptom of a number of other diseases.

T   F   2. Dyspnea is a feeling of air hunger accompanied by labored breathing.

T   F   3. Dyspnea can be a gradual process, or it may occur suddenly.

T   F   4. Twenty percent of the adult U.S. population suffers from some form of chronic obstructive pulmonary disease.

T   F   5. Victims with emphysema are usually cyanotic.

T   F   6. The victim with emphysema usually appears thin and wasted with a barrel-shaped chest.

T   F   7. The chronic-bronchitis-victim uses his neck and chest muscles to assist his breathing.

T   F   8. The signs and symptoms of emphysema and chronic bronchitis often include gasping for air, distended neck veins, leaning forward in an attempt to breathe, and cyanosis.

T   F   9. The number-one goal of COPD emergency care is to enhance oxygenation.

T   F   10. Extrinsic or "allergic" asthma is most often in adults and caused by infection.

T   F   11. Never give asthma victims fluids by mouth.

T   F   12. Status asthmaticus victims should be put in a supine position.

T   F   13. The most common obstructive airway diseases are emphysema, chronic bronchitis and asthma.

T   F   14. Emphysema is a chronic disease that cannot be reversed.

T   F   15. Emphysema and chronic bronchitis are much more common among women.

T   F   16. The number one goal of COPD emergency care is to treat for shock.

T   F   17. One of the three main goals of emergency care for asthma is to treat for shock.

T   F   18. Have a hyperventilation victim breathe into a paper bag.

T   F   19. A typical asthma attack victim will be lying on his side with his legs drawn up in the fetal position.

T   F   20. The major threat to life in a COPD victim is a lack of oxygen.

T   F   21. Dyspnea is defined as a shortness of breath.

T   F   22. About 6,000 people die from asthma each year.

PART II: Multiple Choice   For each question, circle the answer that best reflects an accurate statement.

1. Dyspnea means:
    a. painful, labored breathing.
    b. excess sputum production.
    c. shortness of breath.
    d. fatigue.

2. Which of the following is *not* considered a category of COPD?
    a. emphysema.
    b. asthma.
    c. chronic bronchitis.
    d. atherosclerosis.

3. Status asthmaticus is: (1) a true emergency requiring measures to maintain respirations; (2) a severe, prolonged asthmatic attack; (3) best cared for with the victim in the coma position; (4) is often caused by allergic reaction, respiratory infection, or emotional stress; (5) when the airway becomes obstructed by swelling or mucus.
    a. 1, 2, 4, and 5.
    b. 1, 2, 3, 4, and 5.
    c. 1, 2, and 5.
    d. 1, 2, 3, and 5.

4. Initial care for a person who is hyperventilating includes:
    a. establishing an airway.
    b. encouraging the victim to take rapid shallow breaths.
    c. loosening tight clothing.
    d. showing calmness and reassurance.

5. Anxiety hyperventilation may be treated by:
    a. having the victim breathe at a slower rate.
    b. encouraging the victim to walk rapidly.
    c. having the victim breathe into a plastic bag.
    d. all of these answers.

6. In status asthmaticus:
    a. the victim is not in much danger.
    b. the chest is sunken.
    c. wheezing is very audible.
    d. the victim uses accessory muscles of respiration.

7. Which of the following statements about dyspnea is *not* true?

   a. dyspnea is often caused by chronic lung disease.
   b. dyspnea is a progressive disease.
   c. dyspnea is often caused by chronic heart disease.
   d. dyspnea is often associated with edema in the legs.

8. Which of the following is *not* a symptom of hyperventilation?

   a. slow heart rate.
   b. fainting.
   c. tingling in the hands or feet.
   d. a feeling of weakness.

9. A "pink puffer" has:

   a. emphysema.
   b. congestive heart failure.
   c. diabetes.
   d. chronic bronchitis.

10. Emergency care for COPD victims is aimed primarily at:

    a. causing expectoration of sputum.
    b. enhancing oxygenation.
    c. humidifying the air.
    d. transporting as soon as possible.

11. Victims with chronic obstructive pulmonary disease (COPD) are prone to episodes of:

    a. severe difficulty in breathing.
    b. hyperglycemia.
    c. angina pectoris.
    d. all of these answers.

12. The terms "pink puffers" and "blue bloaters" are used to describe:

    a. newborn victims who are having respiratory difficulties.
    b. victims with heart disease.
    c. victims with chronic obstructive pulmonary disease.
    d. all of these answers.

PART III: Matching: Match the definitions on the right with the correct term on the left.

_____1. Dyspnea

_____2. COPD

_____3. Emphysema

_____4. Chronic bronchitis

_____5. Asthma

_____6. Status asthmaticus

_____7. Pneumonia

_____8. Hyperventilation

A. Pink puffers.

B. Represents a dire medical emergency.

C. Sensation of shortness of breath.

D. Most frequently caused by a bacterial or viral infection.

E. Rapid, deep, abnormal breathing.

F. Characterized by chronic cough, airflow obstruction, or both.

G. Usually brought on by an allergic reaction, respiratory infection, or emotional stress.

H. Blue bloater.

PART IV: What Would You Do If:

1. You are at the home of a middle-aged man and find him sitting on the edge of his bed, gasping for air. He has distended neck veins and audible wheezes and is cyanotic.

2. You are at a college dormitory where you find a woman having an asthma attack. She is fighting to breathe and has audible wheezes. The attack has been severe and prolonged, and the victim is exhausted.

PART V: Practical Skills Check-Off   _____ has satisfactorily passed the following practical skills:
                                          Student's Name

	Date	Partner Check	Inst. Init.
1. Describe and demonstrate how to give emergency care for a victim of chronic bronchitis and emphysema.	__/__/__	☐	_____
2. Describe and demonstrate how to give emergency care for a victim of hyperventilation.	__/__/__	☐	_____

DIABETIC EMERGENCIES

Conservatively estimated, there are more than six million diabetics in the United States. Probably another five million have diabetes but without obvious signs and symptoms; therefore, these victims are completely unaware of their disease. Unfortunately, the first indication of the disease may be a life-threatening medical emergency (such as diabetic coma), and you may not know that diabetes is the cause.

There are two basic types of diabetes: Type I (insulin-dependent, but historically called juvenile diabetes) tends to begin in childhood when a person has little or no ability to produce insulin. Such an individual requires regular insulin injections to maintain body function. Type II (noninsulin-dependent but historically referred to as adult-onset diabetes) tends to develop in adulthood when a person may produce enough insulin but may not be able to utilize it. This type of diabetes is usually controlled by diet and/or oral medication.

CAUSES OF DIABETES

Diabetes seems to be caused by a problem (resulting from injury, infection, or genetic defects) in the tiny **ISLETS OF LANGERHANS**, the area of the pancreas where insulin is formed. **INSULIN** is a hormone needed by the body to facilitate the movement of glucose (sugar) out of the bloodstream, across the cell membrane, and into the cell. Without glucose, the cells are not able to meet their energy needs. Therefore, when insulin is insufficient or absent, as in the case of the diabetic, the blood glucose level increases because it accumulates in the bloodstream (insulin does not move it into the body cells). This causes a paradoxical situation: the diabetic has an extremely elevated blood glucose level but a severely depleted supply of glucose in the cells due to the absence of insulin. All organ systems are affected.

Insulin also prevents amino acids from being used as fuel. Therefore, when insulin levels are too low, proteins are used as fuel, eventually robbing the muscles and vital organs of their mass.

When glucose cannot be used, it builds up in the blood, causing **HYPERGLYCEMIA**, a significant sign of diabetes. The kidneys, whose function is to filter out excesses from the bloodstream and discard them, start spilling sugar into the urine. A large amount of sugar in the urine causes the kidneys to eliminate considerable water simply to wash the sugar away — a condition that leads to **POLYURIA** (frequent passing of large amounts of urine). This combination leads both to the tremendous thirst that affects hyperglycemic diabetics and to the danger of dehydration (Figure 24-1).

Diabetics may lose from 500 to 2,000 calories a day through glucose elimination in the urine, which is why the advanced diabetic is extremely hungry, tends to eat all the time to satisfy his hunger, and still loses weight. The caloric loss also contributes to serious fatigue.

Diabetics face a grave physical situation when their blood glucose level is too high or too low: either condition (hyperglycemia or hypoglycemia) can cause coma, and both can be life-threatening if not treated promptly.

If you encounter a person who is unconscious, look for signs of diabetes: a medical alert tag, bracelet, or card; signs of insulin injection (needle marks in the thigh or abdomen); signs of oral diabetic medication (bottles in the house); signs of poor circulation or amputation of the toes, feet, or lower leg; or other telltale signs of diabetes.

DIABETIC COMA (KETOACIDOSIS AND HYPERGLYCEMIA)

Diabetics who go untreated, who fail to take their prescribed insulin, or who undergo some kind of stress (such as infection) may become comatose with a condition referred to as **DIABETIC COMA** (**KETOACIDOSIS** or **DIABETIC ACIDOSIS**). Diabetic coma, the most frequent cause of hospitalization in diabetics under the age of thirty, is basically a condition of too little insulin and too much blood sugar — in other words, there is not enough insulin to cover the food intake.

Direct causes of imbalance that results in diabetic coma include:

■ Infection — the most common cause of diabetic coma is several days of nonacute, self-limiting infection, such as a viral respiratory infection.

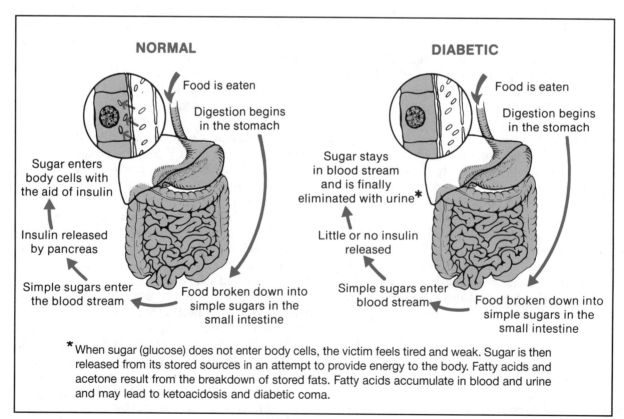

NORMAL

Food is eaten

Digestion begins in the stomach

Sugar enters body cells with the aid of insulin

Insulin released by pancreas

Simple sugars enter the blood stream

Food broken down into simple sugars in the small intestine

DIABETIC

Food is eaten

Digestion begins in the stomach

Sugar stays in blood stream and is finally eliminated with urine*

Little or no insulin released

Simple sugars enter blood stream

Food broken down into simple sugars in the small intestine

*When sugar (glucose) does not enter body cells, the victim feels tired and weak. Sugar is then released from its stored sources in an attempt to provide energy to the body. Fatty acids and acetone result from the breakdown of stored fats. Fatty acids accumulate in blood and urine and may lead to ketoacidosis and diabetic coma.

FIGURE 24-1. Normal versus diabetic use of sugars.

- Failure of the victim to take prescribed insulin, or taking an insufficient amount of insulin.
- Eating too much food that contains or produces sugar.
- Stresses (such as heart attack).

SIGNS AND SYMPTOMS OF DIABETIC COMA

Signs and symptoms of diabetic coma include the following (Figure 24-2):

- Acidosis:
  - Labored respirations and exaggerated air hunger.
  - Sweet or fruity (acetonic) odor on breath.
  - Frequent severe and intense abdominal pain.
  - Varying degrees of responsiveness, from restlessness to complete coma; decreasing levels of consciousness correspond to the degree of dehydration; confusion and disorientation are common.
- Dehydration:
  - Flushed, dry, warm skin.
  - Sunken eyes.
  - Rapid, weak pulse.
  - Intense thirst.
  - Lack of normal skin tone (pinched skin does not return to normal).
  - Anorexia.

- Frequent urination at first; scanty or no urine as dehydration progresses.
  - Dizziness.
  - Irritability.
- Hyperglycemia:
  - Weakness.
  - Weight loss.
  - Fatigue.
- Other symptoms:
  - Abdominal pain, nausea, and vomiting (common).
  - Fever (may occur simultaneously with coma).

The onset of diabetic coma is gradual, developing in most cases over a period of twelve to forty-eight hours. The victim appears extremely ill and becomes sicker and weaker as the condition progresses. If untreated, the victim dies; with treatment, improvement is gradual, occurring six to twelve hours after insulin is administered and metabolic acidosis is treated.

EMERGENCY CARE

To care for diabetic coma, do the following (Figure 24-3):

1. Monitor vital signs carefully every few minutes; rule out heart attack, stroke, or other cardiac emergencies as the cause of the coma.

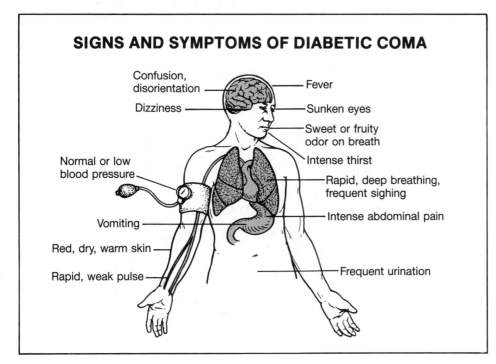

SIGNS AND SYMPTOMS OF DIABETIC COMA

Confusion, disorientation — Fever

Dizziness — Sunken eyes

Sweet or fruity odor on breath

Intense thirst

Normal or low blood pressure

Rapid, deep breathing, frequent sighing

Vomiting

Intense abdominal pain

Red, dry, warm skin

Rapid, weak pulse

Frequent urination

FIGURE 24-2.

Diabetes is a condition in which the body is unable to use sugar normally.
Body cells need sugar to survive.
Insulin in the body permits sugar to pass from the blood stream to body cells.
If there is not enough insulin, sugar will be unable to get to body cells and they
    will starve.
If there is too much insulin, there will be insufficient sugar in the blood stream
    and brain cells will be damaged since they need a constant supply of sugar.

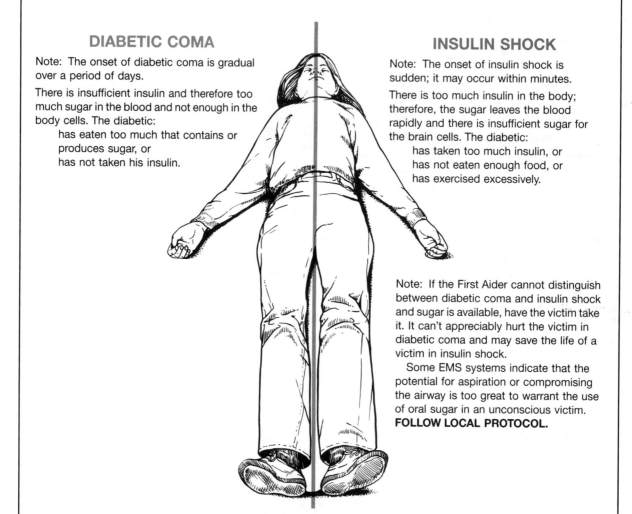

DIABETIC COMA

Note: The onset of diabetic coma is gradual over a period of days.

There is insufficient insulin and therefore too much sugar in the blood and not enough in the body cells. The diabetic:
    has eaten too much that contains or produces sugar, or
    has not taken his insulin.

INSULIN SHOCK

Note: The onset of insulin shock is sudden; it may occur within minutes.

There is too much insulin in the body; therefore, the sugar leaves the blood rapidly and there is insufficient sugar for the brain cells. The diabetic:
    has taken too much insulin, or
    has not eaten enough food, or
    has exercised excessively.

Note: If the First Aider cannot distinguish between diabetic coma and insulin shock and sugar is available, have the victim take it. It can't appreciably hurt the victim in diabetic coma and may save the life of a victim in insulin shock.

Some EMS systems indicate that the potential for aspiration or compromising the airway is too great to warrant the use of oral sugar in an unconscious victim. **FOLLOW LOCAL PROTOCOL.**

EMERGENCY CARE

Activate the EMS system. This victim needs immediate transportation to a medical facility.
Monitor vital signs.
Follow procedures for any comatose victim regarding airway maintenance and artificial ventilation.
Keep victim lying flat with head and shoulders slightly elevated.
If vomiting occurs, put in coma position with head turned to aid draining and prevent aspiration.

This victim desperately needs sugar before brain damage and death occur. Rubbing sugar on the tongue of an unconscious victim should arouse him (use only what the tongue can absorb). Sugar in any form can be given to a conscious victim. He needs immediate transportation to a medical facility. Activate the EMS system.

FIGURE 24-3.

2. Check for signs of head or neck injury. If they are present, care for as indicated.

3. Follow the procedure for any comatose victim with regard to airway maintenance and artificial ventilation. Give CPR support if needed. Be alert for vomiting, and be ready at all times to position the victim on his side with his head turned down to prevent aspiration and allow drainage.

4. Treat the victim for shock. Keep the victim lying down flat or with his head and shoulders elevated slightly unless he is in shock. Make sure that he stays warm. If he is conscious, administer fluids orally (except those that contain sugars or starch). *Follow local protocol.*

5. Activate the EMS system as soon as possible.

6. Continue careful monitoring of vital signs.

7. If you can find them quickly, send any pre-measured insulin vials or bottles with the victim to the hospital; they will help emergency-room personnel determine what kind of treatment is needed.

INSULIN SHOCK (HYPOGLYCEMIA)

Insulin shock occurs when a diabetic has had too much insulin or too little sugar. Insulin shock results from treatment for diabetes, not from the diabetes itself. The glucose moves out of the bloodstream and into the cells more rapidly than it is produced, resulting in an insufficient blood-sugar level to maintain normal brain function. Nerve cells are deprived of glucose, and they die. Because the brain is as dependent on glucose as it is on oxygen, and because the brain is the first organ to react to low blood sugar, permanent brain damage or death can result from insulin shock if emergency care is not given immediately (see Figure 24-4).

Insulin shock has a rapid onset, and it happens more often in children because of their broadly varied activity and diet levels. Insulin shock can be caused by several different factors:

- The diabetic skips a meal but takes the usual amount of insulin.
- The diabetic vomits a meal after taking insulin.
- The victim takes more than the prescribed dosage of insulin, or his normal dosage is accidentally administered in a vein.
- The victim exercises strenuously or excessively.
- The victim is subject to severe emotional excitement or exertion.
- The victim is exposed to severe cold.
- The victim's insulin dosage or diet has been changed, and he does not adapt well to the changes.

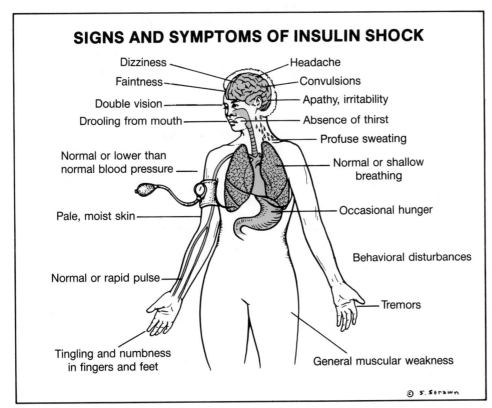

FIGURE 24-4.

Reactions begin five to twenty minutes after the injection of too much insulin, or several hours after other forms of oral medication are taken. The victim appears extremely weak. Insulin shock develops suddenly and progresses rapidly, usually over a period of just a few minutes. *It is a dire medical emergency* that can cause death within a few minutes.

SIGNS AND SYMPTOMS

The signs and symptoms of insulin shock often mimic those of stroke or alcohol or drug intoxication. The most common include (Figure 24-4):

- Headache.
- Extreme muscle weakness and incoordination.
- Hunger.
- Normal or shallow breathing.
- Weakness or paralysis of one side of the body.
- Shakiness (sometimes involving the entire body).
- Normal blood pressure or low blood pressure.
- Normal or rapid pulse; may be full and bounding.
- Double vision and other visual disturbances.
- Apathy, anxiety, combativeness, or irritability.
- Confusion leading to disorientation, eventual unconsciousness, and coma.
- Absence of thirst.
- Profuse drooling from the mouth.
- Tremors.
- Convulsions in late stages.
- Tingling and numbness in the extremities, mostly the fingers and feet.
- Dizziness.
- Diminished levels of consciousness, including fainting.
- Profuse sweating.
- Speech difficulties.
- Disturbances in behavior (the victim may appear to be drunk, hostile, or belligerent).

If you suspect that the victim might be entering a state of insulin shock, ask him two critical questions:

1. Have you eaten today?
2. Have you taken your insulin today?

If the person has taken his insulin but has not eaten, he may be going into insulin shock. If he has eaten but has not taken his insulin, he may be going into diabetic coma. Beware, however, that these guidelines do not always apply.

EMERGENCY CARE

Emergency care for a victim in suspected insulin shock should be as follows:

1. If the victim is conscious, give him orange juice with one to two teaspoons of sugar, soft drinks that contain sugar, sugar cubes, or candy to help increase his blood sugar level.

2. If the victim is unconscious, establish an airway and administer artificial ventilation if necessary. Sprinkle a few grains of granulated sugar underneath the victim's tongue and monitor closely. *Follow local protocol.*

3. If available, place instant glucose between the victim's cheek and gums or under his tongue; place him on his side with his head pointed down to prevent aspiration, and monitor his airway carefully and continuously. He should regain consciousness fairly rapidly, usually within twenty minutes. *Follow local protocol*; this is controversial in some areas.

4. Never give an unconscious person anything to drink.

5. Watch for complications, such as shock or convulsions, and care for appropriately.

6. Activate the EMS system immediately, even if the victim seems to be completely recovered.

Improvement is usually fairly rapid following the administration of sugar, but it is still important to transport the victim to a physician. Do not worry about the amount of sugar given to the victim, as the physician will balance the need for sugar against insulin production when the victim arrives at the hospital.

It is important to note that diabetics are not the only victims who are prone to hypoglycemia. Alcoholics, victims who have ingested certain poisons, and others may develop the same syndrome. Therefore, do not discount the possibility of hypoglycemia in a comatose victim just because he is not known to be a diabetic.

In summary, there are two general rules to remember about emergency care for diabetics:

1. Any victim in coma of unknown cause should receive sugar.

2. Diabetics have trouble with hyperglycemia and hypoglycemia. *When in doubt, give sugar.* You will *not* harm a hyperglycemic victim by giving sugar (the amount administered is trivial compared to what he already has in his blood), but *you may save the life of a hypoglycemic* victim in insulin shock by this emergency care.

| **24** | **SELF-TEST** | **24** |

Student: _____ Date: _____

Course: _____ Section #: _____

PART I: True/False   If you believe that the statement is true, circle the T. If you believe that the statement is false, circle the F.

T   F   1. There are two basic types of diabetes: insulin-dependent and insulin-independent.

T   F   2. Diabetes seems to be caused by a problem in the Islets of Langerhans.

T   F   3. Diabetic coma is the most frequent cause of hospitalization in diabetics.

T   F   4. Diabetic coma is a condition of too little insulin and too much blood sugar in the body.

T   F   5. The most common cause of diabetic coma is stress.

T   F   6. The diabetic-coma victim has intense abdominal pain and a rapid, weak pulse.

T   F   7. The victim in insulin shock appears extremely weak and has profuse sweating.

T   F   8. If a diabetic has taken his insulin and has not eaten, he may go into insulin shock.

T   F   9. Improvement of an insulin-shock victim is usually fairly rapid once sugar has been administered.

T   F   10. If in doubt whether a victim is in diabetic coma or insulin shock, give sugar.

PART II: Multiple Choice   For each question, circle the answer that best reflects an accurate statement.

1. A fruity odor on the breath is often a characteristic of:
   a. stroke.
   b. hypoglycemia.
   c. ketoacidosis.
   d. an ulcer.

2. Which of the following statements about diabetes is true?
   a. another term that may describe insulin shock is hypoglycemia.
   b. a diabetic can suffer from too much insulin and from too little insulin.
   c. diabetes renders the body incapable of metabolizing sugar as an energy source because of lack of insulin.
   d. all of these answers.

3. Which symptom is the characteristic clue indicating diabetic coma?
   a. cherry red lips.
   b. moist, clammy skin.
   c. involuntary muscular twitching.
   d. a sickly, sweet breath odor.

4. The onset of diabetic coma generally occurs:
   a. in five to twenty minutes.
   b. in ten to twelve hours.
   c. in one to two hours.
   d. in twelve to forty-eight hours.

5. The major emergency-care procedure for a victim in diabetic coma is:
   a. to administer insulin.
   b. to treat for shock.
   c. to give a glass of orange juice.
   d. to try to keep him awake.

6. Insulin shock onset generally occurs within:
   a. five to twenty minutes after injection of insulin.
   b. ten to twelve hours after injection of insulin.
   c. twenty-four hours after injection of insulin.
   d. forty-eight hours after injection of insulin.

7. A diabetic person is exhibiting the following signs: rapid, weak pulse; cold, clammy skin; and convulsions. What do these signs indicate?
   a. insulin shock.
   b. diabetic coma.
   c. insulin coma.
   d. diabetic shock.

8. If the First Aider can't distinguish between diabetic coma and insulin shock, what should he do?
   a. nothing, the wrong treatment can be deadly.
   b. treat for shock and activate the EMS system.
   c. give a shot of insulin or put an insulin tablet in the mouth.
   d. assist the victim in taking some type of sugar.

9. What is the emergency care for insulin shock if the victim is unconscious?
   a. administer a glass of orange juice.
   b. do nothing; activate the EMS system immediately.
   c. put an insulin tablet in his mouth or give an insulin shot.
   d. put instant glucose between victim's cheek and gums.

10. Which of the following statements about diabetic coma (hyperglycemia) is *not* true?
   a. diabetic coma is the result of insufficient insulin or too much sugar.
   b. diabetic coma occurs gradually over several days.
   c. diabetic coma is generally a less serious condition than insulin shock.
   d. diabetic coma may be brought about by excessive exercise.

11. Which of the following statements about insulin shock (hypoglycemia) is *not* true?

    a. insulin shock may be brought about by eating too much food.

    b. insulin shock should always be treated by giving the victim sugar.

    c. insulin shock may be caused by excessive exercise.

    d. insulin shock always requires immediate transportation to a medical facility.

12. Which of the following is *not* true about diabetic coma and insulin shock?

    a. the skin is usually red, dry, and warm in diabetic coma; it is usually pale and moist in insulin shock.

    b. the victim is usually intensely thirsty in diabetic coma; insulin shock generally produces an absence of thirst.

    c. rapid, deep breathing and frequent sighing in both diabetic coma and insulin shock.

    d. the pulse may be rapid in either condition.

13. Insulin:

    a. absorbs excess sugar that has been consumed.

    b. converts sugar into glucose in the digestive tract.

    c. permits sugar to pass from the blood into body cells.

    d. all of these answers.

14. An excess of insulin, which may result when a diabetic victim has taken too much insulin, has not eaten, or has over-exercised, is called:

    a. diabetic coma.

    b. diabetic shock.

    c. insulin coma.

    d. insulin shock.

15. A diabetic person is exhibiting the following signs: rapid, weak pulse; cold, clammy skin; and convulsions. What do these signs indicate?

    a. insulin shock.

    b. diabetic coma.

    c. insulin coma.

    d. diabetic shock.

PART III: Matching: Match the correct condition on the right with the description on the left.

Description

_____ 1. Diabetic acidosis.

_____ 2. Too little insulin and too much blood sugar.

_____ 3. A dire medical emergency.

_____ 4. Hunger, headache, and muscular weakness.

_____ 5. Gradual onset.

_____ 6. Diabetic exercises excessively.

_____ 7. Hyperglycemia.

_____ 8. Rapid onset.

_____ 9. Eating too much food that contains sugar.

_____10. Pale, moist skin.

_____11. Labored respirations and acetonic breath odor.

_____12. Victim needs sugar.

_____13. Red, dry, warm skin.

_____14. Hypoglycemia.

_____15. Happens more often in children.

Condition

A. Diabetic coma

B. Insulin shock

PART IV: What Would You Do If:

1. A neighbor frantically calls for help. You respond and find a middle-aged woman unconscious on her bedroom floor. Her husband tells you that she hasn't been very responsive since the previous day and that she complained of abdominal pain. You find her to have flushed, warm, dry skin, acetone breath odor, and a rapid, weak pulse.

2. You respond to a call of a neighbor and find a twelve-year-old child who appears extremely weak. Her skin is pale and moist, she feels faint, has a headache, and is having trouble focusing her eyes. The only other person at home is her brother, who tells you that several hours ago his sister was fine — she had been involved in some foot races and had not eaten yet that day.

PART V: Practical Skills Check-Off _____ has satisfactorily passed the following practical skills:

                                     Student's Name

	Date	Partner Check	Inst. Init.
1. Describe and demonstrate how to give emergency care for diabetic coma and insulin shock.	__/__/__	☐	_____

CHAPTER TWENTY-FIVE

OBJECTIVES

- Learn the common causes of acute abdominal distress and other related gastrointestinal emergencies.
- Identify the signs and symptoms of acute abdominal distress and ruptured esophageal varices.
- Explain special assessment procedures for victims with acute abdominal distress.
- Describe and demonstrate appropriate emergency care for:
  - acute abdominal distress
  - ruptured esophageal varices
  - prolonged vomiting.

ACUTE ABDOMINAL DISTRESS AND RELATED EMERGENCIES

Acute abdominal distress features pain that may stem from the cardiac, gastrointestinal, genitourinary, reproductive, or other systems — or pain that may be referred from elsewhere. The pain due to trauma usually is very localized, and the victim should be able to point to it accurately with one or two fingers unless bleeding is heavy, which usually causes diffuse pain. Pain in the abdomen that is due to organ dysfunction, however, is often vague and may be referred; the victim may point to it with an entire fist or even an open hand, vaguely indicating a larger area of the body.

Because pain can be referred to the abdomen from many different parts of the body, it is extremely difficult to make an accurate assessment of abdominal pain. Your should not attempt such an assessment but concentrate on evaluating the victim's condition and providing necessary supportive care. The information on diseases in this section is presented as background information only.

Several true medical emergencies related to abdominal distress are the danger of aspiration during vomiting and of fatal hemorrhage from ruptured **ESOPHAGEAL VARICES**. These require aggressive care to save lives.

CAUSES OF ABDOMINAL PAIN

According to medical reference guides, there are approximately one hundred different causes of abdominal pain. As an extremely simplified guide, the pain itself often provides clues as to the cause:

- Colicky pain (pain that comes in "waves" separated by a pain-free period) often accompanies an obstruction.
- Pain that shifts position may signal **APPENDICITIS**.

- Sudden, severe pain is often caused by a rupture or perforation.
- Pain that radiates is often due to gallbladder disease (including stones), **KIDNEY STONES**, or **PANCREATITIS**.
- Pain that gradually intensifies is often due to an inflammatory condition that worsens with time.

A common cause of lower abdominal pain on the right side is appendicitis, which often begins as a vague pain across the abdomen and gradually shifts to the right side. Other causes would include muscular strain, intestinal obstruction, or hernia. Pain across the entire lower abdomen or especially at the midline may be caused by **COLITIS** or bowel obstruction. When the pain is mild and not associated with diarrhea, it usually is due to intestinal spasms or excessive intestinal gas. Other causes would include a urinary bladder inflammation, pelvic inflammatory disease, **ECTOPIC PREGNANCY**, and menstrual cramps in females.

SIGNS AND SYMPTOMS OF ABDOMINAL DISTRESS

Any severe abdominal pain should be considered an emergency; any abdominal pain that lasts longer than six hours, regardless of its intensity, should be considered an emergency. A victim with an **ACUTE ABDOMEN** appears very ill; general signs and symptoms of acute abdominal distress may include:

- Abdominal pain (local or diffuse).
- Colicky pain (cramplike pain that occurs in waves).
- Local or diffuse abdominal tenderness.
- Anxiety and reluctance to move.
- Rapid, shallow breathing.
- Rapid pulse.
- Nausea and/or vomiting.
- Low blood pressure.
- Tense, often distended abdomen.
- Signs of shock.
- Signs of internal bleeding: vomiting blood (bright red or coffee-grounds) or blood in the stool (bright red or tarry black).

A victim with acute abdominal distress often positions himself on his side with his knees drawn up toward his abdomen (Figure 25-1).

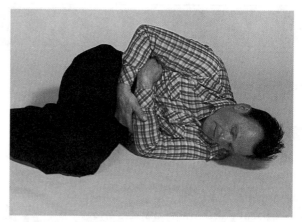

FIGURE 25-1. Typical "guarded" position for victim with acute abdominal distress.

SPECIAL ASSESSMENT PROCEDURES

In assessing a victim with acute abdominal distress, your number-one priority should be to look for signs of shock. Follow these guidelines when assessing this victim:

1. Determine whether the victim is restless or quiet, and whether movement causes pain.
2. See if the abdomen is distended.
3. See if the victim can relax his abdominal wall.
4. Feel the abdomen *very* gently to determine whether it is tense or soft and whether any masses are present (Figure 25-2).
5. Determine whether the abdomen is tender when touched.

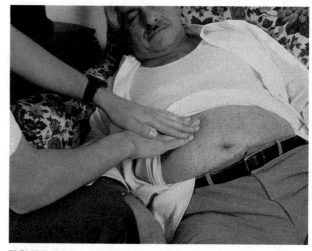

FIGURE 25-2. In the abdominal distress victim, gently determine if the abdomen is tense or soft.

Note: *In a victim with abdominal pain, do not waste time with extensive assessment of the abdomen prior to transporting the victim to a physician or activating the EMS system. Extensive palpation can worsen the pain and aggravate the medical condition that causes it.*

EMERGENCY CARE FOR ACUTE ABDOMINAL DISTRESS

The goals of emergency care for acute abdominal distress are to prevent any possible life-threatening complications (such as shock), to make the victim comfortable, and to arrange transport as quickly as possible for diagnostic care by a physician. Follow these guidelines (Figure 25-3):

1. Keep the airway clear; be alert for vomiting and possible aspiration. If the victim is nauseated, position him on his left side (if it does not cause too much pain) with his head pointed downward to allow drainage if vomiting occurs.

2. Position the victim as comfortably as possible. Allow the victim to determine the most comfortable position unless it interferes with emergency care. Most victims prefer to lie on their side or back with their knees drawn up toward the abdomen.

3. Comfort and reassure the victim (Figure 25-4).

4. *Never give anything by mouth.*

5. Do not give the victim any medications by any route or allow him to take medications himself; medications may mask symptoms and complicate the physician's diagnosis and treatment.

6. Prevent shock; if shock already exists, treat it.

7. Transport the victim to a physician or activate the EMS system as rapidly as possible. Protect the victim from any rough handling.

RUPTURED ESOPHAGEAL VARICES

Esophageal varices — bulging, engorged, and weakened blood vessels lining the wall of the esophagus — can potentially develop in any victim but are most common among heavy alcohol drinkers, victims with liver disease, or victims of **JAUNDICE**. When one or more of these varices rupture, bleeding is profuse and severe and can be fatal within minutes unless the victim has prompt care.

SIGNS AND SYMPTOMS

Look for the following signs and symptoms of esophageal varices:

▪ Vomiting of profuse amounts of bright red blood.

▪ Blood welling up on the back of the throat, with or without vomiting.

▪ Absence of pain or tenderness in the stomach.

▪ Rapid pulse (usually exceeding 120 beats per minute).

▪ Respiratory distress.

▪ Pallor.

EMERGENCY CARE

The victim of ruptured esophageal varices needs rapid blood replacement and surgical procedures aimed at stopping the bleeding. Your first aid priorities are to secure and maintain the airway, prevent aspiration, treat or prevent shock, and activate the EMS system without delay. Follow these guidelines:

1. Immediately secure an open airway.

2. Position the victim on his side with his face pointed downward to allow drainage of blood and saliva. Maintaining a clear airway is critical to the victim's survival.

3. Treat the victim for shock.

4. Activate the EMS system immediately.

Note: *A number of other medical conditions can cause vomiting of blood; gastritis and stomach ulcers are two of the most common. However, while the blood vomited with esophageal varices is dark red in color, the blood vomited from other conditions tends to be the color and consistency of coffee grounds. While these victims need help in maintaining a clear airway and transport for further treatment, their condition is not as rapidly fatal as that of ruptured esophageal varices.*

VOMITING

Vomiting — the stomach's response to an infection, irritation, obstruction, or other disease process — is one of the most common gastrointestinal complaints or emergencies. Most vomiting is caused by self-limiting infection and clears up within a day or two. Vomiting becomes a medical emergency when it is prolonged enough to cause dehydration, when it is aspirated, or when it signals serious medical conditions.

SIGNS & SYMPTOMS

- Abdominal pain, local or diffuse (widespread).
- Abdominal tenderness, local or diffuse.
- Victim is quite anxious, and reluctant to move.
- Rapid, shallow breathing.
- Rapid pulse.
- Nausea and/or vomiting.
- Low blood pressure.
- Victim's position is often lying on one side with legs drawn up to the abdomen.
- When peritonitis is accompanied by hemorrhage, shock may result.
- Bleeding from gastrointestinal tract (from mouth or rectum). Blood in urine. Nonmenstrual vaginal blood.

SPECIAL EXAMINATION PROCEDURES

- Determine whether the victim is restless or quiet and whether movement causes pain.
- Feel abdomen gently to see if it is tense or soft.
- Determine whether the victim can relax the abdominal wall on request.
- Determine whether the abdomen is tender when touched.

EMERGENCY CARE

- The victim needs speedy transportation to a medical facility.
- Keep airway clear and be alert for possible vomiting and subsequent aspiration.
- Comfort and reassure the victim.
- Position the victim comfortably. Allow the victim to determine the most comfortable position unless it interferes with emergency care.
- Record signs and symptoms and victim's account of condition (i.e., time of onset, direction of and characteristics of pain)
- Prevent shock.

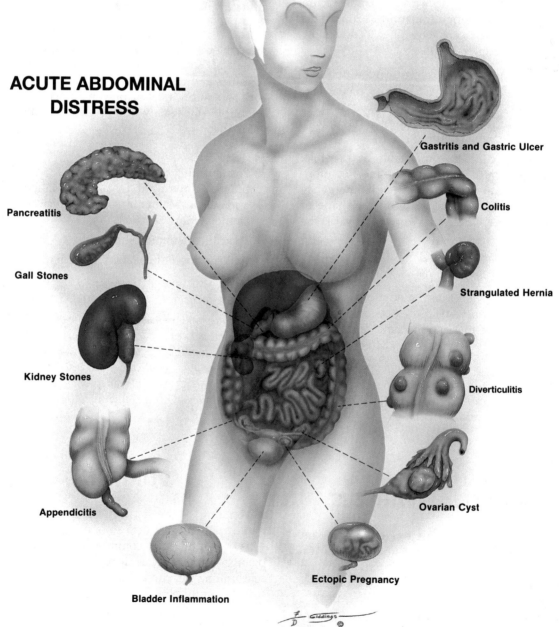

ACUTE ABDOMINAL DISTRESS

Gastritis and Gastric Ulcer

Colitis

Pancreatitis

Gall Stones

Strangulated Hernia

Kidney Stones

Diverticulitis

Appendicitis

Ovarian Cyst

Ectopic Pregnancy

Bladder Inflammation

FIGURE 25-3.

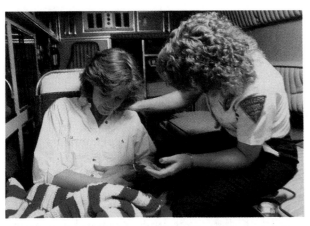

FIGURE 25-4. Reassure and monitor the abdominal-distress victim while waiting for emergency personnel to arrive.

Among the most common of the many causes of vomiting are:

- A viral or bacterial infection involving the stomach or intestinal tract.
- Swallowed foreign objects that obstruct the gastrointestinal tract.
- Peritonitis (severe inflammation of the peritoneal lining).
- Bacteria-contaminated food, creating food poisoning.
- Ingestion of irritants, such as alcohol, certain drugs (such as aspirin), and certain foods.
- Inflammation of the stomach lining (generally caused by too much aspirin, too much alcohol, infection, or stomach ulcer).
- Any disease condition that interferes with the digestive tract's peristaltic contractions (the involuntary, rhythmic contractions or smooth muscle that propel the contents of the gastrointestinal tract along).
- Tumors that obstruct the gastrointestinal tract.
- Forceful vomiting in infants that results when the outlet of the stomach is obstructed or does not function properly.
- Severe fright or intense emotional upset.

Medical emergencies can result when vomiting is prolonged enough to cause substantial fluid loss and **ELECTROLYTE** imbalance (a condition that can develop as rapidly as within twenty-four hours in infants and young children or the elderly). Infants or children who continue to vomit over a period of one day and adults who continue to vomit for several days may lose significant fluid volume and develop electrolyte imbalances serious enough to cause shock.

Another problem occurs when a sleepy, stuporous, semiconscious, unconscious, or comatose victim vomits: the normal gag reflex is depressed or absent, and the victim may aspirate vomitus into the lungs. Because the cough reflex is usually also absent or depressed, the victim does not cough to clear the lungs of the aspirated material. The gastric juices contained in vomitus literally eat away the delicate lung tissue, resulting in rapid tissue destruction, massive infection, and life-threatening pulmonary abscesses.

EMERGENCY CARE

If a victim has vomited enough to cause shock or is in such a condition as to be at high risk of aspiration, follow these guidelines:

1. Take immediate measures to secure an open airway and to maintain it. Place the victim on his left side, his head lower than his feet, and point his head downward to facilitate drainage should vomiting occur.
2. Use the jaw-thrust technique to help keep the airway clear.
3. If the victim has aspirated vomitus, he probably will be breathing rapidly, secreting excessive saliva, and be cyanotic. Assist breathing if necessary. Activate the EMS system immediately. Surgical removal of the aspirated material within thirty to sixty minutes can usually save the victim's life.
4. If the victim has vomited enough to cause shock (signalled by dehydration and a rapid, thready pulse), treat for shock, and transport to a physician or activate the EMS system as soon as possible.

ESOPHAGEAL REFLUX (HEARTBURN)

Esophageal reflux — commonly referred to as heartburn — can be frightening and excruciating for the victim but does not constitute a medical emergency unless it is symptomatic of a serious medical problem, such as myocardial infarction.

Esophageal reflux results when gastric juices spill from the stomach into the esophagus, irritating the esophageal lining. Because the lining does not produce mucus, it cannot protect itself against the corrosive effects of the gastric juices. In most cases, esophageal reflux results in only mild irritation; in extreme cases, deep ulcers or perforations can occur. The resulting pain is called heartburn because of the burning sensation it causes.

The pain, which generally is located beneath the sternum, occurs most often when the person is lying down at night, after he has eaten a heavy meal, or after he has ingested a lot of alcohol. Short, obese people have the highest tendency toward heartburn, as do pregnant women (because of the resulting increase in intra-abdominal pressure). Heartburn is aggravated by straining and lifting and often follows ingestion of certain kinds of foods.

While heartburn may cause problems if perforation results or if it signals other, more serious, medical problems, most cases can be controlled by antacids and changes in the diet. Unless the victim is in danger of developing shock, appears to have a more serious medical problem, or begins to vomit blood, refer him to a physician and limit first aid to reassuring the victim. Make sure that you do not confuse heartburn with cardiac pain; to be certain, assess for cardiac problems.

DIARRHEA
AND CONSTIPATION

Diarrhea is defined as an abnormally large number of loose, watery stools; constipation is defined as stools that are dried, hardened, or extremely difficult to pass. Not medical problems in themselves, diarrhea and constipation are symptomatic of other medical problems that range in seriousness from influenza to cancer.

Among the most common causes of diarrhea are the following:

- Bacterial or viral infections.
- Severe infections (such as dysentary).
- Gastroenteritis and other conditions that irritate the lining of the intestine.
- Parasitic infestations.
- Fecal impaction (obstruction of the intestines caused by dried, impacted stool matter that lodges in the intestinal tract, allowing only liquids to pass).
- Ulcerative colitis and other inflammatory bowel diseases.
- Severe anxiety or stress.
- Extreme emotional reactions.

In itself, diarrhea is rarely a medical emergency. The only cause for concern is when diarrhea has persisted for several days and the victim has become dehydrated or has lapsed into hypovolemic shock as a result of fluid and electrolyte loss.

A victim who is weak, lethargic, dehydrated, and shocky should be treated for shock and transported to a hospital for further treatment.

Chronic constipation occurs most commonly in the elderly, usually as a result of changes in diet and activity level. Those who may have difficulty chewing and swallowing food often rely on a diet of bland, soft foods — which, in turn, tend to produce a small, hard stool that is difficult to pass. Those who are not in good health sometimes stop trying to pass difficult stools, and the fecal matter accumulates in the bowel, causing significant abdominal distension.

As with diarrhea, constipation itself rarely presents a medical emergency. But because chronic constipation can be a symptom of a serious medical disorder — such as cancer of the colon — those complaining of chronic constipation should be seen by a physician.

| **25** | **SELF-TEST** | **25** |

Student: _____ Date: _____

Course: _____ Section #: _____

PART I: True/False   Which of the following may be symptoms of acute abdominal distress? If you believe that the answer is true, circle the T. If you believe that the answer is false, circle the F.

T   F   1. High blood pressure.

T   F   2. Nausea and/or vomiting.

T   F   3. Rapid pulse.

T   F   4. Local or diffuse abdominal tenderness.

T   F   5. Blood in urine

T   F   6. Pain that shifts position.

T   F   7. Colicky pain.

T   F   8. Sudden or severe pain.

T   F   9. In assessing a victim with acute abdominal distress, your number-one priority should be to assess pain.

T   F   10. Allow the abdominal-distress victim to determine the most comfortable position.

T   F   11. The blood vomited with ruptured esophageal varices is the consistency of coffee grounds.

T   F   12. Vomiting becomes a medical emergency when it causes dehydration, when it is aspirated, or when it signals a serious medical condition.

T   F   13. If a victim has aspirated vomitus, he will probably be breathing rapidly, secreting excessive saliva, and be cyanotic.

T   F   14. Esophageal reflux is unconfortable but causes very little pain.

T   F   15. Constipation and diarrhea are often related to dire medical emergencies.

T   F   16. Acute abdominal distress may originate in the cardiac or reproductive systems.

T   F   17. Pain that shifts position may signal appendicitis.

T   F   18. Sudden, severe pain is often caused by a rupture or perforation.

T   F   19. A common cause of lower abdominal pain on the left side is appendicitis.

T   F   20. A victim with an acute abdomen rarely appears ill.

T   F   21. There is usually an absence of pain or tenderness in the stomach with ruptured esophageal varices.

T   F   22. Vomiting is one of the least common gastrointestinal complaints or emergencies.

T   F   23. Esophageal reflux can be excruciating for the victim and constitutes a dire medical emergency.

T   F   24. Diarrhea is rarely a medical emergency.

T   F   25. Chronic constipation occurs most commonly in children.

PART II: Multiple Choice   For each question, circle the answer that best reflects an accurate statement.

1. A victim lying on his side with his knees drawn up, with rapid, shallow breathing and a rapid pulse, who is quiet, anxious, and reluctant to move is likely to be suffering from:
   a. stroke.
   b. insulin shock.
   c. acute abdominal distress.
   d. myocardial infarction.

2. Victims suffering from acute abdominal distress should be allowed to:
   a. determine the most comfortable position for themselves.
   b. drink liquids.
   c. take personal medication.
   d. all of these answers.

3. Pain from acute abdominal distress is often:
   a. colicky.
   b. pain that shifts.
   c. pain that radiates.
   d. all of the above.

4. Which of the following is *not* appropriate emergency care for ruptured esophageal varices?
   a. position the victim to allow drainage from mouth and throat.
   b. treat the victim for shock.
   c. put the victim in a supine position.
   d. activate the EMS system without delay.

5. Which of the following is *not* true about vomiting?
   a. most vomiting is caused by a self-limiting infection.
   b. a medical emergency can develop if vomit is aspirated.
   c. a victim can vomit enough to cause shock.
   d. vomiting is never a serious condition.

6. Any abdominal pain that lasts longer than _____ should be considered an emergency.
   a. 30 minutes.
   b. 6 hours.
   c. 2 hours.
   d. 24 hours.

PART III: What Would You Do If:

1. A victim whom you are assisting complains of lower abdominal pain on the right side that has increased in intensity for the last six hours. The victim is nauseated and anxious.

2. You are at a social gathering where a middle-aged man is vomiting large amounts of bright red blood. The man's wife tells you that he has a history of a drinking problem. He has pale skin and a rapid pulse and is experiencing some respiratory distress.

PART IV: Practical Skills Check-Off

_____ has satisfactorily passed the following practical skills:
Student's Name

	Date	Partner Check	Inst. Init.
1. Describe and demonstrate how to give emergency care for acute abdominal distress.	___ / ___ / ___	☐	_____

EPILEPSY, DIZZINESS, AND FAINTING

Neurological emergencies, basically involving a disturbance in the chemical or electrical activity of the brain, are generally more frightening than they are life-threatening. With quick recognition of the condition and vigorous airway management to prevent oxygen deprivation, you can generally prevent a major medical emergency. A victim who passes from one seizure to another without regaining consciousness first, however, *does* represent a life-threatening medical emergency.

SEIZURES AND EPILEPSY

A seizure is an involuntary, sudden change in sensation, behavior, muscle activity, or level of consciousness and results from irritated, overactive brain cells. Any condition that affects the structural cells of the brain or alters its chemical metabolic balance may trigger seizures.

Evidence suggests that the tendency toward seizures runs in families. More that 12 million Americans suffer seizures each year.

CAUSES OF SEIZURES

A significant cause of seizures is epilepsy, one of the most common and puzzling of central nervous system disorders (Figures 26-1 and 26-2). Epilepsy is a chronic brain disorder characterized by recurrent seizures with or without a loss of consciousness. It includes approximately twenty different seizure disorders. More than 2 million Americans suffer from epilepsy.

TYPES OF SEIZURES

For a complete listing of seizures, see Table 26-1.

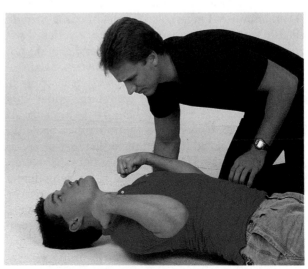

FIGURE 26-1. Epilepsy is one of the most common causes of seizures.

THE VARIOUS CAUSES OF EPILEPTIC SEIZURES

Seizures can occur in anyone as a result of an acute injury to the brain, or a more long-lasting condition involving the brain.

Here are brief explanations of the most common causes of seizures:

- *Toxic* — Seizures can occur as a direct consequence of using drugs or other chemicals or withdrawal from addicting substances, especially alcohol.

- *Metabolic* — Derangements in the body's chemistry may be accompanied by a seizure.

- *Trauma* — A previous injury to the brain could result in scar formation, which can serve as a seizure focus.

- *Infection* — An inflammation of the brain such as that caused by encephalitis.

- *Febrile* — Most commonly seen in children ages six months to three years, these seizures occur in conjunction with a fever. Only in rare cases does this condition cause seizures later in life.

- *Idiopathic* — By definition, this type of seizure arises spontaneously from an unknown cause.

- *Congenital defects of the brain* — Particularly in infants and young children.

- *Brain tumor* — Uncommon, but may have a seizure as its first sign — especially *focal* seizures.

Reprinted from *Mayo Clinic Health Letter*, November 1988 with permission of Mayo Foundation for Medical Education and Research, Rochester, Minnesota.

FIGURE 26-2.

STATUS EPILEPTICUS

While most seizures stop within five minutes (even though the victim may remain unconscious for several minutes longer), status epilepticus is a single seizure that lasts five to ten minutes or a series of seizures that occur in rapid succession and that do not allow for a period of lucidity between seizures. *Status epilepticus is a dire medical emergency;* approximately 1,500 Americans have status-epilepticus seizures a year, and half of them die as a result.

Status epilepticus may result from any worsening of whatever caused the seizures in the first place, or it may occur as a result of a new condition. It is often the result of improper drug therapy for an epileptic victim. Because of the length of the prolonged or recurrent seizures, the brain is deprived of oxygen; irreversible brain damage can result, as well as complications of the cardiac, respiratory, and renal systems. Common complications include cardiac arrhythmias, hypoxia, hyperthermia, and aspiration pneumonia.

SIGNS AND SYMPTOMS / STAGES OF A GRAND MAL SEIZURE

Most seizures are self-limiting (except for status epilepticus), and most last only about five minutes — although the victim may experience residual drowsiness for several hours. The signs and symptoms of a grand mal seizure (including epileptic seizure) occur in stages, and include the following (Figure 26-3):

The Aura

The **AURA** does not "precede" the seizure, as is commonly believed, but is actually a part of the seizure. While many seizures begin with an aura, only about half of those who seize ever experience auras. Generally, the aura lasts only a few seconds and involves a peculiar sensation — such as hallucinations of sight and sound, a peculiar taste in the mouth, a painful sensation in the abdomen, or a sense of movement in some part of the body when no movement actually exists.

As the seizure begins, whether or not an aura exists, the victim usually lets out a loud moan or cry as the chest and abdominal muscles contract rapidly, forcing air out past the closed larynx. The victim then collapses; some muscles are rigid while other are flaccid. While not all victim's experience a loss of consciousness at this point, all experience an altered mental state.

The Tonic Phase

During the tonic phase, which lasts fifteen to twenty seconds, the victim loses consciousness and the eyes roll upward. The tonic phase is characterized by continuous muscular contraction; the body is completely rigid, and the victim does not breathe (since the diaphragm is also seizing). In some victims, the tonic phase may be heralded by a high-pitched cry, increased salivation, dilated pupils, and pupils that are nonreactive to light.

The Hypertonic Phase

The hypertonic phase signals the end of the tonic phase and is characterized by five to fifteen seconds of extreme muscular rigidity and hypertension.

The Clonic Phase

The clonic, or spasm, lasts thirty to sixty seconds and is characterized by muscular rigidity and relaxation that alternate rhythmically in rapid succession.

TABLE 26-1	EPILEPSY: RECOGNITION AND EMERGENCY CARE			
SEIZURE TYPE	**WHAT IT LOOKS LIKE**	**OFTEN MISTAKEN FOR**	**WHAT TO DO**	**WHAT NOT TO DO**
GRAND MAL (Convulsive) (Generalized tonic-clonic)	Sudden cry or moan, rigidity, followed by muscle jerks, frothy saliva on lips, shallow breathing or temporarily suspended breathing, bluish skin, possible loss of bladder or bowel control, usually lasts 2-5 minutes. Normal breathing then starts again. There may be some confusion and/or fatigue, followed by return to full consciousness.	Heart attack. Stroke. Unknown but life-threatening emergency.	Look for medical identification; protect from nearby hazards; loosen ties or shirt collars; place folded jacket under head. Turn on side to keep airway clear. Reassure when consciousness returns. If single seizure lasted less than 10 minutes, ask if hospital evaluation wanted. If multiple seizures, or if one seizure lasts longer than 10 minutes, take to emergency room.	Don't put any hard implement in the mouth. Don't try to hold tongue; it can't be swallowed. Don't try to give liquids during or just after seizure. Don't use artificial ventilation unless breathing is absent after muscle jerks subside or unless water has been inhaled. Don't restrain.
PETIT MAL (Non-convulsive)	A blank stare, lasting only a few seconds, most common in children. May be accompanied by rapid blinking, some chewing movements of the mouth. Child having the seizure is unaware of what's going on during the seizure, but quickly returns to full awareness once it has stopped. May result in learning difficulties if not recognized and treated.	Daydreaming. Lack of attention. Deliberate ignoring of adult instructions.	No emergency care necessary, but medical evaluation should be recommended.	
JACKSONIAN (Simple Partial)	Jerking begins in fingers or toes, can't be stopped by victim, but victim stays awake and aware. Jerking may proceed to involve hand, then arm, and sometimes spreads to whole body and becomes a convulsive seizure.	Acting out bizarre behavior.	No emergency care necessary unless seizure becomes convulsive, then first aid as above.	
SIMPLE PARTIAL (also called sensory)	May not be obvious to onlooker, other than victim's preoccupied or blank expression. Victim experiences a distorted environment. May see or hear things that aren't there, may feel unexplained fear, sadness, anger, or joy. May have nausea, experience odd smells, and have a generally "funny" feeling in the stomach.	Hysteria. Mental illness. Psychosomatic illness. Parapsychological or mystical experience.	No action needed other than reassurance and emotional support.	

(Continued)

TABLE 26-1 EPILEPSY: RECOGNITION AND EMERGENCY CARE (Continued)

SEIZURE TYPE	WHAT IT LOOKS LIKE	OFTEN MISTAKEN FOR	WHAT TO DO	WHAT NOT TO DO
PSYCHOMOTOR (Complex Partial)	Usually starts with blank stare, followed by chewing, followed by random activity. Person appears unaware of surroundings, may seem dazed and mumble. Unresponsive. Actions clumsy, not directed. May pick at clothing, pick up objects, try to take clothes off. May run, appear afraid. May struggle or flail at restraint. Once pattern established, same set of actions usually occur with each seizure. Lasts a few minutes, but post-seizure confusion can last substantially longer. No memory of what happened during seizure period.	Drunkenness. Intoxication on drugs. Mental illness. Indecent exposure. Disorderly conduct. Shoplifting.	Speak calmly and reassuringly to victim and others. Guide gently away from obvious hazards. Stay with person until completely aware of environment. Offer help getting home.	Don't grab hold unless sudden danger (such as a cliff edge or an approaching car) threatens. Don't try to restrain. Don't shout. Don't expect verbal instructions to be obeyed.
MYOCLONIC SEIZURES	Sudden, brief, massive muscle jerks that may involve the whole body or parts of the body. May cause person to spill what they were holding or fall off a chair.	Clumsiness. Poor coordination.	No emergency care needed, but should be given a thorough medical evaluation.	
ATONIC SEIZURES (also called drop attacks)	The legs of a child between 2-5 years of age suddenly collapse under him and he falls. After 10 seconds to a minute, he recovers, regains consciousness, and can stand and walk again.	Clumsiness. Lack of good walking skills. Normal childhood "stage."	No emergency care needed (unless he hurt himself as he fell), but the child should be given a thorough medical evaluation.	
INFANTILE SPASMS	Starts between 3 months and 2 years. If a child is sitting up, the head will fall forward, and the arms will flex forward. If lying down, the knees will be drawn up, with arms and head flexed forward as if the baby is reaching for support.	Normal movements of the baby, especially if they happen when the baby is lying down.	No emergency care, but prompt medical evaluation is needed.	

Source: Epilepsy Foundation of America

GRAND MAL SEIZURES

A Grand Mal Seizure is a sign of an abnormal release of impulses in the brain. It is a physical, not a psychological, disorder.

1
The victim may have an "aura" or premonition which is a part of the seizure. An aura is often described as an odd or unpleasant sensation that rises from the stomach toward the chest and throat.

For some victims the aura is always the same, such as numbness or motor activity (like turning of head and eyes, spasm of a limb) or it may consist of a peculiar sound or taste.

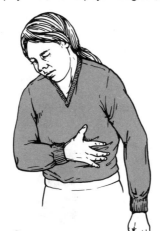

2
Loss of consciousness follows the aura. The forced expulsion of air caused by contraction of the skeletal muscles may cause a high-pitched cry sound. The victim may be pale at this point with possible spasms of various muscle groups, causing the tongue to be bitten.

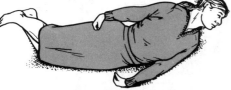

3
The victim will usually fall with convulsions and lose consciousness. Cyanosis may accompany the seizure because breathing stops during the phase of prolonged muscle contraction. Within seconds, the victim will manifest an arched back and alternating contraction and relaxation of movements in all extremities (clonic convulsive movements). Frothing at the mouth occurs, which may be bloody as the result of cheek or tongue biting. The attack usually lasts from about 30 seconds to five minutes. The victim may lose bladder and bowel control.

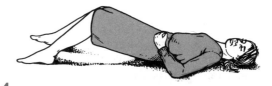

4
Gradually the clonic phase (convulsions) subsides. It is followed by a **postictal state,** characterized by a deep sleep with gradual recovery to a state of transient confusion, fatigue, muscular soreness, and headache. The victim should be encouraged to rest, since activity could precipitate another attack.

EMERGENCY CARE

- If the victim seems to stop breathing, monitor airway and assist ventilation if necessary. The situation becomes life-threatening if the victim passes from seizure to seizure without regaining consciousness (status epilepticus). This situation requires transport and medical attention.
- The major requirements of the First Aider are the ABCs and to protect the victim from hurting himself during a seizure.
- The victim should not be physically restrained in any way unless he is endangering his own welfare.
- Move objects, not the victim.
- Position the victim to allow for drainage and suctioning.
- Loosen tight clothing.
- If status epilepticus occurs or breathing ceases, assist breathing with artificial ventilation. Immediately activate the EMS system.
- Keep victim from being a spectacle.
- Reassure and reorient victim following the seizure.
- Allow him to rest.
- An ambulance is often called for a grand mal seizure, but if the victim responds normally, he may not need transport. If in doubt, always activate the EMS system. Follow local protocol.

FIGURE 26-3.

The arms and legs jerk violently during the clonic phase. Irregular breathing occurs in some, and **APNEA** (absence of breathing) in others, but the apnea, when present, lasts for only about one minute; therefore, resuscitation is not needed. The victim may lose control of bowel and bladder functions and usually produces copious salivation that manifests itself as frothing through clenched jaws. The periods of relaxation gradually become longer until the clonic phase ends, generally signalled by a deep breath followed by irregular, shallow breathing.

Note: *Sometimes fainting is accompanied by jerking of the arms and legs. If the jerking lasts for only a few seconds and the victim regains consciousness with immediate full mental capacity, it was an episode of syncope (fainting), not a seizure.*

Autonomic Discharge

During autonomic discharge, which lasts for a few seconds, the victim experiences hyperventilation, salivation, and rapid heartbeat.

Postictal Stupor

Postictal stupor (sometimes referred to as post-seizure stupor) usually lasts for five to thirty minutes, but it occasionally lasts for several hours. All muscles relax; the victim falls into a deep sleep and experiences pallor. While the victim appears peaceful and relaxed, you should monitor him closely because of the possibility of aspiration of vomitus, leading to respiratory distress.

When the victim awakens from the postictal stupor, he will experience confusion and headache; he will rarely remember the seizure.

EMERGENCY CARE FOR SEIZURES

Although seizures are generally not life-threatening, all who experience a first-time seizure should be evaluated by a physician. Regardless of whether the seizure is the victim's first, observe him carefully throughout. The following specific techniques can help the victim:

1. Stay calm. If the victim is conscious, reassure him. Reassure others who are with the victim, explain what is happening, and try to keep them calm.

2. Stay with the victim until the seizure has passed. If you need help, send someone else to get it. If you leave to get additional help, the victim may injure himself, aspirate, or asphyxiate while you are gone.

3. Help the victim lie down on the floor so that he will not fall and injure himself. Do not move the victim unless he is near a dangerous object that cannot be moved (such as a hot radiator); instead, move objects that are near the victim so that he will not injure himself during the course of the seizure (Figure 26-4). Place padding (such as a folded jacket, a rolled towel, or a pillow) under the victim's head to prevent him from injuring it.

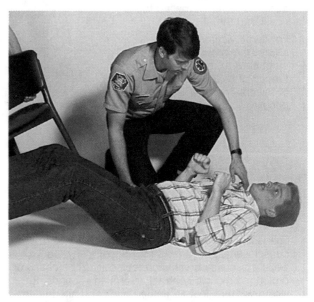

FIGURE 26-4. Move objects away from the seizure victim rather than trying to move him.

4. Never try to force anything between the victim's clenched teeth. Doing so may break the victim's teeth, force his tongue back so that it occludes the airway, cause other injury to the victim, or cause injury to you.

5. Remove or loosen any tight clothing, and remove eyeglasses.

6. Turn the victim on his side (preferably his left side) with his head extended and his face turned slightly downward so that secretions and vomitus can drain quickly out of his mouth. This position also prevents his tongue from falling back and tends to prevent choking (Figure 26-5).

7. Maintain an open airway.

8. If the victim stops breathing, open the airway; remove anything that might impair his breathing, and give artificial ventilation.

9. Watch what you say during the seizure; even though the victim appears asleep or stuporous, he will probably retain his sense of hearing.

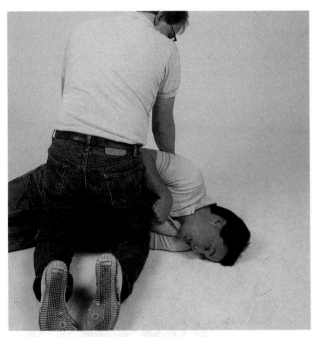

FIGURE 26-5. Position the seizure victim to allow drainage of saliva and vomitus.

10. Do not attempt to restrain the victim unless he is in immediate danger from objects that cannot be moved.

11. If possible, keep the victim from becoming a spectacle. If a screen or other barrier is available, place it around the victim. Ask onlookers and bystanders to leave.

12. Cover the victim with a blanket to keep him warm and to spare him embarrassment once the seizing is over.

13. Following the seizure, reassure and reorient the victim. Speak slowly and calmly in a normal tone of voice. Allow him to rest, and make him as comfortable as possible.

14. Check for and stabilize any injuries that may have occurred during the seizure.

15. If the victim lapses into a second seizure without regaining consciousness from the first one (status epilepticus), activate the EMS system immediately and consider his condition a grave medical emergency. Follow additional guidelines listed below.

16. If the victim is a feverish infant or child, cool the fever with room-temperature (not cold) wet towels or a sponge bath in tepid water. *Follow local protocol.*

17. Never give the victim anything to eat or drink; food or drink may mask symptoms, cause vom-

iting, and interfere with the physician's followup examination.

18. Place the victim in a supine position.

If the victim experiences status epilepticus, *you are dealing with a dire medical emergency.* Your number-one goal is oxygenation. Follow these steps:

1. Place the victim on the floor or bed, away from other furniture. Do not try to restrain him.

2. Clear and maintain his airway. Turn his head sideways to prevent aspiration.

3. Administer artificial ventilation as needed. Even though it can be extremely difficult to administer artificial ventilation to a seizing victim, you must do it — lack of oxygen due to imparied breathing during seizure activity is the most serious threat to life. Monitor for vomiting to prevent aspiration.

4. Carefully monitor vital signs.

5. Activate the EMS system immediately.

DIZZINESS, FAINTING, AND UNCONSCIOUSNESS

Two of the most common medical complaints are dizziness (a term used by victims to describe a broad variety of very different symptoms) and syncope, or fainting. Actually, dizziness and fainting are not medical conditions at all, but are symptoms that can result from a wide variety of diseases.

DIZZINESS

Most victims are not experiencing true dizziness, or vertigo — instead, they may feel woozy, lightheaded (especially when they stand up), or as though they are in a dream. They also may have blurred vision. True vertigo involves a hallucination of motion: the victim feels as though he is spinning around, or more commonly, that the room is whirling in circles. Some feel as though they are being pulled to the ground; others feel that the room has tilted enough so that they can no longer stand up in it. True vertigo is an actual disturbance of the victim's sense of balance.

There are two different types of vertigo, and each causes very different signs and symptoms. Central vertigo, the less common of the two, is also the most serious, because it usually signifies a dramatic medical problem involving the central nervous system. Signs and symptoms of central vertigo include dysfunction of the eye muscles, unequal pupil size, and facial droop. In some cases, central vertigo may mimic a TIA or stroke. Victims with central vertigo do not experience nausea, vomiting, hearing loss, or whirling sensation.

Labyrinthine vertigo, much more common, occurs as a result of disturbance in the inner ear. Victims with labyrinthine vertigo experience nausea, vomiting, rapid, involuntary twitching of the eyeball, and a whirling sensation. Most — if not all — of the symptoms are made worse by even the slightest movement. In an attempt to avoid any movement at all, the victim may appear to be in a coma, with head and neck held rigid, eyes tightly shut, skin pale and sweaty, and heartbeat rapid. Upon assessment, though, you will find that the victim is awake and alert but terrified to move. Some forms of labyrinthine vertigo are hereditary and involve hearing loss; episodes can last for hours and recur over a period of many years.

Management of dizziness is limited to reassuring the victim and positioning him with as little movement as possible. Conduct a thorough assessment to rule out any immediate life-threatening conditions.

FAINTING

Fainting, or syncope, is a transient loss of consciousness that results when, for some reason, the brain is temporarily deprived of adequate oxygen. Some victims feel as though everything is going dark, and then they suddenly lose consciousness. A deathlike collapse follows that puts the body in a horizontal position, allowing blood circulation to the brain to improve. As a result, the victim rapidly regains consciousness. For a few moments after regaining consciousness, the victim may feel confused and anxious; many will not remember the fainting episode at first.

Again, fainting itself is not a disease, but it can be symptomatic of a wide range of conditions and diseases, most commonly severe emotion, fright, certain drugs, profound pain, hypoglycemia, or cardiac arrhythmias.

Some victims have warning signs that they are about to experience syncope. Especially if the syncope is due to extreme emotion or fright, the victim may feel nauseated, lightheaded, weak, cold, and shaky. Some experience deep abdominal pain or a pounding pain in the head.

Fainting in children is often caused by breathholding. Other common causes include hypoglycemia (low blood sugar), dehydration, myocardial infarction, epilepsy, cardiac arrhythmias, congenital heart disease, valvular heart disease, and congenital heart failure.

To care for a fainting victim, follow these guidelines:

1. If the victim has not fainted but tells you that he feels faint, quickly have him lie down; elevate his legs. If he is in a sitting position, have him put his head between his legs (Figure 26-6).

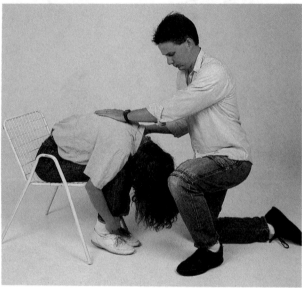

FIGURE 26-6. Have a fainting victim who is in a sitting position put her head between her legs.

2. If the victim has already fainted, keep him in a supine position and elevate his legs ten to twelve inches. If the victim falls against furniture, a wall, or some other obstacle and does not get into a flat position, he will not regain consciousness because the blood flow to his brain will not improve. *Do not allow a person who has fainted to sit up right away;* cerebrovascular accident can result.

3. Until proven otherwise, assume that the brain has been deprived of oxygen. Establish an airway and administer artificial ventilation if necessary. Monitor for possible vomiting.

4. Loosen any tight clothing that may restrict free breathing.

5. Make a rapid assessment for any life-threatening condition that may have caused the fainting; if you determine that the victim has a serious medical condition, initiate appropriate care.

6. Check for any injuries that may have been sustained during the fall, and give appropriate care.

7. If necessary, activate the EMS system; do not allow a victim who has fainted to get up immediately and walk around after regaining consciousness.

| **26** | **SELF-TEST** | **26** |

Student: _____   Date: _____

Course: _____   Section #: _____

PART I: True/False   If you believe that the statement is true, circle the T. If you believe that the statement is false, circle the F.

T   F   1. A seizure is a voluntary, sudden change in sensation, behavior, muscular activity, and level of consciousness.

T   F   2. Epilepsy is a chronic brain disorder.

T   F   3. More than 20 million Americans suffer from epilepsy.

T   F   4. Seizures are always life-threatening.

T   F   5. Grand mal seizures always produce a loss of consciousness.

T   F   6. Jacksonian seizures always involve loss of consciousness.

T   F   7. Status epilepticus is a single seizure that lasts five to ten minutes or a series of seizures that occur in rapid succession.

T   F   8. Irreversible brain damage can result from status epilepticus.

T   F   9. Most seizures are self-limiting and last about five minutes.

T   F   10. The aura precedes the seizure but is not a part of it.

T   F   11. Over 90 percent of those who have seizures experience an aura with each seizure.

T   F   12. During the tonic phase, the victim has five to fifteen seconds of extreme muscular rigidity.

T   F   13. In a postictal stupor, the victim falls into a deep sleep.

T   F   14. Do not attempt to restrain a seizure victim unless he is in immediate danger.

T   F   15. Dizziness and fainting are not medical conditions, but are symptoms.

T   F   16. True vertigo involves a hallucination of motion.

T   F   17. Even though awake and alert, a victim with labyrinthine vertigo may appear to be in a coma.

T   F   18. Fainting is a transient loss of consciousness due to inadequate oxygen to the brain.

T   F   19. Syncope is a very serious form of dizziness.

T   F   20. For a few minutes after regaining consciousness, a fainting victim may feel confused and anxious.

T   F   21. Evidence suggests that the tendency toward seizures runs in families.

T   F   22. Approximately 1,500 Americans have status epilepticus seizures each year.

T   F   23. Ninety percent of victims of status epilepticus seizures will die.

T   F   24. Loss of consciousness follows the aura.

T   F   25. True vertigo is an actual disturbance of the victim's sense of balance.

T   F   26. The number one goal in a status epilepticus emergency is oxygenation.

PART II: Multiple Choice   For each question, circle the answer that best reflects an accurate statement.

1. A characteristic of petit mal seizures is:
   a. convulsive movements of one part of the body.
   b. brief periods where the victim appears to be daydreaming or staring.
   c. loss of consciousness.
   d. repetition of inappropriate acts.

2. Which of the following is *not* a sign of epilepsy?
   a. a clonic phase.
   b. a tonic phase.
   c. an aura.
   d. a catatonic phase.

3. Which of the following emergency-care measures is used when dealing with an epileptic victim?
   a. rush the victim to the hospital; this is a true emergency.
   b. move objects away from the victim which may harm him.
   c. forcibly restrain the victim until his convulsions pass.
   d. force a padded object in between the victim's teeth.

4. The most serious threat in status epilepticus is:
   a. lack of oxygen due to impaired breathing.
   b. fractures.
   c. swallowing the tongue.
   d. dehydration.

5. A grand mal seizure is usually caused by:
   a. loss of consciousness.
   b. psychological stress.
   c. an abnormal release of impulses in the brain.
   d. all of these answers.

6. The most common cause of status epilepticus in adults is:
   a. history of stroke.
   b. failure to take prescribed medication.
   c. history of injury to the head.
   d. high fever.

7. Which of the following is *not* an emergency-care procedure for seizures?
   a. stay calm and reassure the victim.
   b. put a padded object between the victim's teeth.
   c. do not attempt to restrain the victim unless he is in immediate danger.
   d. stay with the victim until the seizure has passed.

PART III: Matching: Match the description at the right with the correct type or phase of seizure at the left.

Types and Phases of Seizures	Description
_____1. Grand mal	A. Begins as convulsive movements in one part of the body, such as a trembling hand or foot, and subsequently spreads to the entire body.
_____2. Petit mal	B. Lasting fifteen to twenty seconds, characterized by continuous muscular contraction.
_____3. Myoclonic	C. Brief periods where the victim appears to be daydreaming or staring; the eyelids may flutter rapidly.
_____4. Psychomotor	D. Characterized by sudden, brief, massive muscle jerks.
_____5. Jacksonian	E. Involves a peculiar sensation that precedes and sometimes warns of an impending epileptic attack.
_____6. Status epilepticus	F. Arched back, alternating contraction and relaxation of movements of all extremities, frothing of the mouth, and clenching of the jaw.
_____7. Aura	G. Starts with blank stare, followed by chewing, followed by random activity.
_____8. Tonic phase	H. A single seizure that lasts 5-10 minutes or a series of seizures that occur in rapid succession.
_____9. Clonic phase	

PART IV: What Would You Do If:

1. You are at a large public gathering and a person suddenly cries out, falls, becomes rigid, and has muscular jerks. He has frothy saliva on the lips and very shallow breathing. In about five minutes the symptoms subside, and within the next thirty minutes the symptoms reappear and subside numerous times.

2. At the same gathering, a person complains of dizziness and nausea. She is shaky, has cool skin, and tells you that she feels faint.

PART V: Practical Skills Check-Off _____ has satisfactorily passed the following practical skills:

Student's Name

	Date	Partner Check	Inst. Init.
1. Describe and demonstrate how to give emergency care to a victim experiencing a grand mal seizure.	___/___/___	☐	_____

CHAPTER TWENTY-SEVEN

OBJECTIVES

- Learn how to deal with children in an emergency.
- Identify how pediatric victims are different from adult victims.
- Know how to obtain a pediatric physical assessment.
- Learn how to give emergency care to a pediatric trauma victim.
- Identify and know how to respond to common emergencies in children, including respiratory distress, airway obstruction, febrile convulsions, cardiac arrest, shock, SIDS, and child abuse/neglect.

PEDIATRIC EMERGENCIES

Every day in the United States, approximately forty-one children die from trauma, and 4,000 more are admitted to hospital emergency rooms with injuries. The leading causes of fatal injuries in children under fourteen are trauma (particularly motor-vehicle accidents), drownings, burns, poisonings, and falls.

Children can be categorized in the following groups:

- "Infant" refers to a child up to the age of twelve months.
- "Child" usually refers to an individual between one and twelve years of age.
- "Adolescent" refers to a person between twelve and eighteen years of age.

However, these categories are not hard-and-fast pigeonholes. Each age group has different emotional and physical characteristics that can complicate your care. Children are *not* just little adults. There are important psychological and physical differences (Figure 27-1). This chapter focuses on those differences to supplement the emergency-care information in other chapters. Remember, however — a breathing problem is a breathing problem; a bleeding wound is a bleeding wound. How you approach it in a baby is a little different from how you approach it in the adult, but the basic emergency care and goals are the same.

ASSESSING THE CHILD

It is difficult to assess pain in children because they lack both the body awareness to describe the exact location of the pain and the vocabulary to describe the nature of the pain. Usually pain, and especially bleeding, is so frightening that they cannot separate the emotional component from the physical. Ask the parents, if possible, how the child usually reponds to pain to get some idea of how typical the reactions are.

During your first look at the child, ask yourself these questions:

- Does he look sick?
- Is he in shock?
- Is he in extreme pain?

With all age groups, follow these general procedures when assessing a child:

1. Perhaps nothing is emotionally harder than a sick or injured child, but prepare yourself

DIFFERENCES BETWEEN CHILDREN AND ADULTS

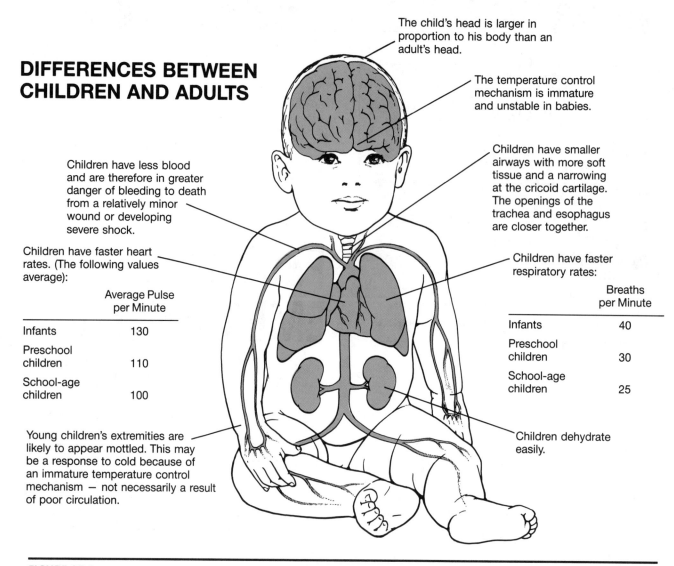

The child's head is larger in proportion to his body than an adult's head.

The temperature control mechanism is immature and unstable in babies.

Children have smaller airways with more soft tissue and a narrowing at the cricoid cartilage. The openings of the trachea and esophagus are closer together.

Children have less blood and are therefore in greater danger of bleeding to death from a relatively minor wound or developing severe shock.

Children have faster heart rates. (The following values average):

	Average Pulse per Minute
Infants	130
Preschool children	110
School-age children	100

Children have faster respiratory rates:

	Breaths per Minute
Infants	40
Preschool children	30
School-age children	25

Young children's extremities are likely to appear mottled. This may be a response to cold because of an immature temperature control mechanism — not necessarily a result of poor circulation.

Children dehydrate easily.

FIGURE 27-1.

psychologically so that you can radiate confidence, competence, and friendliness. Avoid "baby talk." Remember that you are a stranger. Children between one and six seldom like strangers, especially if their parents are not there.

2. Get as close as possible to the child's eye level (Figure 27-2). Sit down next to the child if possible.

3. With children under school age, keep the most painful parts of the assessment for the end.

4. Explain what you are doing in terms they can understand. Follow up on questions. Speak in a calm, quiet voice, and maintain eye contact as much as possible. Even infants will respond to a calm voice, and an apparently unconscious child may actually absorb much of what you say.

5. Involve the parents (or a familiar person) as much as possible. If the case involves an automobile accident and injury to parents, it is still less frightening to a child to be with an injured parent than to be separated. Of course, you must make your decision based on the seriousness of the injury and the necessary emergency care.

6. Be honest. "It will hurt when I touch you here, but it will only last a minute. If you feel like crying, it's okay." Children can tolerate pain if they are prepared for it and are given adequate support.

7. Be gentle. Use all appropriate measures to reduce the amount of pain that a child must endure. If you must restrain a child, be sure that it is

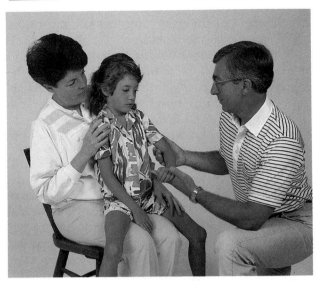

FIGURE 27-2. Establish gentle contact and examine the child visually.

absolutely necessary, and use only the minimum degree to be safe and allow you to provide good care.

TRAUMA

The number-one killer of American children is the automobile. Children may experience trauma while riding bikes, all-terrain vehicles, and motorcycles, even as pedestrians on busy roads and during recreational activities. Basic trauma management in children is the same as for adult basic life support.

1. Establish an airway, and stabilize the cervical spine.
2. Make sure that the child is breathing and has a heartbeat. If not, perform artificial ventilation or CPR.
3. Control bleeding.
4. Treat for shock.
5. Immobilize any neurological and musculoskeletal injuries.

VITAL SIGNS FOR CHILDREN

Check a child's vital signs more frequently than you would an adult's. Pay attention, however, to your subjective impression of the child. Your overall impression of how the child looks and acts can be more important and tell you more about the status of the child than any one vital sign (e.g., the child may be cyanotic, yet still be distracted by toys and cooing).

RESPIRATIONS

Check respirations by placing your hand on the infant/child's stomach. Children breathe faster than adults, with the range of an infant (sixty-four per minute) to an eight-year-old (twenty-three per minute). The key is to take respiratory rates frequently. An increase over the previous rate may be significant. Respiration rates in children alter easily due to emotional and physiological conditions.

PULSE

It is very difficult to feel a carotid pulse in infants and toddlers because their necks are short. To take a pulse the most rapidly, use the radial pulse in a child, but the brachial pulse in an infant. If the radial pulse is not clear, check the brachial pulse above the elbow. Feel for the point on the medial (inside) side of the humerous, mid-shaft in the groove between the biceps and triceps.

Rapid pulse may be caused by shock, fever, or oxygen deficiency. It may also be normal in scared or overly excited children. However, a slow pulse in a child is a worrisome sign. A slow pulse may be caused by pressure in the skull, depressant drugs, or some comparatively rare medical conditions. Ask the parent what is normal for the child.

TEMPERATURE

Children's temperatures are much more important than adult temperatures as warning signals because they can change so quickly. Young children can develop fevers of up to 105 degrees F (40.6 degrees C) rapidly. Causes of high temperature are infection and heatstroke (from being left in a hot car, for instance).

To lower the body temperature (some pediatric physicians are allowing temperatures to remain elevated at a moderate level for a time — *follow local protocol*):

1. Give the child fluids by mouth. *Follow local protocol.*
2. Sponge-bathe the face, hands, feet, etc., or, if necessary, remove the child's clothes and sponge-bathe him in tepid (98 degree F) water. Do not

use alcohol. It may cause hypothermia by cooling the infant off too rapidly.

3. If shivering is induced, stop bathing the child. The body's shivering mechanism will generate more heat than you can dissipate with tepid bathing.

Abnormally low temperatures are signs of shock or some other low metabolic state, near-drowning, or exposure. Treat such cases by doing the following:

1. Passively warm the child by removing wet clothes, and maintain warmth with blankets. Skin contact with a warm individual in an emergency situation may be helpful.

2. Wrap the child in blankets after the initial warming.

3. If the child can swallow, give warm liquids like soup. Be careful — if the gag reflex is absent, the child could choke.

NEUROLOGICAL ASSESSMENT OF CHILDREN

Assessing possible neurological damage in children is similar to the process for adults, but the stimuli must be more simplified. Check for:

▪ Level of consciousness — if the child's consciousness seems lowered, check with the parents to see how typical or unusual this response is.

▪ Pupils — of equal size? Do they respond to light?

▪ Check the head, neck, and chest to observe for signs of trauma.

▪ Response to verbal and/or painful stimuli? Pinch the skin between the child's thumb and forefinger.

▪ Ability to recognize familiar objects and people?

▪ Ability to move extremities purposely?

▪ Clear or bloody fluid draining from ears?

If you suspect neurological damage, keep the child still and quiet, don't allow nonskilled people to move the child, activate the EMS system, and continue to check vital signs.

SPECIAL SITUATIONS FOR CHILDREN

Most emergencies involving children are managed in the same way as those involving adults. However, the different size and physiological development of children mean that you must treat some emergencies differently.

For instance, blunt trauma is the most common injury in children. Quite frequently, a child will be injured severely but will display no early, obvious signs. On accident scenes, try to reconstruct the accident and understand the mechanism of injury.

When you are caring for a child, be aware of the following special conditions and situations:

▪ Small children and infants have heads that are large in proportion to their bodies, making head injuries more likely. Assume cervical damage if a child has an injury above the clavicles, is unconscious, has a mechanism of injury that suggests cervical injury, or has an undefined area of injury.

▪ Because the liver, spleen, and kidneys of children are not as well protected as those of adults, and because they occupy a larger ratio of the abdominal cavity, they are more susceptible to blunt trauma. Children are not as likely as adults to suffer broken ribs but are more likely to have internal chest injuries.

▪ A child's skin surface is large compared to his body mass, making children more susceptible to hyperthermia and dehydration.

▪ Injuries of the extremities, the most common form of pediatric trauma, may also damage the growth plates, with long-term effects that may be a problem when they are adults.

▪ Infants have proportionally large tongues. If a tongue relaxes, it can block the airway.

▪ Infants before the age of nine months cannot yet fully support their own heads. Always support a baby's head when you pick it up.

▪ Most children involved in trauma will have their stomachs enlarged, pressing up on the left side of the diaphragm until the pressure significantly reduces the amount of air that they can breathe. There is a risk of vomiting and potential aspiration. Watch the victim carefully.

▪ You must stop bleeding as quickly as possible, since a comparatively small blood loss in an adult would constitute major bleeding for a child.

▪ Sixty-four percent of bicycle-related deaths in the United States involve children; nearly 90 percent involve motor vehicles, and 50 percent of them occur between Friday afternoon and Sunday evening. Head and neck injuries are involved in three-fifths of all pediatric hospital admissions for bicycle-related injuries.

COMMON EMERGENCIES IN CHILDREN

RESPIRATORY DISTRESS

Respiratory distress can exhaust a child rapidly. In cases of rapid and/or noisy breathing, continue to assess the victim's breathing, and transport him to a medical facility or activate the EMS system.

OBSTRUCTED AIRWAY

Children are more susceptible to respiratory problems than adults because they have smaller air passages and less reserve air capacity.

Follow these steps in caring for an obstructed airway:

1. If the airway is blocked in an older child, roll the child on his side, lift the shoulders, and place a rolled towel underneath them so that the nose is elevated in the "sniffing" position. In a toddler or infant, keep the neck straight, in a neutral position, placing your hand on the forehead, and putting the finger of your other hand just under the infant's chin (Figure 27-3). Hyperextension, standard in older children and adults, may actually reduce the effective size of the airway in a small child or infant.

2. If the airway obstruction is complete, attempt to dislodge the foreign body. Stabilize the head to prevent cervical movement, and attempt to open the airway manually with the most acceptable procedure.

3. Check the child's mouth for foreign objects, and try to remove them with your fingers. *Do not perform blind sweeps*, because you may accidentally

dislodge the foreign object backwards and block the airway.

4. If the child is still not breathing, try to dislodge the obstruction:

   ■ Place a child over one year of age in a supine position and deliver six to ten abdominal thrusts.

   ■ In an infant under one year of age, straddle the baby prone over your arm with the head lower than the trunk, and support the infant's head by firmly holding the jaw. With the heel of your hand, deliver four back blows between the infant's shoulder blades. Place your free hand on the infant's back so that you sandwich him between you hands, then turn him. Place him on your thigh with his head lower than his trunk, and administer four chest thrusts (Figure 27-4).

5. When the foreign body is dislodged, open the airway using the tongue-jaw maneuver, and remove the foreign body with your finger, using a hooking action. Keep the airway open. Transport to the hospital, or activate the EMS system.

6. If the first set of maneuvers fails, repeat the full series once. Transport the victim immediately, or activate the EMS system. Continue to attempt ventilation and to dislodge the object. See Chapter 3 for additional instructions on airway obstruction and artificial ventilation.

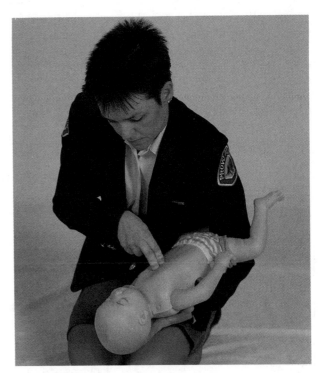

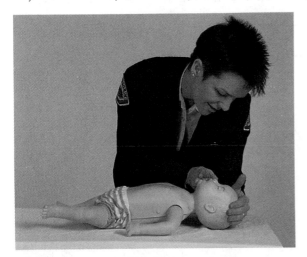

FIGURE 27-3. Airway obstruction may be relieved in an infant or small child by keeping the head in neutral +, not hyperextended.

FIGURE 27-4. Expel a foreign body in an infant with complete airway obstruction by positioning him as shown and applying four chest thrusts.

CARDIAC ARREST

Ninety-five percent of cardiac arrests in children come from airway obstruction and respiratory arrest; the other 5 percent are caused by shock. It is extremely important to prevent both conditions before they become established and to provide breathing assistance.

As with all cases of cardiac arrest, call for help if you are alone. Your goal must be to keep the brain alive. Unless too much time has elapsed between the arrest and artificial ventilation, the child can be neurologically normal, even following comparatively long periods of arrest.

Signs of cardiac arrest in a child are (Figure 27-5):

- Unresponsiveness.
- Convulsions.
- Gasping or no respiratory sounds.
- No audible heart sounds.
- Chest is not moving.
- Pale or blue skin.
- Absent brachial pulse.
- Muscle contractions.

For CPR techniques and emergency care, see Chapter 4.

CONVULSIONS

Convulsions may be caused by any condition that would also produce seizures in adults: head injury, meningitis, oxygen deficiency, drug overdose, and hypoglycemia. Adults seldom have convulsions caused by fever, but children may. The risk of convulsions is high among children up to age two but decreases in children up to age six. Approximately 5 percent of children have febrile convulsions (caused by high fever). Although these childhood convulsions are frightening, they generally leave no adverse permanent effects.

During the seizure, the child's arms and legs become rigid, the back arches, the muscles may twitch or jerk in spasm, the eyes roll up and become fixed, the pupils dilate, and the breathing is often irregular or ineffective; the child may lose bladder and bowel control, and he is completely unresponsive. If the seizure lasts long enough, the skin will turn blue. The spasms will prevent the child from swallowing, and he will push the saliva out of his mouth. He will appear to be frothing at the mouth. If saliva is trapped in the throat, the child will make bubbling or gurgling sounds.

A simple convulsion is self-limiting, ends within fifteen minutes, is grand mal (all muscles involved) in nature, and does not recur. If the child has a single convulsion, all you need to do is maintain an airway and be sure that he does not injure himself. Transport to a medical facility as soon as possible after the single seizure.

Emergency care for childhood *convulsions* is:

1. During a seizure, the tongue may relax and shift backward, decreasing the size of the air passage. To prevent this, turn the child onto his side. This will also help prevent him from breathing fluids into the lungs if he has mucus or is frothing.

2. During the jerky spasm, do not hold the child down, but place him where he will not fall or strike something. A crib with padded sides is excellent; so is a rug on the floor. If a bed does not have sides, watch him to make sure that he does not fall off.

3. Loosen any clothing that is tight and restricting.

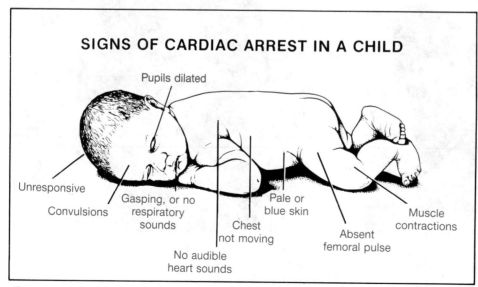

SIGNS OF CARDIAC ARREST IN A CHILD

Pupils dilated

Unresponsive

Convulsions

Gasping, or no respiratory sounds

No audible heart sounds

Chest not moving

Pale or blue skin

Absent femoral pulse

Muscle contractions

FIGURE 27-5.

4. If a child is feverish, sponge him with lukewarm water (98 degrees F).

Repeated or prolonged convulsions can result in death. Activate the EMS system immediately. Only transport to a medical facility if no ambulance is available.

SHOCK

The major causes of shock in children are blood loss, acute infection, and heart failure. These conditions are most commonly caused by major trauma — being hit by a car, or extensive burns.

Newborns will go into shock due to loss of body heat. They cannot shiver or warm themselves through activity (apparent shivering is really due to hypoglycemia), and their surface area is large in relation to their body weight. Be sure to keep infants warm. Remember that all children are more susceptible to hypothermia from shock or blood loss than adults because of their smaller body size. Be sure that they are kept warm.

Signs and symptoms of shock in children are pallor, coldness, sweatiness, low blood pressure, a rapid, thready pulse, lack of vitality, extreme anxiety, or unconsciousness (Figure 27-6).

To provide emergency care for shock:

1. Have the child lie flat.

2. Keep him warm and as calm as possible.

3. Monitor his vital signs often, especially breathing and heart function.

4. Provide aritificial ventilation when indicated.

5. Transport to a medical facility, or activate the EMS system.

SUDDEN INFANT DEATH SYNDROME

Sudden infant death syndrome (SIDS), commonly known as crib death or cot death, is the number-one cause of death among infants between one month and one year of age. About 6,500 babies die of SIDS every year in the United States (two per 1,000 live births). It occurs in both poor and wealthy neighborhoods and in both urban and rural communities.

SIDS cannot be predicted or prevented. It almost always occurs while the baby is sleeping. The typical SIDS case involves an apparently healthy infant, frequently born premature, and usually between the ages of four weeks and seven months, who suddenly dies overnight in his crib. No illness has been present, though the baby may have had recent cold symptoms. There is usually no indication of struggle. Sometimes, though, the child has obviously changed position at the time of death. A red blotchiness of the skin is usually apparent.

MANAGING THE SIDS SITUATION

Do the following in a SIDS emergency:

1. Even if the child is obviously dead, immediately initiate resuscitative efforts. Begin infant CPR, and have someone activate the EMS system.

2. A child may display the obvious characteristics of death (such as rigor mortis); under normal circumstances, you would be required to leave the body undisturbed and contact proper authorities. A SIDS case, however, is not "normal". The extreme emotional condition of the parents makes them victims as much as the infant, and the best first aid is to make them feel that everything possible has been done. Many parents cling to the hope that their infant is not dead and that

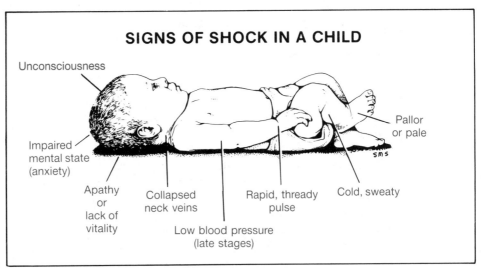

FIGURE 27-6.

he can be resuscitated, even when death is apparent. By starting CPR on the obviously dead child you at least allow the family to have the memory that professional intervention was attempted. Leave no room for "ifs" and "maybe's". *Follow local protocol.*

3. After the ambulance arrives, and ambulance personnel take over, encourage the parents to accompany their baby in the ambulance and offer to stay with children left at home. Support the parents in any way possible.

It is very common for First Aiders to experience emotions after a SIDS call. Ignoring emotions like anxiety, guilt, or anger will not cause them to go away and may have a serious, negative impact on your mental health. A debriefing session after a SIDS case by a professional is very helpful. First Aiders should talk out their feelings with colleagues and spouses, and *not* hold them inside.

CHILD ABUSE AND NEGLECT

Approximately 15,000 cases of child abuse and neglect are reported annually in the United States. However, because child abuse and neglect usually occur in the privacy of the home, no one knows exactly how many children are affected. Child abuse and neglect must be discovered and reported before the child can be protected, and it is generally agreed that this never happens in a majority of incidents.

The adult (usually a parent) who abuses a child often behaves in an evasive manner, volunteering little information or giving contradictory information about what happened to the child. The parent may show outright hostility toward the child or toward the other parent and rarely shows any guilt.

IDENTIFYING ABUSE

Abuse may be physical, emotional, or sexual, or may fall under the category of neglect. Each type of abuse has distinct characteristics — physical and behavioral indicators — that may allow you to identify the child as an abuse victim.

In many cases, a child will be a victim of a combination of physical, emotional, and sexual abuse and neglect. You should generally look for abrasions, lacerations, incisions, bruises, broken bones, multiple injuries in various stages of healing, injuries on both the front and back or on both sides of the child, unusual wounds (such as circular burns), a fearful child, or a child who has injuries to the head, back, and abdomen, including the genitals. Especially look for situations where the injuries do not match the mechanism of injury described by the parents or the victim.

EMERGENCY CARE FOR CHILD ABUSE

If you find yourself in the position of giving first aid to a victim of possible child abuse:

1. Calm the parents and suggest by your actions that you are there to help and render emergency care to the child. Tell them that if the child does happen to be injured, from whatever cause, you are prepared to help with the injuries. Speak in a low, firm voice.

2. Focus attention on the child while you administer emergency care. Speak softly to the child. Call him by his first name. *Do not* ask him to recreate the situation while he is still in the crisis environment, with the abuser still present.

3. Give the needed first aid, request an ambulance if you believe that the child needs a physician's care, and keep your suspicions to yourself. Make careful note, in addition, of all that you have observed at the scene (condition of the home, any objects that might have been used to hurt the child, such as belts or straps).

4. It is *not* your responsibility to confront the parents with the charge of child abuse. You must be tactful and discreet. Being supportive and nonjudgmental with the parents will help them be more receptive to other members of the health-care team.

5. *Always* report your suspicions of child abuse to the proper authorities (emergency-room physician, police).

6. Maintain total confidentiality regarding the incident; do not share it with your family or friends.

TAKE CARE OF YOURSELF

Almost half of the 15,000 children in the United States who die from accidents are pronounced dead either at the scene or at the hospital. The sudden and violent death of a child, either just before you arrive or while you are giving first aid, is emotionally wrenching. As a First Aider, you need to control your emotions so that you can render the best possible assistance and be supportive of other victims. After the case is over, however, you need to deal with those feelings. Talk them out. Find a trusted friend who will listen without cutting you off either to reassure you or give advice about what to do next time.

If you cannot find some way to talk through your feelings and instead try to suppress them, a typical pattern of worry about your own children or nightmares may develop.

| **27** | **SELF-TEST** | **27** |

Student: _____ Date: _____

Course: _____ Section #: _____

PART I: True/False   If you believe that the statement is true, circle the T. If you believe that the statement is false, circle the F.

T   F   1. Don't allow a child victim to have any contact with his parents.

T   F   2. Get as close as you can to the child's eye level.

T   F   3. Children one to six enjoy strangers and will be easy to assess.

T   F   4. Never tell a child the truth about his pain.

T   F   5. Children are more susceptible than adults to respiratory problems.

PART II: Multiple Choice   For each question, circle the answer that best reflects an accurate statement.

1. Children can:
   a. tolerate pain if they are prepared for it.
   b. not tolerate pain without going into shock.
   c. tolerate much higher pain levels if you tell them it shouldn't hurt.
   d. not separate pain and fear.

2. When assessing children, you should:
   a. avoid "baby talk."
   b. keep the most painful parts of the assessment for the end with children under school age.
   c. maintain eye contact as much as possible.
   d. all of these answers are true.

3. In doing an assessment on small children and infants, the First Aider is generally less effective if he:
   a. is gentle.
   b. talks quietly and calmly.
   c. separates the child and the mother.
   d. allows the child to remain with the parents.

4. Which statement concerning child abuse is *not* correct?
   a. focus attention on the child while you administer emergency care.
   b. question the child in the presence of the child's parents.
   c. it is not your responsibility to confront the parents with the charge of child abuse.
   d. you report your suspicions of child abuse to the proper authorities (physician, police).

5. Which of the following is *not* a good procedure for managing a SIDS situation?
   a. immediately initiate resuscitative efforts, depending on local protocol.
   b. encourage the parents to accompany their child in the ambulance.
   c. never discuss a SIDS case with colleagues.
   d. talk out your feelings after dealing with a SIDS emergency.

6. Convulsions in a child up to age two are generally due to:
   a. epilepsy.
   b. fever.
   c. hyperglycemia.
   d. drowning.

7. Which is *not* a correct emergency-care procedure for childhood convulsions?
   a. do not hold the child down.
   b. sponge the child with lukewarm water.
   c. place a hard object in the child's mouth to prevent damage to the teeth or tongue.
   d. place the child on his side to keep the tongue from blocking the airway.

8. The major causes of shock in children are:
   a. blood loss, fever, head injury.
   b. near-drowning, respiratory distress, seizures.
   c. blood loss, acute infection, heart failure.
   d. fever, head injury, epiglottitis.

9. Which of the following is true about SIDS?
   a. SIDS is more common in twins or triplets.
   b. SIDS occurs only in poor, low-income families.
   c. SIDS almost always occurs while the baby is sleeping.
   d. (a) and (c) are correct.

10. Which of the following is *not* true about child abuse/neglect?
    a. abuse may be physical, emotional, or sexual, or may involve neglect.
    b. the adult who abuses a child typically shows guilt and remorse.
    c. signs of child abuse include abrasions, lacerations, and broken bones.
    d. it is not really known how many children are affected by child abuse/neglect.

PART III: Matching: The following steps for emergency care in child trauma are out of order. Place them in the proper order.

_____1. Treat for shock.

_____2. Control bleeding.

_____3. Immobilize neurological injuries.

_____4. Establish an airway.

_____5. Perform necessary CPR.

PART IV: What Would You Do If:

At a motor-vehicle accident, one of the victims is a three-year-old in a safety seat. He is screaming at the top of his lungs, and he has a shallow gash in his thigh from which blood is oozing. His older sister has been thrown from the car and is unconscious. The driver (the father) is staggering up and down the road sobbing.

1. Who would you attend to first and why?

2. How would you approach the child and physically assess him?

3. What would you do to try to calm the child down?

PART V: Practical Skills Check-Off   _____ has satisfactorily passed the following practical skills:
                                                        Student's Name

	Date	Partner Check	Inst. Init.
1. Assessment of an infant-child.	___/___/___	☐	_____
2. Obstructed airway-child.	___/___/___	☐	_____

CHAPTER TWENTY-EIGHT

OBJECTIVES

- Understand the basic anatomy of pregnancy.
- Describe the process of childbirth and the specific stages of labor.
- Know how to assess the need for emergency delivery.
- Know how to assist the mother in delivering the baby and how to care for the baby and mother properly during and after delivery.
- Understand abnormal deliveries and complications of childbirth and know how to give proper emergency care.

CHILDBIRTH AND RELATED EMERGENCIES

The delivery of a baby is a natural function. At times, complications arise that lead to emergency situations outside the hospital setting. The role of the First Aider in a normal delivery is merely to assist the mother and baby. First Aiders should be familiar with the nature, signs, symptoms, and emergency care of normal childbirth and obstetric complications.

ANATOMY OF PREGNANCY

A full-term pregnancy lasts approximately 280 days (ten months) from the first day of the last normal menstrual period. A rule of thumb for calculating the expected delivery date is to subtract three months and add seven days from the first day of the last normal menstrual period.

Figure 28-1 shows the normal structures involved with a full-term pregnancy. The **UTERUS** is a smooth-muscled organ that contains the developing fetus. The special arrangement of smooth muscle and blood vessels in the uterus allows for great expansion during pregnancy, for forcible contractions during labor and delivery, and for rapid contraction after delivery that will constrict blood vessels in the uterus and prevent hemorrhage. During pregnancy, the **CERVIX** (neck of the uterus) contains a mucous

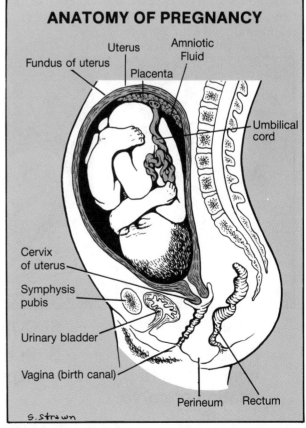

ANATOMY OF PREGNANCY

Uterus
Fundus of uterus
Amniotic Fluid
Placenta
Umbilical cord
Cervix of uterus
Symphysis pubis
Urinary bladder
Vagina (birth canal)
Perineum
Rectum

S. Strawn

FIGURE 28-1.

plug that is discharged during labor. The expulsion of this mucous plug is known as the **BLOODY SHOW**, and appears as pink-tinged mucus in the vaginal discharge.

The **PLACENTA** is a disk-shaped inner lining attached at one surface to the uterus and at the other to the umbilical cord. Rich in blood vessels, the placenta provides nourishment and oxygen from the mother's blood and absorbs waste products from the baby into the mother's bloodstream. After the baby is delivered, the placenta separates from the uterine wall and is delivered as the afterbirth.

The **UMBILICAL CORD** is the unborn baby's lifeline that attaches the baby to the placenta. The cord contains one vein and two arteries. The vein carries oxygenated blood to the fetus, while the arteries carry deoxygenated blood back to the placenta. The structure of the cord and the blood traveling through it at about four miles per hour keep the cord from kinking, which would obstruct the vital blood flow to and from the placenta. When the baby is born, the nerveless cord resembles a sturdy rope; it is about twenty-two inches long and about one inch in diameter.

The **AMNIOTIC SAC**, or bag of waters, is filled with amniotic fluid, in which the baby floats. The amount of fluid varies, usually from 500 to 1,000 milliliters. The plastic-like sac of fluid insulates and protects the baby during pregnancy. During labor, part of the sac usually is forced ahead of the baby, serving as a resilient wedge to help dilate the cervix.

The **BIRTH CANAL** is made up of the cervix and the vagina. Toward the end of a full-term pregnancy, the baby usually has positioned itself head down, with its buttocks toward the upper end of the uterus. The head-down position, with the baby's head already descended through the broad, upper inlet of the mother's pelvis, brings the uterus downward and forward. Mothers can feel the difference and say that the baby has "dropped". This position is most favorable for the baby's passage through the cervix to the vagina.

STAGES OF LABOR

Labor is the term used to describe the process of childbirth. It consists of contractions of the uterine wall that force the baby and, later, the afterbirth (placenta) into the outside world. Normal labor is divided into three stages; the length of each stage varies greatly in different women and under different circumstances (Figure 28-2).

FIRST STAGE (DILATION)

During this first and longest stage, the cervix becomes fully dilated to allow the baby's head to progress from the body of the uterus to the birth canal. Through uterine contractions, the cervix

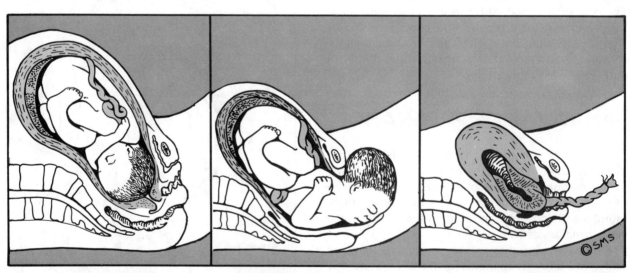

FIRST STAGE:

First uterine contraction to dilation of cervix

SECOND STAGE:

Birth of baby or expulsion

THIRD STAGE:

Delivery of placenta

FIGURE ▪ 28-2.

gradually stretches and thins until the opening is large enough to allow the baby to pass through.

The contractions usually begin as an aching sensation in the small of the back; within a short time, they become cramp-like pains in the lower abdomen that recur at regular intervals. Each contraction lasts thirty to sixty seconds; the pain disappears when the uterus relaxes. At first, the contractions usually occur ten to twenty minutes apart and are not very severe; they may even stop completely for awhile, then start again. Appearance of the mucous plug, discussed earlier, may occur before or during this stage of labor.

Stage one may continue for as long as eighteen hours or more for a woman having her first baby. Women who have had a previous baby may only experience two or three hours of early labor.

SECOND STAGE (EXPULSION)

During this period, the baby moves through the birth canal and is born. Contractions are closer together and last longer — forty-five to ninety seconds. As the baby moves down the birth canal, the mother experiences considerable pressure in her rectum, much like the feeling of a bowel movement. This means that the baby is moving downward.

When the mother has this sensation, she should lie down and get ready for the birth of her child. The tightening and bearing-down sensations will become stronger and more frequent, and the mother will have an uncontrollable urge to push down, which she may do. There probably will be more bloody discharge from the vagina at this point. Soon after the baby's head appears at the opening of the birth canal (**CROWNING**), the shoulders and the rest of the body will follow (Figures 28-3–28-14).

THIRD STAGE (PLACENTAL)

During this stage, the placenta separates from the uterine wall, and the placenta and its attached fetal membranes are expelled from the uterus.

CHILDBIRTH AND THE FIRST AIDER

Childbirth is a natural, normal process, not an illness or disease. It is, however, physically traumatic, and complications can be life-threatening. If you are called to the scene of an imminent childbirth, there are two important first-aid actions:

1. Give the mother calming reassurance. Let her know that you are there to help and that she is going to be okay.
2. Assess the mother to decide if she should be transported to the nearest medical facility, or if she should have the baby at her present location.

The First Aider can decide whether to transport the mother or to prepare for a delivery by asking the mother a few questions and conducting a simple assessment. The mother is usually nervous and apprehensive, so be gentle and kind, showing confidence and support.

Ask these questions:

▪ Have you had a baby before? The birth process will take longer with a first pregnancy, allowing for more transportation time.

▪ Are you having labor pains or contractions? How far apart are they? Contractions thin out and dilate the cervix so that the baby can come through the birth canal. If contractions are five minutes or more apart, transport; two minutes or less apart, do not transport.

▪ Has the amniotic sac (bag of waters) ruptured? If so, when? This usually signifies the end of the first stage of labor, with the birth of the baby not far behind.

▪ Do you feel the sensation of a bowel movement? These are bearing-down sensations that bring the baby through the birth canal. The baby will be born shortly. *Do not* let the mother sit on the toilet.

▪ Do you feel like the baby is ready to be born?

▪ Place the mother on her back with her legs spread and examine the vaginal area. *Do not* touch the vagina. Look to see if the crown of the baby's head, or other presenting part, is pushing out of the vagina. If there is a bulging in the vaginal area, or a part of the head is visible, prepare to deliver the baby where you are.

▪ Never ask the mother to cross her legs or ankles, and never tie or hold her legs together in an attempt to delay delivery. Never try to delay or restrain delivery in any way, since the pressure may result in death or permanent injury to the infant.

During the interview and examination process, make sure that you have sent a *specific* person to phone an ambulance and the mother's physician, if possible.

CHILDBIRTH

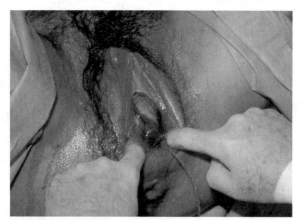

FIGURE 28-3. Early crowning.

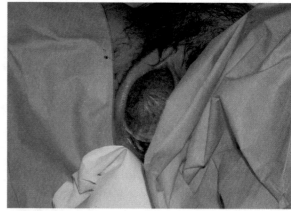

FIGURE 28-4. Late crowning.

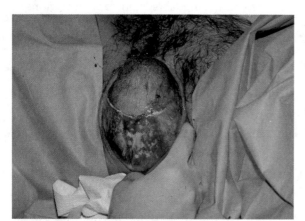

FIGURE 28-5. Head delivering.

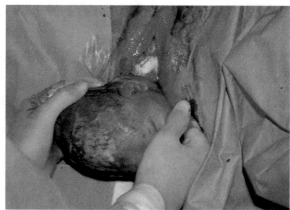

FIGURE 28-6. Head delivers and turns.

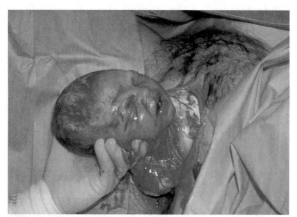

FIGURE 28-7. Shoulders deliver.

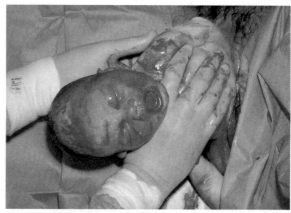

FIGURE 28-8. Chest delivers.

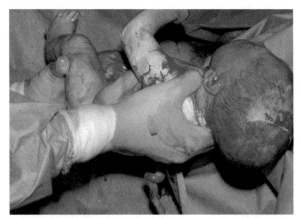

FIGURE 28-9. Infant delivered.

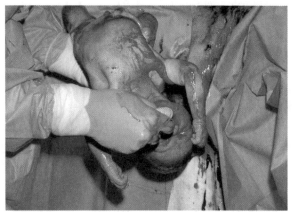

FIGURE 28-10. Suctioning airway.

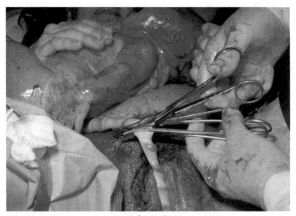

FIGURE 28-11. Cutting of cord.

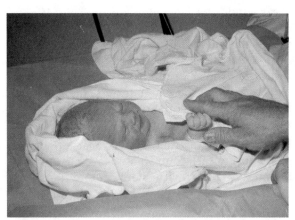

FIGURE 28-12. Wrap the baby after wiping dry with a towel.

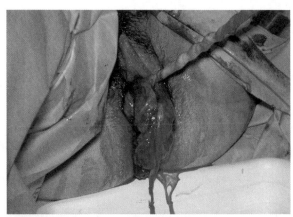

FIGURE 28-13. Placenta begins delivery.

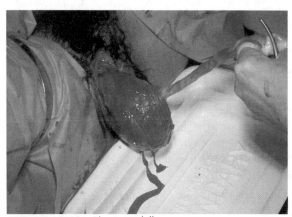

FIGURE 28-14. Placenta delivers.

ASSISTING WITH DELIVERY

1. Be calm. Reassure the mother that you are there to help her with the delivery.

2. Use sterile techniques to the greatest extent possible under the circumstances.

3. Be prepared to administer emergency care to both the mother and the baby, which may include respiratory and cardiac resuscitation for the baby, and shock prevention and control of bleeding for the mother.

4. Ensure the mother's comfort, modesty, and peace of mind as much as possible. Provide a quiet environment, undistracted by children, noise, TV, etc.

5. Have the mother lie across a bed on her back with her knees bent and separated.

6. Remove any clothing that is in the way, and place newspaper, absorbent towels, and other clean material underneath her buttocks.

7. Wear surgical or latex gloves if possible. If not, wash your hands well. Do not place your hands inside the vagina. Inspect the opening of the birth canal (vagina) to determine if the baby's head is visible during contractions. If the exposed area of the baby's head is the size of a fifty-cent piece or larger (crowning), the delivery will probably occur in minutes.

8. Encourage the mother not to bear down or strain during each contraction. Have her breathe in and out rapidly with short panting breaths.

9. *Never* try to hold back the baby's head or tell the mother to hold her legs together to prevent childbirth.

10. As the baby's head begins to emerge, make sure that the amniotic membrane is torn. If not, tear it with your fingernails *before* the baby is born.

11. As the head emerges, gently place one hand over the head and apply gentle pressure to keep the head from suddenly emerging (Figure 28-15).

12. Feel the baby's neck for a possible loop of umbilical cord. If present, slip it over the baby's head (Figure 28-15).

13. Now suction the baby's nose and mouth with a bulb syringe, or wipe out the baby's mouth and nose with facial tissues, gauze, or a clean cloth (Figure 28-15).

14. *Do not* try to push, pull, or turn the baby in any direction.

15. Support the baby's head and neck with your hands, and lift *slightly* upward to help the shoulder emerge (Figure 28-15).

16. Support the body as it emerges, remembering to get a firm hold on the baby.

17. Place the infant at vaginal level and suction the nose and mouth again.

18. Dry the baby immediately and keep it warm. Skin-to-skin contact with the mother will help to warm the baby.

19. Keep the baby's head slightly lower than the rest of its body to facilitate drainage of the throat and mouth.

20. Rub the baby's back and flick the soles of its feet to stimulate the baby's breathing. If there is a mucous obstruction problem, firmly grasp the ankles with your hand, hold the baby upside down, and stroke the baby's neck toward the mouth, then wipe out the mouth.

21. If the baby does not breathe within one minute after birth, begin mouth-to-mouth-and-nose resuscitation. See Chapter 3. Initiate infant CPR if needed. See Chapter 4.

22. Keep the umbilical cord slack, and place the baby with its head extended backward and a pad underneath its shoulders to keep an open airway. The mother can do this by holding the baby on her abdomen if necessary.

23. Try to keep the baby at the same level as the vaginal opening (i.e., between the mother's legs), but be careful that the baby does not fall from this position.

24. Allow the placenta to be born like the baby was (twenty to thirty minutes). Do *not* pull on the cord. To help the mother deliver the placenta, tell her to push or bear down as if she were having a bowel movement.

25. If the area between the mother's vagina and anus is torn and bleeding, treat it like an open wound (direct pressure with gauze or sanitary pads).

26. Place two sanitary napkins over the vaginal and **PERINEAL** area, touching only the outer surface and placing the napkins from the vagina toward the anus. Help the mother place her thighs together to hold the napkins in place.

27. The umbilical cord does not have to be cut; in fact, it can stay intact for up to two days if necessary without undue concern. After the placenta is born, place it in a plastic bag along with three-quarters of the umbilical cord. Loosely bind the top of the plastic bag.

28. Elevate the mother's feet if necessary.

29. Locate the uterus again, and massage the lower abdomen to help contract the uterus, thereby controlling bleeding. Rub with a circular

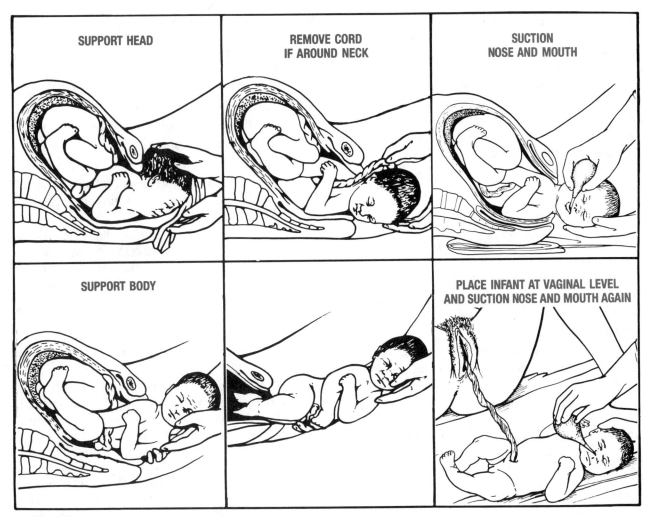

FIGURE 28-15.

motion, using the flat of your four fingers cupped around the uterus, until you feel it firm up. Encourage the mother to nurse the baby, because this will help to control bleeding by stimulating contraction of the uterus.

30. Continue to give the mother comfort and emotional support.

31. Cover the mother and baby for warmth. Remember — complications are more likely to develop in a cold, stressed infant. Prepare both for transportation to the hospital. The adequately wrapped baby should be transported in the mother's arms.

32. Jot down any important information that the physician at the hospital should know about, i.e., time of delivery, appearance and color of amniotic fluid, cord around neck, etc.

33. Tag the mother and baby with tape around their wrists, and write the mother's name on both, with the sex of the baby and the time of delivery.

34. Make sure that the mother and baby, along with the placenta in a plastic bag, are properly transported to the hospital. Transportation by ambulance is best.

OTHER EMERGENCY DELIVERIES

You may need to assist at a birth at a roadside, at an accident scene, or under other emergency conditions. Basically, try to follow the procedures as outlined previously, adapting as needed to the emergency situation.

■ Shield the mother from onlookers. Try to keep her as warm and comfortable as possible.

■ If no sterile equipment is available, use the cleanest items that you have — towels or part of the mother's clothing. If newspapers are available, place some underneath the mother. When possible, place a raincoat or blanket underneath her if she must lie on the ground.

▪ If the mother is in an automobile accident and lying on the seat, have her place one foot on the floorboard.

▪ In an emergency situation, do not try to wipe away secretions from the vagina, since you may contaminate the birth canal.

▪ Be sure to record the time of birth.

COMPLICATIONS OF PREGNANCY

If complications occur, do the following:

▪ If the cord is wrapped tightly around the baby's neck, immediately clamp or tie it in two places and cut it.

▪ If an arm, leg, or shoulder emerges first, do *not* pull. Transport the mother to the hospital immediately.

▪ If the buttocks emerge first (breech birth) (Figure 28-16), support the emerging body. *Do not* pull. Place two fingers into the vagina to locate and pull down slightly on the baby's mouth. If the baby does not emerge, transport immediately.

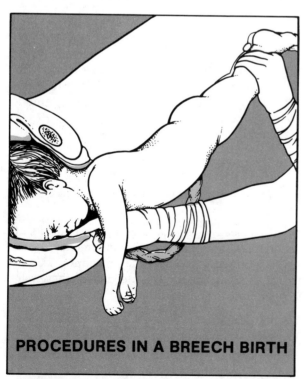

PROCEDURES IN A BREECH BIRTH

FIGURE 28-16.

▪ If a cord emerges before the baby (prolapsed cord), put your hand into the vagina and gently push the baby's head back until a pulse is felt in the umbilical cord. Stay in this position and transport immediately.

▪ In cases of spontaneous abortion:
— Provide basic life support for the woman.
— Give her care for shock.
— Call an ambulance as soon as possible.
— Have any passed tissue or evidence of blood loss (bloody sheets, towels, underwear) taken to the hospital.

▪ A common condition affecting about one out of every twenty mothers is **TOXEMIA OF PREGNANCY**. It occurs most frequently in the last trimester and is most likely to affect women in their twenties who are pregnant for the first time. The two stages of toxemia are:

— **PREECLAMPSIA**: A previously normal pregnant woman develops one or more of the signs or symptoms.

— **ECLAMPSIA**: In addition to any or all of the other signs and symptoms, the woman has convulsions, a sudden fever, and irritated reflexes. Eclampsia is one of the most severe complications of pregnancy. The death rate for mothers is from 5 to 15 percent; for babies, it is about 25 percent. Death can occur from cerebral hemorrhage, respiratory arrest, renal failure, or circulatory collapse. During a seizure, the placenta can separate from the uterine wall.

▪ Eclampsia can usually be prevented if you keep the mother quiet, which will aid in keeping her blood pressure down. If you encounter a toxemic woman:

— Contact her physician and the ambulance service immediately.

— Position the victim on her left side; this will allow her to breathe easier, thus supplying the baby with more oxygen.

— Keep the victim as calm and quiet as possible.

— Continually check the victim's vital signs until the ambulance team arrives and takes over.

| **28** | **SELF-TEST** | **28** |

Student: _____   Date: _____

Course: _____   Section #: _____

PART I: True/False   If you believe that the statement is true, circle the T. If you believe that the statement is false, circle the F.

T   F   1. Emergency childbirth is just that — measures that should be taken under an emergency when it is impossible for the mother to reach a hospital or physician.

T   F   2. If the woman is having her first child and the visible part of the baby's head is smaller than a fifty-cent piece, the birth is probably about twenty miutes away, and you should try to transport her if a hospital is close by.

T   F   3. If you are close to a medical facility and the birth begins, instruct the woman to clamp her legs tightly together and try to keep the baby's head inside the birth canal.

T   F   4. If the baby doesn't breathe within a minute after birth, the First Aider should give mouth-to-mouth-and-nose resuscitation, and should begin infant CPR if necessary.

T   F   5. It is important to take the placenta to the hospital with the mother and baby.

T   F   6. It is *not* essential for the First Aider to cut the umbilical cord.

T   F   7. After delivery, gentle massage of the uterus helps to control the mother's bleeding.

T   F   8. The mother and baby should always be taken to the hospital after the birth.

T   F   9. A gentle pull on the baby as it is being born will give a more efficient delivery.

T   F   10. An umbilical cord that is wrapped around the baby's neck must be quickly, but gently, removed.

PART II: Multiple Choice   For each question, circle the answer that best reflects an accurate statement.

1. If the baby's head emerges from the birth canal and the amniotic sac is still unbroken, you should:
    a. wait for the baby to emerge completely.
    b. tear the bag with your fingers so that the fluid can drain.
    c. carefully puncture the bag, taking care not to injure the baby.

2. A woman should be given immediate help instead of transport when her labor contractions are regularly spaced:
    a. five minutes apart.
    b. three minutes apart.
    c. two minutes or less apart.
    d. one minute apart.

3. A baby should be breathing within how much time after birth?
    a. ten seconds.
    b. one to two minutes.
    c. five minutes.
    d. thirty to forty-five seconds.

4. In order to decide whether to transport the mother prior to delivery, the First Aider should:
    a. ask the mother if she is having her first baby.
    b. examine the mother for signs of crowning.
    c. ask the mother if she feels as if she has to move her bowels.
    d. all of the above.

5. As the baby's head emerges, you should:
    a. push gently on top of the head.
    b. pull gently on top of the head.
    c. apply downward pressure.
    d. guide and support the head.

6. If the baby does not begin to breathe by itself, you should:
    a. start mouth-to-mouth-and-nose resuscitation, and begin infant CPR if necessary.
    b. hyperextend its neck.
    c. use the Holgar-Nielsen method of resuscitation.
    d. turn the baby upside down and gently shake it.

7. To make a final decision about delivery at the scene:
    a. ask the woman how far apart her contractions are.
    b. examine the vaginal opening for signs of crowning.
    c. feel the woman's abdomen for signs of movement.
    d. check the perineum for signs of bulging.

8. If a First Aider starts for the hospital with the mother and the delivery starts during the trip, the First Aider should:
    a. stop and prepare for the delivery.
    b. have the woman hold her legs together tightly.
    c. pack the vaginal opening with sanitary napkins.
    d. place the hand firmly against the vaginal opening.

9. Labor is divided into _____ stages.
    a. 2.   c. 4.
    b. 3.   d. 1.

10. The longest stage of labor is likely the:
    a. first stage (dilation).
    b. second stage (expulsion).
    c. third stage (placental).
    d. all stages are about equal in length.

11. The purpose of uterine contractions in the first stage of labor is to:
    a. dislodge the placenta and stimulate pelvic expansion.
    b. force extra oxygenated blood to the baby and move the baby through the birth canal.
    c. stretch the cervix to allow the baby to pass through.
    d. sluff off excess blood and nutrients from the uterine wall to provide the baby with extra nutrients for the birth ordeal.

12. The developing baby is attached by the umbilical cord to the:
    a. cervix.
    b. placenta.
    c. amniotic sac.
    d. perineum.

13. The umbilical cord contains:
    a. one vein and one artery.
    b. one vein and two arteries.
    c. two veins and one artery.
    d. two arteries.

14. There are three cases in which you should *not* try to transport a mother who is about to deliver to the hospital. They include all *except*:
    a. when you have no transportation available.
    b. when the hospital or doctor cannot be reached.
    c. when the delivery can be expected within five minutes.
    d. if the mother requests you to act as the midwife or physician.

15. If you think you have time to transport the mother to the hospital, do *all but one* of the following:
    a. keep the mother lying down.
    b. allow the mother to go to the toilet immediately before you leave.
    c. never ask the mother to cross her legs in an attempt to delay delivery.
    d. have the mother bend her knees and spread her thighs apart so that you can watch for crowning.

16. Crowning indicates:
    a. the position of the baby is incorrect for delivery.
    b. the baby's head can be seen at the opening of the birth canal.
    c. the bag of waters is not broken.
    d. lack of oxygen in the baby.

17. As the delivery is imminent, have the mother:
    a. pant with the contractions.
    b. push as hard as she can.
    c. hold her breath for 15-second intervals.
    d. take slow, deep breaths.

PART III: Matching: Match the descriptions with the proper stage of childbirth.

Stages of Labor	Descriptions
Stage 1	A. The placenta is "born."
Stage 2	B. Contractions occur and the "bag of waters" breaks.
Stage 3	C. The baby is born.

PART IV: What Would You Do If:

You are at a neighboring apartment where a woman is in labor. The hospital is thirty minutes away. She suddenly says, "The baby's coming — *now!*" This is her sixth child.

1. What questions would you ask the mother?

2. What preparations would you make for childbirth?

3. How would you assist with the childbirth?

CHAPTER TWENTY-NINE

OBJECTIVES

- Understand the various burn classifications and how they relate to the anatomy of the skin.
- Identify the characteristics of first-, second-, and third-degree burns and be able to calculate the extent of burns using the Rule of Nines.
- Explain how to assess the severity of burns and describe appropriate burn management for thermal burns.
- Identify the signs and symptoms of inhalation injuries and describe appropriate emergency care.
- Recognize the various types of chemical burns and describe appropriate emergency care.
- Understand how electrical energy and lightning can injure the body and describe appropriate emergency care for electrical shock and lightning injuries.

BURN EMERGENCIES

TYPES OF BURN INJURIES

More than two million burn accidents occur each year in the United States. Of those who are burned (in fires, by chemicals, by the sun, in automobile accidents, or in other kinds of accidents), more than 12,000 die as a result of their burns, and almost one million require long-term hospitalization. Burns are a leading cause of accidental death in the United States.

Burns can be complex injuries. In addition to the burn itself, a number of other functions may be affected. Since burns injure the skin, they impair the body's normal fluid/electrolyte balance, body temperature, body thermal regulation, joint function, manual dexterity, and physical appearance (Figure 29-1).

Children under the age of six receive more burns than people in any other age group. The most common kind of burn is a **SCALD** (Figure 29-2). Toddlers pull pans of boiling water off of stoves. People scurrying to get dinner on the table trip over an infant crawling across the floor and dump a steaming cauldron of soup all over the infant. People misjudging the temperature of bath water dip babies into steaming tubs and turn faucets of scalding water on soapy arms and legs. In terms of injury and death, scald burns are the most severe.

Second to scalds in this age group are **CONTACT BURNS** (Figure 29-3). An eighteen-month-old who is just learning to walk needs to support his shaky steps, and he will lean against a radiator, oven door, woodburning stove, or other hot object as readily as he will lean against a sofa. There are other kinds of burns, too, as houses catch on fire and parents do not wake up. Small children sometimes chew on electrical cords sustaining severe electrical burns (Figure 29-3).

Children from the ages of three to eight still suffer most from scald burns — and still in the kitchen and

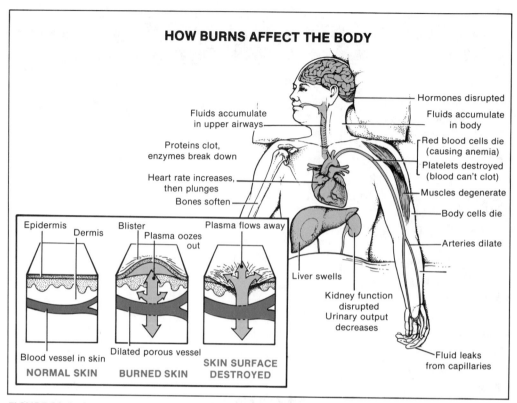

FIGURE 29-1. Burns may cause shock by damaging surface tissue and dilating underlying blood vessels, which may lead to extensive loss of plasma.

bathtub — but they also have discovered matches and cigarette lighters. Some like to fix breakfast for themselves and end up igniting pajamas on stove tops. Some use their teeth to pry stubborn electrical cords out of wall sockets. Children nine to twelve may play with gunpowder and gasoline; others stand nearby and watch. All may be hurt in the resulting explosion.

In adolescence, flame injury is the most serious burn risk. There are automobile accidents — steam burns from radiators, eye burns from battery acid, flaming gasoline from rear-end collisions. Concerned with their appearance, teenagers misuse sunlamps.

Young adults who have joined the work force become vulnerable to the whole range of industrial

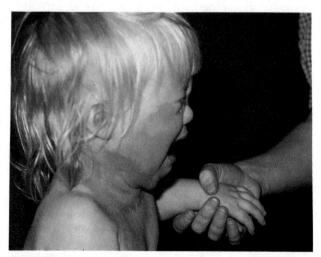

FIGURE 29-2. Scalds are the most common causes of burns in children under eight years of age.

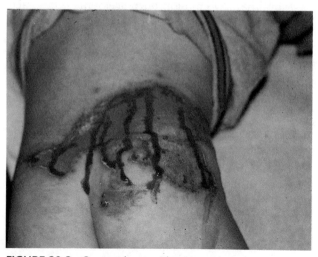

FIGURE 29-3. Contact burn with a steam iron.

burns — flame, chemical, and electrical. Those in the twenty to forty-four age group are often worried, preoccupied, and troubled, and as a result, they are not careful.

In adults forty-five to sixty years of age, matches, stoves, and smoking materials are the most common sources of ignition. Those over sixty have lost some valuable reflexes and abilities, and they are the most vulnerable of all.

Depending on the type of accident that caused the fire or burn, there is often associated trauma. Most frequently, you will see burn victims with internal injury, blunt trauma, head injury, multiple fractures, and serious lacerations.

The seriousness of a burn is determined by the following factors:

- Degree of the burn.
- Percentage of the body burned.
- Severity of the burn.
- Location of the burn.
- Accompanying complications (such as pre-existing physical or mental conditions).
- Age of the victim.

DEGREE OF THE BURN

Burns are classified by degree of damage to the skin and underlying tissues. (See Figures 29-4–29-11.)

FIRST-DEGREE BURNS

First-degree burns can be caused by a flash, a flame, a scald, or the sun. They are the most common and the most minor of all burns. The skin surface is dry; no blisters or swelling occur. The skin is reddened and extremely painful, but the epidermal layer is the only one affected (Figures 29-12 and 29-13). First-degree burns heal in two to five days with no scarring. Peeling of the outer epidermal layer usually occurs, and some temporary discoloration may result.

SECOND-DEGREE BURNS

Second-degree burns result from contact with hot liquids or solids, flash or flame contact with clothing, direct flame from fires, contact with chemical substances, or the sun. The skin appears moist and mottled, and it ranges in color from white to cherry red. The burned area is blistered and extremely painful. The epidermis and dermal layers of skin are usually burned, and damage may result to some fat domes of the subcutaneous (fatty tissue just underneath the skin) layer (see Figures 29-12 and 29-13).

Second-degree burns are considered minor if they involve less than 15 percent of the body surface in adults and less than 10 percent in children. When 15 to 30 percent of an adult's body surface or 10 to 20 percent of a child's body surface is involved, a second-degree burn is considered moderate. The burn is considered severe if it involves the face, hands, feet, or genital area. A second-degree burn is considered critical if it involves more than 30 percent of the total body surface in an adult and 20 percent in a child.

Healing of a minor second-degree burn usually requires five to twenty-one days; if infection occurs, healing time usually takes longer.

THIRD-DEGREE BURNS

Third-degree, or full thickness burns, are the most serious, resulting from contact with hot liquids or solids, flames, chemicals, or electricity. The skin becomes dry and leathery; charred blood vessels are often visible. The skin is a mixture of colors: white (waxy-pearly), dark (khaki-mahogany), and charred. While a third-degree burn may be very painful, the victim often feels little or no pain, because the nerve endings have been destroyed (see Figures 29-12 and 29-13). The burn extends through all dermal layers and can involve subcutaneous layers, muscles, organs, and bone. (In some areas, a burn that involves the muscle and bone is classified as a fourth-degree burn.)

Third-degree burns are considered minor if they occur on less than 2 percent of the body surface. Moderate burns involve 2 to 10 percent of the body surface. Third-degree burns are classified as critical if they occur on more than 10 percent of the total body surface, if there is any involvement of the face, hands, feet, or genital area, or if the burns are caused by chemicals or electricity.

Third-degree burns that cover small areas require weeks to heal, while larger burns usually require skin grafting and take months or years to heal completely.

PERCENTAGE OF BODY BURNED: THE RULE OF NINES

The Rule of Nines (Figure 29-14) can be used to calculate quickly the amount of skin surface that has received burns. It can help you to quickly understand the severity of a burn.

TYPES OF BURNS

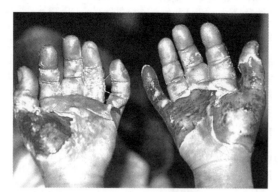

FIGURE 29-4. Second- and third-degree burns.

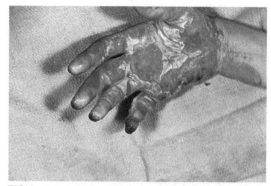

FIGURE 29-5. Third-degree flare burns.

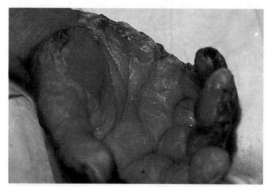

FIGURE 29-6. Second- and third-degree burns.

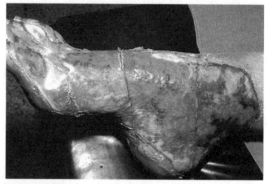

FIGURE 29-7. Second- and third-degree burns.

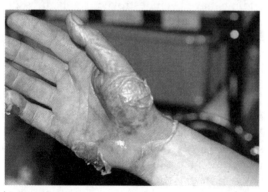

FIGURE 29-8. Second-degree burn.

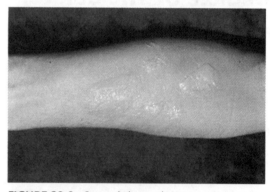

FIGURE 29-9. Second-degree burn.

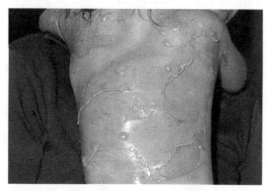

FIGURE 29-10. Second-degree burn.

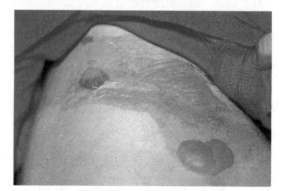

FIGURE 29-11. Second-degree burn.

BURNS CLASSIFICATION

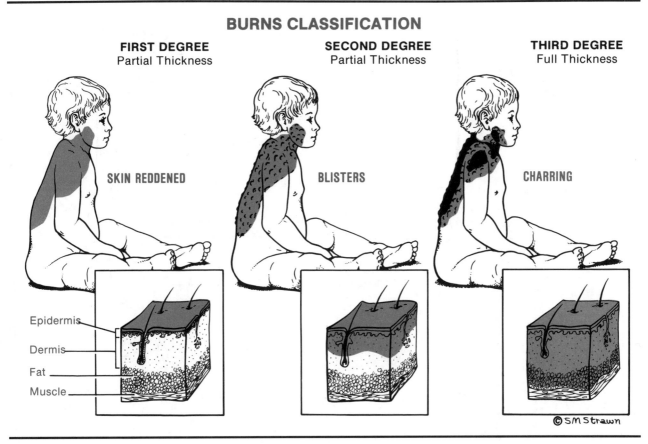

FIRST DEGREE Partial Thickness	**SECOND DEGREE** Partial Thickness	**THIRD DEGREE** Full Thickness
SKIN REDDENED	BLISTERS	CHARRING

Epidermis
Dermis
Fat
Muscle

©SMStrawn

FIGURE 29-12.

SKIN LAYERS AND STRUCTURES

DEGREE OF BURN

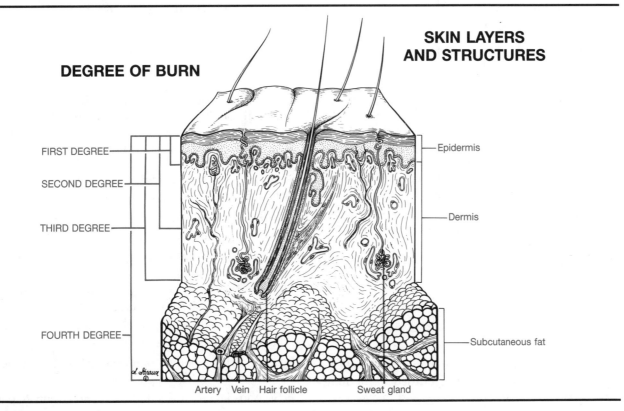

FIRST DEGREE
SECOND DEGREE
THIRD DEGREE
FOURTH DEGREE

Epidermis
Dermis
Subcutaneous fat

Artery   Vein   Hair follicle   Sweat gland

FIGURE 29-13. Classification of burns according to the depth of tissue involvement.

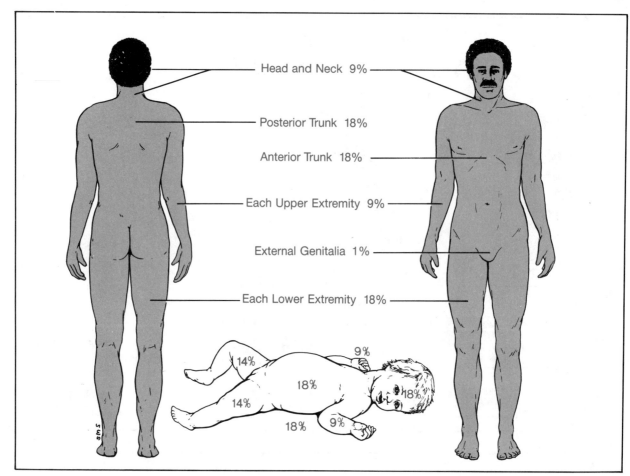

FIGURE 29-14. The Rule of Nines: A method for estimating percentage of body surface involved with burns. The body surface is divided into regions, each of which represents 9% or a multiple of 9% of the total surface, except in infants.

The Rule of Nines divides the body into regions, each of which represents 9 percent of the total body surface (or a multiple of 9 percent). Head and neck compose 9 percent; anterior (front) trunk, 18 percent; posterior (back) trunk, 18 percent; each upper extremity, 9 percent; the genital area, 1 percent; and each lower extremity, 18 percent. For infants and children, the same percentages may be used with the exception of the head and legs. Appearance, sensation, and circulation around the burn can also help you to classify burns.

SEVERITY OF THE BURN

Most burn wounds are a combination of classifications; that is, part of the skin is burned to the first degree, part to the second degree, and maybe part to the third degree.

A full-thickness burn (third degree) is one that burns through all layers of skin into the subcutaneous tissues; first- and second-degree burns, going through only part of the skin, are referred to as partial-thickness burns.

In general, the following burns are considered critical (Figure 29-15):

- Burns that are complicated by respiratory tract injuries or other major injuries or fractures.
- Third-degree burns involving the face, hands, feet, or genital area.
- Third-degree burns that cover more than 10 percent of an adult's body surface.
- Third-degree burns that cover more than 2 to 3 percent of a child's body surface.
- Second-degree burns that cover more than 30 percent of an adult's body surface.
- Second-degree burns that cover more than 20 percent of a child's body surface.

CRITICAL BURNS

NOTE: The general condition of the victim must also be considered. For example, a moderate burn in an aged or critically ill person might be serious.

CRITICAL BURNS are burns complicated by respiratory tract injury and other major injuries or fractures.

THIRD-DEGREE burns involving the critical areas of the face, hands, feet, or genitalia.

SECOND-DEGREE burns covering more than 30% of the body surface.

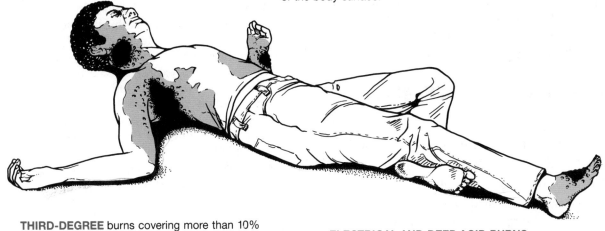

THIRD-DEGREE burns covering more than 10% of the body surface.

ELECTRICAL AND DEEP ACID BURNS

BURNS in victims with underlying physical or medical conditions.

FIGURE 29-15.

- First-degree burns that cover more than 75 percent of the body surface.
- Most chemical burns.
- Most electrical burns.
- Burns in victims who have serious underlying medical conditions, such as diabetes, seizure disorders, or hypertension.

In general, the following burns are classified as moderate:

- Third-degree burns that cover from 2 to 10 percent of an adult's body surface, excluding the face, eyes, ears, hands, feet, and genital area.
- Second-degree burns that cover between 15 and 30 percent of an adult's body surface.
- First-degree burns that cover between 50 and 75 percent of an adult's body surface.
- An uncomplicated burn that covers between 10 and 20 percent of a child's body surface in the second degree.

- Critical burns that do not have complicating factors.

In general, the following burns are classified as minor:

- Second-degree burns covering less than 15 percent of the total body surface of an adult.
- Second-degree burns covering less than 10 percent of the total body surface of a child.
- First-degree burns that involve less than 20 percent of an adult's or child's body surface.

Remember — even *minor* burns of the face, eyes, ears, hands, feet, or genital area need immediate care and transport to a hospital.

LOCATION OF THE BURN

Certain areas of the body are more critically damaged by burns than others, and it is essential that you recognize which areas represent the greatest hazard.

Burns on the face or neck should be seen by a physician immediately because of possible burns to the eye area or respiratory complications. Check the eyes to make sure that no injury has occurred. Then assess whether respiratory damage is present.

Other locations of burns that are particularly critical include the hands, feet, and external genitalia. Any burn to the upper body is more serious than a burn of similar extent and degree on the lower body. Victims with burns in any of these areas should be transported to a hospital or burn center immediately.

BURN MANAGEMENT

The first priority in emergency care is to prevent further injury. The problems most often associated with burns are:

- Airway or respiratory difficulties.
- Related musculoskeletal injuries.
- Loss of body fluids, contributing to shock.
- Pain contributing to shock.
- Anxiety contributing to shock.
- Swelling.
- Infection due to destruction of skin tissue.

Care of a burn and associated injuries must start immediately — preferably at the moment of burning. Unfortunately, this early emergency care is too often administered by terrified but well-meaning family, friends, or bystanders. Sometimes even the burn victim himself will attempt to care for the burn. One reason why burns are so often critically damaging or even fatal is that some individuals who administer early emergency care are poorly informed about methods of care. Instead of helping the victim, they hinder or even hurt him. Remember: a First Aider does not *treat* a burn; he merely cares for the burn until the victim can be transported to a hospital or burn center for thorough treatment.

EMERGENCY CARE

Your first priority is to prevent further injury to the victim or injury to others. Emergency care for specific burns will be discussed later in this chapter. Regardless of the type of burn, use the following general guidelines in administering care:

1. Remove the victim from the source of the burn. This seems extremely simple, but it is surprising how many fail to do this. If the victim was burned by a fire, take him as far away as possible without inflicting further injury. Get him far enough away so that he does not inhale smoke. If the burn resulted from the victim lying in a puddle of petroleum by-product or strong chemical, take him out of the puddle. If he was struck by lightning, get him to shelter.

2. Eliminate the cause of the burn. Again, this is simple logic. Put out the fire. Wash away the chemicals. (Greater details on this follow.) Immerse scald or grease burns in cold water to stop the burning (Figure 29-16). If the victim's clothes are on fire, roll him on the ground until the flames are extinguished, douse him with water, and remove all clothing (including items that tend to retain heat, such as jewelry and shoes). Never cover a burn with dirt in an attempt to extinguish flames unless it's the only available thing. If you successfully eliminate the cause of the burn, you can help prevent someone else at the scene from sustaining a burn injury.

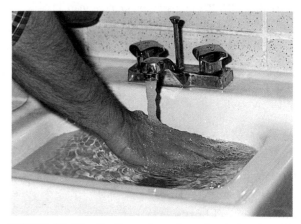

FIGURE 29-16. Cooling a burn by submerging in cold running water.

3. Assess the victim's vital signs — airway, breathing, and circulation — as you would for any injury.

4. Assess for respiratory/cardiac complications. Check the victim thoroughly to determine whether breathing or heartbeat have stopped. If the victim is still breathing, look for signs of injury to the respiratory system. Be especially alert for wheezing or coughing as the victim breathes, for sooty or smoky smell on his breath, for particles of soot in his saliva, and for burns of the mucous membranes in his mouth and nostrils. If any of these signs are present, immediately assist breathing. Even though the victim does

not manifest actual breathing difficulty at the time he receives the burn, remember that respiratory injuries frequently do not manifest themselves until twelve to twenty-four hours after the actual injury. This type of victim requires hospitalization.

5. Cover the burn with a sterile burn dressing or sheet.

6. Activate the EMS system as soon as possible.

INHALATION INJURIES

More than half of all fire-related deaths are caused by smoke inhalation; 80 percent of those who die in residential fires do so because they have inhaled heated air, smoke, or other toxic gases — not because they have been burned to death. Suspect inhalation injury in any victim of thermal burn, especially if the victim was confined in an enclosed space at any time during the fire.

Three causes of inhalation injury accompany burns:

▪ Heat inhalation.

▪ Inhalation of toxic chemicals or smoke.

▪ Inhalation of carbon monoxide (the most common burn-associated inhalation injury).

Most of the damage done to the upper airway is a result of heat inhalation — mucous membranes and linings get scorched, and edema partially blocks the airway. The severity of the inhalation injury is determined by the products of combustion (what was burned), the degree of combustion (how completely the materials were burned), the duration of exposure (how long the victim was exposed to the smoke or gases), and whether the victim was in a confined space.

Because edema and other damage can be progressive, the inhalation injury may appear to be mild at first but may become more severe. Depending on the materials that were burned and the length of the victim's exposure to the fire, symptoms may occur within a few minutes but may not appear for many hours.

Specific signs and symptoms of upper-airway injuries are (Figure 29-17):

▪ Singed nasal hairs.

▪ Burned specks of carbon in the sputum.

▪ A sooty or smoky smell on the breath.

▪ Respiratory distress accompanied by restriction of chest-wall movement, restlessness, chest tightness, difficulty in swallowing, hoarseness, coughing, cyanosis, and noisy breathing.

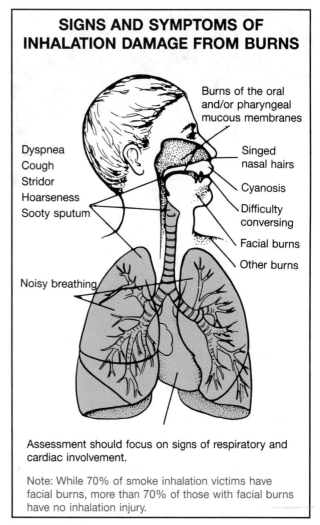

SIGNS AND SYMPTOMS OF INHALATION DAMAGE FROM BURNS

Burns of the oral and/or pharyngeal mucous membranes

Dyspnea
Cough
Stridor
Hoarseness
Sooty sputum

Singed nasal hairs

Cyanosis

Difficulty conversing

Facial burns

Other burns

Noisy breathing

Assessment should focus on signs of respiratory and cardiac involvement.

Note: While 70% of smoke inhalation victims have facial burns, more than 70% of those with facial burns have no inhalation injury.

FIGURE 29-17.

▪ You may be able to see actual burns of the oral mucosa (Figure 29-18).

Assume respiratory injury if in doubt, especially if facial burns are present.

More critical respiratory injury results from the inhalation of noxious chemicals, carbon-monoxide fumes, or smoke. Noxious fumes can result from the burning of a number of ordinary household objects, such as carpets, draperies, wall coverings, floor coverings, upholstery, and lacquered wood veneer on furniture. There are almost three hundred toxic substances that result from burning wood alone.

When noxious fumes are inhaled, mucosa in the lungs swell and break, leaking fluid into the nearby alveolar spaces and damaging the cilia. Mucous builds up and plugs the air passages. The final result is reduced oxygen exchange that can eventually lead to death if left untreated.

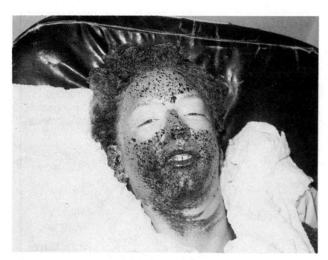

FIGURE 29-18. Facial inhalation burn.

Carbon-monoxide poisoning is the major cause of death at the scene of a fire. Even when carbon-monoxide does not cause death, it can cause long-term neurological damage by depriving the brain of oxygen (while the damage will not be apparent for several days, its onset is usually rapid after that). Almost everything gives off carbon-monoxide when it burns. Carbon-monoxide is colorless, odorless, and tasteless, making it extremely difficult to detect. Carbon-monoxide is especially hazardous among sleeping victims, who simply never wake up.

Since burns usually do not alter levels of consciousness, assume that any burn victim who is unconscious is suffering from carbon-monoxide poisoning (see Chapter 18, "Poisoning Emergencies"). Even if the victim is conscious but complains of headache and weakness, nausea and/or vomiting, and loss of manual dexterity, or if he seems confused, lethargic, irrational, or reckless, immediately assume that carbon-monoxide poisoning has occurred. *Very* late signs and symptoms may include a cherry-red coloring of the unburned skin, changes in coloration of the mucous membranes (usually to bright cherry red), unconsciousness, and obvious neurological damage. Do not rely on any one of these signs or symptoms to lead you in a sure direction. Cherry-red discoloration may not occur until after death, for example, so you should not wait for it as an indication in a victim.

Victims who have sustained severe respiratory injury may experience no change in skin color and no unusual signs of injury in the chest area. The signs and symptoms listed above can be a clue, as can burns of the head, neck, or upper body and changes in the level of consciousness.

EMERGENCY CARE

Take the following measures to prevent further respiratory complications:

1. Place the victim in an upright position to allow for easier breathing if vital signs and injuries do not contraindicate it.
2. If respiratory distress occurs, maintain an adequate airway.
3. Remove the victim as far as possible from the source of the burn — especially if it is a fire. Try to situate him so that he is breathing fresh air and has no danger of inhaling more smoke.
4. Mouth-to-mouth ventilation may be required to help him initiate his own clear breathing. Clear all foreign particles from the airway.
5. Remove any clothing that may restrict chest movement or breathing. Remove neckties and necklaces if they have not burned and if they are not sticking to the skin.
6. Activate the EMS system immediately.

THERMAL AND RADIANT BURNS

Thermal burns are caused by flame or radiant heat, including sunburn and scalding.

EMERGENCY CARE

Emergency care should always begin by removing the victim from the source of the burn or extinguishing the source itself. Unless specified otherwise, do the following regardless of the degree of burn:

1. Put out the fire and extinguish burning clothing.
2. After assuring airway and breathing, remove any smoldering clothing that does not stick to the burned skin, and remove any shoes or jewelry that may retain heat. Be sure that they do not stick to the skin. If clothing adheres to the skin, cut carefully around it, but do not try to remove it forcefully.
3. First-degree burns should be immersed in cool water (see Figure 29-16); place a cool compress on burns located on the trunk or face. Whenever possible, make a moist compress with sterile gauze and clean water; whatever you use, both water and dressings must be as clean as possible. Remoisten dressings periodically to keep them damp but not soaked (Figure 29-19). *Note: Some physicians do not recommend wet burn dressings for any type of burn — follow local protocol.* Cover the

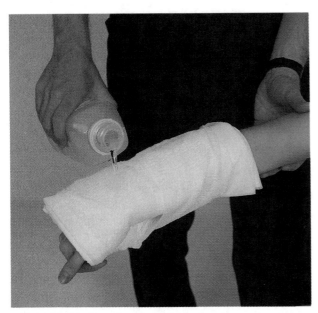

FIGURE 29-19. Remoistening a burn dressing.

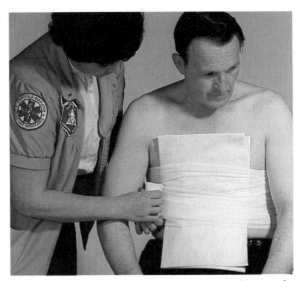

FIGURE 29-21. Application of bulky burn dressing for moderate and critical burns.

burned area with a sterile dressing or other clean woven materials, such as sheets or towels; do not use material that might adhere or disintegrate (See Figure 29-20 for a burn-care kit). Never use ice, ointments, or any other covering on any type of burn. For all but the most superficial first-degree burns, transport the victim to a hospital or activate the EMS system.

4. Second-degree burns should be immersed in cool water and covered with cool compresses within thirty minutes of occurrence. Moderate and critical burns should be covered with a bulky, dry dressing and loosely bandaged in place (Figures 29-21 and 29-22). This emergency care can substantially reduce swelling and provide significant pain relief. Never try to rupture blisters over the burn; if you accidentally break a blister, keep it as sterile as possible.

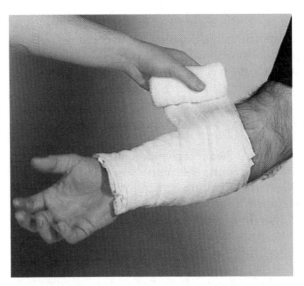

FIGURE 29-22. In moderate and critical burns, cover with a thick, clean, dry dressing and loosely bandage in place.

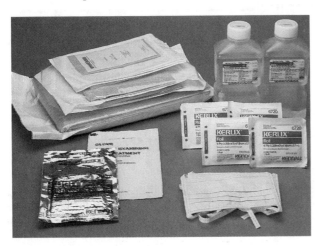

FIGURE 29-20. Burn-care kit.

5. Protect the victim from heat loss and possible hypothermia by covering him with a dry blanket, avoiding exposure to drafts. Burn victims have had their body's normal thermal regulatory system disrupted, and they can lose heat rapidly.

6. Anticipate respiratory problems if burns are present around the face (especially if nasal hairs or openings are singed), if the victim has been unconscious in a burning area, or if the victim has been exposed to smoke or hot gases. Any burn victim can rapidly develop respiratory complications. *Assume that inhalation injury has occurred until proven otherwise.*

7. Take appropriate measures to prevent shock.

Once you have completed initial emergency care, examine the victim for any obscured damage. Especially examine the eyes for burns or other injury, the pulses in all extremities (since swelling can act as a tourniquet), and all limbs (to determine possible fractures or lacerations). Remove any other jewelry, belt buckles, or glasses that might constrict the body in the event of swelling.

Thermal burns in infants and small children pose a special problem, because their body surface is much larger in proportion to their total body mass. Therefore, potential fluid losses are massive, and the onset of shock rapid. Wrap a burned baby in a moist, sterile sheet, and cover him with enough blankets to keep him warm. Activate the EMS system immediately, and maintain the airway while waiting for emergency personnel.

SCALDING

Cover scald burns (Figures 29-23–29-25) with a cool, moist, sterile dressing. Transport the victim to a hospital or activate the EMS system. Do not apply ointment, grease, or butter to the scalded area.

SUNBURN

Sunburn, the most common type of burn, should be cared for with cool compresses if the burn is first degree. Transport any victim to a hospital who has developed blistering or who has experienced obvious fluid loss. Intensity of the burn will depend on factors such as whether the victim's skin was wet, whether the wind was blowing, and at what altitude the victim was when the burn was sustained. Burns in redheaded, blond, or fair-skinned victims will likely be more critical than those in brunettes.

CHEMICAL BURNS

Speed is essential for chemical burns, the more quickly you can remove the source of the burn and initiate care, the less severe the burn will be. Any chemical burn is considered particularly severe if it involves the eyes, face, hands, feet, genital area, or large areas of tissue anywhere on the body (Figure 29-26).

EMERGENCY CARE

Prior to beginning emergency care, make sure that it is safe to approach the victim; if not, wait for trained rescue personnel to arrive. During each step of rescue, make sure that you protect yourself from contamination.

1. If possible, immediately don latex or rubber gloves to prevent injury to yourself, and begin to flush the burned area vigorously and forcefully with water; if the victim is at home, the shower or garden hose is ideal. Irrigate the area continuously for at least *twenty minutes* under a steady stream of water, and make sure that no particles of chemical remain. There are three important exceptions to this rule:

   - Lime powder creates a corrosive substance when mixed with water; keep the lime powder dry, brush it off the victim's skin, and remove the victim's clothing if there is lime powder on it. Then flush with water (Figures 29-27 and 29-28).

   - Phenol (carbolic acid) should be washed off with alcohol prior to irrigating the burn with water. If alcohol is not available or if you are not sure it is phenol, immediately irrigate with water. *Follow local protocol.*

SCALD INJURIES

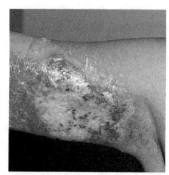

FIGURE 29-23. Scald burn.

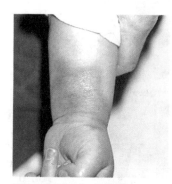

FIGURE 29-24. Scald burn.

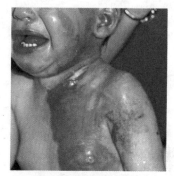

FIGURE 29-25. Third-degree scald burn.

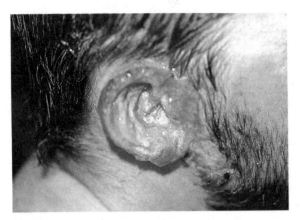

FIGURE 29-26. Chemical burn.

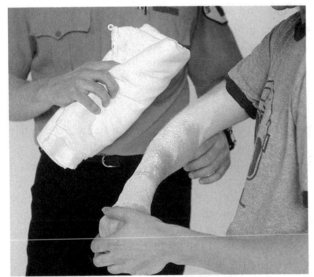

FIGURE 29-27. Lime powder should be brushed off the skin before flushing with water.

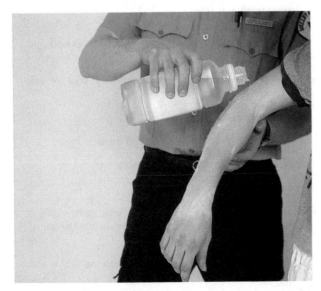

FIGURE 29-28. After brushing off lime powder, flush with water.

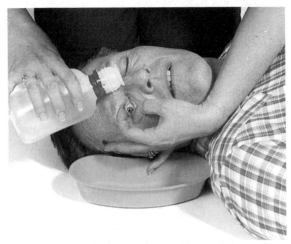

FIGURE 29-29. Flushing a chemical burn of the eye.

■ Concentrated sulfuric acid produces heat when mixed with water and may cause greater burn injuries unless flushed vigorously with a hose or in a shower.

2. While flushing, remove the victim's clothing, shoes, and stockings and any other items of jewelry or apparel that might be contaminated with the chemical. Take care not to contaminate your own skin, eyes, or clothing with the substance.

3. After you remove the victim's clothing, continue flushing his entire body for about thirty minutes. Do not waste time trying to find an antidote — flushing with water is more effective and most available.

4. Make sure to flush the eyes if any chemicals splash into them (Figure 29-29). Have the victim remove contact lenses if he is wearing them, because they prevent thorough irrigation of the eye. Use a faucet or hose running on low pressure; you might also use a pan, a bucket, a cup, or a bottle. Be sure to irrigate well underneath the lids, and flush for at least twenty minutes. Never use a chemical antidote in the eyes. See Chapter 14, "Eye Injuries."

5. When flushing is complete, cover the area with a sterile dressing.

6. Do not make the mistake of trying to neutralize a burned area with alkali or acid solutions. You may guess wrong about the content of the chemical agent that caused the burn, and you may worsen the burn by attempting to neutralize it. You may also miscalculate the quantity needed to neutralize it. Worst of all, neutralization reactions generate heat that can extend the depth of tissue damage and intensify the injury.

7. Activate the EMS system as soon as possible.

The most common types of chemical injury result from acids and alkalis (e.g., lye). Oxidizing agents destroy tissue, reducing agents denature the body protein, and desiccants cause dehydration and excessive heat in bodily tissues. Depending on the chemical agent, burns from chemicals damage much more than just skin surface; underlying tissue damage is usually great and is intensified by failure to act quickly and irrigate properly. If possible, get the name of the chemical involved and send the container to the hospital with the victim.

ELECTRICAL BURNS

Approximately 3,000 electrical injuries each year in the United States cause burns, and approximately 40 percent of all victims die as a result of their injuries. While lightning accounts for approximately 25 percent of all electrical-burn injuries, it only causes fewer than two hundred deaths per year in the United States. Approximately 3 percent of all serious burn injuries are caused by electrical accidents, and approximately 90 percent of the victims of electrical burns are male.

Understanding electrical burns is critical; it will not only help you to aid a victim, but it may also save your own life.

PROTECTING YOURSELF AND THE VICTIM

Follow these guidelines when approaching an accident that involves downed power lines or other electrical hazards:

- Look for downed wires whenever an accident has involved a vehicle that has struck a power pole. How can you tell if a line might be downed and hidden in the grass or brush? Carefully look at the next pole down the line, and count the number of power lines at the top crossarm — there should be the same number of lines at the top crossarm of the damaged pole. If there aren't, watch out! If it is dark, use a flashlight or spotlight to inspect the poles and surrounding area (Table 29-1).

- *Never* attempt to move downed wires! Only authorized repairmen from the power company should be allowed to touch a high-voltage wire; they have the skill and the proper equipment (including high-voltage rubber gloves and fiberglass prods).

- Call for help from the power company *immediately* upon observing a downed power line.

- If a downed power line is lying across a wrecked vehicle, *do not touch the vehicle*, even if the victims inside are seriously injured. You will most likely die if you touch it. If the victims inside are conscious, shout to them and warn them not to leave the vehicle — if they touch the ground and the car at the same time, the current will kill them.

TABLE 29-1	RULES FOR DOWNED POWER LINES
	1. If any lines are suspected of being down, notify the power company and request an emergency crew. Then notify all rescue personnel of possible danger.
	2. Inspect the emergency scene. If there is a possibility of a downed line or weakened pole, do not proceed in your vehicle, and do not leave your vehicle until you have inspected the surrounding area.
	3. If the vehicle is in contact with the line, stay inside and wait for the power company crew.
	4. When entering an area, if the soles of your feet tingle, go no further. You are entering an energized area.
	5. A downed power line should be assumed to be live unless the power company crew says otherwise.
	6. Remember that vehicles, guardrails, metal fences, etc., conduct electricity.
	7. If a vehicle is in contact with a live wire, maintain a safe distance, and tell victims to remain in the vehicle until the power company crews can assist. Never have a victim attempt to jump clear of a vehicle unless there is immediate danger of explosion or fire.
	8. Remember that hurried actions in an emergency situation involving downed power lines can jeopardize the victim and the rescuer.
	9. **Never attempt to move a high-voltage power line.**

- If the car begins to burn and the victims inside are at risk of dying in the fire, instruct them to open the car door and jump as far as they can away from the car. In any case, it is critical that they *not touch the car and the ground at the same time.*

- If a downed power line is in the area but is *not* near or touching the vehicle, proceed as usual with emergency care.

- Relatively low voltages, such as household 120 volts, can cause burns to tender tissue such as the mouth (when a child chews on an electrical cord, for example — see Figure 29-30). However, many victims of electrocution (such as swimmers when a poolside radio falls into the water) will show no visible signs of injury.

- The best clue for scene evaluation is to make a visual sweep for power cords that may be routed to a tool that the victim may still be holding. (Remember, a power tool does not have to be "on" to present a shock hazard!) If you have a possible pool-drowning victim, check quickly in the water for electrical cords or hazards. Before entering the water to remove the victim, brush the ends of the fingers of one hand very lightly against the water. If you feel a tingle, turn all the power off at the main switch before putting even a toe in the water.

- If a victim has been found in a bathtub with a radio, portable heater, or other appliance that has energized the water, be sure that you *pull the plug of the appliance* before you touch the victim. A victim also may be found leaning across a kitchen counter with one hand in the sink (which is grounded) and the other on some appliance (toaster, mixer, etc.). The shock did not come from the sink; the sink only completed the circuit. The shock came from the appliance, when an accidental connection occurred, causing the metal parts to become energized with respect to ground. The cure is simply to *pull the plug* to remove the shock hazard before starting victim care.

SIGNS AND SYMPTOMS OF ELECTROCUTION

If you are unsure whether or not a person has been shocked, examine him for signs and symptoms of electrocution:

- Dazed and confused condition.
- Obvious and severe burns on the skin surface.
- Unconsciousness.
- Weak, irregular, or missing pulse.
- Shallow, irregular, or missing breathing.
- Possibility of multiple severe fractures due to intense muscular contractions.

EFFECTS OF ELECTRICAL SHOCK ON THE BODY

The following effects occur in electrical shock (Figure 29-31):

- Because alternating current produces severe muscular contractions, the victim may be violently thrown clear of the electrical source, but in his fall, he may sustain fractures, lacerations, or head injuries. The muscular contractions cause the blood pressure to skyrocket suddenly, resulting in minute spots of brain hemorrhage, hemorrhage involving other organs, or eye disorders (one or both eyes may be severely bloodshot).

- Temporary paralysis may occur due to extensive neurological damage involving the cells through which the current passes. Because of paralysis, respiration may cease.

- The effects of an electrical shock on the heart may lead to complete cardiac arrest or permanent tissue damage.

- The kidneys, spinal cord, and brain often are severely damaged.

- True electrical burns are caused by the passage of an electrical current through the skin after contact with a conductor. The entry wound is usually a blood-deprived, whitish-yellow, coagulated area; at times it may appear charred or depressed, with initially well-defined edges. The exit wound is usually dry with depressed edges; it normally looks as if the electrical current exploded as it left

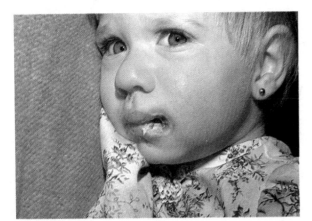

FIGURE 29-30. Electrical burn caused by chewing on an electrical cord.

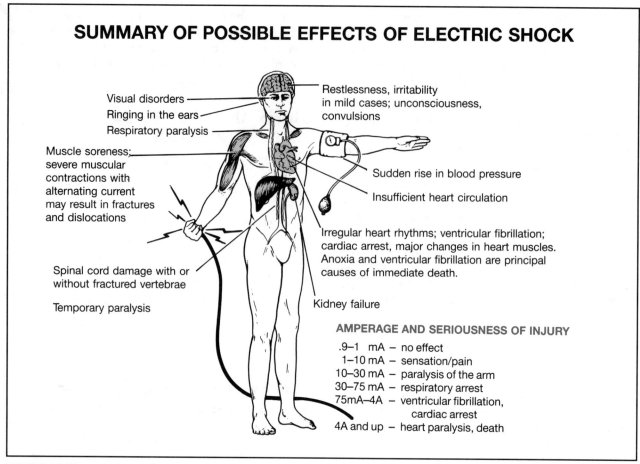

SUMMARY OF POSSIBLE EFFECTS OF ELECTRIC SHOCK

Visual disorders

Ringing in the ears

Respiratory paralysis

Restlessness, irritability in mild cases; unconsciousness, convulsions

Muscle soreness; severe muscular contractions with alternating current may result in fractures and dislocations

Sudden rise in blood pressure

Insufficient heart circulation

Irregular heart rhythms; ventricular fibrillation; cardiac arrest, major changes in heart muscles. Anoxia and ventricular fibrillation are principal causes of immediate death.

Spinal cord damage with or without fractured vertebrae

Temporary paralysis

Kidney failure

AMPERAGE AND SERIOUSNESS OF INJURY

.9–1 mA – no effect

1–10 mA – sensation/pain

10–30 mA – paralysis of the arm

30–75 mA – respiratory arrest

75mA–4A – ventricular fibrillation, cardiac arrest

4A and up – heart paralysis, death

FIGURE 29-31.

the body. Skin damage may vary from small circular spots to large areas of charred destruction (Figure 29-32).

- Because electrical currents generate heat, tissue destruction is usually deep (Figure 29-33). What may appear to be a small surface burn usually extends far below the surface of the skin. Blood vessels supplying the skin are often destroyed, and blood clots may be seen for some distance surrounding the original wound. A limb that appears to be only minimally damaged may become deprived of blood in a few days and, finally gangrenous.

- Additional complications of electrical injury — some of which may not appear immediately — include nerve damage, severe pain along the nerve channels, spinal-cord lesions and injuries, cardiac abnormalities, rapid heartbeat that lasts for several weeks, respiratory infection, death of muscle tissue, muscle lesions, delayed hemorrhage, gastric or duodenal ulcers, bleeding in the gastrointestinal tract, and acute kidney failure.

- If a woman is pregnant, the fetus is especially susceptible to electrical current, since the placenta and amniotic fluid provide little resistance. Even a minor shock can be serious to a fetus; the change in fetal heartbeat can cause stillbirth. Any woman who sustains even a slight shock should be monitored closely throughout her pregnancy.

EMERGENCY CARE

Do the following to care for a victim of electrical shock:

1. Your first priority is to protect yourself while you get the victim away from the source of electrocution. Follow instructions given earlier in this chapter. Do *not* approach the victim if you cannot do so safely; instead, call for appropriate help.

2. If possible, immobilize the victim's spine before you move him; he probably has suffered spinal damage, since electrical injury usually throws a victim.

ELECTRICAL BURNS

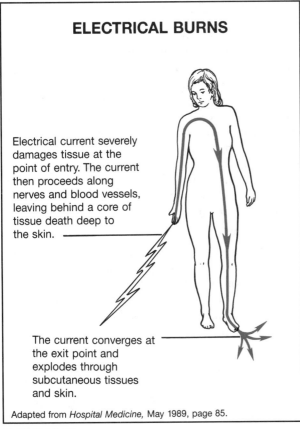

Electrical current severely damages tissue at the point of entry. The current then proceeds along nerves and blood vessels, leaving behind a core of tissue death deep to the skin. ─────

The current converges at the exit point and explodes through subcutaneous tissues and skin.

Adapted from *Hospital Medicine*, May 1989, page 85.

FIGURE 29-32.

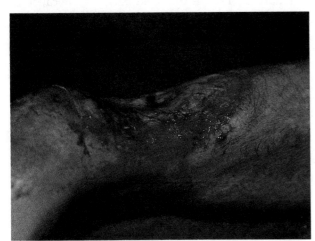

FIGURE 29-33. Deep third-degree electrical burn.

3. Start CPR immediately if indicated (the victim has no carotid pulse), even if you are unsure about the extent of injury. Most electrical-injury victims — even those in full arrest — can be successfully resuscitated with vigorous CPR. An electrocuted victim's heart may start up again on its own, but it is essential that you reduce the time when breathing is absent; therefore, begin CPR immediately.

4. Assess and care for any burns; cool burn sites and apply moist, sterile dressings.

5. Treat the victim for shock.

6. A victim sustaining electrical shock may become hysterical and start to run around in circles, behaving erratically. Force him to lie down and keep quiet; maintain his body temperature.

7. Activate the EMS system immediately. **Note:** If the victim is conscious and his condition is not urgent, provide basic burn care for entrance and exit wounds and splint fractures.

LIGHTNING INJURIES

While approximately one-third of all those struck by lightning die as a result, approximately two-thirds can be revived. The following (in rank order) are places where people are killed by lightning most often: open fields, under trees, on or near water, near tractors/heavy equipment, on golf courses, and at telephones. The person may be struck directly by the lightning, or the lightning may "splash" off an adjacent object that was struck directly. The longer the victim is in contact with the lightning, the more serious the injury. A victim who has been struck by lightning does *not* hold a charge, so it is safe to handle and treat this victim.

Always assume that a victim of lightning strike has sustained multiple injuries; most are knocked down or thrown, so also assume spinal injury. In addition to related injuries, the victim of lightning strike generally has sustained injury to the following body systems:

- The nervous system: In almost all instances of lightning strike, the victim becomes unresponsive; few actually remember being struck. Even after consciousness returns, the nervous system is affected, and there may be a full spectrum of changes. Some victims suffer partial paralysis, and occasionally, paralysis of the respiratory system causes sudden death. Fixed and dilated pupils are a normal reaction.

- The sensory system: Some victims experience a loss of sight or hearing; others lose the ability to speak. Most victims regain their speech, hearing, and sight (usually to full capacity) within several days. A *little* blood coming from the ears is normal after a lightning strike, since the tympanic membranes are often ruptured. This does not necessarily indicate skull fracture or head injury.

- The skin: Lightning causes a burn that typcially is mottled, feathery, or patchy, appearing in a scattered pattern over the skin and looking like tiny flowers. In some cases, the burn may be red, mottled, white, swollen, or blistered. The feathery burn usually fades and disappears within forty-eight to seventy-two hours (Figures 29-34 and 29-35).

- The heart: Cardiac damage is common in lightning strikes. The heart is often in the line of current; the most serious injury occurs when the current crosses the heart. The lightning strike itself can disrupt the heart's rhythm, but ensuing complications are what generally lead to full cardiac arrest or fibrillation. In some cases, the coronary arteries may undergo spasm.

- The vascular system: Within seconds following the lightning strike, the victim may become unresponsive, appear white and mottled, have cool arms and legs, and lose pulses. If the injury is moderate, the conditions probably will correct themselves quickly; in cases of severe injury, blood may coagulate, and tissues in the arms and legs may die, leading to amputation.

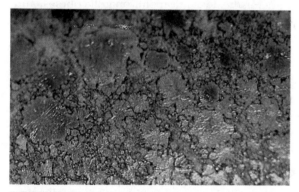

FIGURE 29-34. Lightning burn.

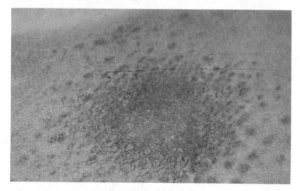

FIGURE 29-35. Lightning burn.

Emergency Care

Immediate care consists of restoring and maintaining breathing and circulation. Such measures should be continued even if the victim appears lifeless — victims of lightning have been resuscitated as long as thirty minutes after the strike without any residual damage. If the strike occurred in an open area, quickly move the victim to a protected area to reduce the chance of a second strike. If a group has been struck by lightning, care for the apparently dead first. Those who display vital signs will probably recover spontaneously, even though burns will require further care.

Initially, do the following:

1. Survey the entire scene. Assess what happened, and make sure that the victim is free from further injury. For example, remove any debris that has fallen on him, move him away from sources of electricity, and so on. Persons who are struck by lightning are safe to handle — it is impossible to get electrocuted by touching him.

2. Assess breathing and circulatory status. Begin artificial ventilation or CPR to maintain breathing and heartbeat. *The key to survival is early, vigorous prolonged resuscitation efforts.* Make those efforts even if the victim appears to be dead! Once breathing and circulation are initiated, monitor breathing and pulse continuously — the victim may arrest again. In administering artificial ventilation, do not tilt the head backward because of the possibility of spinal injury. Hold the head in a neutral position, and bring the jaw forward gently.

3. Stabilize the victim's neck to prevent aggravating a possible cervical-spine injury. If possible, move the victim to dry ground after stabilizing his neck.

4. Check skin color.

5. If the victim is conscious, check movement in all the extremities.

6. Assess the victim for open wounds or fractures, and provide appropriate care.

7. Activate the EMS system immediately.

| **29** | **SELF-TEST** | **29** |

Student: _____ Date: _____

Course: _____ Section #: _____

PART I: True/False   If you believe that the statement is true, circle the T. If you believe that the statement is false, circle the F.

T   F   1. More than half of all fire-related deaths are caused by smoke inhalation.

T   F   2. Most of the damage done to the upper airway is a result of inhalation of carbon monoxide.

T   F   3. Common signs and symptoms of upper-airway injury from inhalation include burned specks of carbon in the sputum, hoarseness, coughing, and cyanosis.

T   F   4. Carbon-monoxide poisoning is the major cause of death at the scene of most fires.

T   F   5. First-degree thermal burns should be immersed in cool water.

T   F   6. Second-degree burns should not be immersed in cool water.

T   F   7. Chemical burns should be continuously irrigated for at least twenty minutes.

T   F   8. A lime-powder burn should be treated like other chemical burns.

T   F   9. Lightning causes more deaths than any other type of electrical burn.

T   F   10. As many as 70 percent of smoke-inhalation victims have facial burns.

T   F   11. Victims of lightning have been resuscitated as long as thirty minutes after a strike without residual damage.

T   F   12. If a group has been struck by lightning, care for the apparently dead first.

T   F   13. While approximately two-thirds of all those struck by lightning die as a result, approximately one-third can be revived.

T   F   14. Always assume that a victim of a lightning strike has sustained multiple injuries.

PART II: Multiple Choice   For each question, circle the answer that best reflects an accurate statement.

1. The First Aider's first action at a burn accident should be to:
   a. remove the victim from the source of the burn.
   b. examine the victim for respiratory or cardiac complications.
   c. determine the severity of the burn.
   d. open and maintain the victim's airway.

2. The first step in caring for a first-degree burn is usually to:
   a. transport the victim to a medical facility as soon as possible.
   b. cover the area with a moist, bulky dressing.
   c. apply grease or petroleum jelly to the area.
   d. submerge the burned area in cold water.

3. Immersion of second-degree thermal-burn areas in cold water can:
   a. reduce swelling.
   b. relieve pain.
   c. prevent infection.
   d. a and b are correct.

4. Emergency care for a chemical burn caused by dry lime is to:
   a. flush the lime with running water.
   b. apply a neutralizer to the lime.
   c. first brush the dry lime from the victim's skin, hair, and clothing.
   d. apply an occlusive bandage.

5. What should be done when caring for most chemical burns?
   a. neutralize the area with alkali or acid solutions.
   b. remove clothing while flushing the area with water.
   c. locate an antidote before treating; water may intensify the reaction.
   d. cover the area with a dry, sterile gauze.

6. Immediate care in the case of a lightning victim should consist of:
   a. determine the victim's reaction to pain.
   b. treatment for shock.
   c. getting the victim under cover.
   d. restoring and maintaining breathing and heartbeat.

7. According to the Rule of Nines, which of the following areas is estimated to comprise 9 percent of the body area?
   a. one leg.
   b. back of trunk.
   c. front of trunk.
   d. one arm.

8. In a serious burn case, pain is best relieved by the exclusion of air from a burn through the application of a:
   a. burn spray.
   b. thick, clean, dry dressing.
   c. thick, petroleum-based burn ointment.
   d. soybean-oil-base burn ointment.

9. Which of the following causes the most damage in upper-airway inhalation injury accompanying burns?
   a. heat.
   b. noxious chemicals.
   c. carbon monoxide.
   d. smoke.

10. What care should be given if clothing or debris is sticking to a burn that is not severe?
    a. remove it carefully.
    b. soak the involved area in cool salt water.
    c. leave it alone.
    d. scrub the involved area with a soft brush and water.

11. Which of the following comes first in emergency care of an electrical-burn victim?
    a. separate the victim carefully from the electrical source.
    b. CPR.
    c. opening an airway.
    d. locating entrance and exit wounds.

12. In reference to the Rule of Nines, the infant's head area represents what percent of total body area?
    a. 4½%.
    b. 9%.
    c. 15%.
    d. 18%.

13. What should a First Aider do if he comes across a downed power line lying across a wrecked vehicle?
    a. instruct conscious victims to attempt to jump from the vehicle.
    b. tell conscious victims to stay inside the vehicle and wait for a power company crew.
    c. tell victims to turn on the ignition and move the vehicle.
    d. throw blanket or jacket over the line, and instruct conscious victims to leave the vehicle.

14. Possible effects of electric shock include:
    a. ringing in the ears.
    b. visual disorders.
    c. kidney failure.
    d. all of the above.

15. Lightning accounts for approximately _____ of all electrical burn injuries.
    a. 5%.   c. 25%.
    b. 15%.   d. 40%.

16. Which of the following statements about lightning is *not* true?
    a. some victims temporarily lose their speech, hearing, and sight.
    b. lightning rarely causes a burn to the skin.
    c. the first priority in treating these victims is to restore breathing and circulation.
    d. heart damage is a common result of lightning injuries.

PART III: Matching: Match the severity of burn at the left with the correct description at the right.

A. Critical

B. Moderate

C. Minor

_____ 1. Third-degree burns between 2 and 10 percent of the body of an adult (excluding face, hands, and feet).

_____ 2. Burns complicated by respiratory-tract injury and/or fractures.

_____ 3. First-degree burns that cover more than 75 percent of the body surface.

_____ 4. Second-degree burns between 15 to 25 percent of an adult's body surface.

_____ 5. Second-degree burns over less than 15 percent of an adult's body surface.

_____ 6. Third-degree burns involving more than 10 percent of an adult's body surface.

_____ 7. Second-degree burns covering more than 30 percent of an adult's body surface.

_____ 8. Third-degree burns that cover more than 2 to 3 percent of a child's body surface.

_____ 9. Third-degree burns that involve face, hands, feet, or genital area.

_____10. First-degree burns involving 50 to 75 percent of an adult's body surface.

_____11. Second-degree burns covering less than 10 percent of a child's body surface.

PART IV: What Would You Do If:

1. A ten-year-old boy was playing with gasoline and received burns on his abdomen and lower extremities.

2. An industrial worker has dry lime powder spilled over his whole body.

3. A teenage boy is hit by lightning on a golf course. He is not breathing and has no detectable carotid pulse.

PART V: Practical Skills Check-Off _____ has satisfactorily passed the following practical skills:
                                              Student's Name

	Date	Partner Check	Inst. Init.
1. Describe and demonstrate how to care for first- and second-degree burns of the extremities.	___/___/___	☐	_____
2. Describe and demonstrate how to care for a lime-powder burn.	___/___/___	☐	_____

CHAPTER THIRTY

OBJECTIVES

- Understand how the body attempts to maintain normal temperature and how the body can lose heat.
- Recognize the causes, signs, and symptoms of heat stroke, heat exhaustion, and heat cramps.
- Describe appropriate emergency care for heatstroke, heat exhaustion, and heat cramps.
- Identify the causes, signs, and symptoms of hypothermia and frostbite.
- Describe the appropriate emergency care for hypothermia and frostbite.

HEAT AND COLD EMERGENCIES

Heat and cold produce a number of different injuries. Critical to your ability to care for those injuries is a basic understanding of the way in which the body maintains its temperature and how it physiologically adjusts to extremes in heat and cold.

HOW THE BODY MAINTAINS EQUILIBRIUM

The human body stubbornly defends its constant core temperature of 98.6° F. Obviously, if this temperature is to be maintained, heat loss must equal heat production. This equilibrium is maintained by variations in the blood flow to the outer part of the body: when the core temperature rises, vessels near the skin dilate,, and the blood brings increased heat to the skin, where it is dissipated by radiation and convection (Figure 30-1). This works only as long as the skin temperature is lower than the temperature of the outside environment. What happens when the temperature of the air approaches or exceeds the temperature of the skin? Heat loss by radiation or convection is impossible, and the body relies on dissipation through evaporation of sweat. But the sweat mechanism also has its limits. The normal adult can sweat only about one liter per hour and can sweat at that rate for only a few hours at a time. In addition, sweating only works if the relative air humidity is low; sweat evaporation ceases entirely when the relative humidity reaches 75 percent.

Since body temperature is actually a measure of heat content or storage, a fall in temperature indicates a decrease, while a rise denotes an increase in the total heat content of the body. A normal-sized, unclothed man can reach and maintain thermal equilibrium in a room with a temperature of 86° F. He retains only that amount of heat generated by his basic metabolic processes and does not need to utilize any of his reserve mechanisms of heat loss. For persons wearing normal indoor clothing, the optimum comfort range is considered to be 70° to 80° F., with relative humidity between 40 and 60 percent.

HOW THE BODY LOSES HEAT

The body loses heat through radiation, conduction, convection, and evaporation of moisture (Figure 30-2).

HEAT REGULATION UNDER NORMAL DEMAND

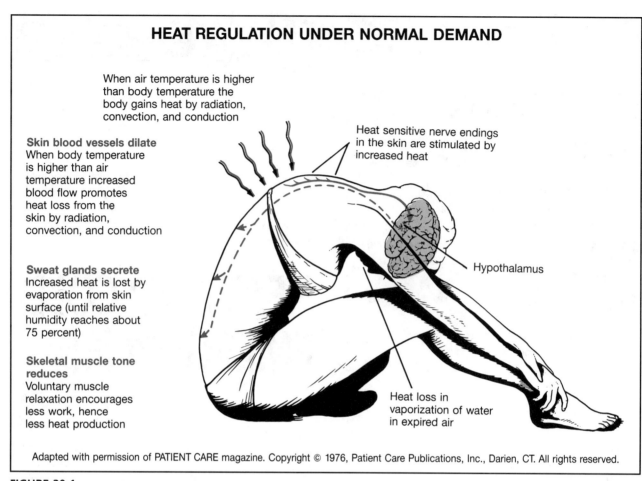

When air temperature is higher than body temperature the body gains heat by radiation, convection, and conduction

Skin blood vessels dilate
When body temperature is higher than air temperature increased blood flow promotes heat loss from the skin by radiation, convection, and conduction

Sweat glands secrete
Increased heat is lost by evaporation from skin surface (until relative humidity reaches about 75 percent)

Skeletal muscle tone reduces
Voluntary muscle relaxation encourages less work, hence less heat production

Heat sensitive nerve endings in the skin are stimulated by increased heat

Hypothalamus

Heat loss in vaporization of water in expired air

FIGURE 30-1.

RADIATION

Radiation, the most significant method of heat loss, involves the transfer of heat from the surface of one object to the surface of another without physical contact. Heat loss from radiation varies considerably with environmental conditions. In a temperate climate and under normal conditions, a person loses about 60 percent of his heat production by radiation. Most heat loss is from the head (approximately 50 percent), hands, and feet. At temperatures of 90° F., however, radiation loss will probably drop to zero; in subzero temperatures, loss of heat through radiation will skyrocket.

CONDUCTION AND CONVECTION

Conduction and convection, less important methods of heat loss in temperate climates, are major considerations in cold regions. By conduction, the cold air in immediate contact with the skin is warmed. The heated molecules move away, and

cooler ones take their place. Those, in turn, are warmed, and the process starts all over again. Any process that speeds movement of the air — such as wind — also speeds the cooling process.

The phenomenon of convection has been incorporated into the concept of windchill (Figure 30-3). A unit of windchill is defined as the amount of heat that would be lost in an hour from a square meter of exposed skin surface with a normal temperature of 91.4° F. In essence, the windchill factor combines the effects of the speed of the wind and the temperature of the environment into a number that indicates the danger of exposure. When the windchill factor is −10, the temperature is bitterly cold; at −20, exposed flesh may freeze; at −70, exposed flesh will freeze in less than one minute; and at −95, exposed flesh will freeze in less than thirty seconds. For instance, flesh will freeze in less than one minute in only ten-mile-per-hour winds if the temperature is forty degrees below zero.

Conduction is the method of heat loss in waterchill. Water conducts heat 240 times more quickly

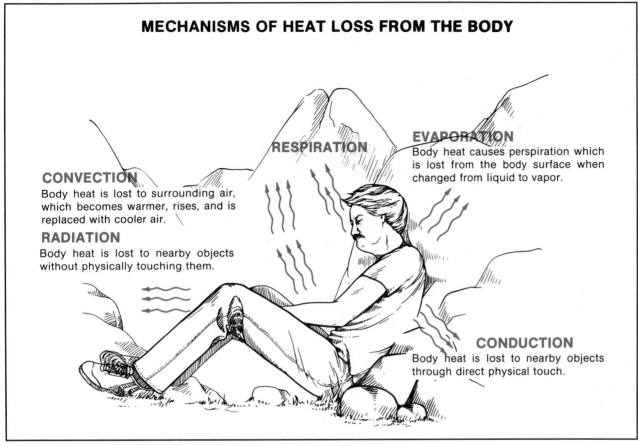

MECHANISMS OF HEAT LOSS FROM THE BODY

RESPIRATION

EVAPORATION
Body heat causes perspiration which is lost from the body surface when changed from liquid to vapor.

CONVECTION
Body heat is lost to surrounding air, which becomes warmer, rises, and is replaced with cooler air.

RADIATION
Body heat is lost to nearby objects without physically touching them.

CONDUCTION
Body heat is lost to nearby objects through direct physical touch.

FIGURE 30-2. The illustration assumes that a wet, poorly dressed climber has taken shelter in a crevasse or among cold, wet rocks.

than air. This means that wet clothing conducts heat away from the body at a much higher rate than dry clothing. A person whose clothing is wet, then, is in exceptional danger of losing heat. The wet clothing pulls heat away from the body more rapidly than the body can produce it.

Heat loss by conduction also occurs when a person inhales cold air and exhales warm air, when water and food are taken into the digestive tract, and when waste materials (urine and feces) are eliminated.

EVAPORATION

Loss of heat by evaporation of perspiration is usually more massive in hot weather; it slows down when the air is humid. In cold climates, the only loss from perspiration is due to wearing improper clothing. When the temperature of the air equals or exceeds the temperature of the skin, body heat must be eliminated through evaporation.

HOW THE BODY CONSERVES HEAT

How does man conserve body heat? Since approximately 80 to 85 percent of all heat loss occurs from the body surface, any reduction in skin temperature should conserve body heat. The skin is heated in three ways: (1) blood rushes to the surface of the skin from internal organs; (2) hair erects, thickening the layer of warm air trapped immediately next to the skin; and (3) little or no perspiration is released to the skin surface for evaporation (Figure 30-4). Therefore, the ways in which man remains cool are restricting blood flow to the skin, limiting the amount of body hair, and wearing only one layer of clothing.

Blood flow is also increased to the skin surface when the body becomes overheated. When vessels at the skin surface dilate, the heat in the blood is taken to the skin surface, where it is lost through radiation and convection. Additional heat is lost through perspiration and respiration.

WIND CHILL INDEX

WIND SPEED MPH	WHAT THE THERMOMETER READS (degrees F.)											
	50	40	30	20	10	0	−10	−20	−30	−40	−50	−60
	WHAT IT EQUALS IN ITS EFFECT ON EXPOSED FLESH											
CALM	50	40	30	20	10	0	−10	−20	−30	−40	−50	−60
5	48	37	27	16	6	−5	−15	−26	−36	−47	−57	−68
10	40	28	16	4	−9	−21	−33	−46	−58	−70	−83	−95
15	36	22	9	−5	−18	−36	−45	−58	−72	−85	−99	−112
20	32	18	4	−10	−25	−39	−53	−67	−82	−96	−110	−121
25	30	16	0	−15	−29	−44	−59	−74	−88	−104	−118	−133
30	28	13	−2	−18	−33	−48	−63	−79	−94	−109	−125	−140
35	27	11	−4	−20	−35	−49	−67	−82	−98	−113	−129	−145
40	26	10	−6	−21	−37	−53	−69	−85	−100	−116	−132	−148

Little danger if properly clothed	Danger of freezing exposed flesh	Great danger of freezing exposed flesh

FIGURE 30-3.

Source: U.S. Army

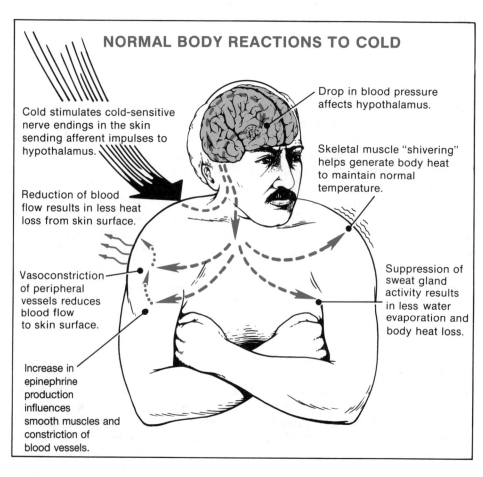

NORMAL BODY REACTIONS TO COLD

Cold stimulates cold-sensitive nerve endings in the skin sending afferent impulses to hypothalamus.

Drop in blood pressure affects hypothalamus.

Skeletal muscle "shivering" helps generate body heat to maintain normal temperature.

Reduction of blood flow results in less heat loss from skin surface.

Vasoconstriction of peripheral vessels reduces blood flow to skin surface.

Suppression of sweat gland activity results in less water evaporation and body heat loss.

Increase in epinephrine production influences smooth muscles and constriction of blood vessels.

FIGURE 30-4.

HOW CLOTHING AFFECTS THERMAL EQUILIBRIUM

Clothing provides thermal resistance to heat loss; that thermal resistance is expressed in "clo" units. One clo is defined as the equivalent to normal indoor clothing and is the amount of clothing insulation required to keep a resting/sitting person with average metabolism indefinitely comfortable in an environment of 70° F. with an air movement of twenty feet per minute and a relative humidity of less than 50 percent. Clothing acts as insulation because it traps air between its fibers; one inch of fabric is roughly equivalent to four clo.

In cold weather, most people wear more layers of clothing than they need while they are working and less than they need while they are resting. Heat loss needs to be increased when the body is active and decreased when it is inactive. The pattern of clothing employed by most people defeats both those purposes.

Clothes serve an important role in relation to perspiration. In the summer (or in hot weather), they act as a barrier to evaporation or perspiration, thereby frustrating the coolant system designed by the body. In cold weather, a person wearing too many layers of clothing perspires heavily, and the layer of clothing next to the skin remains wet. This causes the person to lose heat 240 times faster than if the clothing remained dry.

HYPERTHERMIA (HEAT-RELATED INJURY)

Heat-related injuries fall into three major categories: heatstroke, heat exhaustion, and heat cramps. Heat emergencies are most frequent on days when the temperature is 95 to 100° F., when the humidity is high, and when there is little or no breeze. Most highly susceptible to heat injuries are the following people:

- Athletes.
- Workers who labor outdoors or near furnaces or ovens.
- Those who are in poor physical condition.
- The chronically ill.
- Those who are not acclimated.
- Those with weak cardiovascular systems.
- Those who are using certain drugs (such as diuretics).
- Alcoholics.
- The obese.
- Burn victims.
- The elderly.
- Children.

Most heat injuries occur early in the summer season, before people have acclimated themselves to the higher temperatures. The heat and humidity risk scale (Figure 30-5) indicates when problems are most likely to occur.

HEATSTROKE

Heatstroke, a true life-threatening emergency, has a mortality ranging from 20 to 70 percent. Heatstroke is sometimes called sunstroke, although the sun is not required for its onset. The condition results when the heat-regulating mechanisms of the body break down and fail to cool the body sufficiently. The body becomes overheated, the body temperature rises to between 105 and 110° F., and no sweating occurs in about half the victims. Because no cooling takes place, the body stores increasingly more heat, the heat-producing mechanisms speed up, and eventually the brain cells are damaged, causing permanent disability or death.

There are two basic kinds of heatstroke. Classic heatstroke, in which people lose the ability to sweat, generally affects the elderly or the chronically ill during a heat wave. Exertional heatstroke, in which victims retain the ability to sweat, is accompanied by physical exertion and muscle stress (Figure 30-6).

Heatstroke most seriously affects the aged; infants and children (who sweat less, generate more heat, and have a smaller body surface); debilitated, malnourished, and inexperienced athletes; those who have a prior history of heatstroke; or those who are short, stocky, and heavily muscled. Drug abusers are especially susceptible, especially those who use barbiturates and hallucinogens. Even healthy individuals, when overexerted, can fall victim. Young people who suffer from heatstroke may not completely lose the ability to sweat, and their skin may be moist and hot instead of characteristically dry.

Heatstroke commonly occurs during times of high temperatures combined with high humidity and low wind velocity.

Signs and Symptoms

Heatstroke is indicated by the following signs and symptoms (Figure 30-7):

- Temperature of 105° F. or higher.

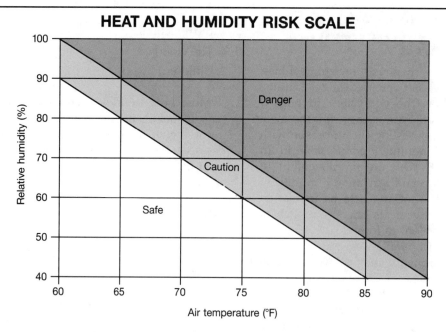

HEAT AND HUMIDITY RISK SCALE

FIGURE 30-5. The risk of illness is increased when heat and humidity produce dangerous conditions. Lower temperatures with high humidity can also cause the body's temperature to rise.

- Hot, reddish skin; skin can be wet or dry, since approximately half of all heatstroke victims sweat profusely.
- An initially rapid, strong pulse of 160 or more, continuing rapid but becoming weak as damage progresses.
- Initially constricted pupils, later becoming dilated.
- Tremors.
- Mental confusion and anxiety; victims may show unusual irritability, aggression, combative agitation, or — in the extreme — psychotic or hysterical behavior.
- Initially deep, rapid breathing that sounds like snoring; breathing becomes shallow and weak as damage progresses.
- Headache.
- Dry mouth.
- Shortness of breath.
- Loss of appetite, nausea, or vomiting.
- Increasing dizziness and weakness.
- Decreased blood pressure.

- Convulsions, sudden collapse, and possible unconsciousness; *all* heatstroke victims have compromised levels of consciousness, ranging from disorientation to coma.
- Seizures.

Victims may lapse into a coma, become delirious, and die. About 4,000 Americans die of heatstroke each year; 80 percent of those deaths occur among people over the age of fifty. Heatstroke is the second most common cause of death among high school athletes (second only to spinal-cord injury). Untreated, all victims die. The longer care is delayed, the more permanent and disabling the damage, particularly to the central nervous system.

Emergency Care

Emergency care of heatstroke is aimed at *immediate* cooling of the body. *Act fast;* do whatever is necessary to cool the body. The priority of emergency care is to remove the victim from the source of heat when possible; other top priorities include

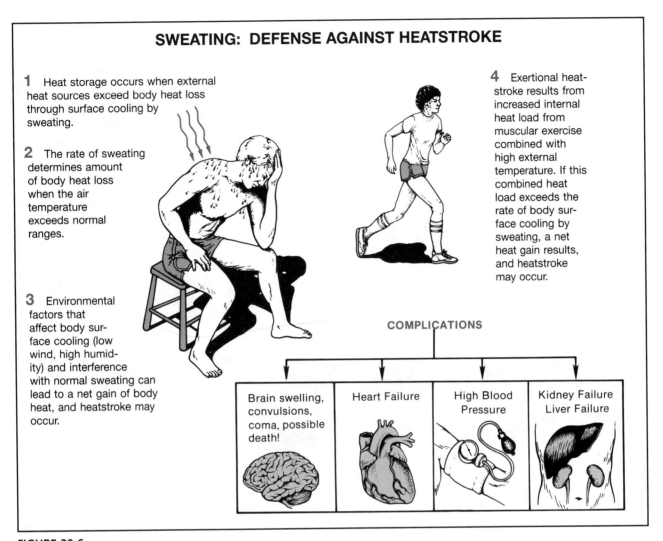

SWEATING: DEFENSE AGAINST HEATSTROKE

1 Heat storage occurs when external heat sources exceed body heat loss through surface cooling by sweating.

2 The rate of sweating determines amount of body heat loss when the air temperature exceeds normal ranges.

3 Environmental factors that affect body surface cooling (low wind, high humidity) and interference with normal sweating can lead to a net gain of body heat, and heatstroke may occur.

4 Exertional heatstroke results from increased internal heat load from muscular exercise combined with high external temperature. If this combined heat load exceeds the rate of body surface cooling by sweating, a net heat gain results, and heatstroke may occur.

COMPLICATIONS

Brain swelling, convulsions, coma, possible death!

Heart Failure

High Blood Pressure

Kidney Failure Liver Failure

FIGURE 30-6.

airway, ventilation, oxygenation, circulation, and transport. To give emergency care:

1. Remove the victim when possible from the source of heat, and establish an airway.

2. Remove as much of the victim's clothing as possible or reasonable, pour cool water over his body (avoiding his nose and mouth), fan him briskly, and shade him from the sun if he is still outdoors. Place cold packs under the victim's arms, around his neck, and around his ankles to cool the large surface blood vessels (Figure 30-8). Simple ice packs or hyperthermia blankets will not effectively lower temperature when used alone; use a variety of methods. Wrapping a wet sheet around the victim's body and then directing an electric fan at the victim are also good ways of cooling (Figure 30-9). Use slower cooling if the victim starts to shiver, since shivering

produces heat. Continue until his temperature falls below 103° F.

3. When the victim's body temperature has dropped to 102° F., take measures to prevent chilling. Monitor temperature carefully throughout emergency care, taking the temperature every five minutes with a thermometer that records up to 108° F. Keep working to reduce the temperature. If the victim's temperature does not drop to below 100° F., hyperthermia could recur.

4. Elevate the victim's head and shoulders slightly during cooling, and make sure that he is comfortable.

5. Never give the victim stimulants or hot drinks.

6. Because heatstroke involves the entire body, a number of complications may result from the

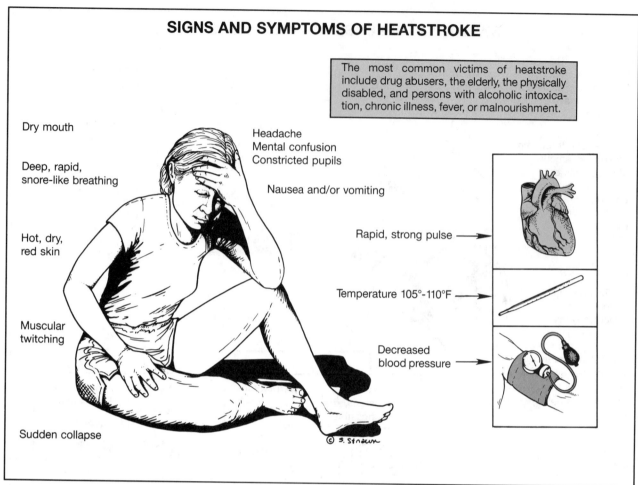

FIGURE 30-7.

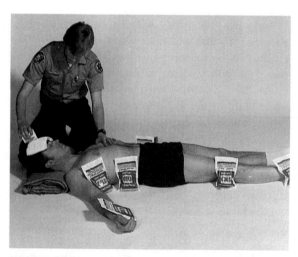

FIGURE 30-8. Use cold applications on the head and body to cool a victim of heatstroke.

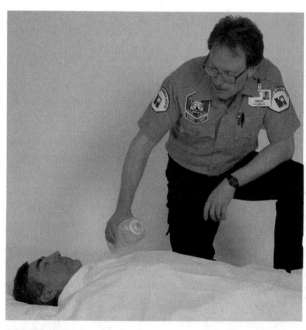

FIGURE 30-9. Wrapping a heatstroke victim in a wet sheet and directing a fan at the victim are good ways of cooling.

ailment itself or from necessary care. Be prepared to care for the following complications as cooling proceeds:

▪ Convulsions. Tremors and convulsions tend to accompany rapid cooling and, because convulsions produce great body heat, they can impair treatment. Convulsions are most likely to occur once the body cools to 104° F.

▪ Aspiration of vomitus. Vomiting commonly accompanies convulsions caused by cooling techniques. Position the victim for easy drainage.

7. If you succeed in lowering the core body temperature at least four degrees Fahrenheit over a thirty- to sixty-minute period, discontinue active cooling measures while transporting or waiting for emergency personnel. The body usually will continue to cool spontaneously. Monitor core temperature every ten minutes to make sure that temperature keeps dropping.

8. Watch the victim closely and maintain normal body temperature. If hyperthermia recurs before emergency personnel arrive, begin cooling procedures again. The core temperature must drop below 100° F. and must stay that low before the danger has passed.

9. If you are transporting the victim, run the vehicle's air-conditioning system at maximum capacity if possible. If that is not possible, wrap the victim in wet sheets and direct a fan at him.

10. *Always* activate the EMS system for a victim of heatstroke, even if you are able to lower the body temperature; a victim of heatstroke always needs hospital care.

HEAT EXHAUSTION

Heat exhaustion, the most common heat injury, occurs in an otherwise fit person who is involved in extreme physical exertion in a hot, humid environment. It results from a serious disturbance of the blood flow, similar to the circulatory disturbance of shock. Heat exhaustion is, in fact, a mild state of shock brought on by the pooling of blood in the vessels just below the skin, causing blood to flow away from the major organs of the body. Due to prolonged and profuse sweating, the body loses large quantities of salt and water. Heat exhaustion can also occur among the elderly or the infirm, who have too little salt even without activity. When the water is not adequately replaced, blood circulation diminishes, affecting brain, heart, and lung functions. Heat exhaustion is sometimes, though not always, accompanied by heat cramps due to salt loss.

There are two basic kinds of heat exhaustion:

▪ Salt-depletion, in which unacclimatized individuals exert themselves and drink enough water but do not replace the salt.

▪ Water-depletion, which usually occurs among the elderly or chronically ill who do not drink enough water during extreme heat. This type of heat exhaustion is characterized by extreme anxiety and agitation, intense thirst, headache, weakness, fever, muscular incoordination, and decreased sweating.

The most critical problem in heat exhaustion is dehydration.

Signs and Symptoms

Primary signs and symptoms of heat exhaustion are much like flu symptoms. They can include the following:

▪ Headache, giddiness, and extreme weakness.

▪ Nausea and possible vomiting.

▪ Dizziness and faintness.

▪ Profuse sweating.

▪ Loss of appetite.

▪ Fatigue.

▪ Diarrhea.

▪ Collapse and unconsciousness (usually brief).

▪ Below-normal body temperature or normal body temperature; in occasional cases, body temperature may be slightly elevated.

▪ Dilated pupils.

▪ Weak and rapid pulse.

▪ Rapid, shallow breathing.

▪ Pale, cool, sweaty skin, usually ashen gray in color.

▪ Possible heat cramps or muscular aches.

▪ Inelastic skin.

▪ Difficulty in walking.

Heat Exhaustion Versus Heatstroke

While the signs and symptoms of heat exhaustion may seem similar to those of heatstroke to the casual observer, there are some distinct differences that will help you make the correct evaluation (Figure 30-10).

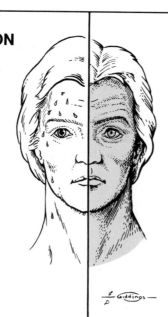

HEAT EXHAUSTION

- Moist and clammy skin, usually pale

- Pupils dilated

- Normal or subnormal temperature

- Weak, dizzy or faint

- Headache

- No appetite, nausea

HEATSTROKE

- Dry hot skin, usually red

- Pupils constricted

- Very high body temperature

- Coma or near coma

- Pulse strong and rapid

FIGURE 30-10.

The two most reliable and distinct differences are the condition of the skin and the body temperature. In heatstroke, the skin is flushed and hot to the touch; victims experiencing heat exhaustion usually have wet or clammy, pale, cool skin. Body temperature in a heatstroke victim can soar to above 106° F.; in a victim of heat exhaustion, it usually stays at normal or sometimes even dips below normal.

Emergency Care

To give emergency care to a victim of heat exhaustion:

1. Move the victim to a cool place away from the source of heat, but make sure that he does not become chilled. Apply cold, wet compresses to his skin, and fan him lightly.

2. Have the victim lie down (Figure 30-11). Raise his feet eight to twelve inches, and lower his head to

help increase blood circulation to the brain. Remove as much of the victim's clothing as possible, and loosen what you cannot remove. Help make the victim as comfortable as possible.

3. If the victim is fully conscious, administer cool water at the rate of one-half glassful every fifteen minutes for one hour (Figure 30-12).

4. If the victim is unconscious, remove his clothing and sponge him off with cool water.

5. If the victim vomits, stop giving him fluids and activate the EMS system immediately. (This is usually the only instance in which a heat-exhaustion victim will require hospitalization.)

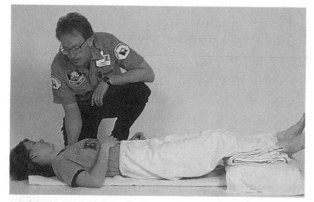

FIGURE 30-11. Have the heat-exhaustion victim lie down with feet elevated.

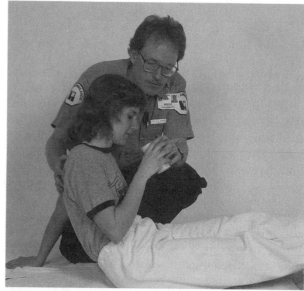

FIGURE 30-12. If the heat-exhaustion victim is fully conscious, administer cool water.

6. Take the victim's temperature every ten or fifteen minutes; activate the EMS system as soon as possible. If the victim's temperature is above 101° F. or rising, activate the EMS system.

HEAT CRAMPS

Heat cramps are the least common and least serious heat injury. They are muscular spasms that occur when the body loses too much salt during profuse sweating, when not enough salt is taken into the body, when calcium levels are low, and when too much water is consumed. Occasionally, heat cramps can be caused by overexertion of muscles or inadequate stretching or warmup. Heat cramps can be mild or extremely painful. When the body becomes low on salt and water, the victim interprets it as thirst. To quench his thirst, he consumes large quantities of water without replacing the salt. Heat cramps usually occur in the arms, legs, or abdomen (the major complaint may be severe abdominal pain) and are often a signal of approaching heat exhaustion.

Hot weather is not necessarily requisite to heat cramps. A person who exercises strenuously in cold weather and perspires may develop heat cramps if he drinks water but does not replace salt. Heat cramps result when blood-calcium levels are too high in proportion to blood-sodium levels. In order to function properly, the muscles need a strict balance of water, calcium, and sodium; whenever that balance is disrupted, regardless of temperature, heat cramps may result.

Signs and Symptoms

Signs and symptoms of heat cramps can include (Figure 30-13):

- Severe muscular cramps and pain, especially of the legs, calves, and abdomen.
- Faintness and dizziness.
- Exhaustion or fatigue.
- A stiff, boardlike abdomen.
- Possible nausea and vomiting.
- Normal mental status and consciousness level.

Emergency Care

To care for a victim with heat cramps:

1. If the victim is in a hot environment, remove him from the heat immediately.

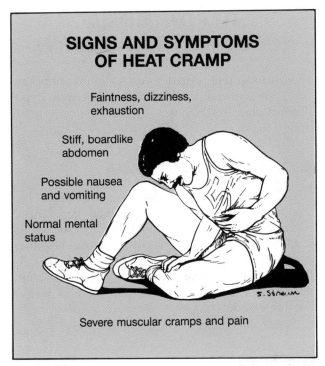

SIGNS AND SYMPTOMS OF HEAT CRAMP

Faintness, dizziness, exhaustion

Stiff, boardlike abdomen

Possible nausea and vomiting

Normal mental status

Severe muscular cramps and pain

FIGURE 30-13.

2. Administer sips of saltwater at the rate of one-half glassful every fifteen minutes. Dilute one teaspoon of salt or one boullion cube in one quart of water, or use a commercial product with a low glucose content. Do *not* give the victim salt tablets.

3. Do *not* massage the cramping muscles; massage may actually increase the pain. To relieve pain, try gently stretching the involved muscle groups. Manipulate or push the knotted muscle mass back to its normal position. *Follow local protocol.*

4. Explain to the victim what happened to him — and why — so that he can avoid a recurrence. Assure the victim that nothing is critically wrong with him; some individuals fear a blood clot or muscle tear. Help the victim remain calm and relaxed, since relaxation will speed recovery. The victim should avoid exertion of any kind for twelve hours because heat cramps can recur. If the victim resists restricted activity, you may have to arrange transport for him to prevent heatstroke or heat exhaustion. Finally, advise the victim to salt food more heavily and to increase fluid intake until all cramping stops.

5. Follow local protocol regarding activating the EMS system. Generally, you should activate the EMS system if the victim has other injuries or illnesses, if other symptoms develop, or if the victim worsens and/or does not respond to care.

HYPOTHERMIA (COLD-RELATED INJURY)

Major injuries related to extreme cold temperatures are general hypothermia, immersion hypothermia, and frostbite.

GENERAL HYPOTHERMIA

General hypothermia, the most life-threatening cold injury, affects the entire body with generalized severe cooling. Mortality from general hypothermia is as high as 87 percent. Hypothermia can be either acute (occurring suddenly, as when someone falls through ice) or chronic (developing gradually from prolonged exposure to wind, cold, or cool water) See Table 30-1.

There are three categories of general hypothermia that are determined by core body temperature:

- Mild hypothermia (90-95° F.).
- Moderate hypothermia (82-89.9° F.).
- Severe hypothermia (less than 82° F.).

Cases have been documented in which victims have survived with a core temperature as low as 64.4° F. In general, thermal control is lost once the body temperature is lowered to 95° F. and the body is no longer in thermal balance. Coma occurs when the body's core temperature reaches approximately 79° F.

General hypothermia usually is due to immersion in extremely cold water or to overall exposure without ensuing frostbite. However, it can happen indoors, and it does not necessarily require cold weather. Extremely low temperatures are not

TABLE 30-1	ACCIDENTAL HYPOTHERMIA			
Predisposing Factors	Signs Others See	Symptoms Victim Feels	Prevention	Emergency Care
Poor physical condition Failure to eat and drink enough Little body fat Inadequate clothing (wool is best) Lack of shelter from snow, rain, wind Wetness (from perspiration or precipitation) Exhaustion	Coordination loss; slow, stumbling pace Speech distortion Forgetfulness Lack of judgment; irrational ambition Overactive imagination; possible hallucinations Blue, puffy skin Dilated pupils of eyes Slow, shallow breathing Confusion, stupor, possible unconsciousness	Violent shivering, with muscle tension Fatigue Feeling of extreme cold or numbness Loss of coordination; stumbling, thick speech, disorientation Rigidity of muscles after shivering stops Blue, puffy skin Pulse slow, irregular, or weak	Rest and eat before exertion Nibble on high-energy food continuously while on trail Wear windproof outer clothing, wool underneath Carry emergency camping equipment Make camp immediately if storm, injury, or loss of direction occurs Keep moving; this keeps the body producing heat; if camped, use isometric exercises	MINIMIZE HEAT LOSS: Protect victim from cold Place insulating pad between victim and ground Remove wet clothing; wrap in dry clothing and/or blankets Keep victim dry ADD HEAT: Have victim get into sleeping bag with another person Give warm liquids Apply heat, using warmed stones wrapped in cloth, heat packs, or hot water in a canteen Keep physical contact with others for body heat Have victim breathe warm, moist air

Adapted from: Brent Q. Hafen and Brenda Peterson, *First Aid for Health Emergencies*, West Publishing Co., 1980, p. 248.

necessary to induce hypothermia — it can occur in temperatures as high as 65° F., depending on the windchill factor, and at temperatures well above freezing. Most cases result when the temperature is about 60° F. or less. Wetness — either from water or perspiration — always compounds the problem; exhaustion also affects any case of hypothermia. Always consider hypothermia in any victim of trauma in cold weather.

Some of the contributing factors to hypothermia, even in the absence of thermal stress, include the following:

- Use of drugs: Some drugs, such as alcohol, may render the person unable or unwilling to seek shelter; hypothermia is common among alcoholics. Any substance that alters perception or judgment can lead to hypothermia.

- Surgery.

- Water activities: Swimmers, divers, and boaters in cold water are especially prone to hypothermia. Any victim of a near-drowning should be treated for hypothermia, since the core cools first.

- Disease: Some existing diseases or conditions will render an individual more prone to hypothermia. They include any circulatory disease, diabetes, hypoglycemia, infection, cancer, and stroke.

- Trauma: Massive loss of blood resulting from physical trauma may induce hypothermia. Accidents during swimming and water skiing are very likely to produce hypothermia if drowning does not occur. Any injury or blow to the head, neck, and spine can also disturb the body's thermoregulatory capability.

- Extremes of age: Premature babies, children under one year of age, and the elderly are particularly susceptible. Delayed circulation, less body fat, lessened physical activity, poor diet, poor appetite, and decreased metabolism all make the elderly more susceptible.

- Immobility.

Basically, hypothermia occurs when the body loses more heat than it produces. Death can occur within two hours of the first signs and symptoms (Figure 30-14). As body cooling progresses, hypothermia manifests itself in five stages:

1. Shivering (an attempt by the body to generate heat).

2. Indifference, sleepiness, apathy, and listlessness.

3. Decreased level of consciousness with a glassy stare and possible freezing of the extremities.

4. Decreased vital signs with slow pulse and slow respiration rate.

5. Death.

Hypothermia can occur with little warning. Initial reactions to cold, of course, are shivering and "goosebumps," but in hypothermia, these are not enough to maintain body temperature.

Signs and Symptoms

General signs and symptoms of hypothermia include (Figure 30-15):

- Trembling on one side of the body without shivering (shivering does not occur if body temperature goes below 90° F.).

- Uncontrollable fits of shivering.

- Vague, slow, slurred, and thick speech.

- Amnesia, memory lapses, and incoherence.

- Poor judgment.

- Staggering gait.

- Postural dizziness.

- Muscular rigidity in later stages.

- Skin color ranging from cyanosis to waxen; skin often appears gray and bloodless.

- Disorientation and mental confusion.

- Sluggish pupils.

- Apathy.

- Semi-rigid skin.

- Bloated face.

- Increased blood pressure, heart, and respiratory rates at first; decreased heart and respiratory rates, irregular heartbeat, weak, shallow, or absent pulse and respiration as hypothermia progresses.

- Dehydration.

- Low blood pressure.

- Drowsiness and/or stupor; unresponsiveness to verbal or painful stimuli.

- Apparent exhaustion; inability to get up after rest.

- Unconsciousness, deep coma with severe hypothermia.

Note: The above symptoms are not in any order of progression; for a progressive list of symptoms, see Figure 30-16.

How the victim looks and acts depends in part on the severity of the hypothermia. If the core temperature is above 90° F., the patient will probably shiver

STAGES OF HYPOTHERMIA
(General Body Cooling)

1. **Shivering** (a response by the body which generates heat) does not occur below a body temperature of 90°F.

2. **Apathy** and decreased muscle function, first fine motor and then gross motor functions.

3. **Decreased level of consciousness** with a glassy stare and possible freezing of the extremities.

4. **Decreased vital signs** with slow pulse and slow respiration rate.

5. **Death**

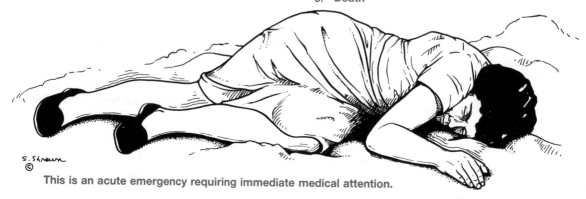

S. Shraun ©

This is an acute emergency requiring immediate medical attention.

EMERGENCY CARE

- Keep the victim dry and remove wet clothing.
- Apply external heat to both sides of the victim using whatever heat sources are available, including the body heat of rescuers.
- If the victim is conscious and in a warm place, have him breathe warm, moist air if available.
- Monitor respirations and pulse and provide artificial ventilation and CPR as required. No one is dead until warm and dead.
- Do not give hot liquids by mouth.
- Do not allow victim to exercise.
- Handle the victim gently.

If less than 30 minutes from medical facility:
1. Prevent further heat loss.
2. Handle with care.
3. Activate EMS system.

If more than 30 minutes from a medical facility:
1. Prevent further heat loss.
2. Handle with care.
3. Follow rewarming techniques discussed in this chapter. Follow local protocol.
4. Prepare for CPR.
5. Activate the EMS system.

There is disagreement among some experts regarding the temperature used for rewarming cold injuries. It is important that you follow local protocol.

FIGURE 30-14.

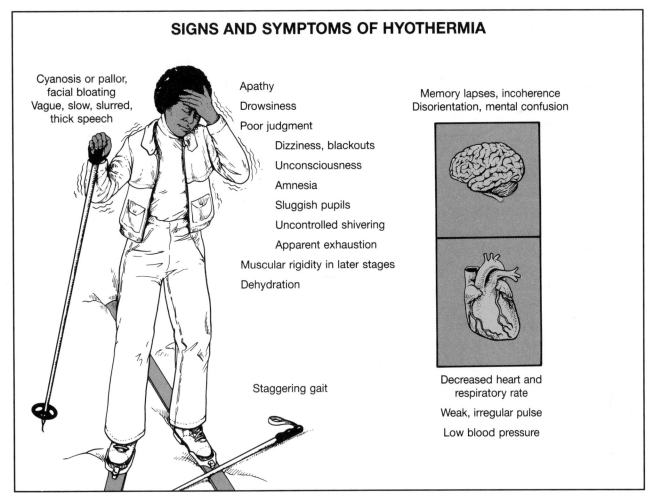

SIGNS AND SYMPTOMS OF HYOTHERMIA

Cyanosis or pallor, facial bloating Vague, slow, slurred, thick speech

Apathy

Drowsiness

Poor judgment

Dizziness, blackouts

Unconsciousness

Amnesia

Sluggish pupils

Uncontrolled shivering

Apparent exhaustion

Muscular rigidity in later stages

Dehydration

Staggering gait

Memory lapses, incoherence Disorientation, mental confusion

Decreased heart and respiratory rate

Weak, irregular pulse

Low blood pressure

FIGURE 30-15.

violently and complain of being very cold. While the victim will be able to answer questions and will have almost normal thinking abilities, he may be slower than normal in responding to questions and commands. He will most likely be oriented as to where and who he is and what day and time it is. He will probably be able to move around quite normally but may be slightly uncoordinated and unable to perform simple tasks requiring manual dexterity, such as unzipping a zipper or tying shoes.

When core temperature drops below 90° F., the victim will be disoriented about who he is, where he is, and what day it is. His speech may not make much sense; he may become confused and withdrawn. The victim may not be able to care for himself, and he may even do senseless or wrong things in his confusion. His muscles may be stiff, even resembling rigor mortis; he may be uncoordinated, unable to perform physical tasks, and stumble when he tries to walk. When the core temperature

reaches the low 80s, he will probably drift into unconsciousness.

Most victims with a core temperature above 90° F. will survive with emergency care; those with a lower core temperature require extreme care in handling and rapid transport to a hospital.

Emergency Care

The basic principles of emergency care for hypothermia include preventing heat loss, rewarming the victim as quickly and safely as possible, and remaining alert for complications (see Figure 30-14).

Some general guidelines apply to emergency care for hypothermia victims, whether they are wet or dry, on land or in water. Victims in seemingly unlikely situations can be hypothermic. Hypothermia can be a complication even when the weather is warm and the victim is dry.

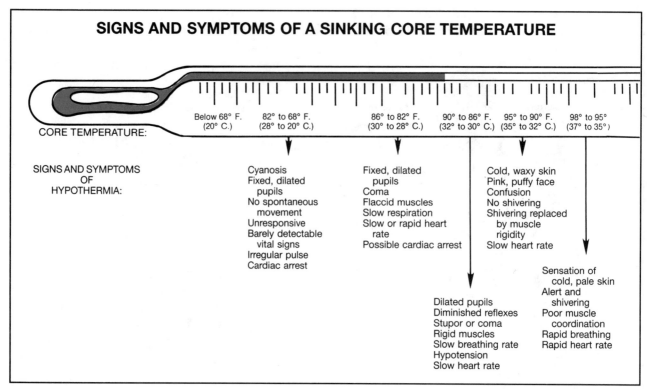

FIGURE 30-16.

The most basic guideline and top priority is to *never allow the victim to stay in a cold environment.* Insulate him from the cold however you can: use wool blankets, plastic sheets, newspapers, plastic air-bubble packing material, or a sleeping bag; prewarm a sleeping bag by lying in it. Insulate the victim from the ground up; get something underneath him as quickly as possible. Do everything possible to prevent further heat loss.

Whenever possible, keep the victim in a horizontal position; it helps prevent shock and increases blood flow to the brain. If you are transporting a hypothermia victim out of the mountains, injuries should be directed uphill. Elevate the victim's head if he has sustained head or chest injuries, if he has shortness of breath, if he has symptoms of myocardial infarction, or if the terrain is extremely steep.

To give emergency care, follow these general guidelines:

1. Handle the victim *very* gently and do not allow the victim to exert himself.

2. Be aware that when a victim is removed from the water, he can experience a drastic drop in blood pressure. This can be rapidly fatal.

3. Check the vital signs.
   - Vital signs are slowed in hypothermia victims, so measure for one full minute to make an accurate assessment.
   - Open the airway, and restore breathing and circulation if necessary by administering CPR.
   - *Before* you begin CPR, make sure that there is *no* pulse. In severe hypothermia, a victim may breathe only three or four times a minute; a heartbeat of only five to ten beats per minute is enough to sustain life in a hypothermic victim. A slow pulse is tolerable if breathing is also slow. If you cannot detect pulse or respiration, but an unconscious victim shows any movement at all, assume that there is some cardiac activity, and do not perform CPR.

4. If possible, place the victim in a warm, draft-free environment. Prevent further heat loss by insulating the victim:
   - Insulate the head as well, since as much as 70 percent of the body's heat can be lost this way.
   - Do not allow the victim's skin to be exposed to wind, cold air, or water spray.

- If the victim can be sheltered in a warm, windless place, *gently* remove wet clothing and replace it with dry. Wrap the victim in dry blankets. The vigorous movement of removing wet clothing may cause ventricular fibrillation. Instead, layer dry clothing and coverings on top of the wet.

- If dry clothing or coverings are not available, press as much water as possible out of the wet clothes and cover them with plastic sheeting to insulate.

- If the victim is wearing a coat or jacket, have him put his arms next to his body instead of in the sleeves.

5. If a victim is *not* shivering, do not try to rewarm him; instead, activate the EMS system or transport him immediately to a hospital, keeping his head lower than his feet. If the victim is conscious and shivering, begin rewarming. *Add heat gradually and gently;* the slower, the safer. As a general rule, keep the victim's extremities protected against the cold, but do not warm the extremities. During rewarming, insulate the skin against direct contact with heated objects; hypothermic skin burns easily. General methods of rewarming include the following:

   - Passive external rewarming, for victims with mild to moderate hypothermia, consists of simply removing the victim from the cold environment and insulating him against further heat loss. Wrap him in dry blankets or sleeping bags. In most cases, the body will begin to rewarm itself. Monitor the victim carefully. *Passive external rewarming is all you should do if the victim can be transported to a hospital within a reasonable amount of time.*

   - Active external rewarming can be dangerous to the victim and should be done *only if you cannot arrange transport immediately. Follow local protocol.* It is essential that you monitor the victim closely. To rewarm, apply heat packs, hot water bottles, or an electric blanket to the victim to *add* heat. Heat packs should be applied to the groin, neck, and lateral chest and should not exceed 110° F. Protect the skin from burns. *Never* immerse the victim in a tub of hot water or in a hot shower. You can also wrap the victim in a sleeping bag with another person, avoiding contact with the arms and legs and providing body-trunk contact only. Remember — active external rewarming should be done only if the victim cannot be transported to a hospital quickly.

6. *Never* rub or manipulate the extremities; you can force cold venous blood into the heart, resulting in cardiac arrest.

7. Never give the victim coffee or alcohol.

8. Administer fluids to the victim only after uncontrollable shivering stops and the victim has a clear level of consciousness; he should be able to swallow and cough.

9. Assess the victim for other injuries, such as frostbite and fracture. Give emergency care accordingly.

10. Try to keep the temperature of the room and/or the vehicle constant throughout emergency care and/or transport. Continue to monitor vital signs carefully.

11. Activate the EMS system immediately. Transport to a hospital is the most important factor.

SEVERE HYPOTHERMIA

Signs and Symptoms

Signs and symptoms of severe hypothermia are a little different, as is emergency care. Signs and symptoms include:

- Core temperature less than 82° F. (oral temperature less than 90° F.).
- Extremely low respiration, heart rate, and blood pressure, progressing to apnea and pulselessness.
- Absence of shivering, even though the victim is extremely cold.
- Fruity, acetone odor on the breath.
- Gross errors of judgment.
- Fixed, dilated pupils.
- Deep coma.
- Deathlike appearance.

Severe, life-threatening hypothermia can make a victim appear clinically dead. He may be in a coma, be cold to the touch, have fixed and dilated pupils, be in shock, have slow or no reflexes, breathe only once or twice per minute, be stiff (like rigor mortis), and assume a fetal position. The key in hypothermia is that *a person is not dead until he is warm and dead. Always* assume that the victim is still alive.

Emergency Care

Initiate the following care for severe hypothermia:

1. *Do not* allow any physical exertion; the victim should not move at all. Any movement can cause sudden death.

2. *Never* try to rewarm a severely hypothermic victim. Wrap him in blankets to insulate against heat loss, but do not apply any heat source, such as hot water bottles or electric blankets.

3. Handle the victim with great care.

4. Assess vital signs over a two-minute period. If there is no heartbeat after two minutes, initiate CPR. *Note:* There is controversy about the use and rate of CPR for severe hypothermia; follow local protocol.

5. Use gentle mouth-to-mouth or mouth-to-nose ventilation if the victim is not breathing. Rapid mouth-to-mouth breathing can trigger cardiac arrest.

6. If you are less than fifteen to thirty minutes from a medical facility, do not take time to care for the victim; transport to a hospital *immediately* or activate the EMS system. While waiting for emergency personnel, continually monitor vital signs, and handle the victim with extreme caution.

HYPOTHERMIA IN THE ELDERLY

The elderly probably account for nearly half of all victims of hypothermia. The likeliest victims are the very old, the poor who are unable to afford adequate housing or heating, and those whose bodies do not respond normally to cold. The greatest risk is to the aged whose temperature regulation is defective; they may not shiver, and therefore cannot conserve body heat when they need it the most. The elderly are also more likely to be taking medication, and they typically already have a lower core temperature. They cannot feel temperature changes as easily, often have chronic illness, and are usually on a fixed income. They tend to have less body fat and an inadequate diet and lead a sedentary lifestyle.

Signs and symptoms of hypothermia in the elderly include:

- Facial bloating; skin color pale and waxy, at other times oddly pink.

- Absence of shivering, but skin feels cold to the touch.

- Irregular, slow heartbeat; slurred speech; shallow, very slow breathing that may be barely discernible.

- Low blood pressure.

- Drowsiness, perhaps lapsing into coma. The lower the body temperature, the more likely the victim will be unconscious.

Always consider the possibility of hypothermia in an unconscious elderly victim. In addition to other guidelines already mentioned, *never* use a hot bath with an elderly victim.

IMMERSION HYPOTHERMIA

Immersion hypothermia — a lowering of the body temperature that occurs as a result of immersion in cold water — should be considered in all cases of accidental immersion. Immersion in cold water can cause breathing abnormalities and muscular dysfunction.

Body temperature drops to equal the water temperature within ten minutes; body temperature drops twenty-five to thirty times faster in water than in air of the same temperature. When the water is 50° F. or lower, death can occur within a few minutes. Therefore, emergency care is vital and consists of getting the victim out of the water immediately. Most deaths in cold water (75° F. or less) are due to rapid loss of body heat, leading to unconsciousness and, in some cases, drowning and heart failure. Hypothermia in this instance is likely to become fatal when body temperature drops to 94° F.

Immersion hypothermia can creep up unnoticed on divers and swimmers as body temperature drops. Extra fat layers tend to insulate individuals from cooling. Pound per pound, adult women have greater heat-loss resistance in cold water than men. Similarly, adults last longer than children, and girls have more resistance than boys. Insulating layers of clothing are important, too, so *never* remove clothing from a person in the water.

Victims who have been in the water for some time should be lifted in a horizontal position. Do not allow the victim any rapid activity in the water; turbulence and activity decrease survival time by 75 percent. Instruct the victim to make as little effort as possible to keep afloat until you can reach him.

Once the victim is out of the water, follow these guidelines:

1. Keep the victim still and quiet. The coldest blood is in the extremities; if the victim walks, moves, or struggles, the coldest blood will circulate rapidly to the heart, dropping core temperature by as much as 6° F.

2. Remove the victim's wet clothing carefully and gently if he can be sheltered in a warm place out

of the wind. Do not let the victim struggle to help you.

3. Handle the victim very gently; never rub or massage him.

4. Protect the victim from cold air or water spray. Dress him in dry clothing, his arms next to his body instead of in sleeves. If no dry clothing is available, use any insulation material — even dry newspapers. Cover the insulation with a water-proof material, such as plastic sheeting. Insulate the victim from the ground up.

5. Protect the victim from the wind. If no shelter is available, position other people around him to keep him sheltered.

6. Never give hot liquids by mouth, and never give alcoholic beverages.

7. Follow rewarming techniques described under general hypothermia.

8. Activate the EMS system immediately.

If a victim in the water cannot be rescued immediately, instruct him verbally to exert himself as little as possible. He should keep his head and face out of the water, cross his legs under water to decrease heat loss, and do as little as necessary to stay afloat. If there are several in the water, have them form a tight circle with their chests together to maintain heat (Figure 30-17).

FROSTBITE (LOCAL COOLING)

Frostbite, the literal freezing of body tissue, often accompanies hypothermia. In those cases, care of the hypothermia always takes precedence. Frostbite — which most commonly affects the hands, feet, ears, nose, and cheeks — occurs when ice crystals form between the cells of the skin, and then grow by extracting fluid from the cells. Circulation is obstructed, causing additional damage to the tissue affected.

Factors that increase the likelihood of frostbite include:

■ Any kind of trauma; always check for frostbite in trauma victims who are injured in cold weather.

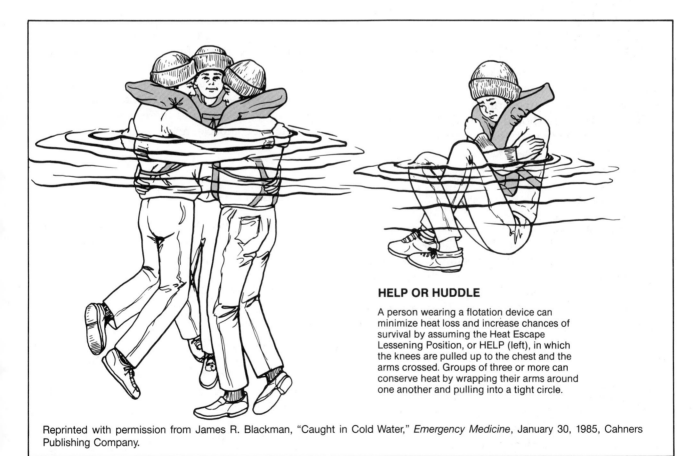

HELP OR HUDDLE

A person wearing a flotation device can minimize heat loss and increase chances of survival by assuming the Heat Escape Lessening Position, or HELP (left), in which the knees are pulled up to the chest and the arms crossed. Groups of three or more can conserve heat by wrapping their arms around one another and pulling into a tight circle.

Reprinted with permission from James R. Blackman, "Caught in Cold Water," *Emergency Medicine*, January 30, 1985, Cahners Publishing Company.

FIGURE 30-17.

- Age; the elderly and the newborn are most susceptible.
- Tight or tightly laced footwear.
- Use of alcohol during exposure to cold (alcohol lowers the ability to conserve heat.)
- Wet clothing.
- High altitudes.
- Loss of blood.
- Race; blacks are three to six times more likely to get frostbite.

Stages of Frostbite

There are three general stages of frostbite (Figure 30-18).

Incipient

Sometimes called "frost nip," incipient frostbite usually only involves the tips of the ears, the nose, the cheeks (over the cheekbones), the tips of the toes or fingers, and the chin. The victim is usually unaware that he has frost nip and will not realize it until someone tells him that his skin looks blanched or white. Incipient frostbite comes on slowly and is painless while developing; at first the skin is reddened, then it becomes white. Incipient frostbite develops after direct contact with a cold object, cold air, or cold water. Nipped fingers can be rewarmed by holding them in the armpits or on someone's abdomen. The skin should *not* be rubbed. The area will tingle slightly as it thaws and as circulation improves.

Superficial

Superficial frostbite involves the skin and the tissue just beneath the skin. While the skin itself is firm, white, and waxy in appearance, the tissue beneath it is usually soft. As the area thaws, it may become purple or mottled blue and may tingle and burn after initially becoming numb. The area usually swells during thawing.

Deep

In deep frostbite, the tissue beneath the skin is solid to the touch; it may involve the entire hand or foot. The skin is mottled or blotchy and ranges in color from white to grayish-blue. Deep frostbite is an extreme emergency and can result in permanent tissue loss (Figure 30-19).

Degrees of Frostbite

The four degrees of frostbite can generally be assessed by the color and appearance of the skin; however, these changes may appear over several days, making assessment difficult. In blacks or other individuals with dark skin, note blistering and swelling, not color change.

1. **First-degree.** During injury, first-degree frostbite causes the skin to become white and plaquelike. After rewarming, the skin is red, hot, and dry; there will be itching, burning, and swelling.

2. **Second-degree.** During injury, second-degree frostbite causes the skin to become white; there will be blisters filled with clear fluid. After rewarming, the clear blisters become filled with straw-colored fluid; there will be swelling and intense burning as the skin thaws (Figure 30-20).

3. **Third-degree.** In third-degree frostbite, the skin becomes discolored and fails to blanch with pressure. The skin may be covered with deep, small blisters that are filled with dark fluid. After rewarming, some tissue dies; the blisters become filled with bloody fluid, and there is generally severe swelling.

4. **Fourth-degree.** During injury, fourth-degree frostbite involves a full-thickness freeze, including the bone and muscle; the skin color may range from white to deep purple, and there is no pain, swelling, or blistering. After rewarming, no feeling is present, and there is significant death of the skin, muscle, and bone.

Emergency Care

The key to emergency care for frostbite is to *never* thaw the tissue if there is any possibility of refreezing. General guidelines for care include the following (*follow local protocol*):

1. Remove the victim immediately, if possible, from the cold environment.

2. If the tissue is still frozen, keep it frozen until you can initiate care. *Never* initiate thawing procedures if there is any danger of refreezing — keeping the tissue frozen is less dangerous than submitting it to refreezing.

3. Protect the injured area from friction or pressure. Remove any constricting clothing or jewelry. If clothing is frozen to the skin, leave it; remove it after thawing.

STAGES OF FROSTBITE

1. INCIPIENT (Frost Nip)
Affects tips of ears, nose, cheeks, fingers, toes, chin - skin blanched white, painless

FROSTBITE is localized cooling of the body.

- 70% of the body is composed of water.
- When the body is subjected to excessive cold, the water in the cells can freeze; resulting ice crystals may even destroy the cell.
- Never rub the skin of a victim with frostbite; rubbing can result in permanent tissue damage.

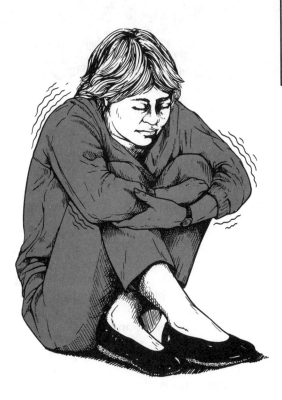

2. SUPERFICIAL
Affects skin and tissue just beneath skin; skin is firm and waxy, tissue beneath is soft, numb, then turns purple during thawing.

3. DEEP
Affects entire tissue depth; tissue beneath skin is solid, waxy white with purplish tinge.

1. Emergency care for Incipient Frostbite:
The skin can be warmed by applying firm pressure with a hand (no rubbing) or other warm body part, by blowing warm breath on the spot, or by submerging in warm water.

2. Emergency care for Superficial Frostbite:
Treatment includes providing dry coverage and steady warmth. Submerging in warm water is also helpful.

3. Emergency care for Deep Frostbite:
This victim needs immediate hospital care. Dry clothing over the frostbite will help prevent further injury. Submerging in warm water can help thaw. Rewarm by immersion in water heated to 100°-110° F, and maintain body core temperature. The frostbitten part should not be rubbed or chaffed in any way. The part should not be thawed if the victim must walk on it to get to the medical facility. Do not delay activating the EMS system for rewarming. *Follow local protocol.*

FIGURE 30-18.

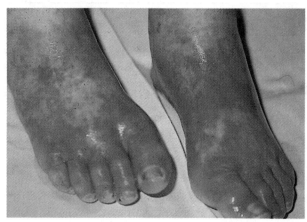

FIGURE 30-19. Deep frostbite.

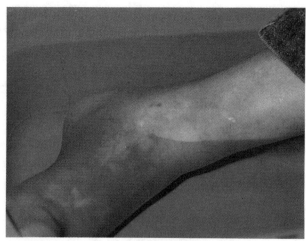

FIGURE 30-21. Thaw the frostbitten part rapidly in water just above body temperature (100°-110°F.).

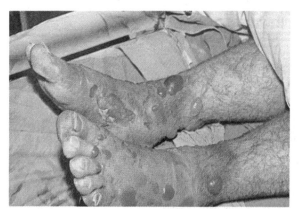

FIGURE 30-20. Second-degree frostbite.

6. Keep rewarming until the color no longer improves. The affected area should turn deep red or bluish, and the skin should be soft and pliable. Rewarming to this point may take as long as thirty or forty minutes, depending on the severity of the frostbite. *Never* attempt to rewarm the area by rubbing or massaging, and never rub a frostbitten area with snow or alcohol. Do not delay transportation for rewarming. *Follow local protocol.*

7. Once the skin is thawed, any solution that comes in contact with it must be sterile.

8. Activate the EMS system, or transport the victim as quickly as possible, preferably while continuing the rewarming process. *All* victims of frostbite require hospitalization.

9. During transport to a hospital or while waiting for emergency personnel, monitor vital signs, keep the victim warm, and elevate affected parts. Protect affected tissue from further injury or irritation. Cover the affected part with a blanket for warmth, but do not allow direct contact with the injured tissue. Place sterile cotton or gauze between affected toes and fingers; do not break blisters or treat them with salve, ointment, or bandages.

4. It is a mistake to thaw frostbitten tissue gradually; thaw the tissue *rapidly* in water just above body temperature (approximately 38°-44° C. or 100°-110° F.) (Figure 30-21). Check the water temperature with a thermometer and keep the water warm by adding warm water; never heat the cooled water with any type of flame or electric unit. The heat must be evenly distributed and kept constant. *Never use dry heat* — it is too difficult to control the temperature. Slow rewarming leads to tissue loss, and water that is too hot may add burn injury to the frostbite. *Follow local protocol.*

5. Rewarming is extremely painful; the victim may want to take analgesics (aspirin or nonaspirin products) to help relieve pain during rewarming. *Follow local protocol.*

10. If feet are involved, do not allow the victim to walk.

| **30** | **SELF-TEST** | **30** |

Student: _____ Date: _____

Course: _____ Section #: _____

PART I: True/False   If you believe that the statement is true, circle the T. If you believe that the statement is false, circle the F.

T   F   1. Heatstroke commonly occurs during times of high temperatures combined with low humidity and low wind velocity.

T   F   2. About 4,000 Americans die each year of heatstroke.

T   F   3. Emergency care of heatstroke is aimed at immediate cooling of the body.

T   F   4. If heatstroke is nonexertional, remove the victim's clothing, moisten the skin with cool water, and, if possible, direct a fan at the skin.

T   F   5. Heat exhaustion is the most common heat injury.

T   F   6. The most critical problem in heat exhaustion is dehydration.

T   F   7. Heat exhaustion is always accompanied by heat cramps.

T   F   8. In heat exhaustion, the skin is flushed and hot, and in heatstroke, the skin is cool and pale.

T   F   9. Do not give a heat-exhaustion victim fluids by mouth.

T   F   10. Heat cramps are the least common and least serious heat injury.

T   F   11. Heat cramps occur only in hot weather.

T   F   12. Death can occur within two hours of the first signs and symptoms of hypothermia.

T   F   13. Once body-core temperature drops below 90° F., the hypothermia victim will be disoriented, confused, and withdrawn.

T   F   14. Hypothermia can be a complication even when the weather is warm.

T   F   15. Whenever possible, keep a hypothermia victim in a sitting position.

T   F   16. If a hypothermia victim is not shivering, do not try to rewarm him.

T   F   17. Active rewarming of hypothermia victims should always be attempted before transporting to a hospital.

T   F   18. Never try to rewarm a severely hypothermic victim.

T   F   19. The elderly account for nearly half of all victims of hypothermia.

T   F   20. A victim of immersion hypothermia should be encouraged to increase physical activity.

T   F   21. Always thaw a frostbitten part even if there is a possibility of refreezing.

T   F   22. Frostbite should be thawed gradually.

T   F   23. If possible, use dry heat to thaw frostbitten parts.

PART II: Multiple Choice   For each question, circle the answer that best reflects an accurate statement.

1. Which of the following is *not* a means for the body to lose heat?
   a. evaporation.
   b. osmosis.
   c. convection.
   d. radiation.

2. The phenomenon of conduction has been incorporated into the concept of _____.
   a. windchill.
   b. evaporation.
   c. perspiration.
   d. hyperthermia.

3. What is the most important characteristic of heatstroke?
   a. profuse perspiration.
   b. dizziness.
   c. very hot and dry skin.
   d. painful muscle cramps or spasms.

4. Which of the following is the most important emergency-care procedure for victims of heatstroke?
   a. treat for shock.
   b. replace lost body fluids.
   c. cool body any way possible.
   d. give victim salt-and-sugar water.

5. The two most distinct differences between heatstroke and heat exhaustion are:
   a. pulse rate and presence of perspiration.
   b. skin condition and pupil reaction.
   c. body temperature and presence of perspiration.
   d. body temperature and skin condition.

6. The victim suffering from heat exhaustion can be identified by which of the following:
   a. hot, dry, flushed skin.
   b. cool, moist skin, shallow breathing.
   c. cool, dry skin, dizziness, headache.
   d. hot, moist skin, labored respirations, slow pulse.

7. A heat exhaustion victim needs to be hospitalized if:
    a. he is vomiting and cannot replenish salt or fluid by mouth.
    b. he feels dizzy or nauseated.
    c. he experiences a loss of appetite.
    d. his body temperature falls below normal.

8. Which of the heat-related emergencies listed below is the most serious?
    a. heat exhaustion.   c. heat cramps.
    b. heatstroke.   d. all are equally serious.

9. Who is the *least* likely to suffer from immersion hypothermia (pound for pound)?
    a. female children.   c. adult men.
    b. male children.   d. adult women.

10. Which of the following is *not* a procedure for care of an immersion-hypothermia victim?
    a. handle victim very gently.
    b. encourage the victim to walk around to increase circulation.
    c. remove the victim's wet clothing.
    d. protect the victim from the wind.

11. In cases where the hypothermia victim cannot get medical care immediately, the first priority is to:
    a. administer CPR.
    b. monitor vital signs.
    c. prevent further heat loss.
    d. rewarm the victim as quickly as possible.

12. The first stage of hypothermia is:
    a. shivering.   c. indifference.
    b. sleepiness, apathy.   d. exhaustion.

13. For which of the following reasons should a frostbitten part be left frozen?
    a. assessment has not been confirmed.
    b. pain becomes severe as thawing takes place.
    c. there is a possibility of refreezing.
    d. acclimatization needs to be increased.

14. A frostbitten part should be rewarmed:
    a. by rubbing.
    b. with water between 100 and 110° F.
    c. with heat from a fire or stove.
    d. with water between 75 and 85° F.

PART III: Matching: Match the type of emergency at the left with the correct signs/symptoms and emergency care at the right.

Type of Emergency	Signs/Symptoms and Emergency Care
A. Heatstroke	_____ 1. Pale and clammy skin.
B. Heat exhaustion	_____ 2. Firm, waxy, white skin.
C. Heat cramps	_____ 3. Apply firm pressure with a hand or other warm body part.
D. Frostbite	_____ 4. A dangerous medical emergency.
E. Hypothermia	_____ 5. Hot, flushed, dry skin.
	_____ 6. Painful abdomen.
	_____ 7. Body temperature can reach 106° F.
	_____ 8. Do not rub or chafe.
	_____ 9. Give sips of cool saltwater.
	_____10. Keep the victim dry and replace wet clothing.
	_____11. Slow, slurred, thick speech.
	_____12. Wrap in wet sheet.
	_____13. Sweating mechanisms fail.
	_____14. General cooling of entire body.
	_____15. May require CPR.

PART IV: What Would You Do If:

1. A middle-aged man who is playing baseball on a hot and humid day becomes dizzy and weak. He has moist, pale, clammy skin, complains of a headache, and is nauseous.

2. You arrive at a winter campout area and find a victim who is confused and disoriented. He has a stumbling gait, and his face appears bloated and cyanotic. He also seems irrational, and his speech is thick and slurred.

PART V: Practical Skills Check-Off   _____ has satisfactorily passed the following practical skills:
Student's Name

	Date	Partner Check	Inst. Init.
1. Describe and demonstrate how to give appropriate emergency care for heatstroke and heat exhaustion.	___/___/___	☐	_____
2. Describe and demonstrate how to give appropriate emergency care for a hypothermia and frostbite.	___/___/___	☐	_____

CHAPTER THIRTY-ONE

OBJECTIVES

■ Understand how drowning and near-drowning occur and identify the mechanism of injury that occurs with different types of drowning.

■ Describe appropriate emergency care for near-drowning victims.

■ Describe and demonstrate proper handling and stabilization techniques for water emergencies.

WATER EMERGENCIES

Nearly 9,000 people die each year in the United States from water accidents. This statistic is especially tragic, because a number of the deaths could be prevented with prompt and proper care. Many victims of water-related emergencies can be saved by some of the simple essentials of basic life support, such as removing them from the water and positioning them to allow drainage of the airway.

DROWNING AND NEAR-DROWNING

Drowning is defined as death from suffocation due to submersion (Figure 31-1); near-drowning is survival, at least temporarily (twenty-four hours), from near-suffocation due to submersion. Drowning is the third leading cause of accidental death in the United States. Among adults, alcohol intoxication is a factor in approximately 45 percent of all drownings. Five times as many males drown as females; male drowning mortality peaks at fifteen to nineteen years of age, with the highest female mortality appearing at the preschool ages of one to four. In addition, approximately 80,000 near-drowning incidents occur each year in the United States. See Table 31-1.

The major causes of drowning are:

■ Becoming exhausted while swimming, skin diving, or attempting a rescue.

■ Losing control and getting swept into water that is too deep.

■ Losing a support (sinking or capsizing of a boat).

■ Getting trapped or entangled while in the water.

■ Using drugs or alcohol prior to entering the water.

■ Suffering seizures while in the water.

■ Using poor judgment while in the water.

■ Suffering hypothermia.

■ Suffering trauma.

■ Suffering a diving accident.

■ Lack of supervision of children.

WHAT HAPPENS IN DROWNING AND NEAR-DROWNING

The key to saving a near-drowning victim is understanding what happens to the victim and applying proper resuscitation techniques.

Fresh-Water Versus Saltwater Drowning

In fresh-water drowning, water passes through the lungs into the bloodstream and may cause marked **HEMODILUTION** or overhydration. The degree of hemodilution, however, is directly dependent on the volume of water aspirated, and only rarely is enough taken in to reduce the sodium in the blood

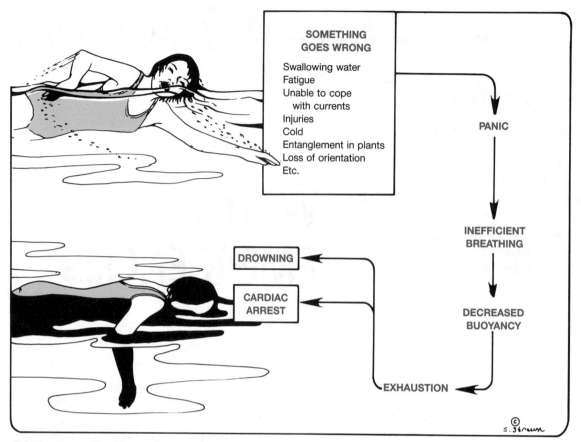

FIGURE 31-1. The effect of panic in water accidents, where panic can often contribute to the death of the person who loses self-control.

sufficiently to cause death. More commonly, simple asphyxia is the cause of death (Figure 31-2).

In saltwater drowning, salt from the aspirated water causes loss of large amounts of fluid from the circulation into the lungs. The salt draws body fluids from the cells into the lungs, resulting in pulmonary edema and death.

The basic differences between fresh-water and saltwater drownings are related to the salt content of the body fluid compared to that of the water. In saltwater drowning, the water is saltier than body fluids, so water "leaves" the blood and enters the lungs to dilute the salt concentration. The air in the lungs mixes with the fluids and forms a frothy foam, which acts as a barrier to oxygen diffusion.

In fresh-water drowning, there is less salt in the water than in the body fluids, so the water "leaves" the lungs and enters the blood. This causes serious chemical imbalances in the blood, may rupture red blood cells, and interferes with oxygen exchange and delivery.

"Wet" Verus "Dry" Drowning

"Wet" drowning occurs when fluid is aspirated into the lungs; "dry" drowning occurs when a severe muscle spasm of the larynx cuts off respiration but does not allow aspiration of a significant amount of fluid into the lungs. Approximately 10 to 40 percent of all drownings are estimated to be "dry."

Warm-Water Versus Cold-Water Drowning

There is a significant difference between warm-water and cold-water drownings. Warm-water victims are more acidotic (chemically imbalanced). Cold-water immersion causes what is known as the diving reflex; facial immersion in cold water causes the blood to be diverted from the extremities and concentrated in circulation to the heart, lungs, and

TABLE 31-1	PREVENTING NEAR-DROWNING ACCIDENTS

Three caveats apply to the vast majority of drowning and near-drowning incidents (see table).

- *Children should be under constant supervision if a lake, pool, or pail of water of any size is nearby.*
- *Water sports and alcoholic beverages never mix.*
- *Life preservers or life jackets should always be worn when boating.*

Where people drown

Type of water or site	Drownings (%)
Salt water	1-2
Fresh water	98-99
Swimming pools	
Private	50
Public	3
Lakes, rivers, streams, storm drains	20
Bathtubs	15
Buckets of water	4
Fish ponds or tanks	4
Toilets	4
Washing machines	1

Adapted with permission from Orlowski JP: Drowning, near-drowning, and ice-water submersions. *Pediatr Clin North Am* 1987;34(1):77.

These and other standard water safety precautions for swimming, diving, and boating should be made clear and repeated frequently.

Effective prevention in children requires constant supervision and common sense. A young child can find and fall into water in just a minute or two — less time than anyone would realize he or she is gone unless attention is continuous — and fences are not always effective in keeping children out of places where they should not go. A fence may appear to enclose a pool completely, but the gate may not be self-closing or the lock may be broken. The vast majority of children who drown in swimming pools do so in the backyards of their own homes, usually in the later afternoon on summer weekends. And isn't it sensible to require that baby sitters know CPR?

Programs that claim to "drown-proof" or teach young children to swim are controversial, and many experts feel they provide a false sense of security. The American Academy of Pediatrics does not recommend teaching children younger than 3 years of age to swim, although some regional programs take children as young as 6 months. Drown-proofing programs fail — studies indicate that a significant number of children have submersion accidents despite their training — because the sequential patterning approach used to teach the very young child in a structured environment engenders, in effect, learned helplessness. The cues a child learns in the class or pool setting are missing in the real-life crisis.

A large number of adult drowning victims have detectable levels of blood alcohol. Swimmers should be warned about diving in shallow or unexplored water. Boating precautions should be heeded by all boaters. Seizure disorders are an important but easily overlooked risk factor in persons of all ages.

brain. The diving reflex can also be precipitated by fear. The diving reflex is more pronounced, and cooling is more rapid, in the young. In water at or below 68° F., the body's metabolic requirements are only about half of normal, reducing the need for oxygen and protecting the vital organs.

USING RESCUE BUOYS

If you need to perform rescues around large bodies of water, always carry a rescue buoy and swimming fins. The buoy is usually made of aluminum or polyurethane and is attached to a six-foot towline with a nylon or canvas strap on the opposite side to slip over your shoulder. This, in essence, becomes a towline for the rescuer. The proper methods for rescue will not be discussed here but may be obtained from the Council for National Cooperation in Aquatics and the National Surf Life Saving Association of America.

STABILIZATION IN AND REMOVAL OF THE VICTIM FROM THE WATER

It is important that you properly stabilize the victim in the water and remove him carefully. The American National Red Cross suggests that the victim not be removed from the water until a backboard or other rigid support can be used to splint him. Many water-accident victims may be found floating facedown and must be rolled onto their back. To turn a victim, follow these general guidelines. See Figures 31-3–31-5 and accompanying instructions for specific techniques. *Always follow local protocol.*

1. Avoid any bending or twisting of the neck and torso.
2. Keeping the victim's head and body aligned, place one of your hands in the middle of his back, your arm directly over his head, and your forearm along his spine.

DROWNING

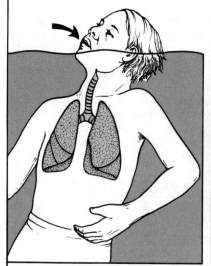

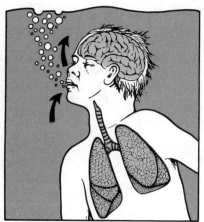

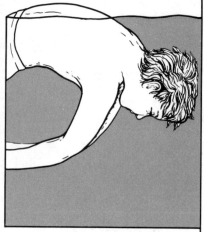

Drowning is a major source of accidental death and can be a result of cold, fatigue, injury, disorientation, intoxication, etc., or of the victim's own limited swimming ability.

The drowning victim struggles to inhale air as long as possible, but eventually he goes beneath the water where he must exhale air and inhale water.

Loss of consciousness, convulsions, cardiac arrest and death follow.

In about 10% of all drownings, a muscle spasm of the larynx closes the victim's airway, causing him to die of asphyxiation without ever inhaling water.

FIGURE 31-2.

3. Place your other hand under his jaw, and your forearm on his sternum.

4. Slowly and carefully, keeping the body and head aligned, rotate the victim in the water. If you are in deep water, float the victim to more shallow water if possible before attempting to rotate and rescue him.

5. Float a rescue device next to the victim. With one rescuer at the head and one at the foot of the victim, lower the device beneath the victim and allow it to come up slowly until the victim is fully supported. Properly align the device and immobilize the victim to the device at the chest, waist, hips, above the knees, below the knees, at the forehead, and at the feet. Use a scoop stretcher; aluminum, plastic, or wooden backboard; water ski; surfboard; picnic bench; ironing

board; or other device to immobilize the victim (Figure 31-6).

6. Do not attempt to move the victim from the water until he is immobilized; however, emergency procedures, such as mouth-to-mouth ventilation, can be accomplished in the water while the victim is in a neutral position.

7. After initial rescue procedures, immediately initate life-saving care. Never assume that a victim is dead.

HEAD- AND SPINAL-INJURED PATIENTS

Today, increasingly more head and spinal injuries are occurring from water accidents, such as diving

HEAD-AND-BACK SUPPORT TECHNIQUE

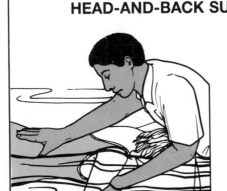

1. Keeping the victim's head and body aligned, place one of your hands in the middle of his back, your arm directly over his head.

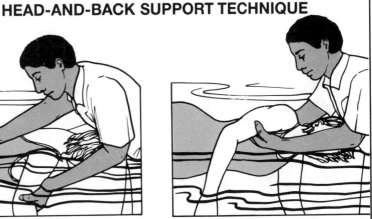

2. Place your other hand under the victim's upper arm, near the shoulder.

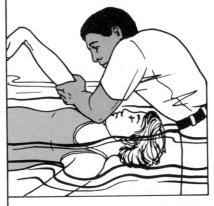

3. Slowly and carefully, keeping the body and head aligned, rotate the victim over in the water by lifting the shoulder up and rotating it over.

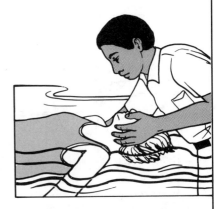

4. If you suspect a spinal injury, do not attempt to move the victim from the water until a spineboard can be used to immobilize the spine. Other emergency procedures — such as mouth-to-mouth resuscitation — can be accomplished while the victim is supported in a neutral position in the water.

5. Use a spineboard or other rigid support — such as a water ski, a surfboard, a picnic bench, an ironing board, or a wooden plank — to immobilize the spine. Slide it underneath the victim and let it float up until it is snugly against the victim's back. Use several large towels to secure the victim to the spineboard if you do not have anything else. Never try to support the victim's spine with anything that might bend or break, such as an air mattress or a styrofoam float.

FIGURE 31-3. Steps involved in turning a drowning or near-drowning victim from a face-down position to the back.

HEAD-AND-CHIN SUPPORT TECHNIQUE

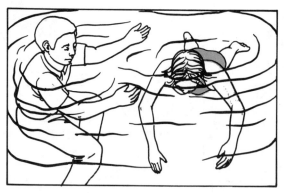

1. The rescuer approaches from either side of the victim.

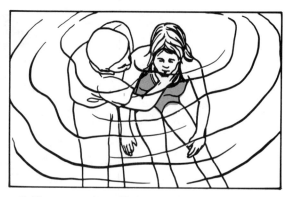

2. The rescuer places his forearm along the length of the victim's sternum. The hand of the forearm that is against the victim's chest supports the victim's chin. The thumb of that hand is on one side of the victim's chin, and the fingers are on the other side.

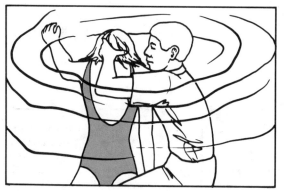

3. The rescuer's other forearm is simultaneously placed along the length of the victim's spine. The hand of this arm supports the victim's head at the base of the skull by using the thumb on one side of the head and the fingers on the other side. Both of the rescuer's wrists are locked, and the forearms are squeezed together with inward and upward pressure.

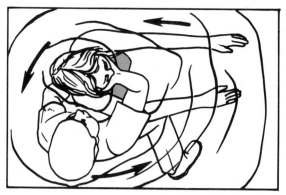

4. To turn the victim to a face-up position, the victim is rotated toward the rescuer.

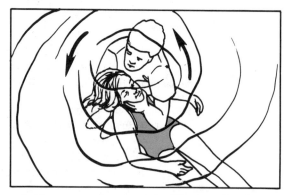

5. The rescuer submerges during this step and surfaces when the victim is face-up in the water. This step may be performed while standing in place or while moving in a headfirst direction. This movement must be done slowly to prevent any movement of the rescuer's arms and hands and also to reduce any drastic twisting of the victim's hips and legs.

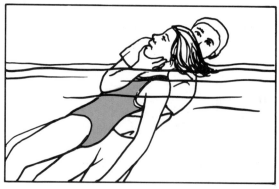

6. The victim can be supported or towed to shallow water in this position.

FIGURE 31-4.

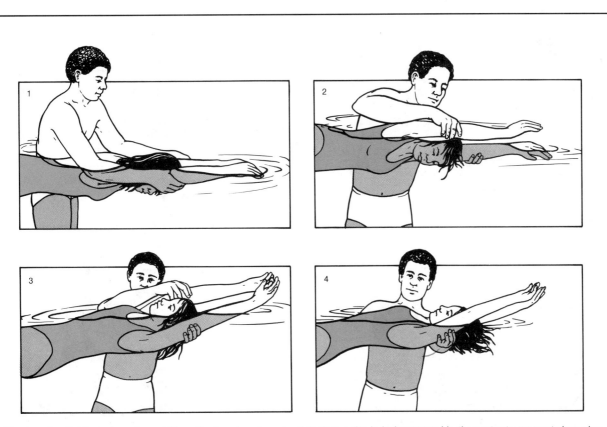

The head splint technique immobilizes the head and neck while the victim is being turned in the water to prevent drowning. To perform the head splint, the rescuer extends the victim's arms alongside the head. The victim's upper arms are then pressed against the head to create a splint. With the water at chest level, the rescuer should move the victim forward to a horizontal position (1). The rescuer should continue to move the victim forward, while rotating the victim's torso toward himself (2, 3), bringing the victim's head to rest in the crook of the arm until help arrives (4). Notice in the figure that during the rotation of the victim, the rescuer lowers himself until the water is at shoulder level.

Adapted from: Pat Samples, Spinal Cord Injuries: "The High Cost of Careless Diving," *The Physician and Sportsmedicine*, July 1989.

FIGURE 31-5.

injuries. Unless you are specifically trained in water rescue, these five basic rules should be used when aiding a possible head- or spinal-injured victim in the water:

1. Do not remove the injured victim from the water.

2. Keep the injured afloat on his back.

3. Wait for help.

4. Always support the head and neck level with the back.

5. Maintain the airway and support ventilation in the water.

EMERGENCY CARE

Dr. Philip Boysen says, "The care provided a victim of near-drowning during the first few minutes at the scene probably determines outcome more than anything else."

In the absence of suspected neck or spinal injury, resuscitation of near-drowning victims differs little if at all from standard CPR techniques. Be sure to assess for associated injuries or illness, including drug/alcohol abuse, cardiac arrest, airway obstruction, hypothermia, head injury, spinal injury, or internal injury. To give emergency care:

1. Obviously, you must reach the victim, with due concern for your own safety. Reach and pull, throw a line to the victim, or tow him in. As a last resort, go into the water yourself. *Never go into the water if you cannot swim or have not been trained in water-rescue techniques.*

2. After reaching the victim, establish an airway and initiate ventilations, even before the victim is removed from the water. Use mouth-to-mouth or mouth-to-nose ventilations. Do not waste time trying to remove water from the victim's lungs prior to attempting ventilation; do *not* use the

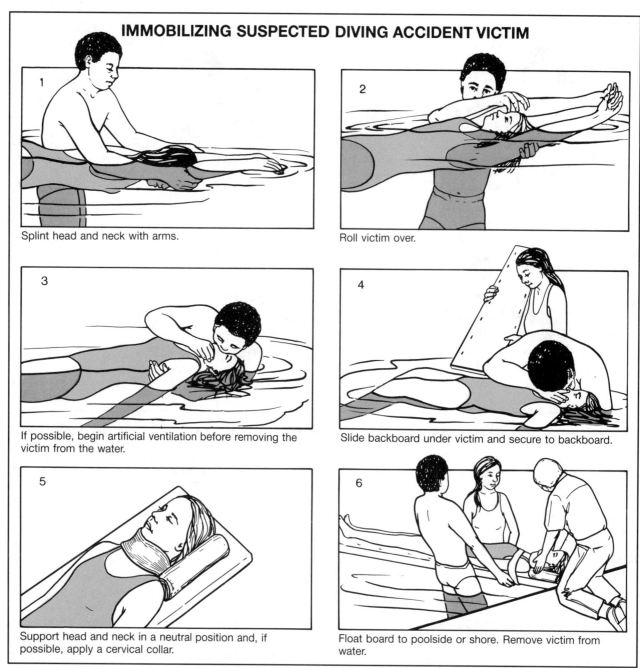

IMMOBILIZING SUSPECTED DIVING ACCIDENT VICTIM

1. Splint head and neck with arms.

2. Roll victim over.

3. If possible, begin artificial ventilation before removing the victim from the water.

4. Slide backboard under victim and secure to backboard.

5. Support head and neck in a neutral position and, if possible, apply a cervical collar.

6. Float board to poolside or shore. Remove victim from water.

FIGURE 31-6. Immobilizing suspected diving accident victim, using a backboard or firm flat object like a door. Follow local protocol.

Heimlich maneuver in an attempt to force water out the victim's lungs. *Follow local protocol.*

3. Suspect cervical injury, and take proper precautions as described.

4. After the victim has been removed from the water, quickly determine whether there is a pulse, and begin CPR if necessary. If you can feel the carotid pulse within sixty seconds, do not begin CPR. Clear the airway as necessary.

5. Treat for hypothermia.

6. Activate the EMS system as soon as possible. *Always* arrange to have a near-drowning victim transported to a hospital, even if you think that the danger has passed. A near-drowning victim can develop secondary complications (such as pulmonary edema) and die up to seventy-two hours after the incident. (Approximately 15 percent of all drowning deaths are due to secondary complications.)

| **31** | **SELF-TEST** | **31** |

Student: _____ Date: _____

Course: _____ Section #: _____

PART I: True/False   If you believe that the statement is true, circle the T. If you believe that the statement is false, circle the F.

T   F   1. Death from drowning always results from a victim inhaling water, and a drowning victim's lungs always contain water.

T   F   2. Warm-water and cold-water drowning are virtually the same.

T   F   3. The physiological processes that occur during drowning in fresh water and salt water are completely different.

T   F   4. The Heimlich maneuver is an effective way of forcing water from a drowning victim's air passages.

T   F   5. If you suspect that a drowning victim has sustained a neck or back injury, you should move him carefully from the water before strapping him to a backboard.

T   F   6. A drowning victim may still die up to two days following successful resuscitation, so close monitoring (preferably in a hospital) is essential.

T   F   7. If a victim is in trouble near a deck or the pool's edge, it is always best to rescue by getting into the water yourself.

T   F   8. In salt-water drowning the water "leaves" the lungs and enters the blood.

T   F   9. A spinal-injury victim who is in the water should be removed from the water immediately, then splinted on the shore.

T   F   10. A major cause of drowning is inadequate supervision of children.

T   F   11. Most drownings occur in salt water.

T   F   12. Over half of fresh-water drownings occur in lakes or rivers.

T   F   13. The care provided a victim of near-drowning the first few minutes at the scene is probably the major determinant of whether the victim recovers.

T   F   14. In the head-splint technique, when the victim is being rotated, it is important for the rescuer to be out of the water as far as possible.

T   F   15. The diving reflex causes blood to be shunted from the body core into the extremities.

T   F   16. Approximately 10 to 40 percent of all drownings are estimated to be "dry."

T   F   17. The American Pediatric Academy does not recommend teaching children younger than three years of age to swim.

T   F   18. Among adults, alcohol intoxication is a factor in only a few drownings.

T   F   19. A near-drowning victim should always be transported to a hospital, even if he appears to have fully recovered.

T   F   20. Fifteen percent of all drowning deaths are due to secondary complications.

T   F   21. Do not attempt to remove a suspected spine injured victim from the water until he has been immobilized.

T   F   22. Approximately 5,000 near-drowning incidents occur each year in the U.S.

PART II: What Would You Do If:

1. You are at a mountain lake and a child is seen floating face-down twenty to thirty feet offshore.

PART III: Practical Skills Check-Off   _____ has satisfactorily passed the following practical skills:
                                                          Student's Name

	Date	Partner Check	Inst. Init.
1. Demonstrate the head-and-back support technique, the head-and-chin support technique, and the head-splint technique.	__/__/__	☐	_____
2. Demonstrate how to care for and immobilize a near-drowning victim before removing him from the water.	__/__/__	☐	_____

PSYCHOLOGICAL EMERGENCIES AND DISASTERS

Effective emergency care requires not only an understanding of the nature and care of psychological emergencies, but also of the normal emotional responses to illness and injury experienced by victims. Everyone involved in a critical illness or injury — the victim, the family, bystanders, and even health professionals — responds to stresses that occur naturally in such emergencies. You can deal effectively with these responses, both in others and in yourself, only if you understand and anticipate the reactions.

PRINCIPLES OF PSYCHOLOGICAL EMERGENCY CARE

Physical emergency care is tangible — it is band-aging wounds, splinting bones, or restoring breathing. Psychological emergency care does not benefit from tangible properties. You cannot readily see the comfort that you provide to a husband who loses his wife in an apartment building fire. It is hard to immediately gauge the results of caring for a child who is depressed because a flood destroyed her home.

Stating the principles behind psychological emergency care — tangible principles that should guide First Aiders — can help make emotional emergency care more understandable.

■ Every person has limitations. In an emergency involving psychological crises, every person — including yourself — is susceptible to emotional injury.

■ Each person has a *right* to his feelings. Each person reacts individually to the environment. A person who is emotionally or mentally disturbed does not want to feel that way, but at that particular time, those feelings are valid and real. Those suffering an emotional crisis simply need help to pull themselves together. Psychological care means that you are accepting and helpful, not critical or judgmental.

- Each person has more ability to cope with crisis than he thinks he has. A person who is under severe emotional stress will believe he has lost total control. For every manifestation of crazed emotion, some strength is probably left within.

- Everyone feels some emotional disturbance when involved in a disaster or when injured. A relatively minor hand injury may seem of little consequence to you, but it could ruin the career of a concert violinist.

- Emotional injury is just as real as physical injury. Unfortunately, physical injury is visual, so people more readily accept it as being real. You would not expect a man to walk one month after having his leg amputated in an industrial accident, yet too many times, the victim suffering emotional trauma is expected to act normal immediately.

GOALS OF PSYCHOLOGICAL EMERGENCY CARE

Psychological emergency care should be planned and developed with four goals in mind:

- To help the injured person begin functioning normally again as soon as possible.

- Even when the victim cannot be returned to normal quickly, to minimize as much as possible his psychological disability.

- To decrease the intensity of his emotional reaction until professional medical help is available.

- To keep the victim from hurting himself or others.

EMOTIONAL RESPONSES OF VICTIMS

Although victims' reactions to critical illness or injury are largely determined by mechanisms that they already have developed, most of these reactions will follow common patterns. Victims usually become aware of painful or unpleasant sensations, and sometimes of decreased energy and strength, when they become ill. The common response to this awareness is anxiety.

Feelings of loss of control are common among ill or injured persons. They may feel helpless in knowing that they are completely dependent on someone else, often a stranger, whose experience and ability they cannot evaluate easily. Victims whose self-esteem depends on their being active, independent, and aggressive are particularly prone to anxiety.

Victims often respond to discomfort or limitation of activity by becoming resentful and suspicious. They may vent this anger on the First Aider by becoming impatient, irritable, or excessively demanding. Remember that the victim's anger stems from fear and discomfort, not from anything you have done. You should be aware that once victims begin to see themselves as ill or injured, the signs and symptoms depicted in Figure 32-1 may occur.

In addition, victims usually will have uncomfortable feelings about being helped by a stranger. Some victims may consider the physical assessment a humiliating invasion of privacy. Therefore, try to establish a relationship with the victim during an initial interview, then conduct the physical assessment. Assess the victim in an efficient, businesslike manner, and continue talking with the victim during the entire procedure.

VICTIM ASSESSMENT IN PSYCHOLOGICAL EMERGENCIES

The assessment should begin as soon as you begin talking with the victim. Note the victim's general appearance and clothing and whether he is neat or disheveled. Also note the victim's rate of speech. If it is slowed, it may suggest depression or some kind of intoxication. If it is rapid and pressured, it may suggest mania or the presence of stimulants. Keep the following questions in mind when assessing these victims:

- Is the victim expressing rage or hostility?
- Is the victim easily distracted?
- Are the victim's responses appropriate?
- Is the victim alert and able to communicate coherently?
- Is the victim's memory intact?
- What is the victim's mood?
- Does the victim seem abnormally depressed, elated, or agitated?
- Does the victim appear fearful or worried?
- Does the victim show evidence of disordered thought, such as disturbances in judgment, delusions (false ideas), or hallucinations (seeing or hearing things that are not there)?
- Has the victim tried to hurt himself or others?

SIGNS AND SYMPTOMS OF PSYCHOLOGICAL EMERGENCIES

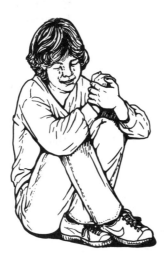

FEAR
May be afraid of a person or persons, activity or place.

ANXIETY
Not related to any specific person, place or situation.

CONFUSION
May be preoccupied with fears or imaginary attacks.

BEHAVIORAL DEVIANCE
Radical change in lifestyle, values, relationships, etc.

ANGER
Inappropriate anger directed at an inappropriate source usually brief but destructive.

MANIA
Unrealistically optimistic — unwarranted risks and poor judgement.

DEPRESSION
May range from crying to inability to function to threatened suicide. Often has feelings of hopelessness, helplessness, unworthiness, and guilt.

WITHDRAWAL
Loses interest in people or things that were previously considered important.

LOSS OF CONTACT WITH REALITY
Has trouble distinguishing or identifying smells, sounds, and sights in the real world from those in an imaginary world.

One or more of the above symptoms may indicate a psychological emergency. These may also be accompanied by physical signs and symptoms such as sleeplessness, loss of appetite, loss of sex drive, constipation, crying, tension, irritability.

FIGURE 32-1.

■ Is the victim withdrawn? (Generally, victims in psychological distress do not want to help themselves, nor do they want help from others (Figure 32-2).)

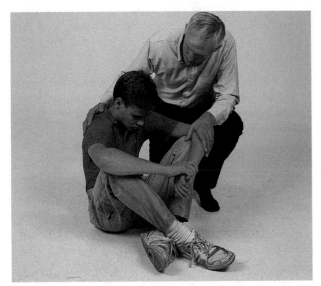

FIGURE 32-2. Victims in psychological distress may be withdrawn and may not want to help themselves, nor want help from others.

Initial questions should be direct and specific to establish whether the victim is alert, oriented, and able to communicate. Collect only information that is crucial to immediate emergency care. In general, seriously disturbed victims should be seen by a physician who can decide whether they need to be hospitalized.

PHYSICAL DISORDERS THAT RESEMBLE PSYCHOLOGICAL DISTURBANCES

Occasionally, you will encounter a victim who displays the signs and symptoms of a psychological disturbance but who is in fact suffering from a physical illness or injury. It is critical that you assess each victim (an exception, of course, would be the extremely paranoid or violent victim who obviously does not have a life-threatening problem), because ignoring a life-threatening problem or serious illness could cause the victim to die while you are trying to care for a nonexistent psychological disorder.

Just because you smell alcohol on a victim's breath, do not automatically assume that he is drunk. Persons in diabetic coma may appear to be drunk, and you may, indeed, smell alcohol on their breath. A victim who appears to be drunk could have hit his head on something.

Another way in which psychological trauma is related to physical condition is the fact that psychological trauma often follows (or is a result of) physical injuries.

Diabetes, seizure, severe infections, metabolic disorders, head injuries, hypertension, stroke, alcohol, and certain drugs all may cause disturbed behavior.

GENERAL GUIDELINES FOR CRISES AND PSYCHOLOGICAL EMERGENCIES

When dealing with the emotionally disturbed, follow these general guidelines (Figure 32-3):

- Be prepared to spend time with the victim. You must be able to talk to the person and learn what is bothering him.

- Be as calm and direct as possible. Most emotionally disturbed individuals are terrified of losing self-control. You will elicit the best cooperation possible if you show the victim through your actions that you have confidence in his ability to maintain control (Figure 32-4).

- Identify yourself clearly. Tell the victim exactly who you are and what you are trying to do.

- Do not rush the victim to the hospital unless some medical emergency dictates the need for life-saving care. Instead, take your time.

- Talk to the victim alone. Often, a victim hesitates to talk in front of relatives or friends because he is ashamed and does not want to lose their respect. Sometimes *they* may be the source of the problem — a fact that the victim cannot divulge in their presence.

- Sit with the victim while you talk to him. Never tower above him. Most victims with psychological disorders have problems relating to others, especially authority figures.

- Be interested in the victim's story, and empathize, but do not be over sympathetic. Treat the victim as if you expect him to improve and recover.

- Never be judgmental. The victim is convinced that his feelings are accurate. They are real to him, no matter how ridiculous they may appear to you.

- Be honest. Reassure the victim sincerely; give supportive information that is truthful. Do not make promises that you cannot keep.

- Make a definite plan of action, a technique that helps to reduce the victim's anxiety.

- Do not require the victim to make decisions.

- Encourage the victim to participate in some motor activity, a technique that further reduces anxiety. Let the victim do as many things as possible.

- Stay with the victim at all times.

- Never assume that it is impossible to communicate with a victim until you have tried.

- When you talk to the victim, ask questions that are direct and specific. This will enable you to measure his level of consciousness and contact with reality. Do not confuse the victim by asking complicated questions. However, avoid asking questions that can be answered with a "yes" or "no." Give the victim a chance to explain his situation. His method of explanation may help you in assessment.

- If a victim is extremely fearful or violent, skip the physical assessment unless you have serious suspicions of a physical problem that will require immediate attention.

- Do not be afraid of silences. They may seem intolerably long, but maintain an attentive and relaxed attitude.

- As you talk to the victim, encourage him to communicate. Let the victim know that you are interested in what he has to say and that you would like to learn more.

- As you talk to the victim, point out something in his behavior or conversation that will help you direct the conversation in ways helpful to you. Do this only if the victim seems to be wandering; never interrupt while he is trying to express a thought.

- Do not foster unrealistic expectations. For instance, do not listen to the story and then say, "You have nothing whatsoever to worry about." Instead, find out what the victim's strengths are, and reinforce them.

- Respect the victim's personal space. Some people will be able to tolerate you if you sit close and touch them; others prefer to maintain a distance and do not like to be touched.

COMMUNICATING IN PSYCHOLOGICAL EMERGENCIES

The main consideration in giving psychological emergency care is to develop confidence and rapport with the victim by:

- Identifying yourself.
- Expressing your desire to help.
- Using understandable language.
- Maintaining eye contact.
- Listening intently and being empathetic.
- Acting interested and concerned.
- Giving calm and warm reassurance.
- Not invading victim "space" until it is comfortable.
- Never using any physical force unless the victim is a threat to himself or others.
- Never lying to or misleading the victim.
- Not engendering false hope.
- Not judging, criticizing, arguing, or being overly sympathetic.
- Explaining the situation to the victim and your plan of action, letting him know that you are in control.
- Avoiding stock phrases like "everything will be o.k."

VICTIMS WITH SPECIAL COMMUNICATION NEEDS

Geriatric

- Do not assume senility or lack of understanding.
- Use victim's name.
- Check for hearing deficiency.
- Allow extra time for response.
- Ask victim what makes him most comfortable.

Pediatric

- May be frightened.
- May be modest.
- Move slowly.
- Explain procedures.
- Use simple terms.
- Allow child to keep toy, blanket, etc.
- Be honest about pain caused by procedure.
- Dolls may be useful to demonstrate procedure.
- Parents and siblings may be useful to help calm and explain.

Deaf

- Determine if victim can read lips.
- Position self properly.
- Use interpreter if necessary and possible.
- Use common signs:
  - sick
  - hurt
  - help
  - etc.
- Use written messages.

Blind

- Determine if victim has hearing impairment.
- Do not shout.
- Explain incident and procedures in detail.
- Lead victim if ambulatory, alerting to obstacles.

Non-English Speaking

- Use interpreter if available.
- Use gestures.
- Refer to illustrated charts.

Confused and/or Developmentally Disabled

- Determine level of understanding.
- Speak at appropriate level.
- Wait for delayed response.
- Speak as you would to any adult.
- Evaluate understanding and re-explain if necessary.
- Listen correctly.

FIGURE 32-3.

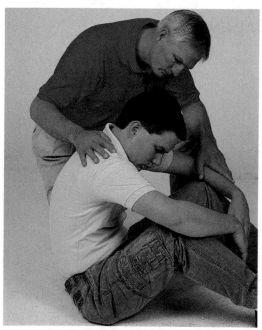

FIGURE 32-4. When dealing with a psychological emergency, be calm and show through your actions that you have confidence in the victim's ability to maintain control of himself.

- Do not abuse or threaten.

- Do not let the victim get you angry. Remain kind and calm. You may be upset by what the victim says to you, but do not react in any way.

- Avoid any kind of excitement.

- If the victim is severely disturbed and has become violent, call the police. Never attempt physical restraint; wait for professional help.

- If the environment or the scene of the accident is especially hectic, remove the victim from the scene before you try to question or calm him. The victim will probably remain disturbed as long as the environment is chaotic.

- Communicate confidence in yourself. Move with assurance.

- If the victim disagrees with you, do not argue. Instead, point out that there are many different ways to view a situation; admit that you might be wrong.

- Carefully explain the situation to the victim, and explain your plan of action step by step to avoid apprehension or fear.

- Always call for professional help in a serious psychological emergency.

VICTIMS WHO ARE CHILDREN

When a child is involved in a psychological emergency, you will need to revise your procedure slightly. A child may be unable to talk about problems directly; you might be able to work around the problem by using techniques such as storytelling, game-playing, or picture-drawing, which help to establish rapport. If the child refuses to talk, watch as he interacts with others, and try to ascertain the extent of the problem. Use the following guidelines:

- Make the assessment short; a child has a short attention span.

- Even though you want to protect the child or shield him from unpleasant facts, do not lie. If you have to tell him something unpleasant, do it gently and gradually.

- You might need to suggest some possible feelings to the child before he will be able to tell you exactly how he feels.

- Do not think that the capacity for violence is absent just because you are working with a child. Children can be especially prone to suicide and homicide; many adults mistakenly brush off a child's destructive tendencies.

- Remember that a child, more than any other victim, is likely to be frightened, not only by the ordeal itself but by the appearance of strangers.

- Protect a child's modesty.

- Move slowly, and carefully explain what you are doing in simple terms that a child can understand. Move in reverse order, toe to head, so that you can build a level of confidence before examining more threatening areas.

- Take a child's age group into consideration. Children aged one to three will suffer special anxiety from being separated from parents; be especially gentle, and allow the child to keep a favorite toy or blanket during assessment if possible. Children aged three to six tend to become especially upset over injury; cover even slight external wounds with dressings or bandages so that the child cannot see them. Children of elementary-school age are particularly concerned about modesty; take extra measures to help them remain modest and covered at all times during assessment.

- Be honest about any pain that might be caused by a procedure.

- Use dolls when appropriate to explain a procedure.

- Use a friendly tone of voice.

VICTIMS WITH SPECIAL COMMUNICATION NEEDS

At times you may need to help victims who have special communication needs. These victims may include children (see "Victims Who Are Children"), the elderly, the deaf, the blind, the non-English-speaking, and the confused and/or developmentally disabled. The number-one rule is to avoid stereotyping. Regardless of the victim's communication difficulties, use his name (first or last) in addressing him. Refer to Figure 32-3 for specific guidelines.

SUICIDE

Suicide is any willful act designed to end one's own life. Men are more often successful at suicide, but women make three times as many attempts. More than half of all suicides are committed with firearms; among nonsuccessful attempts, the most common methods are drug ingestion and wrist slashing. Suicide is now the tenth leading cause of death in the United States among all ages and the second leading cause of death among college-age students. Even with these staggering statistics, many researchers believe that suicide is vastly underreported due to the stigma surrounding it.

Typically, a suicide attempt occurs when a person's close emotional attachments are in danger, when he loses a significant family member or friend, or when he is seriously ill. Suicidal people often feel unable to manage their lives, and they frequently lack self-esteem. *Every suicidal act or gesture should be taken seriously, and the victim should be evaluated by a mental health professional.* Always activate the EMS system in an attempted suicide.

Many suicide victims make last-minute attempts to communicate their intentions; most do not really want to die but use the suicidal attempt as a way to get attention, receive help, or punish someone. Commonly, family members and friends will note a complete turn-around in the person's mood. Such a change commonly occurs for a person who has decided on suicide, because it represents a solution to his problems.

Figure 32-5 provides an excellent summary of suicidal emergencies and how to deal with them. The more you study the information, the better you will be able to assist in this type of psychological emergency.

RAGE, HOSTILITY, AND VIOLENCE

Violence is generally an attempt to gain security or control; many psychological-emergency victims become assaultive or violent. The angry, violent victim may be ready to fight with anyone who approaches, and he may be difficult to control. The anger may be a response to illness, and the aggressive behavior may be the victim's way of coping with feelings of helplessness. Violence can be precipitated by victim mismanagement (real or perceived), psychosis, alcohol or drug intoxication, fear, panic, or head injury.

In approaching any psychological-emergency scene, visually locate the victim before you physically approach him. Determine whether he is disoriented, whether drugs or alcohol are involved, and whether the victim has a gun or other weapon. In these circumstances, it is always best to summon the police and wait for their arrival.

See Figures 32-6 and 32-7 for detailed information on assessing and dealing with disruptive and aggressive victims.

MASS CASUALTIES AND DISASTERS

When the situation involves multiple casualties, such as an automobile accident with several victims or a natural disaster (tornado, flood, earthquake), people may become dazed, disorganized, or overwhelmed. The American Psychiatric Association has identified five possible types of reactions in such situations (Figure 32-8):

1. **Normal reaction.** In multiple-casualty situations, the normal reaction consists of signs and symptoms of extreme anxiety, including sweating, shaking, weakness, nausea, and sometimes vomiting. Individuals experiencing this type of response may recover completely within a few minutes and can be helpful if given clear instructions.

2. **Blind panic.** In this type of reaction, the individual's judgment seems to disappear completely. Blind panic is particularly dangerous because it may lead to mass panic among others.

3. **Depression.** The individual who remains motionless and looks numbed or dazed is depressed. It is important to give such a person a task to perform in order to bring him back to reality.

SUICIDAL EMERGENCIES

MISCONCEPTION	FACT
People who talk about suicide don't commit suicide	Eight out of ten people who commit suicide have given definite warnings of their intentions. Almost no one commits suicide without first letting others know how he feels.
You can't stop a person who is suicidal. He's fully intent on dying.	Most people who are suicidal can't decide whether to live or die. Neither wish is necessarily stronger.
Once a person is suicidal, he's suicidal forever.	People who want to kill themselves are only suicidal for a limited time. If they're saved from feelings of self-destruction, they often can go on to lead normal lives.
Improvement after severe depression means that the suicidal risk is over.	Most persons commit suicide within about 3 months after the beginning of "improvement," when they have the energy to carry out suicidal intentions. They also can show signs of apparent improvement because their ambivalence is gone — they've made the decision to kill themselves.
If a person has attempted suicide, he won't do it again.	More than 50% of those who commit suicide have previously attempted to do so.

ASSESSING LETHALITY

Age and sex: incidence of suicide is highest in adolescents (ages 15 to 24) and in persons age 50 and over. Men succeed at suicide more often than women.

Plan: Remember these points:
Does the victim have a plan? Is it well thought out?
Is it easy to carry out (and be successful)?
Are the means available? (For example, does the victim have pills collected, or a gun?)
A detailed plan with availability of means carries maximum lethality potential.

Symptoms: What is the victim thinking and feeling?
Is he in control of his behavior? (Being out of control carries higher risk.)
Alcoholics and psychotics are at higher risk.
Depressed people are most at risk at the onset and at decline of depression.

Relationships with significant others: Does the victim have any positive supports?
Family, friends, therapist? Has he suffered any recent losses? Is he still in contact with people? Is he telling his family he's made his will? Is he giving away prized possessions?

Medical history: People with chronic illnesses are more likely to commit suicide than those with terminal illnesses. Incidence of suicide rises whenever a victim's body image is severely threatened — for example, after surgery or childbirth.

The goal is to shift the intensity of a suicidal act from a desire to commit suicide to conflict over the need to commit suicide. The following guidelines can help:
- Specifically talk to the victim about his intent.
- Ask the victim how serious he is about killing himself.
- Ask what his concerns are about taking his life. He will probably have some conflict.
- Ask why he thinks suicide is the answer to his problems.
- Ask what other alternatives the victim has considered and what problems block the choice of the other alternatives.
- Ask what hope the victim has — even if it seems remote or blocked.
- By this time you may have helped decrease the intensity of the victim's need to commit suicide, even though it may be temporary.
- Always get professional help.
- A suicidal victim should be transported to the hospital for evaluation even though he says everything is okay. Police assistance may be necessary.

FIGURE ▪ 32-5.

DISRUPTIVE AND AGGRESSIVE VICTIMS
Assessing the Situation

Any behavior that presents a danger to the victim or others or that delays or prevents appropriate care is disruptive and may precipitate a psychological emergency. Common causes of disruptive behavior include stress-induced hysteria; aggression, alcohol or drug problems; neurological trauma; metabolic imbalances; organic brain syndromes; psychological disorders.

Assessing the Situation

- What information do you have from the situation — what happened?
- Is the environment (emotional, social, and/or physical) dangerous to you and/or others?
- Does the victim seem agitated, elated, depressed, or restless?
- Has he already demonstrated aggressive or violent behavior?
- Does he talk loudly and in a sarcastic way?
- Does he use vulgar language?
- Is he easily provoked to anger?
- Does he have a limited attention span?
- Does the victim seem to be out of control or disoriented?
- Does he seem to be afraid or panicky?
- Does he have a weapon?
- Is there evidence of alcohol or drug use?
- Is a domestic disturbance involved?
- Has criminal activity occurred?

If you answer **yes** to several or most of the above questions, use extreme caution. If possible, try not to control or suppress the victim's behavior. Rather, allow him to express his feelings. Remember — the most effective way to deal with a victim who exhibits aggressive and/or violent behavior is to reduce the crisis and prevent further disruptive behavior. **Probably the safest thing to do in these situations is to call the police.**

FIGURE 32-6.

4. **Overreaction.** The person who talks compulsively, jokes inappropriately, and races from one task to another, usually accomplishing little, is overreacting.

5. **Conversion hysteria.** The person's mood may shift rapidly from extreme anxiety to relative calmness. The person may convert anxiety to some bodily dysfunction. This reaction can result in hysterical blindness, deafness, or paralysis.

Observe the following guidelines in dealing with mass-casualty situations (see also Figure 32-9):

1. Identify yourself. Strive to remain self-assured and sympathetic, and act businesslike.

2. Care for serious physical injuries immediately, and reassure anxious victims or bystanders.

3. Keep spectators away from the victims, but do not leave the victims alone. If all rescue personnel are busy dealing with physical injuries,

assign a responsible bystander to stay with any person showing unusual behavior.

4. Assign tasks to bystanders to keep them occupied. Feeling that they are useful and responsible will lessen their anxiety greatly.

5. Respect the right of victims to have their own feelings. Make it apparent that you understand the victims' feelings. Do not try to tell the victims how they should feel.

6. Accept victims' physical and emotional limitations. Fear and panic are as disabling as physical injuries, and some people are able to deal with anxiety better than others. Do not try to force victims to deal with more than they seem able to cope with. Help victims to recognize and use their remaining strength and lessen their anxiety.

7. Accept personal limitations. In mass-casualty situations, realize that there are limits as to what can be done. Do not overextend yourself, and provide more effective care by establishing priorities.

DISRUPTIVE AND AGGRESSIVE VICTIMS
Management Guidelines

Remember — your first task is to protect yourself and others.

Don'ts	Do's
■ Don't put yourself in a position of danger.	■ If danger exists, create a safe zone and wait for assistance (police and/or emergency units).
■ Don't attempt to diagnose, judge, label, or criticize the victim.	■ Keep bystanders outside of safe zone.
■ Don't isolate yourself from other helpers.	
■ Don't isolate yourself with a victim who has a record of potential violence.	■ Remove any person or object from the environment that seems to be triggering the victim's aggression.
■ Don't disturb a victim with emergency care or taking vital signs any more than is necessary.	■ Convey a sense of helpfulness rather than hostility or frustration.
	■ Establish voice control by asking bystanders what the problem is loud enough so that the victim can hear you.
■ Don't turn your back on the victim.	■ Identify yourself.
■ Don't position yourself between the victim and the only doorway.	■ Let the victim know what you expect.
■ Don't forget that disturbed victims' moods can fluctuate rapidly.	■ Present a comfortable, confident, and professional manner.
■ Don't reject any of the victim's complaints — acknowledge them.	■ Ask the victim his name and what the problem is.
■ Don't threaten, lie, bluff, or deceive the victim.	■ Listen to, but do not take personal or respond to insults and abusive language.
■ Don't take insults personally.	■ Be honest.
■ Don't rush into action.	■ Speak in short sentences with simple ideas and explanations.
■ Don't show hostility toward the victim's words or actions.	■ Remain relaxed and confident.
■ Don't appear aggressive or defensive.	
■ Don't be overly friendly.	■ Adjust your physical distance from the victim to a safe range — at first no closer than approximately ten to fifteen feet — move closer only after adequate assessment and it appears that it's safe to do so.
■ Don't sound authoritarian or demanding when you speak to the victim.	■ Respect the victim's difficulty in self-control. Tell him that you are aware of the problem of dealing with it, and acknowledge the victim's attempt to deal with it.
■ Don't attempt to restrain a victim unless you have adequate assistance to do so safely. It is best to call the police.	■ Acknowledge the victim's complaints — you do not have to agree, but acknowledge that he has a reason to be upset.
	■ Use gestures and other nonverbal messages carefully. They may communicate the opposite of what you intend. A disturbed victim may interpret friendliness and smiling as an attempt to trick him.
	■ If your preventive actions fail to reduce hostile, violent, and combative behavior, the victim is in control and it may be necessary to restrain the victim to protect him and others.
	■ Assess the victim's strengths.
	■ Make certain that you have a plan and sufficient help to prevent injury to the victim and yourself.

Note: If you help at the scene of a criminal act, your first concern is to care for the injured victim(s).
- Always cooperate with law enforcement personnel.
- Disrupt or touch as little evidence as possible.
- If the victim is moved, mark the original body position.
- Provide reassurance and emotional support. Common victim responses include outrage, disbelief, withdrawal, hysteria, and depression.

FIGURE 32-7.

EMOTIONAL REACTIONS IN MASS CASUALTIES AND DISASTERS

Reaction	Signs and Symptoms	Do's	Don'ts
Normal	Fear and anxiety Muscular tension followed by trembling and weakness Confusion Profuse perspiration Nausea, vomiting Mild diarrhea Frequent urination Shortness of breath Pounding heart These reactions usually dissipate with activity as the person organizes himself	Normal reactions usually require little emergency care Calm reassurance may be all that is necessary to help a person pull himself together Watch to see that the individual is gaining composure, not losing it Provide meaningful activity Talk with the person	Don't show extreme sympathy
Panic (blind flight of hysteria)	Unreasoning attempt to Loss of judgment — blindness to reality Uncontrolled weeping or hysteria often to the point of exhaustion Aimless running about with little regard for safety Panic is contagious when not controlled. Normally calm persons may become panicked by others during moments when they are temporarily disorganized	Begin with firmness Give something warm to eat or drink Firmly, but gently, isolate him from the group. Get help if necessary Show empathy and encourage him to talk Monitor your own feelings Keep calm and know your limitations	Don't brutally restrain him Don't strike him Don't douse him with water Don't give sedatives
Overactive	Explodes into flurry of senseless activity Argumentative Overconfident of abilities Talks rapidly — will not listen Tells silly jokes Makes endless suggestions Demanding of others Does more harm than good by interfering with organized leadership Like panic, overactivity is contagious if not controlled	Let him talk and ventilate his feelings Assign and supervise a job that requires physical activity Give something warm to eat or drink	Don't tell him he is acting abnormally Don't give sedatives Don't argue with him Don't tell him he shouldn't act or feel the way he does
Underactive (daze, shock, depression)	Cannot recover from original shock and numbness Stands or sits without talking or moving Vacant expression Emotionless "Don't care" attitude Helpless, unaware of surroundings Moves aimlessly, slowly Little or no response to questioning Pulls within self to protect from further stress Puzzled, confused Cannot take responsibility without supervision	Gently establish contact and rapport Get him to ventilate his feelings and let you know what happened Show empathy Be aware of feelings of resentment in yourself and others Give him warm food or drink Give and supervise a simple, routine job	Don't tell him to "snap out of it" Don't give extreme pity Don't give sedatives Don't show resentment
Severe physical reaction (conversion hysteria)	Severe nausea Conversion hysteria — the victim converts his anxiety into a strong belief that a part of his body is not functioning (paralysis, loss of sight, etc.). The disability is just as real as if he had been physically injured	Show interest Find a small job for him to take his mind off the injury Make him comfortable and summon medical aid Monitor your own feelings	Don't say, "There's nothing wrong with you" or, "It's all in your head" Don't blame or ridicule Don't call undue attention to the injury Don't openly ignore the injury

Source: American Psychiatric Association

FIGURE 32-8.

GENERAL GUIDELINES FOR DISASTER MANAGEMENT

While each disaster presents individual problems, there are some guidelines that are general and that will usually apply to any disaster you may be called to respond to:

1 Don't let yourself become overwhelmed by the immensity of the disaster. Administer aid to those who need it. Carefully evaluate the injuries, and determine which victims should be treated first. Then set about administering the aid, treating victims one by one. This will help you maintain some calm and feel that you are making progress, despite the immensity of the disaster.

2 Obtain and distribute information about the disaster and the victims. The families of victims deserve accurate information about both the disaster and the victims themselves.

3 Reunite the victim with his family as soon as possible. There are two benefits of this: first, emotional stress will be lessened once the victim is with family members. Second, family members may be able to provide you with critical medical history that may affect your ability to treat the victim.

4 Encourage victims who are able to do necessary chores. Work can be therapeutic, and should be used to help the victim get over his own problems. Help the victim devise a schedule to perform his own daily routines like he did before the disaster.

FIGURE 32-9.

REACTIONS OF FIRST AIDERS

First Aiders are not immune to the stresses of emergency situations. When dealing with the critically ill and injured, you may experience a wide range of feelings, some of which are unpleasant. You may feel irritated by the family or the victim's demands, be anxious when faced with life-threatening injuries, become defensive at implications that you are not competent to handle emergencies, and become sad in response to tragedy. Although these feelings are natural, it is best not to express them during an emergency. Furthermore, if you give an outward appearance of calmness and confidence, it will help to relieve the anxiety of those on the scene.

TRIAGE

All the medical knowledge in the world, and all the finest care by a First Aider, is of no avail if priorities are not ordered properly. It is critical that you know which victims of a multiple-victim accident or disaster require emergency care first. Your ability to save lives depends upon your assessment of the victims and upon triage — the ability to classify which victims require attention and care the

most desperately, and which victims can wait without being endangered. (See Figures 32-10 – 32-12.)

CONDUCTING THE TRIAGE

Triage should be completed by the most experienced First Aider as soon as the scene is secured (that is, traffic is controlled, the fire is out, and so on). The key is for the triage First Aider to not stop at one victim and become preoccupied with a bloody wound or shock, but to move through the victims to complete the triage. This sets the stage for the next arriving rescuers, who can focus on caring for salvageable victims. Many victims experience an injury that does not show on the surface but that is more devastating to life than many observable injuries.

The triage rescuer should quickly evaluate each victim's condition, categorizing and prioritizing for care and applying the ABCs (airway/breathing/circulation) on a limited basis (depending on the availability of triage and emergency-care personnel) until triage is completed. The following evaluation order should be followed:

1. Ask a *conscious* victim the following questions:
   - Where do you hurt? A response may indicate if the victim can hear and understand and may reveal the condition of his thought processes.

THREE-LEVEL TRIAGE METHOD

Injury Priority	Injury Description
LIFE-THREATENED (Highest Priority)	Critically injured but can recover if treated immediately.
URGENT (Second Priority)	Seriously injured; may die without further treatment.
DELAYED (Lowest Priority)	Noncritical injuries or minor wounds.
Note: DEAD — morgue in different location	Victims requiring vigorous care for cardiac arrest should be treated as dead.

FIGURE 32-10.

TWO-LEVEL TRIAGE METHOD

Injury Priority	Injury Description
IMMEDIATE (First Priority)	Includes those who have critical injuries that threaten life but are salvageable; those requiring immediate medical care (within five to fifteen minutes) to survive.
DELAYED (Second Priority)	Includes those who are seriously injured but are not life-threatened; those whose injuries are minor and treatment can be delayed; and those who are very critically injured — non-salvageable or dead. Also includes those with no injuries or only minor injuries requiring emergency care.

FIGURE 32-11.

■ Are you allergic to anything, and have you had any serious illness recently? This tests the victim's recall and thinking processes.

■ Were you unconscious at any time? This question may reveal possible head injuries and help to recall the immediate past.

■ Do you have any medical illnesses, such as diabetes? Have you taken any medication or drugs/alcohol within the past six hours? Do you hurt anywhere specifically? Are you experiencing any vision, hearing, balance, or other abnormal problems? Do you have feeling in your arms and legs? (Pinch each limb prior to asking.) How long since you last ate?

2. The *unconscious* victim needs the following specific priority assessment. Perform it within thirty seconds.

■ Open airway by tilting back the head or lifting the chin and supporting the neck, if there is a suspected neck injury.

■ Listen for breathing and any possible airway obstruction.

■ If airway obstruction is present, perform the Heimlich maneuver with the victim lying on his back.

■ Check chest movement and mouth for breathing.

■ If breathing is absent, perform mouth-to-mouth ventilation.

■ Check the carotid pulse for heartbeat and circulation. If you find no pulse, tag the victim and move on to the next triage victim unless other triage personnel are available.

■ Hemorrhage should be controlled quickly by direct pressure or a dressing/pressure bandage and elevation. Remember — you give only limited emergency care. You cannot afford to wait six to seven minutes for the blood to clot.

■ The victim now needs to be marked or tagged according to the seriousness and kinds of injuries involved.

TRIAGE SUMMARY

Triage means sorting multiple casualties into priorities for emergency care or for transportation to definitive care. Priorities are usually given in three levels as follows: In a two-level system, the Lowest and Second Priorities would be in the delayed category and the highest priority maintains that immediate status.

LOWEST PRIORITY

- Fractures or other injuries of a minor nature
- Obviously mortal wounds where death appears reasonably certain
- Cardiac arrest (if sufficient personnel are not available to care for numerous other victims)
- Follow local protocol

SECOND PRIORITY

- Burns
- Major or multiple fractures
- Back injuries with or without spinal cord damage

HIGHEST PRIORITY

- Airway and breathing difficulties
- Cardiac arrest if sufficient personnel available
- Uncontrolled or suspected severe bleeding
- Severe head injuries
- Severe medical problems: poisoning, diabetic and cardiac emergencies, etc.
- Open chest or abdominal wounds
- Shock

PROCEDURES

1. The most knowledgeable First Aider arriving on the scene first must become triage leader.

2. Primary survey should be completed on all victims first. Correct immediate life-threatening problems.

3. Ask for additional assistance if needed.

4. Assign available manpower and equipment to priority one victims.

5. Arrange for transport of priority one victims first.

6. If possible, notify emergency personnel and/or hospital(s) of number and severity of injuries.

7. Triage rescuer remains at scene to assign and coordinate manpower, supplies and vehicles.

8. Victims must be reassessed regularly for changes in conditon.

FIGURE 32-12.

| **32** | **SELF-TEST** | **32** |

Student: _____ Date: _____

Course: _____ Section #: _____

PART I: True/False   If you believe that the statement is true, circle the T. If you believe that the statement is false, circle the F.

T F   1. Sit while talking to a victim with a psychological disorder.

T F   2. When talking to a victim, ask questions that are direct and specific to measure the victim's level of consciousness and contact with reality.

T F   3. Do *not* allow silences when talking with psychological victims.

T F   4. Do *not* leave a victim of psychological emergencies alone.

T F   5. When dealing with children, story-telling, game-playing, or picture-drawing will help establish rapport.

T F   6. It is appropriate to lie to a child to protect him from unpleasant facts.

T F   7. Suicidal threats from children don't need to be taken seriously.

T F   8. Few people have as much ability to cope with crisis as they think they do.

T F   9. Feelings of loss of control are common among ill or injured persons.

T F   10. Victims often respond to discomfort or limitation of activity by becoming resentful and suspicious.

T F   11. People under severe emotional stress usually feel like they are in total control.

T F   12. Victims in psychological distress may not want help from others.

T F   13. Most suicidal acts are gestures that don't have to be taken seriously.

T F   14. Violent behavior is often an attempt to gain control.

T F   15. Burns are in the highest priority of care in triage procedures.

PART II: Multiple Choice   For each question, circle the answer that best reflects an accurate statement.

1. First Aiders should observe all of the following guidelines when dealing with mass-casualty situations *except*:
    a. strive to remain self-assured and conduct themselves in a businesslike manner.
    b. recognize the responsibility to provide care to every victim and overextend themselves to see that it is provided.
    c. assign tasks to bystanders to keep them occupied.
    d. make it apparent that victims' anxious feelings are understood, and reassure them.

2. How should the First Aider handle emotional reactions in mass casualties and disasters?
    a. show extreme sympathy.
    b. douse the person with water.
    c. firmly but gently isolate the person from the group.
    d. administer mild sedatives.

3. Which of the following is *not* a general guideline for disaster management?
    a. obtain and distribute information about the disaster and the victims.
    b. reunite the victim with his family as soon as possible.
    c. help the victim devise a schedule to perform his daily routines.
    d. treat every victim you come to before going on to someone else.

4. A victim who is talking compulsively and joking inappropriately is exhibiting which type of emotional reaction?
    a. normal.
    b. panic.
    c. overactivity.
    d. conversion hysteria.
    e. underactivity.

5. Which guideline for psychological first aid is *not* correct?
    a. establish rapport with the victim.
    b. encourage the victim to talk out feelings and fears.
    c. use the slapping technique to bring an emotionally distraught victim around.
    d. encourage an exhausted person to rest and sleep.

6. All of the following are principles of psychological emergency care *except*:
    a. every person has limitations.
    b. emotional trauma is less serious than physical trauma.
    c. every person has a right to his own feelings.
    d. everyone feels emotional disturbance as a result of physical injury.

7. In dealing with a mentally disturbed person, you should:
    a. use strong physical force to restrain the victim before something serious happens.
    b. do whatever you can to calm the victim down.
    c. lie to the victim if you have to to calm him.
    d. not let the victim talk too much — he may get more upset.

8. What is a sound practice when dealing with suicidal individuals?
   a. trust rapid recoveries.
   b. try to shock the victim out of a suicidal act.
   c. show the person you are disgusted with his actions.
   d. ask the victim directly about suicidal thoughts.

9. What physical illness is most likely to lead the First Aider to suspect a psychological disturbance?
   a. cardiac arrest.
   b. epilepsy.
   c. diabetic coma.
   d. shock.

10. Which guideline for communicating in a psychological emergency is *not* correct?
   a. maintain eye contact.
   b. give warm and calm reassurance.
   c. be overly sympathetic to show you care.
   d. do not judge, criticize, or argue with a victim.

11. Which of the following is *not* true for children experiencing a psychological emergency?
   a. may be unable to talk about the problem directly.
   b. may be especially prone to homicide or suicide.
   c. often concerned with modesty.
   d. less likely to be frightened than other victims.

12. Which of the following is *not* a management guideline for the disruptive victim?
   a. position yourself between the victim and the only doorway.
   b. present a comfortable, confident, professional manner.
   c. adjust your physical distance from the patient to a safe range.
   d. let the victim know what you expect.

13. To evaluate an unconscious victim for purposes of triage, check the following:
   a. breathing, bleeding, burns.
   b. bleeding, pulse, head injury.
   c. breathing, pulse, shock.
   d. breathing, pulse, bleeding.

14. Triage specifically means:
   a. giving emotional support and reassurance to victims.
   b. mobilizing available rescue personnel and services at the disaster site.
   c. establishing a general plan for the community to follow in case of a disaster.
   d. assessment of the injured and separation into categories according to the severity of injuries so treatment can proceed.

15. Which one of the following is not in the highest triage priority?
   a. airway and breathing difficulties.
   b. severe bleeding.
   c. fractures.
   d. open chest wound.

PART III: Matching: Match the type of reaction at the left with the correct definition at the right.

Types of Reactions		Definitions
_____ 1. Normal reaction	A.	Mood may shift rapidly from extreme anxiety to relative calmness.
_____ 2. Blind panic	B.	The individual remains motionless and looks numbed and dazed.
_____ 3. Depression	C.	Extreme anxiety, including sweating, shaking, weakness, nausea, and sometimes vomiting.
_____ 4. Overreaction	D.	Judgment seems to disappear completely.
_____ 5. Conversion hysteria	E.	Person talks compulsively, jokes inappropriately, and races from one task to another, usually accomplishing little.

PART IV: What Would You Do If:

1. You are a pedestrian at a busy downtown intersection where a person is wandering dangerously among the traffic and seems to be oblivious to what is going on around him. He's anxious and withdrawn and is talking to himself. He also seems to be very fearful of something.

2. A child of about five years of age is injured (not seriously — a few abrasions and small lacerations) in a pedestrian/auto accident. She is crying and is very upset. There is no adult at the scene who knows the child.

PART V: Practical Skills Check-Off   _____ has satisfactorily passed the following practical skills:
Student's Name

	Date	Partner Check	Inst. Init.
1. Demonstrate in a role-playing situation an understanding of the general guidelines for the management of crises and psychological emergencies.	___/___/___	☐	_____
2. Demonstrate the proper triage evaluation procedure for a conscious victim.	___/___/___	☐	_____

CHAPTER THIRTY-THREE

LIFTING AND MOVING VICTIMS

OBJECTIVES

- Learn the general guidelines for lifting and moving victims.
- Recognize the circumstances and types of moves that can be used in an emergency.
- Describe and demonstrate how to use the various lifts, carries, and equipment in moving victims.

The need for First Aiders to move victims varies in different circumstances and localities. When possible, immobilizing and moving victims should be left to emergency-medical-care personnel.

Always Follow Local Protocol

After receiving emergency care, an injured person often requires transportation and handling. It is the responsibility of the First Aider to see that the victim is transported in such a manner that will prevent further injury and that will not subject the victim to unnecessary pain or discomfort. Improper handling and careless transportation often add to the original injuries, increase shock, and endanger life. If possible, handling and transportation should be left to the professional emergency teams.

Under normal circumstances, a victim should not be moved until a thorough assessment has been made and emergency care has been rendered. A seriously injured person should be moved in a position that is least likely to aggravate injuries. Various methods for carrying a victim can be used in emergencies, but the stretcher is the preferred method of transportation. When a stretcher is unavailable or impractical, other means may be employed.

While speed is important in a few cases, it is always more important to accomplish the handling and transfer in a way that will not injure the victim further.

The photo series in this chapter will review the various lifts and moves.

MOVING VICTIMS — GENERAL GUIDELINES

1. If you find a victim in a face-down position, move him to an assessment position after doing the ABC assessment and checking for possible neck and spinal injury (Figures 33-1–33-6).

2. Provide all necessary emergency care. Fractures, including those of the neck and back, should be splinted.

3. Move a victim only if there is immediate danger, such as:

   - Fire or danger of fire.
   - Explosives or other hazardous materials are involved.
   - It is impossible to protect the accident scene.
   - It is impossible to gain access to other victims in a vehicle who need life-saving care.

   Only in a "threat-to-life" situation should a victim be moved before the ABCs are completed.

4. If it is necessary to move a victim, the speed with which he is moved will depend on the reason for

MOVING VICTIM INTO ASSESSMENT POSITION

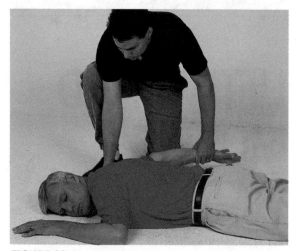

FIGURE 33-1.

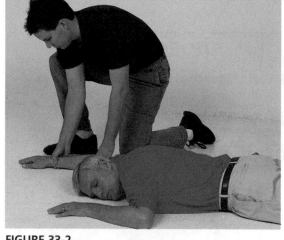

FIGURE 33-2.

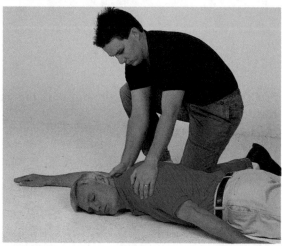

FIGURE 33-3.

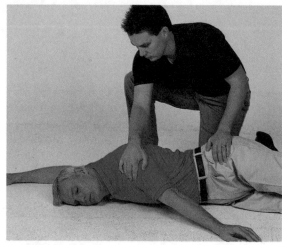

FIGURE 33-4.

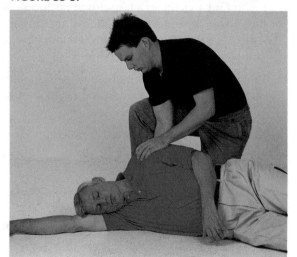

FIGURE 33-5.

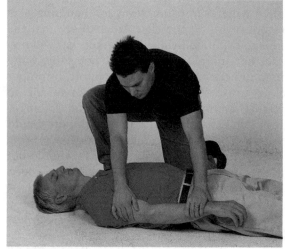

FIGURE 33-6.

Moving victim from a face-down position to an assessment position after doing the ABC assessment and checking for possible neck injury. First, the First Aider moves the victim's nearer arm above the head; he then places one hand behind the victim's head and neck and the other hand on the distant shoulder; he rolls the victim toward the First Aider by pulling the shoulder. Once the victim is flat, the extended arm is brought back to the side.

moving him. For example, an emergency move would be required if there is a fire. The victim would need to be pulled away from the area as quickly as possible. See Figures 33-7–33-10 for emergency moves. However, if a victim needs to be moved only to gain access to other victims in a vehicle, due consideration should be given to his injuries before and during movement.

WHEN TO MAKE AN EMERGENCY MOVE

Normally, top priority in emergency care are maintaining the victim's airway, breathing, circulation, and spinal status and controlling hemorrhage. But when the scene of the accident is unstable, threatening your life as well as that of the victim, your priority changes — you must first move the victim. *Follow local protocol.*

Under life-threatening conditions, you need to move the victim without taking normal precautions, like splinting. You may have to risk injury to the victim in order to save his life. *You should make an emergency move only when no other options are available.*

Obviously, there are several situations in which you should not enter the scene at all until law-enforcement personnel have secured it. You must avoid increasing the size or scope of an emergency by becoming a victim yourself, especially when other rescuers will need to risk their lives in order to help you.

Consider an emergency move under the following conditions:

- Uncontrolled traffic: If you do not have the immediate resources to direct traffic away from the accident victim, move the victim to safety as quickly as possible.

- Physically unstable surroundings: Immediately move a victim out of an environment that poses an immediate threat to life, such as a vehicle that you cannot stabilize and is in danger of toppling off an embankment.

- Exposure to hazardous materials: When a victim is directly exposed to substances that can cause grave injury or death, move him immediately. A common example is a victim who is lying in gasoline spilled from an overturned vehicle.

- Fire: Fire should always be considered a grave threat, not only to the victims, but to the rescuers.

- Hostile crowds: Crowds are at the very least a nuisance — but when you sense that onlookers

EMERGENCY MOVES

- The major danger in moving a victim quickly is the possibility of spine injury.

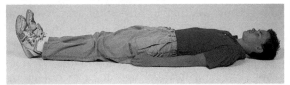

FIGURE 33-7.

- In an emergency, every effort should be made to pull the victim in the direction of the long axis of the body to provide as much protection to the spine as possible.
- It is impossible to remove a victim from a vehicle quickly and, at the same time, provide protection for his spine.

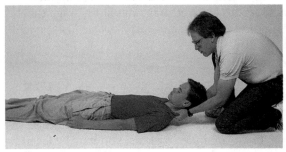

FIGURE 33-8.

- If the victim is on the floor or ground, he can be dragged away from the scene by tugging on his clothing in the neck and shoulder area.

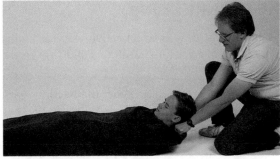

FIGURE 33-9.

- It may be easier to pull the victim onto a blanket and then drag the blanket away from the scene.
- Such moves are emergency moves only. They do not

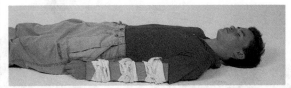

FIGURE 33-10.

- Where possible, all injuries should be immobilized as much as possible prior to movement.
- All injuries should be protected as much as possible during movement.

are becoming unruly or hostile, move the victim to a safer place immediately.

■ Weather conditions: Move a victim immediately if you cannot minimize or control his exposure to dangerous weather in any other way. Generally, the victim is in a dangerous situation if the weather is very cold (especially if the victim is wet), very hot (especially if the victim is lying on asphalt), or windy enough to turn objects into projectiles.

When you need to move a victim immediately — such as when he is in danger of an explosion, collision, fall, fire, or hazardous-material spill — immobilizing the spine may waste precious time. However, there are several safe ways to move a victim even under emergency conditions. They include the blanket drag, the shirt drag, the sheet drag, and the fireman's carry. *Follow local protocol.*

ONE-MAN TECHNIQUES

Although two or more persons should be available to move injured victims, you may be faced with a situation of moving a victim by yourself. This is often necessary in a life-threatening situation — a flood, fire, or building collapse.

THE BLANKET DRAG

The blanket drag is an effective way for a single rescuer to move a victim to safety. Follow these steps (Figure 32-11):

1. Spread a blanket alongside the victim; gather about half the blanket into lengthwise pleats.

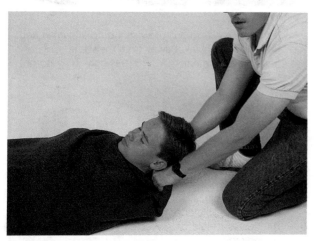

FIGURE 33-11. Blanket drag.

2. Roll the victim away from you onto his side, and tuck the pleated part of the blanket beneath him as far as you can.

3. Roll the victim back onto the center of the blanket, preferably on his back; wrap the blanket securely around him.

4. Grab the part of the blanket that is beneath the victim's head, and drag the victim toward you. If you need to traverse a stairway, keep the body parallel to the overall angle of the stairway and keep the victim's body from bouncing on the steps.

5. If you do not have a blanket, roll the victim onto a coat and drag him to safety.

THE SHIRT DRAG

If the victim is wearing a shirt, use it to support his head and to pull him. Follow these guidelines (Figure 32-12):

1. Fasten the victim's hands or wrists loosely together, and link them to his belt or pants. You need to prevent the victim's arms from flopping toward you or slipping out of the shirt.

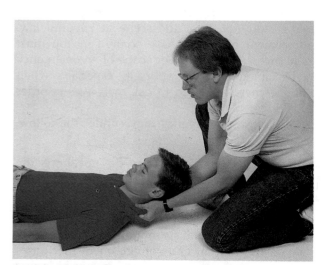

FIGURE 33-12. Shirt drag.

2. Grasp the shoulders of the victim's shirt under the head to form a support.

3. Using the shirt as a "handle," pull the victim toward you. Be careful not to strangle the victim; the pulling power should engage the axillas, not the victim's neck.

4. The shirt drag cannot be used if the victim is wearing only a tee-shirt.

THE SHEET DRAG

Sheets can be used in many ways to move victims; one of the easiest is the sheet drag, or the fashioning of a drag harness out of a sheet. Follow these guidelines (Figure 33-13):

1. Fold a sheet several times lengthwise to form a narrow, long "harness."

2. Lie the folded sheet centered across the victim's chest at the nipple line.

3. Pull the ends of the sheet under the victim's arms at the axillas and behind the victim's head; twist the ends of the sheet together to form a triangular support for the head, being careful not to pull the victim's hair.

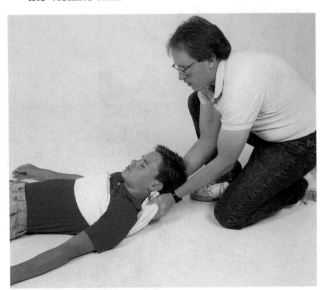

FIGURE 33-13. Sheet drag.

4. Grasping the loose ends of the sheet, pull the victim toward you.

5. The sheet drag can also work well to slide a victim out of a car and onto a board when you need to move him head-first.

THE FIREMAN'S CARRY

The fireman's carry is not as safe as most groundlevel moves because it places the victim's center of mass high — usually at the rescuer's shoulder level — and because it requires a fair amount of strength. If you need to move the victim over irregular terrain, however, it can be a better choice than a drag. Unless it is a life-or-death situation, do not attempt a fireman's carry if the victim has fractures of the extremities or suspected spinal injury.

To perform the fireman's carry, follow these steps (Figure 33-14–33-17):

1. Position the victim on his back, with both knees bent and raised. Grasp the back sides of the victim's wrists.

2. Stand on the toes of both of the victim's feet. Lean backward, pulling the victim up and toward you. As the victim nears a standing position, crouch slightly and pull him over your right shoulder.

3. Stand upright.

4. Pass your right arm between the victim's legs and grasp the victim's arm that is nearest your body.

5. The fireman's carry can also be accomplished with an assisting rescuer.

THE FIREMAN'S CARRY

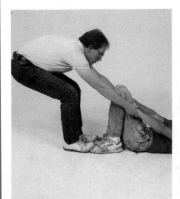

FIGURE 33-14.

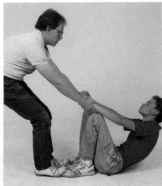

FIGURE 33-15.

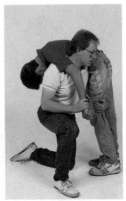

FIGURE 33-16.

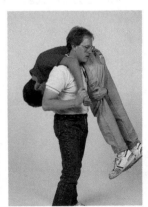

FIGURE 33-17.

OTHER EMERGENCY MOVES

Other emergency moves include the piggyback carry (Figures 33-18–33-19), the one-rescuer crutch (Figure 33-20), the one-rescuer cradle carry (Figure 33-21), the fireman's drag (Figure 33-22), the shoulder drag (Figure 33-23), and the foot drag (Figure 33-24).

OTHER EMERGENCY MOVES

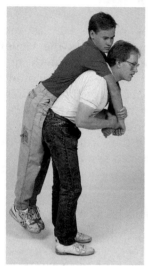

FIGURE 33-18.

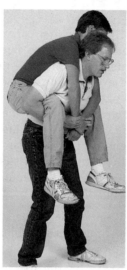

FIGURE 33-19. Piggyback carry.

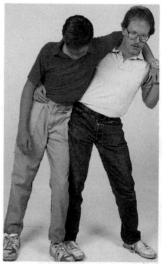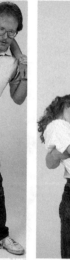

FIGURE 33-20. One-rescuer crutch.

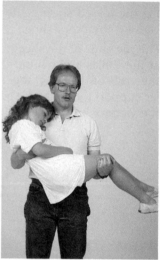

FIGURE 33-21. One-rescuer cradle carry.

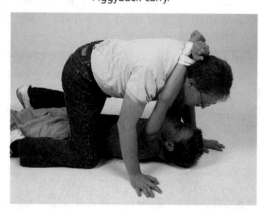

FIGURE 33-22. Fireman's drag.

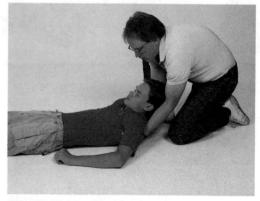

FIGURE 33-23. Shoulder drag.

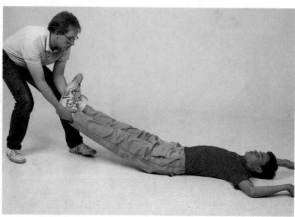

FIGURE 33-24. Foot drag.

TWO- AND THREE-MAN TECHNIQUES

SEAT CARRIES (TWO RESCUERS)

Follow these guidelines:

1. Raise the victim to a sitting position.

2. Each First Aider steadies the victim by positioning an arm around his back.

3. Each First Aider slips his other arm underneath the victim's thighs, then clasps the wrist of the other First Aider. One pair of arms should make a seat, the other pair a backrest (Figures 33-25–33-27).

4. Slowly raise the victim from the ground. Make sure that you move in unison.

In another method, the First Aiders form a seat with four hands, and the victim supports himself by placing his arms around the First Aiders' necks (Figures 33-28–33-30).

TWO-RESCUER SEAT CARRY

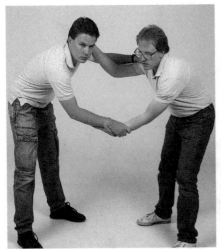

FIGURE 33-25.

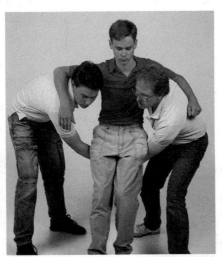

FIGURE 33-26.

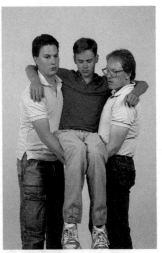

FIGURE 33-27.

Alternate Method of Seat Carry

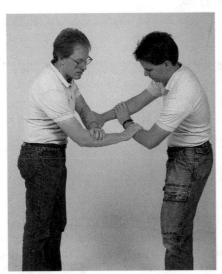

FIGURE 33-28.

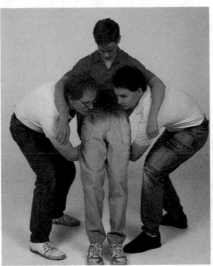

FIGURE 33-29.

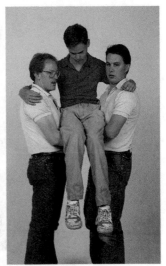

FIGURE 33-30.

EXTREMITY LIFT (TWO RESCUERS)

Never use the extremity lift when the victim has back injuries. If you do not suspect an injury of this type, proceed as follows (Figures 33-31 and 33-32):

1. One First Aider kneels at the victim's head; the other kneels beside the victim's knees.

2. The First Aider at the victim's head places one hand under each of the victim's shoulders; the second First Aider grasps the victim's wrists.

3. The First Aider at the victim's knees pulls the victim to a sitting position by pulling on the victim's wrists; the First Aider at the victim's head assists by pushing the victim's shoulders and supporting the victim's back.

4. The First Aider at the victim's head slips his hands under the arms and grasps the victim's wrists.

EXTREMITY LIFT

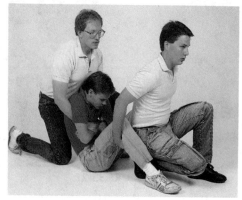

FIGURE 33-31.

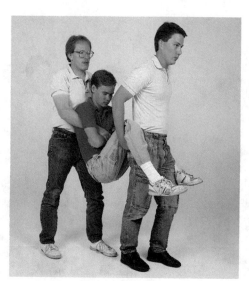

FIGURE 33-32.

CHAIR LITTER CARRY

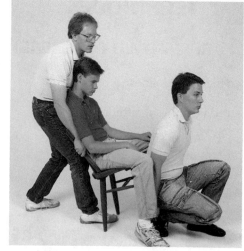

FIGURE 33-33.

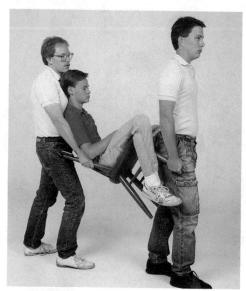

FIGURE 33-34.

5. The First Aider at the victim's knees slips his hands beneath the victim's knees.

6. Both First Aiders crouch on their feet.

7. Both First Aiders simultaneously stand in one fluid motion.

CHAIR LITTER CARRY

If the victim does not have contraindicating injuries, and if a chair is available, sit the victim in the chair. One First Aider then carries the back of the chair while the other carries the legs; the chair itself is used as a litter (Figures 32-33 and 32-34). Be sure the chair is sturdy enough to support the weight of the victim.

FLAT LIFT AND CARRY (THREE RESCUERS)

The three-rescuer flat lift and carrry is an effective way to move a severely injured victim. Be careful of backstrain, however. If there is no spinal injury, use the following technique (Figures 33-35–33-38):

1. Three First Aiders line up on one side of the victim. The tallest stands at the victim's shoulders, another stands at his hips, and another at his knees.

2. Each First Aider kneels on the knee closest to the victim's feet, on the least injured side.

3. The First Aider at the victim's shoulders works his hands underneath the victim's neck and shoulders; the First Aider at the hips works his hands underneath the victim's hips and pelvis; the First Aider at the knees works his hands underneath the victim's knees.

4. In unison, raise the victim to knee level and slowly turn the victim toward all three First Aiders until the victim rests on the bends of their elbows. *Follow local protocol.*

5. In unison, all three rise to a standing position. Walk with the victim to a place of safety or to the stretcher.

6. To deposit the victim on the stretcher, simply reverse the procedure.

One of the great advantages of the three-rescuer flat lift and carry is that it enables you to move the victim through narrow passages and down stairs. The procedure can also be done with four men, positioning First Aiders at the victim's head, chest, hips, and knees. Support is then given to the head, chest, hips, pelvis, knees, and ankles.

THE CANVAS LITTER/ POLE STRETCHER

Canvas litters (Figure 33-39) have been used by armies worldwide for at least two centuries. The modern tubular-framed, vinyl-coated nylon version accommodates victim's weighing up to 350 pounds.

Canvas litters work well when a victim can be log-rolled but do not work as well when the victim has

THREE-RESCUER FLAT LIFT AND CARRY

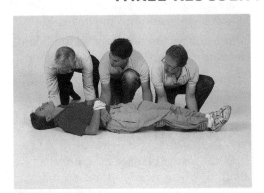

FIGURE 33-35.

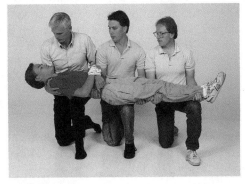

FIGURE 33-36.

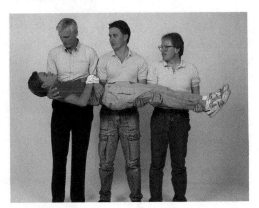

FIGURE 33-37.

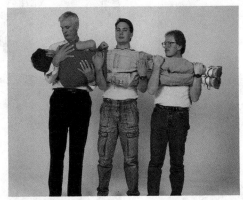

FIGURE 33-38.

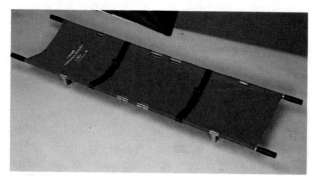

FIGURE 33-39. Pole stretcher.

to be moved lengthwise. They generally should not be used when spinal immobilization is necessary unless they are used with a long backboard.

BACKBOARDS

Backboards (Figures 33-40 and 33-41) are some of the rescuer's most versatile tools.

There are several ways to get a victim onto a backboard, and the method you choose will depend on whether you need to immobilize the spine and how the victim is positioned.

If you need to immobilize the spine, manually support the victim's head and neck in normal anatomic position. Maintain that manual support until the victim is supine on the backboard. If possible, apply a rigid extrication-type cervical collar to the victim's neck. What you do next depends on the victim's position. *Follow local protocol.*

If the victim is sitting (see Chapters 12 and 13 for the use of backboards):

1. Approach the victim from behind; slide the board carefully behind his back.

2. Tell the victim to lean against the board; anchor the bottom of the board with your knee to keep it from shifting position.

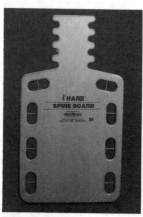

FIGURE 33-40.
Short backboard.

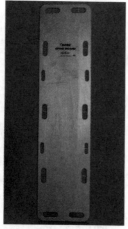

FIGURE 33-41.
Long backboard.

3. Slowly tilt the board backward, maintaining manual support of the victim's head and neck. As the victim becomes supine, slide his lower body onto the board. Move in several short steps instead of one long one.

If the victim is recumbent (see Chapters 12 and 13):

1. Logroll the victim onto the board or slide him lengthwise, depending on the space.

2. Carefully maintain manual support of the head and neck.

If the victim is supine (see Chapters 12 and 13):

1. Bring the board to within arm's reach.

2. Grasp the victim's forearm closest to you, and lie it across the victim's chest.

3. Grasp the elbow of the same arm. With your other hand, grasp the trouser-leg of the victim's knee on the same side, bringing the knee into a raised position. Grasp the knee.

4. Holding onto the victim's elbow and knee, push away from you while a second rescuer gently rotates the head in the same direction.

5. With the victim on his side, examine his back. Then pull the backboard toward you and place it on edge against the victim's back. Roll the victim toward you and onto the board.

6. Strap the victim securely to the board, using at least three straps and preferably four.

If the victim is in a prone position, logroll him onto a spine board. *Follow local protocol.*

BLANKET STRETCHER

You can use a blanket as a stretcher when space is limited or you need to traverse stairs or cramped corners. Use a blanket only if you suspect no back, or pelvic injuries, or a fractured skull. *Follow local protocol.*

Any blanket used as a stretcher should be strong, free of holes, and in good condition. It must be large enough to support the victim's entire body; if you are not sure, test it by trying it out on a rescuer. If the weather is cold, you might use two blankets instead of one, wrapping alternating folds of the blankets around the victim for warmth.

To use a blanket as a stretcher (Figures 33-42–33-47):

1. Logroll or slide the victim onto the center of the blanket.

2. Tightly roll the side edges of the blanket toward the victim; these rolled edges will form handholds.

── BLANKET LIFT AND CARRY ──

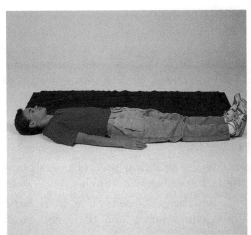

FIGURE 33-42.

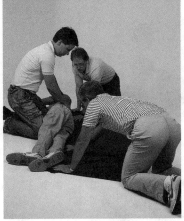

FIGURE 33-43.

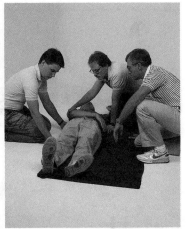

FIGURE 33-44.

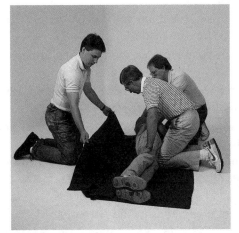

FIGURE 33-45.

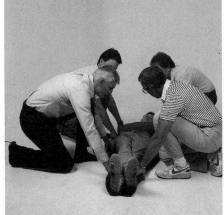

FIGURE 33-46.

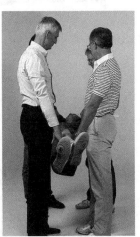

FIGURE 33-47.

3. Position as many rescuers around the victim as needed to distribute the hands evenly. Lift and carry the victim smoothly and evenly.

IMPROVISED STRETCHERS

A satisfactory stretcher may be improvised with a blanket, canvas, brattice cloth, or a strong sheet, and two poles or pieces of pipe, seven to eight feet long. To construct an improvised stretcher using two poles and a blanket, proceed as follows (Figures 33-48–33-50):

■ Place one pole about one foot from the center of the unfolded blanket.

■ Fold the short side of the blanket over the pole.

■ Place the second pole on the two thicknesses of the blanket about two feet from the first pole and parallel to it.

■ Fold the remaining side of the blanket over the second pole. When the victim is placed on the blanket, the weight of the body secures the poles.

Cloth bags or sacks may be used for stretcher beds. Holes should be made in the bottoms of bags or sacks so that the poles may be passed through them. Enough bags or sacks should be used to produce the required length of the bed. A stretcher may also be made from three or four coats or jackets. The sleeves should be turned inside out with the jacket fastened and the sleeves inside the coat. A pole should be placed through each sleeve.

IMPROVISED STRETCHER

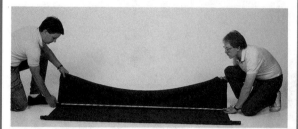

FIGURE 33-48.

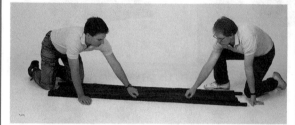

FIGURE 33-49.

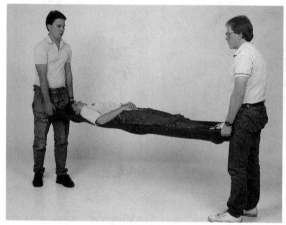

FIGURE 33-50.

STRETCHER TRANSPORTATION

When the canvas stretcher is to be used to transport a victim, care should be taken to see that the crosspieces are locked in place. Any stretcher should be tested to determine serviceability immediately prior to placing an injured person on it. This should be done by placing an uninjured person weighing as much or more than the victim on the stretcher. The stretcher is then lifted waist high and lowered to the ground. Once the stretcher has been tested, it should be padded with a blanket or similar material.

When lifting a victim for stretcher transportation, it is preferable to have four or more persons lift. If only four persons are available and a spinal injury is not suspected, the following method is recommended:

- Each of the four bearers rests on the knee nearest the victim's feet. Three of the bearers position themselves on the victim's least injured side, at the victim's knees, at the hips, and at the shoulders. The fourth bearer is positioned at the victim's hips on the opposite side from the others.
- The hands of the bearer at the shoulders are placed under the victim's neck and shoulders.
- The hands of the bearer at the knees are placed under the victim's knees and ankles.
- The other two bearers each place their hands under the victim's pelvis and the small of the back.
- The four bearers slowly lift the victim, keeping the body level.
- The victim is rested on the knees of the three bearers on the same side.
- The fourth bearer places the stretcher under the victim.
- The bearer who has placed the stretcher assumes his original position.
- The victim is lowered gently to the stretcher and covered with a blanket.
- The bearers position themselves one at each end and one at each side of the stretcher, facing the victim.
- All bearers grasp and lift the stretcher.
- The two bearers in the center shift one hand toward the victim's feet and support this end, while the bearer at the victim's feet turns around to a marching position.
- The victim usually is transported feet first, so that the bearer at the victim's head can constantly monitor the victim's condition (Figure 33-51).

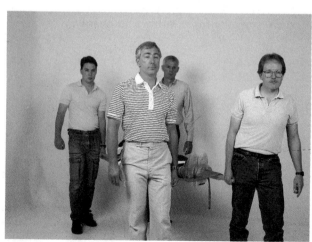

FIGURE 33-51.

| **33** | **SELF-TEST** | **33** |

Student: _____ Date: _____

Course: _____ Section #: _____

PART I: True/False   If you believe that the statement is true, circle the T. If you believe that the statement is false, circle the F.

T   F   1. All necessary emergency care usually should be provided before moving a victim.

T   F   2. Only in a "threat-to-life" situation should a victim be moved before the ABCs are completed.

T   F   3. In an emergency move, every effort should be made to pull the victim in the direction of the long axis of the body.

T   F   4. The major danger in moving a victim quickly is the possibility of spinal injury.

T   F   5. The extremity lift is a good lift to use if the victim has back injuries.

T   F   6. The three-rescuer flat lift is not a good move to use in a severely injured victim.

T   F   7. One of the disadvantages of the three-rescuer flat lift and carry is that it does not enable you to move the victim through narrow passages.

T   F   8. A canvas or pole stretcher generally should not be used when spinal immobilization is necessary unless it is used with a long backboard.

T   F   9. A blanket stretcher is a good method to use when moving a spinal-injured victim.

T   F   10. When lifting a victim for stretcher transportation, it is preferable to have four or more persons lift.

T   F   11. A victim should be transported head-first on a stretcher.

T   F   12. The blanket drag is an effective way for a single rescuer to move a victim to safety.

T   F   13. The sheet drag cannot be used if the victim is wearing only a tee-shirt.

T   F   14. The fireman's carry is considerably safer to use than most other ground-level moves.

T   F   15. It is impossible to remove a victim from a vehicle quickly and at the same time provide protection for the spine.

T   F   16. A victim should usually not be moved until a thorough assessment has been made.

T   F   17. A sheet drag should never be used to slide a victim out of a car.

T   F   18. If you find a victim in a face-down position immediately move him into the assessment position before doing the ABC check.

PART II: Multiple Choice   For each question, circle the answer that best reflects an accurate statement.

1. Two or more rescuers can use a blanket to transport an injured victim safely as long as the victim does not have:
    a. a fractured pelvis.
    b. a spinal injury.
    c. a skull fracture.
    d. any of the above.

2. When carrying a victim on a litter, how many rescuers should ideally lift and carry?
    a. two.
    b. three.
    c. four or more.
    d. eight.

3. Why should an injured person be carried feet-first when being transported by litter?
    a. being able to see where he is going will calm him.
    b. the litter bearer at the rear will be better able to observe the victim.
    c. the litter bearer at the rear can protect the victim from being hit by flying debris.
    d. the victim's body weight will be more evenly distributed.
    e. a victim should not be carried feet-first.

4. An injured person may be moved by a First Aider only if the victim's position:
    a. puts him in danger of developing shock.
    b. endangers his life.
    c. is inconvenient for giving first aid.
    d. prevents him from receiving first aid.

5. If you are using a clothes drag to move an injured victim, move him by pulling him on his:
    a. back, feet first.
    b. back, head first.
    c. stomach, feet first.
    d. stomach, head first.

6. Where do the rescuers kneel to perform the three-man lift and carry?
    a. on the knee nearest the victim's head on the injured side.
    b. on their right knees and on both sides of the victim.
    c. on the knee nearest the victim's feet and on the least injured side.
    d. on the knee nearest the victim's feet and on both sides.

7. When is it appropriate to move a victim away from the emergency site before giving emergency care?
   a. when there is danger of fire or explosion.
   b. when the victim is blocking another victim who needs life-saving care.
   c. when it is impossible to protect the scene.
   d. alll of these answers.

8. A victim who is slightly injured may be moved by one rescuer using the:
   a. crutch method.
   b. fireman's carry.
   c. shoulder drag.
   d. extremity lift.

9. Victims usually should be positioned _____ when transporting them on a stretcher.
   a. over the heads of the bearers.
   b. on the side.
   c. feet-first.
   d. head-first.

10. Which of the following statements are true about moving victims?
    1) pull in the direction of the long axis of the body.
    2) a victim in a face-down position should be left in that position.
    3) never drag a victim by his clothing.
    4) a stretcher is the preferred method of transportation.
    a. 2 and 3.
    b. 1, 2, and 3.
    c. 1 and 4.
    d. 1, 2, 3, and 4.

11. The correct sequence for moving a victim into an assessment position is:
    a. extend the victim's near arm above his head, place the rescuer's hand behind the victim's head, grasp the victim's far shoulder with the opposite hand, and roll the victim toward the rescuer.
    b. extend both of the victim's arms above his head, support the victim's neck, and roll the victim away from the rescuer.
    c. position both of the victim's arms at his sides, and roll the victim in one unit toward the rescuer.
    d. straighten the victim's arms and legs, position his head toward the rescuer, and roll the victim in one unit toward the rescuer.

12. A two-rescuer seat could be used when the victim is:
    a. conscious, but needs support.
    b. unconscious.
    c. suspected of having a neck injury.
    d. unconscious, with unknown injuries.

13. If the move is a nonemergency move, you should:
    a. treat for shock before moving the victim.
    b. complete emergency care before attempting to move the victim.
    c. only move the victim if it is inconvenient to give first aid.
    d. unconscious, with unknown injuries.

14. The primary consideration in an emergency move is protection of the:
    a. head.
    b. extremities.
    c. heart.
    d. spine.

15. What is the greatest danger associated with moving a victim too quickly?
    a. hemorrhage
    b. cardiac arrest.
    c. spinal injury.
    d. shock.

PART III: What Would You Do If:

1. It is necessary to move a severely injured trauma victim who is unconscious; other rescuers are available.

2. It is necessary to move an unconscious victim away from a burning automobile.

PART V: Practical Skills Check-Off

_____ has satisfactorily passed the following practical skills:
Student's Name

	Date	Partner Check	Inst. Init.
1. Demonstrate five one-man techniques for moving victims.	__/__/__	☐	_____
2. Participate in a demonstration of three two-man techniques for moving victims.	__/__/__	☐	_____
3. Participate in a demonstration on how to lift and/or move a victim with three or more rescuers.	__/__/__	☐	_____

CHAPTER THIRTY-FOUR

OBJECTIVES

- Understand that extrication can be hazardous and dangerous and is best left to carefully trained professionals if possible.

- Understand the major goals and principles of extrication.

- Learn how to stabilize a vehicle, gain access to a victim, stabilize and disentangle him, and properly prepare the victim for removal.

- Learn about specialized extrication situations.

VEHICLE STABILIZATION AND VICTIM EXTRICATION

EXTRICATION

The term "extricate" means to disentangle or free from entrapment. Extrication is the process of removing a victim or victims from a dangerous, life-threatening situation. Two important factors to consider concerning extrication are:

1. Does the victim *really* need to be moved now? Is the victim's life in danger if you do not move him, or can you give emergency care to the trapped victim and wait for a trained rescue team with proper equipment?

2. If the victim *has* to be moved immediately, plan and prepare well, and practice safety-first.

If you decide that the victim does not need to be rescued immediately and a rescue team will be arriving soon, do the following:

- Control the hazards and stabilize the accident scene (shut off engines, put out flares, douse fires, etc.). Allow no smoking because of the possibility of spilled gasoline.

- Gain access to the victim, if possible, and if safe to do so.

- Give ABCs and other emergency care to stabilize the victim.

- Remain with the victim until the rescue team arrives.

Bystanders can be helpful or a hindrance. One of the First Aiders should be responsible for telling bystanders what to do. Give bystanders specific instructions on how to help you, or to stay out of the way so that they do not interfere or run the risk of becoming injured themselves.

FIND ALL OF THE VICTIMS

Care first for all victims who can be located immediately, then scour the area (ditches, bushes, etc.) for any victim who may be hidden. Use a systematic approach so that no victims are missed.

- If a passenger is conscious and coherent, ask how many people were in the car.

- Question witnesses about whether someone left the site or whether a passerby took a victim away.

- In cases of high impact, search the vehicle and area carefully, especially in ditches and tall weeds. A victim can even be wedged under the dashboard.

- Look for tracks in the earth or snow. A victim who can free himself from the vehicle may leave to get help, or wander aimlessly.

DANGERS AT ACCIDENT SCENES

If a car is on fire and fire-fighting personnel have not yet arrived, decide if you can remove the passengers quickly enough or whether you should fight the fire. If the passengers are not trapped, move them first. If they cannot be extricated quickly, deal with the fire.

Any accident with a possible power-line involvement is potentially dangerous. Assume that all downed lines are live, and call for expert assistance as soon as you arrive at the scene. Park your vehicle at a safe distance from a downed power line. Warn any bystanders to stand clear, and tell victims to stay inside their vehicles. Persons inside a vehicle with an electrical line contacting it are safe, because the tires provide insulation. Quickly contact the electric company to shut off power and handle downed lines, etc. Do *not* try to handle a live wire by yourself.

STABILIZING THE VEHICLE

After all possible outside hazards are controlled, make the rescue setting as safe as possible. Suspect any vehicle as being unstable until you have made it stable, regardless of how it may have come to rest after the collision. Suspect that a vehicle is *not* stable if it is on a tilted surface (such as a hill), if part of it is stacked on top of another vehicle, or if it is on a slippery surface such as ice, snow, or spilled oil. Vehicles that have come to rest on their side or roof should also be considered unstable. Even when the vehicle is upright and appears to be stable, use blocks or wedges at wheels to prevent unexpected rolling. Chock wheels tightly against the curb when possible.

OVERTURNED VEHICLE

To stabilize an overturned vehicle, place a solid object — such as a wheel chock, spare tire, cribbing, or timber — between the roof and the roadway. If necessary, use the vehicle's bumper jack to angle the vehicle against the solid object until the vehicle is stable. Hook a chain to the vehicle's axle, then loop the chain around a tree or post. Any vehicle that can be moved easily during extrication or victim care needs to be stabilized by the placement of cribbing or step-blocks under the frame, and by clipping the valve stems of the tires. Excess motion of the vehicle could prove fatal for a victim with severe spinal injuries and may injure the rescue team.

UPRIGHT VEHICLES

One of the first steps in stabilizing a vehicle that rests on all four wheels is simply to place the gear selector in park or, on a standard shift, into reverse. Another immediate stabilization technique is to cut the valve stems so that the car rests on the rims, thus reducing the amount of vehicle movement.

TOOLS AND EQUIPMENT NEEDED

It is important to be prepared in case a rescue squad is not available. Basic tools that can be used include: hammer, screwdriver, chisel, crowbar, pliers, linoleum knife, work gloves and goggles, shovel, tire irons, wrenches, knives, car jacks, and ropes or chains. Ingenuity and creative thought can put these basic tools to work in a safe, effective way.

GAIN ACCESS TO THE PATIENT

Use the following procedures if you need to use force in gaining access.

DOORS

Attempt to open the door nearest the victim by using the door handle. If the doors are locked, try to open the lock by either having a person in the car do so, or by using a coat hanger or other device between the door frame and window. Routinely unlock all other doors when you gain entrance to the vehicle to allow access by other rescuers. If the doors cannot be opened, determine the best point of entry and proceed accordingly.

WINDOWS

Windows of vehicles usually are made of tempered glass (Figures 34-1 and 34-2); rear and side windows are designed to break into small granules. Cover the victim with a heavy safety blanket at the earliest opportunity (Figure 34-3).

Locate the window farthest from the victim, and give a quick, hard thrust in the lower corner with a spring-loaded punch, screwdriver, or other sharp object. If you have time and the correct materials, put strips of broad tape or a sheet of contact paper over the glass to prevent the broken pieces from

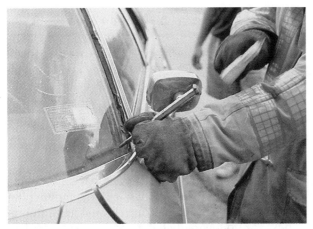

FIGURE 34-1. Tempered glass should be shattered with a sharp tool. Strike tool with a hammer in a lower corner close to the door.

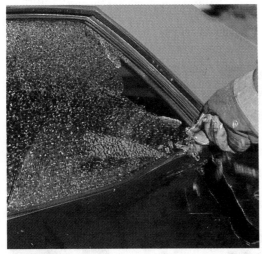

FIGURE 34-2. Tempered glass — usually found in side and rear windows.

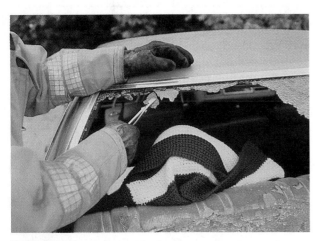

FIGURE 34-3.

spraying onto the victim. Use your gloved hand to carefully pull the glass outside the vehicle. Clear all glass away from the window opening.

Before you crawl in, drape a heavy tarp or blanket over the door edge and the interior of the car just below the window.

STABILIZE THE VICTIM

As soon as you are able to gain access to the victim, do the following:

1. Conduct a quick but thorough primary survey to determine the extent of injuries.

2. If more than one victim is involved, complete triage.

3. Perform the ABCs.

4. Correct life-threatening problems (Figure 34-4).

5. Provide other emergency care as needed.

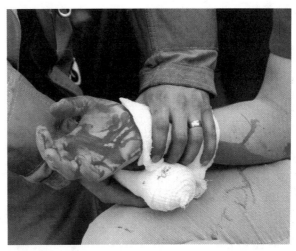

FIGURE 34-4. Perform a victim assessment and give needed emergency care in the car.

6. On occasion, you may need to move the victim quickly and immediately, such as when the vehicle is on fire, before you can immobilize him with a rigid support, such as a spineboard. Cut any jammed seat belts. If there is any possibility of a cervical-spine injury, immobilize the victim's spine using the horse-collar technique, which is one of the easier methods of one-person rescue in a life-and-death situation (Figure 34-5). Used when the victim is sitting, take a standard blanket and roll it lengthwise until it is approximately

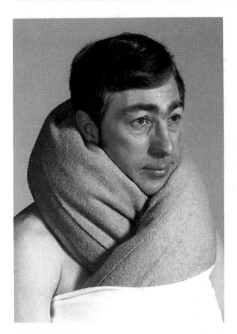

FIGURE 34-5. Improvised cervical collar or horse-collar.

four to six inches across. Reach in with one hand and provide gentle immobilization while placing the blanket behind the victim's head, allowing both long ends to fall across his chest. Pass the blanket across his chest from one side to the other. Place gentle tension on both long ends, then pass the ends under opposite arms. Gather the blanket behind the victim, and rotate him from the seat into your arms. The horse collar also provides support of the head and neck without taking the time to place a cervical collar on the victim.

7. Stabilize the victim(s) before you move them by:
   - bandaging all wounds.
   - splinting all fractures.
   - giving psychological support.

8. After the victim(s) have been stabilized and moved, continue to check for:
   - open airway.
   - breathing.
   - circulation or pulse.
   - bleeding is controlled.
   - normal victim temperature.

PROPER SPLINTING

Very often, victims in need of extrication have possible neck and back injuries. In any accident situation, assess for neck and back injuries by:

1. Asking what happened, where does it hurt, and where is there no feeling?
2. Feel along the neck and back for muscle spasms, deformities, and painful areas.
3. See if the victim can grip your hands with his hands or wiggle his toes. Difficulty in moving the arms, legs, or head; a feeling of weakness, numbness, or no feeling below the injury; or complete paralysis all indicate neck or back injuries involving the spinal cord.

If you suspect a neck or back injury, a backboard and cervical support should be used to stabilize and transport the victim (Figure 34-6). For more information on the use of backboards, see Chapter 33, "Lifting and Moving Victims."

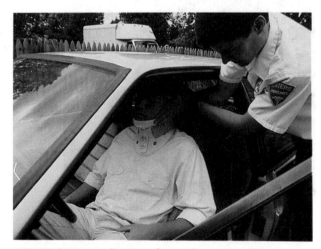

FIGURE 34-6. Application of a rigid cervical collar.

Once the cervical support and short backboard have been applied (refer to Chapter 33), the victim may be placed on a long backboard. This can be done by putting the victim's head, trunk, and legs in a straight line position (always holding neck and head in alignment with body) and then sliding the victim onto a long backboard (Figures 34-7–34-9).

REMOVING A VICTIM ON SEAT OF VEHICLE

When a victim is lying down on the seat of a car, urgent first aid should be administered before

── REMOVING A VICTIM WITH A LONG BOARD ──

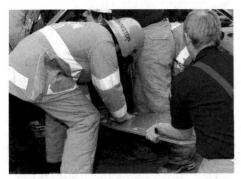

FIGURE 34-7. A victim with a possible spinal injury is stabilized in the vehicle. The end of a long board is then securely placed next to the seat.

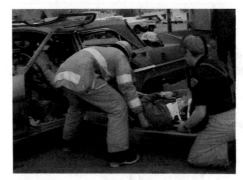

FIGURE 34-8. Slowly and carefully move victim to a prone position, and slide him onto the long board.

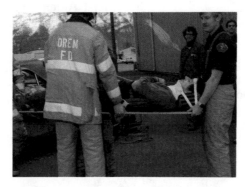

FIGURE 34-9. Carefully lift and remove victim.

moving unless there is immediate danger. The following steps should be considered:

1. One First Aider maintains a slight and gentle traction on the victim's head so that it is maintained in a normal straight line with the body.

2. Apply a cervical collar.

3. Another First Aider carefully moves the victim's legs and body into alignment while head traction is maintained. While two First Aiders maintain body alignment and head traction, another First Aider, preferably two, move the victim slightly away from the seat to allow a long backboard to be slipped beneath the victim's back (Figure 34-10).

4. Ease the victim back against the backboard. When the First Aider at the victim's head gives a signal, the other First Aiders push and hold the victim snugly against the backboard until the backboard and victim are lying flat on the seat (Figure 34-11).

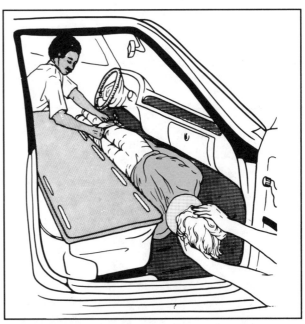

FIGURE 34-10. Keeping head, neck, and legs in proper alignment in preparation for applying long backboard.

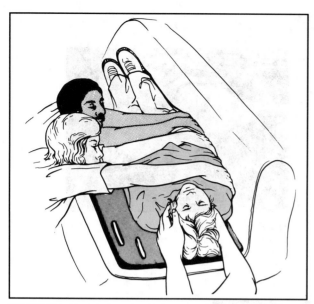

FIGURE 34-11. Moving the victim onto the long backboard.

5. Secure the victim to the backboard and remove him from the car.

6. If a victim is found lying face down, give urgent first aid without moving him any more than necessary. If the victim must be turned over in order to administer first aid, follow guidelines discussed in Chapter 33.

REMOVING A VICTIM LYING ON FLOOR OF VEHICLE

Sometimes a victim is in a space, such as under the steering wheel, dashboard, or on the floor, that does not allow for sliding a backboard into place. If this is the case, place the backboard flat on the seat. One First Aider keeps the head and neck in alignment with the body, while another First Aider maintains alignment of the feet and legs. This can be accomplished more easily if the victim's legs are secured together with a bandage. While the two First Aiders maintain the victim's body alignment, another First Aider(s) is able to reach over the seat and get a secure hold on the victim's clothing at the waist, hip, and thigh area. At a signal from the First Aider who is maintaining head and neck alignment, all the First Aiders lift the victim — while body alignment is maintained — onto the backboard. The victim is then secured to the backboard. The victim is then secured to the backboard before being moved again.

| **34** | **SELF-TEST** | **34** |

Student: _____   Date: _____

Course: _____   Section #: _____

PART I: True/False   If you believe that the statement is true, circle the T. If you believe that the statement is false, circle the F.

T   F   1. Bystanders are always a hazard in extrication situations.

T   F   2. Suspect any vehicle as being unstable until you have made it stable.

T   F   3. A part of stabilizing a victim is to splint all fractures.

T   F   4. Slight, gentle in-line traction should be placed on a victim's head before a cervical collar is applied.

T   F   5. When a First Aider gains access to an accident victim, he should first establish an open airway.

T   F   6. All outside hazards need to be controlled before a rescuer enters a wrecked vehicle.

T   F   7. Extricate means to quickly pull a person out of a wrecked vehicle.

T   F   8. Bystanders should be given instructions on how to help, or stay out of the way.

T   F   9. Do not worry about a downed power line unless it is sparking.

T   F   10. Stabilize a vehicle with a standard shift by placing the transmission into first gear.

T   F   11. Select a window to break closest to the victim so you will have immediate access to him.

T   F   12. The horse-collar technique is used to immobilize a possible fractured neck.

PART II: Multiple Choice   For each question, circle the answer that best reflects an accurate statement.

1. Cars that are upside down or lying on their side should be:
    a. turned upright.
    b. taken apart.
    c. stabilized as is.
    d. not touched.

2. What is the first step if a windshield or rear window must be removed to gain access to the victim?
    a. remove chrome trim around the window.
    b. cover the victim with a blanket or other covering.
    c. cut the top and sides of rubber moulding.
    d. strike the window with a sharp instrument.

3. Once the First Aider has gained access to the victim, he should next:
    a. check for breathing and heartbeat.
    b. control severe bleeding.
    c. splint fractures.
    d. treat for shock.

4. When a victim is lying down on the seat of a car, what is the first step involved in removing him?
    a. move the legs and body into alignment.
    b. maintain slight and gentle traction on the victim's head.
    c. apply a cervical collar.
    d. move the victim slightly away from the seat.

5. Extrication means:
    a. picking and sorting of the injured.
    b. gaining access to an accident scene.
    c. moving and transporting the injured.
    d. disentangling or freeing a trapped victim.

6. What should the First Aider do if the victim does not need to be rescued immediately and a rescue team will be arriving soon?
    a. control the hazards and stabilize the accident scene.
    b. gain access to the victim if possible.
    c. give emergency care to stabilize the victim.
    d. all of the above.

7. At the scene of an accident, an automobile has hit a utility pole, causing an electrical wire to fall across the top of the car. The First Aider notes there are two apparently uninjured persons inside. What should he do first?
    a. remove the downed wire.
    b. set flares around the area.
    c. notify the utility company.
    d. direct the victims not to touch any metal in the car or attempt to get out.

8. What part of the vehicle should you check first for the possibility of gaining access to a trapped victim?
    a. windows.
    b. floor.
    c. roof.
    d. doors.

9. Important principles to remember in gaining access and extricating victims include: (1) although the first impulse is often to remove the victim from the wreckage, it is generally better to remove the wreckage from the victim; (2) make every effort not to further injure the victim during attempts to gain access; (3) cervical or thoracic fractures should be suspected in any unconscious victim; (4) in gaining access, try the easiest approach first.

   a. 1, 2, 3, and 4.
   b. 2, 3, and 4.
   c. 2 and 4.
   d. 1, 2, and 4.

10. The First Aider should search for injured victims of an automobile accident in which of the following places?

   a. wedged under the dashboard.
   b. tall weeds.
   c. ditches.
   d. all of these answers.

PART III: What Would You Do If:

A sixty-five-year-old driver has run his vehicle into a parked car, then skewed sideways into traffic where his car was broadsided on the passenger side. When you arrive, he is unconscious and pale and slumped into the steering wheel. He is not wearing a seat belt. Both doors are jammed, but the window on the passenger's side is knocked out.

1. What two important factors concerning extrication would you first consider?

2. If you decided that the driver doesn't need to be rescued immediately and a rescue team will be arriving soon, what would you do?

3. How would you gain access to the victim?

PART IV: Practical Skills Check-Off

_____ has satisfactorily passed the following practical skills:
          Student's Name

	Date	Partner Check	Inst. Init.
1. Gained access to a victim.	_/_/_	☐	_____
2. Gave ABCs and other emergency care to stabilize the victim.	_/_/_	☐	_____
3. Created and positioned an improvised cervical collar.	_/_/_	☐	_____

GLOSSARY OF TERMS

A

ABD dressings: one of many names for large, thick-layered, bulky pads used for quick application to stem profuse bleeding.

Abdominal breather: a victim whose chest does not seem to move during respiration, but his abdomen does.

Abdominal cavity: the space bounded by the abdominal walls, the diaphragm, and the pelvis; contains most of the organs of digestion.

Abrasion: a scraped or scratched skin wound.

Absorption: passage of a substance through a membrane into blood.

Acceleration-deceleration injury or accident: injury caused by the sudden acceleration and deceleration of the head as the brain is slapped back and forth by the skull and then rebounds.

Acetaminophen: pain reliever used as an aspirin substitute as it is less likely to cause gastric irritation.

Activated charcoal: powdered charcoal that has been treated to increase its powers of absorption; used as a general-purpose antidote.

Acute: having rapid onset, severe symptoms, and a relatively short duration.

Acute abdomen: a term indicating the presence of some abdominal process that causes the sudden irritation of the peritoneum and intense pain.

Adam's apple: the projection on the anterior surface of the neck, formed by the thyroid cartilage of the larynx.

Addiction: the state of being strongly dependent upon some agent; drugs, tobacco, for example.

Adipose tissue: fatty tissue.

Advanced cardiac life support (ACLS): the use of adjunctive equipment, cardiac monitoring, defibrillation, intravenous lifeline, and drug infusion.

AIDS: acquired immune deficiency syndrome; a fatal disease first noted in 1978 and caused by a virus. It is spread through direct contact with the blood, semen, or oral secretions of infected individuals.

Air splints: a double-walled plastic tube that immobilizes a limb when sufficient air is blown into the space between the walls of the tube, to cause it to become almost rigid.

Airway: the route for passage of air and/or gases into and out of the lungs.

Alcoholism: addiction to alcohol; overuse that affects the individual's health and social functioning.

Alkaline: having a pH greater than 7.0; in human physiology, having a pH greater than 7.35.

Alveolus: a cavity; specifically, the socket holding a tooth; or a terminal air sac of the lung.

Ammonia: an agent frequently used in pesticides, medications, and common household products.

Amnesia: loss of memory.

Amniotic sac: a thick, transparent sac that holds the fetus suspended in the amniotic fluid.

Amputation: complete removal of an appendage.

Anaphylactic shock: an exaggerated allergic reaction with severe bronchospasm and vascular collapse, which may be rapidly fatal.

Anatomy: the structure of the body, or the study of body structure.

Angina pectoris: a spasmodic pain in the chest, characterized by a sensation of severe constriction or pressure on the anterior chest; associated with insufficient blood supply to the heart; aggravated by exercise or tension and relieved by rest or medication.

Anoxia: without oxygen; a reduction of oxygen in body tissues below required physiology levels.

Anterior: situated in front of, or in the forward part of; in anatomy, used in reference to the ventral or belly surface of the body.

Antihistamines: a drug that helps counteract the effects of allergic-type reactions.

Antiseptic: any preparation that prevents the growth of bacteria.

Aorta: the largest artery in the body, originates at the left ventricle and terminates at the bifurcation of the iliac arteries.

Apex: the peak, top or highest point.

Aphonic: loss of voice.

Apnea: absence of respiration.

Appendage: any subordinate organ or external part, for example, a leg, arm.

Appendicitis: inflammation of the vermiform appendix.

Arterial pulse (pressure) points: points where an artery passes over a bony prominence or lies close to the skin; at these points the artery can be palpated and the arterial pulse taken.

Arterial system: all of the arteries considered together.

Arteries: a blood vessel, consisting of three layers of tissue and smooth muscle, that carries blood away from the heart.

Arteriosclerosis: a generic name for several conditions that cause the walls of the arteries to become thickened, hard, and inelastic.

Artificial ventilation: movement of air into and out of the lungs by artificial means.

Aseptic: sterile; free of bacteria.

Asphyxia: suffocation; a condition characterized by hypercarbia and hypoxemia.

Aspiration: to inhale materials into the lungs.

Atherosclerosis: a common form of arteriosclerosis caused by fat deposits in arterial walls.

Atria: either of the two upper chambers on each side of the heart that receive blood from the veins and in turn force it into the ventricles.

Aura: a premonitory sensation of impending illness, usually used in connection with an epileptic attack.

Avulsion: an injury that leaves a piece of skin or other tissue either partially or completely torn away from the body.

Axilla: the armpit.

B

Back blows: sharp blows delivered with the First Aider's hand over the victim's spine between the scapulae to relieve upper airway obstruction.

Backboard: *see* Spineboard.

Bactericide: an agent capable of killing bacteria.

"Bad trip": a drug episode resulting in a state of intense anxiety or panic.

Bandage: a material used to hold a dressing in place.

Bandage compress: a folded cloth or pad used for applying pressure to stop hemorrhage or as a wet dressing.

Barbiturates: a class of drugs that produce a calming, sedative effect.

Basic life support: maintenance of the ABCs (airway, breathing, and circulation) without adjunctive equipment.

Battle's sign: a contusion on the mastoid process of either ear; sign of a basilar skull fracture.

Biological death: present when irreversible brain damage has occurred, usually after 3-10 minutes of cardiac arrest.

Birth canal: the vagina and the lower part of the uterus.

Black eye: a discoloration of the skin or flesh around an eye, resulting from a sharp blow or contusion.

Bleeder: in surgery, a small blood vessel that is bleeding profusely; also, a hemophiliac victim.

Blood clots: *see* Clot.

Blood pressure: the pressure exerted by the pulsatile flow of blood against the arterial walls.

Blood volume: the total amount of blood in the heart and blood vessels; represents 8 to 9 percent of body weight in kilograms.

Bloody show: the mucous and bloody discharge signaling the beginning of labor.

Blunt trauma: injury caused by impact of a blunt object, such as a rounded stone, in contrast to that caused by a sharp object such as a knife.

Botulism: food poisoning caused by *Clostridium botulinum* toxin.

Bounding pulse: unusually strong pulse.

Brachial artery: the artery of the arm that is the continuation of the axillary artery, that in turn branches at the elbow into the radial and ulnar arteries.

Brachial pulse: pulse produced by compressing the major artery of the upper arm; used to detect heart action and circulation in infants.

Brain: organ in the skull that controls all bodily functions and is the seat of consciousness.

Brain stem: the stem-like portion of the brain that connects the brain with the spinal cord; includes the pons, medulla, and mesencephalon.

Bronchospasm: severe constriction of the bronchial tree.

Bruise: an injury that does not break the skin but causes rupture of small underlying blood vessels with resulting tissue discoloration; a contusion.

Burn pads: one of many names for large, thick-layered, bulky pads used for quick application to stem profuse bleeding.

C

Cafe coronary: common name for incident where people choke to death on a foreign object obstructing the upper airway.

Capillaries: the very small blood vessels that carry blood to all parts of the body and the skin. Capillaries are a link between the ends of the arteries and the beginning of the beginning of the veins.

Capillary refill: a method of assessing the adequacy of circulation to the extremities. Gentle pressure is exerted on the nail bed until the underlying tissue whitens, then pressure is released, and the time for return of the pink color is observed.

Carbon dioxide: CO_2; a colorless and odorless gas that neither supports combustion nor burns; a waste product of aerobic metabolism; in combination with water (H_2O)-, forms carbonic acid (H_2CO_3).

Carbon monoxide: CO; a colorless, odorless, and dangerous gas formed by the incomplete combustion of carbon; it combines four times as quickly with hemoglobin than oxygen; when in the presence of heme, replaces oxygen and reduces oxygen uptake in the lungs.

Cardiac arrest: the sudden cessation of cardiac function with no pulse, no blood pressure, unresponsiveness.

Cardiac compression: a technique of external heart massage to restore the pumping action of the heart.

Cardiac muscle: the heart muscle.

Cardiogenic shock: the inability of the heart to pump adequate amounts of blood to perfuse the vital organs.

Cardiopulmonary arrest: cessation of cardiac and respiratory activity.

Cardiopulmonary resuscitation (CPR): application of artificial ventilation and external cardiac compression in victims with cardiac arrest to provide an adequate circulation to support life.

Carotid artery: the principal artery of the neck, palpated easily on either side of the thyroid cartilage.

Carotid pulse: pulse taken at the carotid artery.

Cat-scratch fever: a benign, subacute, regional lymphadenitis resulting from the scratch or bite of a cat or a scratch from a surface contaminated by a cat; it is marked by a primary papular eruption at the site of inoculation which may develop into a small ulcer.

Cellulitis: a spreading redness and swelling of the skin usually caused by infection.

Central nervous system: the portion of the nervous system consisting of the brain and spinal cord.

Cerebral thrombosis: thrombosis of a cerebral vessel, which may result in cerebral infarction.

Cerebrospinal fluid: fluid secreted by cells in cavities within the cerebrum. It circulates through the membranes that cover and protect the brain and spinal cord.

Cerebrovascular accident (CVA): sometimes called stroke or apoplexy; the sudden cessation of circulation to a region of the brain, due to thrombus, embolism, or hemorrhage.

Cervical collar: a device used to immobilize and support the neck.

Cervical spine: that portion of the spinal column consisting of the seven vertebrae that lie in the neck.

Cervical vertebrae: the first seven vertebrae of the spinal column that lie in the neck.

Cervix: the lower portion, or neck, of the uterus.

Chest thrust: a series of manual thrusts to the chest to relieve upper airway obstruction.

Chief complaint: the problem for which a patient seeks help, stated in a word or short phrase.

Chlorine: a greenish-yellow, incombustible, poisonous gas that is highly irritating to the respiratory organs.

Chronic: of long duration, or recurring over a period of time.

Chronic obstructive pulmonary disease (COPD): a term comprising chronic bronchitis, emphysema, and asthma; an illness that causes obstructive problems in the airways.

Circulatory system: the body system consisting of the heart and blood vessels.

Clamping injury: usually involves a finger, or part of the hand, which has been strangled or stuck in a hole and cannot be readily extracted or has been extracted with damage.

Clavicle(s): the collarbone; attached to the uppermost part of the sternum at a right angle, and joins the scapular spine to form the point of the shoulder.

Clinical death: a term that refers to the lack of signs of life, when there is no pulse and no blood pressure; occurs immediately after the onset of cardiac arrest.

Closed-chest compression: external cardiac massage.

Closed wound: a wound in which the skin is not broken.

Clostridium perfringens: anaerobic bacteria that can cause food poisoning in cooked food held without proper refrigeration.

Clot: a semi-solidified mass, as of blood or lymph, also called a coagulum.

Coccygeal spine: *see* Coccyx.

Coccyx: the lowest part of the backbone; composed of three to five small, fused vertebrae; also called the tailbone.

Colitis: inflammation of the colon.

Comatose: in a state of coma.

Compensatory shock: the first stage of shock.

Compound fracture(s): an open fracture; a fracture in which there is an open wound of the skin and soft tissues leading down to the location of the fracture.

Compress (compression dressing): a folded cloth or pad used for applying pressure to stop hemorrhage or as a wet dressing.

Compulsive drug use: preoccupation with the procurement and use of a drug.

Concussion: a jarring brain injury resulting from a head blow or fall.

Congestive heart failure (CHF): excessive blood or fluid in the lungs or body tissues caused by the failure of the ventricles to pump blood effectively.

Conjunctivitis: inflammation of the conjunctiva.

Connective tissue: the tissue that binds together and supports the various structures of the body.

Constrict: to make smaller by drawing together or by squeezing.

Contact burns: a burn caused by touching either a hot surface or a live electrical circuit.

Contamination: contact with an unsterile object or infective agent.

Continuity: an unbroken, connected whole.

Contract: to draw together or to shorten.

Contusions: a bruise; an injury which causes a hemorrhage into or beneath the skin, but does not break the skin.

Cornea: the transparent structure covering the pupil.

Coronary artery disease: progressive narrowing and eventual obstruction of the coronary arteries by the atherosclerotic process.

Costal: pertaining to the ribs.

Coup-contrecoup: a type of head injury causing contusion or bruising of the brain.

CPR: cardiopulmonary resuscitation.

Cravat: a special type of bandage made from a large triangular piece of cloth and folded to form a band; used as a temporary dressing for a fracture or wound.

Crepitus: a grating sound heard and a sensation felt when the fractured ends of a bone rub together.

Cricoid cartilage: a firm ridge of cartilage that forms the lower part of the larynx.

Crossed-finger technique: method to open clenched jaw.

Croup: the general term for a group of viral infections that produce swelling of the larynx.

Crowning: the stage of birth when the presenting part of the baby is visible at the vaginal orifice.

Cryotherapy: to treat with cold.

Culture: the cultivation of mircooganisms, such as bacteria, for scientific study.

Cyanosis: blueness of the skin due to insufficient oxygen in the blood.

D

Decapitation: the removal of the head.

Decelerating aortic injury: a possible laceration of the aorta caused by a victim being hurled into an immovable object such as a dashboard.

Decompression: removal of compression or pressure.

Defibrillation: application of an unsynchronized DC electrical shock to terminate ventricular fibrillation.

Dehydration: loss of water and electrolytes; excessive loss of body water.

Delirium tremens (DTs): a form of insanity, often temporary, caused by alcohol poisoning; characterized by sweating, tremor, great excitement, precordial pain, anxiety, and mental distress; occurs usually following heavy alcohol intake.

Depress: to decrease the force or activity.

Depressant: an agent that lowers functional activity, a sedative.

Dermatitis: inflammation of the skin.

Diabetes: a general term referring to disorders characterized by excessive urine excretion, excessive thirst, and excessive hunger.

Diabetic acidosis: a variety of metabolic acidosis produced by accumulation of ketone bodies resulting from uncontrolled diabetes mellitus.

Diabetic coma: result of an inadequate insulin supply that leads to unconsciousness, coma, and eventually death unless treated.

Diaphragm: a large skeletal muscle which is a major component in the act of respiration and which separates the chest cavity from the abdominal cavity.

Dilate: to expand and enlarge.

Direct pressure: force applied directly on top of a wound to stop bleeding.

Dislocation: the state of being misaligned; the displacement of the ends of two bones at their joint so that the joint surfaces are no longer in proper contact.

Disoriented: the loss of proper bearings, or a state of mental confusion as to time, place, and identity.

Distal: farther from any point of reference; generally, the point of reference is the heart.

Distended: inflated or enlarged.

Dorsalis pedis artery: an artery located in the top back of the foot.

Dressing: protective covering for a wound, used to stop bleeding and to prevent contamination of the wound.

Drug abuse: the self-administration of a drug or drugs in a manner not in accord with approved medical or social patterns.

Dyspnea: difficulty in breathing, with rapid, shallow respirations.

Dysrhythmias: disturbances in the cardiac rhythms.

E

Ecchymosis: blood under the skin causing a black and blue mark, bruise.

Eclampsia: a toxic condition of pregnancy, causing convulsions and coma, associated with hypertension, edema, and proteinuria.

Ectopic pregnancy: a pregnancy in which the fetus is implanted elsewhere than in the uterus, e.g. in the fallopian tube or in the abdominal cavity; produces abdominal pain, bleeding.

Edema: a condition in which fluid escapes into the body tissues from the vascular or lymphatic spaces and causes local or generalized swelling.

Electrocardiogram (ECG or EKG): a graphic tracing of the electrical currents generated by the process of depolarization and repolarization of the myocardial tissues.

Electrolyte: a substance whose molecules dissociate when put into solution.

Embolism: the sudden blocking of an artery or vein by a clot or foreign material which has been brought to the site of lodgement by the blood current.

Embolus: any foreign matter, as a blood clot or air bubble, carried in the bloodstream.

Epiglottis: the lidlike cartilaginous structure overhanging the superior entrance to the larynx and serving to prevent food from entering the larynx and trachea while swallowing.

Epiglottitis: a bacterial infection occurring in children, marked by swelling of the epiglottis, high fever, pain on swallowing, and drooling; airway obstruction can result with great rapidity.

Epilepsy: a chronic brain disorder marked by paroxysmal attacks of brain dysfunction, usually associated with some alteration of consciousness, abnormal motor behavior, psychic or sensory disturbances; may be preceded by aura.

Epinephrine: adrenalin; hormone and drug that has powerful beta stimulating properties, used in the treatment of asthma, anaphylaxis, asystole, and fine ventricular fibrillation.

Esophageal varices: dilated veins in the wall of the esophagus that develop in patients with liver disease. If these enlarged veins rupture, subsequent bleeding can be fatal.

Esophagus: the portion of the digestive tract that lies between the pharynx and the stomach.

Evert: to turn inside out, to turn outward.

Evisceration: internal organs exposed to the outside through a complete break in the abdominal wall.

Exhalation: the act of breathing out; expiration.

External ear: all of the ear external to the tympanic membrane.

External maxillary artery: artery anterior to the angle of the mandible on the inner surface of the lower jaw that contributes much of the blood supply to the face.

F

Fallopian tubes: the bilateral tubes extending from the ovaries to the uterus.

Femoral artery: the principal artery of the thigh, a continuation of the iliac artery; supplies blood to the lower abdominal wall, the external genitalia, and the lower body extremities; pulse may be palpated in the groin area.

Femoral pulse: located approximately two fingerbreadths inferior to the midpoint line between the anterior superior iliac spine and the pubic symphysis.

Femur: the bone that extends from the pelvis to the knee; the longest and largest bone of the body; the thigh bone.

Fever: an elevation of body temperature beyond normal.

Fibrin: fibrous protein material formed and utilized to produce a blood clot.

Fibula: the smaller of the two bones of the lower leg.

Finger sweep: technique to remove a foreign object from the oropharynx so that it does not reenter the airway.

Flaccid: a term meaning soft, limp, without any muscular tone.

Flail chest: a condition in which several ribs are broken, each in at least two places; or a sternal fracture or separation of the ribs from the sternum producing a free-floating segment of the chest wall that moves paradoxically on respiration.

Flank: the part of the body below the ribs and above the ilium.

Flutter pulse: repetitive, regular, and rapid beating of the heart.

Foreign object: not normally a part of the body.

Foreskin: the fold of skin covering the glans penis.

Fracture: a break or rupture in a bone.

avulsion: an indirect fracture caused by avulsion or pull of a ligament.

comminuted: a fracture in which the bone is shattered, broken into small pieces.

compression: a fracture produced by compression, e.g. vertebral fracture.

depressed: a fracture of the skull in which a fragment is depressed.

greenstick: an incomplete fracture, the bone is not broken all the way through; seen most often in children.

impacted: a fracture in which the ends of the bones are jammed together.

longitudinal: a break in a bone extending in a longitudinal direction.

oblique: a fracture in which the break crosses the bone at an angle.

spiral: a fracture in which the break line twists around and through the bone.

transverse: a fracture in which the break line extends across the bone at right angle to the long axis.

Frostbite: damage to the tissues as a result of prolonged exposure to extreme cold.

G

Gallbladder: the sac located just beneath the liver that concentrates and stores bile.

Gangrene: local tissue death as a result of an injury or inadequate blood supply.

Gastric distention: inflation of the stomach caused when excessive pressures are used during artificial ventilation or when several breaths are administered in rapid succession.

Gastrointestinal tract: the digestive tract, including stomach, small intestine, large intestine, rectum, and anus.

Gauze: a light, open-meshed fabric of muslin or similar material.

General purpose dressing: one of many names for large, thick-layered, bulky pads used for quick application to stem profuse bleeding.

Genitalia: the external sex organs.

Glaucoma: a disease that produces increased pressure within the eyeball; can lead to blindness.

Globe: the eyeball.

Glucose: a simple sugar.

Good Samaritan laws: laws written to protect emergency care personnel which require a standard of care to be provided in good faith, to a level of training, and to the best of ability.

Groin: the inguinal region; junction of the abdomen and the thigh.

Ground splint: asking the patient to keep his prone body very still as if it were splinted to the ground.

H

Habituation: a situation in which a victim produces a tolerance to a drug and becomes psychologically dependent on the drug.

Head-tilt/chin-lift maneuver: opening the airway by tilting the victim's head backward and lifting the chin forward, bringing the entire lower jaw with it.

Heart attack: a layman's term for a condition resulting from blockage of a coronary artery and subsequent death of part of the heart muscle; an acute myocardial infarction; a coronary.

Heart disease: abnormal condition of the heart or heart and circulation.

Heat burns: *see* thermal burns.

Heat exhaustion: prostration caused by excessive loss of water and salt through sweating; characterized by cold, clammy skin and a weak, rapid pulse.

Heat stroke: life-threatening condition caused by a disturbance in temperature regulation; characterized by extreme fever, hot and dry skin, delirium, or coma.

Heimlich maneuver: also known as manual thrust; a system developed by Heimlich to remove a foreign body from the airway.

Hematoma: localized collection of blood in the tissues as a result of injury or a broken blood vessel.

Hemodilution: an increase in the volume of blood plasma resulting in reduced concentration of red blood cells.

Hemophilia: an inherited blood disease occurring mostly in males, characterized by the inability of the blood to clot.

Hemoptysis: coughing up of bright red blood.

Hemorrhage: abnormally large amount of bleeding.

Hemorrhagic shock: a state of inadequate tissue perfusion due to blood loss.

Hemothorax: an accumulation of blood in the chest cavity.

Hepatitis B: hepatitis caused by a virus that is spread through blood-to-blood contact (transfusion, needle stick), mucous membrane (saliva or sputum contact), or sexual contact. It is a serious disease with long-term side effects. Signs and symptoms are nausea, vomiting, fatigue, abdominal pain, and jaundice.

Hernia: the abnormal protrusion of any organ through an opening into another body cavity; most common in the inguinal hernia where a loop of intestine descends into the inguinal canal in the groin.

Humerus: the bone of the upper arm.

Hyperglycemia: abnormally increased concentration of sugar in the blood.

Hypertension: high blood pressure, usually in reference to a diastolic pressure greater than 90-95 mm Hg.

Hyperthermia: greatly increased body temperature.

Hyperventilation: an increased rate and depth of breathing resulting in an abnormal lowering of arterial carbon dioxide, causing alkalosis.

Hypoglycemia: an abnormally diminished concentration of sugar in the blood; insulin shock.

Hypothermia: decreased body temperature.

Hypovolemic shock: decreased amount of blood and fluids in the body.

I

Iliac crest: the highest point of the hipbone.

Impaled object: an object which has caused a puncture wound and which remains embedded in the wound.

Incision: an open wound with smooth edges.

Incontinence: inability to prevent the flow of urine or feces.

Infection: an invasion of a body by disease-producing organisms.

Infectious: capable of being transmitted by infection.

Inflammation: a tissue reaction to disease, irritation, or infection, characterized by pain, heat, redness, and swelling.

Ingestion: intaking of food or other substances through the mouth.

Inhalation: the drawing of air or other gases into the lungs.

Insulin: a hormone secreted by the islets of Langerhans in the pancreas; essential for the proper metabolism of blood sugar.

Insulin shock: not a true form of shock; hypoglycemia caused by excessive insulin dosage, characterized by sweating, tremor, anxiety, unusual behavior, vertigo, and diplopia; may cause death of brain cells.

Intestines: the portion of the alimentary canal extending from the pylorus to the anus.

Intrathoracic: within the thorax.

Intravenous: within or into a vein.

Inverted: turned inside out or upside down.

Involuntary muscle: muscles that function without voluntary control; smooth (as opposed to skeletal) muscles.

Irregular pulse: one in which the beats occur at irregular intervals.

Irreversible shock: the final stage of shock.

Irrigation: cleansing by washing and rinsing with water or other fluids.

Islets of Langerhans: clusters of cells in the pancreas that produce insulin.

J

Jaundice: yellow color of the tissues seen in liver disease.

Jaw thrust maneuver: a procedure for opening the airway, wherein the jaw is lifted and pulled forward to keep the tongue from falling back into the airway.

Joint: the juncture where two bones come in contact.

ball-and-socket: a type of synovial joint in which a spheroidal surface on one bone (the ball) moves within a concavity (the socket) on the other bone, as in the hip bone.

freely movable: a synovial joint, a special form of articulation permitting more or less free movement.

hinge: a joint that allows angular movement only.

immovable: fibrous joint, one in which the components are connected by fibrous tissue.

limited motion: a joint that cannot be moved through a full range of motion.

pivot: a uniaxial joint in which one bone pivots within a bony or an osseoligamentous ring.

Joint capsule: a fibrous sac that, with its synovial lining, encloses a joint.

K

Kerlix: a type of self-adhering roller material.

Ketoacidosis: a condition arising in diabetics where their insulin dose is insufficient to their needs; fat is metabolized, instead of sugar, to ketones; characterized by excessive thirst, urination, vomiting, and hyperventilation of the Kussmaul type.

Kidneys: the paired organs located in the retroperitoneal cavities that filter blood and produce urine, also act as adjuncts to keep a proper acid-base balance.

Kidney stone: stones that pass from the kidney and into the ureter where they cause excruciating pain until they enter the bladder.

Kling: a type of self-adhering roller material.

L

Laceration: a wound made by tearing or cutting of body tissues.

Laryngeal edema: fluids invading the tissues of the larynx causing swelling.

Laryngectomy: the surgical removal of the larynx.

Laryngospasm: severe constriction of the larynx, often in response to allergy or noxious stimuli.

Larynx: the voice box.

Ligament: tough band of fibrous tissues which connects bones to bones about a joint or supports any organ.

Light burns: burns resulting from concentrated sources of light, i.e. a welding torch or the sun.

Liver: the large organ in the right upper quadrant of the abdomen that secretes bile, produces many essential proteins, detoxifies many substances, and stores glycogen.

Lividity: redness caused by blood pooling in the dependent parts of the body that is seen 15 to 30 minutes after death.

Locomotion: movement or the ability to move from one place to another.

Logroll: a method of rolling the body as a complete unit.

Long bones: a bone that has a longitudinal axis of considerable length consisting of a shaft and an extended portion at each end that is usually articular.

Lumbar spine: the lower part of the back formed by the lowest five non-fused vertebrae.

M

"March" fracture: *see* Fatigue fracture.

Maxillofacial: the lower half of the face.

Mechanism of injury: factors involved in producing the injury.

Medic Alert: identification system for patients with hidden medical condition.

Metabolic acidosis: excessive amounts of lactic and other organic acids in the body.

Metabolism: the conversion of food into energy and waste products.

Microorganisms: minute living organisms, usually microscopic.

Midline: the median line or plane of the body.

Mortal: subject to death, destined to die.

Mouth-to-mouth ventilation: the preferred emergency method of artificial ventilation when adjuncts are not available.

Mouth-to-nose ventilation: artificial ventilation in which the First Aider's lips make a seal around the victim's nose as the First Aider exhales into the victim's nose. The victim's mouth is kept closed, although sometimes the lips are spread apart during the exhalation by the victim.

Multitrauma dressings: one of many names for large, thick-layered, bulky pads used for quick application to stem profuse bleeding.

Musculature: the muscular system of the body, or a part of the system.

Musculoskeletal system: all the collective bones, joints, muscles, and tendons of the body.

Myocardial infarction: the damaging or death of an area of heart muscle resulting from a reduction in the blood supply reaching that area.

Myocardium: heart muscle.

N

Narcotics: drugs used to depress the central nervous system, thereby relieving pain and producing sleep.

Nausea: an unpleasant sensation, vaguely referred to the epigastrium and abdomen, often culminating in vomiting.

Nerve: a cordlike structure composed of a collection of fibers that convey impulses between a part of the central nervous system and some other region.

   cranial: the twelve pairs of nerves connected with the brain.

   spinal: the thirty-one pairs of nerves arising from the spinal cord.

Nervous system: the brain, spinal cord, and nerve branches from the central, peripheral, and autonomic systems.

   autonomic (involuntary): the portion of the nervous system concerned with regulation of the activity of cardiac muscle, smooth muscle, and glands.

   cerebrospinal (voluntary): that portion of the nervous system consisting of the brain and spinal cord.

Neurogenic shock: shock caused by massive vasodilation and pooling of blood in the peripheral vessels to a degree that adequate perfusion cannot be maintained, resulting from loss of effective nervous control of blood vessels.

Neurological: of or relating to the branch of medical science dealing with the nervous system and its disorders.

Neurovascular: pertaining to both nervous and vascular elements; pertaining to the nerves that control the caliber of blood vessels.

Nosebleed: hemorrhage from the nose.

O

Obstructed airway: a blockage or obstruction in the airway which impairs respiration.

Occiput: the back of the skull.

Occlude: to close off or stop up; obstruct.

Occlusive dressing: a watertight dressing for a wound.

Ocular: pertaining to the eye.

Open fracture: a fracture exposed to the exterior; an open wound lies over the fracture.

Open wound: a wound in which the affected tissues are exposed by an external opening.

Opiate: technically, one of several alkaloids derived from the opium poppy plant.

Orbital fracture: fracture of the skull bone around the eye socket.

Orbits: the bony, pyramid-shaped cavities in the skull that hold the eyeballs.

Oriented: the determination of one's position with respect to space and time.

Oropharynx: area behind the base of the tongue between the soft palate and upper portion of the epiglottis.

Orthopedic: pertaining to the correction of deformities.

Ovaries: the female gonad in which eggs and female hormones are produced.

Overdose: amount of medicine, drug, etc. in excess of that prescribed.

Oxygen: a colorless, odorless, tasteless gas essential to life and comprising 21 percent of the atmosphere; chemical formula O_2.

P

Pallor: a paleness of the skin.

Palmar: corresponding to the palm of the hand.

Palpate: to examine by feeling and pressing with the palms and fingers.

Palpation: the act of feeling with the hand for the purpose of determining the consistency of the part beneath, in physical diagnosis.

Pancreas: a large gland, 6 to 8 inches long, that secretes enzymes into the intestines for digestion of foods. It also manufactures insulin, which is secreted into the bloodstream.

Pancreatitis: an inflammation of the pancreas.

Paradoxical breathing: associated with flail chest, where a loose segment of chest wall moves in the opposite direction to the rest of the chest during respiratory movements.

Paralysis: loss or impairment of motor function of a part due to a lesion of the neural or muscular mechanism.

Partial neck breather: one who has had a tracheotomy, an incision into the windpipe.

Patella: a small, flat bone that protects the knee joint; the kneecap.

Pathogen: any disease producing microorganism or material.

Pediatric: relating to children; medical practice devoted to the care of children up to age 15.

Pelvic girdle: the large, bony structure supporting the abdominal and pelvic organs, made up of the two innominate bones that arise in the area of the last nine vertebrae and sweep around to form a complete ring.

Penicillin: powerful antibiotic used in treatment of a wide variety of infections.

Penis: the male organ of urinary discharge and copulation.

Perfusion: the act of pouring through or into; the blood getting to the cells in order to exchange gases, nutrients, etc. with the cells.

Perineum: the pelvic floor and associated structures occupying the pelvic outlet.

Periosteum: the dense, fibrous tissue covering the bone.

Physical dependence: habituation or use of a drug, or other maneuver, because of its physiologic support, and because of the undesirable effects of withdrawal.

Physiology: the study of body functions.

Placenta: a vascular organ attached to the uterine wall that supplies oxygen and nutrients to the fetus; also called the afterbirth.

Plasma: the fluid portion of the blood, retains the clotting factors, but has no red or white cells.

Platelet: a small cellular element in the blood that assists in blood clotting.

Pleura: a continuous serous membrane that lines the outer surfaces of the lungs and the internal surface of the thoracic cavity.

Pleural cavities (space): the potential space between the parietal and visceral pleura.

Pneumothorax: an accumulation of air in the pleural cavity, usually entering after a wound or injury that causes a penetration of the chest wall or laceration of the lung.

Polyuria: a condition of excessive urination.

Posterior: situated in the back of or behind a surface.

Posterior tibial artery: the artery located posterior to the medial malleolus, supplies blood to the foot.

Preeclampsia: the condition that precedes eclampsia, or toxemia of pregnancy, characterized by hypertension, edema, and seizures.

Pressure bandages: a bandage with which enough pressure is applied over a wound site to stop bleeding.

Pressure points: one of several places on the body where the blood flow of a given artery can be restricted by pressing the artery against an underlying bone.

Primary survey: the process of finding and treating the most life-threatening emergencies first, dealing with breathing, heartbeat, and profuse bleeding.

Progressive shock: the second of the three stages of shock.

Psychogenic shock: a shocklike condition due to excessive fear, joy, anger, or grief.

Psychological dependence: dependence of a drug, or other therapeutic maneuvers, because of its support to the victim's psyche, rather than to his physiologic function.

Pubic bones: the anterior inferior part of the hip bone on either side.

Pulmonary edema: condition of the lungs when the pulmonary vessels are filled with exudate and foam, usually secondary to left heart failure.

Pulse: the rhythmic expansion and contraction of an arterial wall caused by ventricular systole and diastole.

Puncture wounds: a result of any sharp object that pierced the skin.

Pupil: the small opening in the center of the iris.

Pupillary: pertaining to the pupil.

R

Rabid: having or pertaining to rabies.

Rabies: viral disease of the CNS transmitted by the bite of an infected animal, invariably fatal unless treated before symptoms appear; also called hydrophobia from the supposed aversion of the victim to water.

Raccoon's sign: also called "coon's eyes;" bilateral symmetrical periorbital ecchymoses seen with skull fracture.

Radial artery: one of the major arteries of the forearm; the pulse is palpable at the base of the thumb.

Radial pulse: pulse taken where the radial artery crosses the distal end of the radius, that is, near the base of the thumb.

Radius: the bone on the thumb side of the forearm.

Red blood cells: an erythrocyte; the cell that carries oxygen from alveoli to cell.

Reduce: to restore a part to its normal position.

Relative skin temperature: the quickest and most common type of temperature taken in the field; accomplished by touching the back of the hand to the victim's skin to monitor for abnormally high or low temperatures.

Respiration: the act of breathing; the exchange of oxygen and carbon dioxide among the tissues, lungs, and atmosphere.

Respiratory: related to breathing or respiration.

Respiratory arrest: the cessation of breathing.

Respiratory system: a system of organs that controls the inspiration of oxygen and the expiration of carbon dioxide.

Responsive: acting or moving due to the application of a stimulus.

Retinal detachment: the sensory portion of the retina separates from the choroid.

Rigor mortis: stiffening of a person's body and limbs shortly after death.

Roller bandage: a strip of rolled-up material used for bandages.

Rupture: a tear or dissolution of continuity; a break of any organ or tissue.

S

Sacral spine: the lower part of the spine formed by five fused vertebrae.

Sacrum: part of the lower spine formed by five fused vertebrae.

Salicylates: any salt of salicylic acid.

Salmonella: an organism related to that of typhoid fever which produces intestinal upsets.

Scald: burn or injury caused by hot liquid or steam.

Scapula: shoulder blade.

Scarring: the marking resulting from being scarred.

Scrotum: a pouch of thickened skin hanging at the base of the penis, containing the testicles and their accessory ducts and glands.

Secondary survey: a head-to-toe evaluation of a victim to determine injuries.

Septic shock: a shock developing in the presence of, and as a result of, severe infection.

Septicemia: a systemic disease associated with the presence and persistence of pathogenic microorganisms or their toxins in the blood.

Septum: a dividing wall or partition, usually separating two cavities.

Serum: the liquid portion of the blood containing all of the dissolved constituents except those used for clotting.

Shock: a state of inadequate tissue perfusion that may be a result of pump failure (cardiogenic shock), volume loss or sequestration (hypovolemic shock), vasodilation (neurogenic shock), or any combination of these.

Sign: bodily evidence of disease found on physical examination.

Sinusitis: inflammation of a sinus.

Skeleton: the hard, bony structure that forms the main support of the body.

    appendicular: the bones of the limbs.

    axial: the bones of the cranium, vertebral column, ribs, and sternum.

Sling: a triangular bandage applied around the neck to support an injured upper extremity; any wide or narrow material long enough to suspend an upper extremity by passing the material around the neck; used to support and protect an injury of the arm, shoulder, or clavicle.

Smooth muscle: a nonstriated muscle found in the walls of the internal organs and blood vessels; generally not under voluntary control.

Sniffing position: the position for endotracheal intubation with the neck flexed and the head extended.

Snowblindness: obscured vision caused by sunlight, reflected off snow.

Soft tissue: the nonbony and noncartilaginous tissue of the body.

Spinal cord: the cord of nerve tissues extending from the brain down the length of the spine.

Spine board: a device used primarily for transporting victims with suspected or actual spinal injuries.

Spleen: the largest lymphatic organ of the body; located in the left upper quadrant of the abdomen.

Splint: any support used to immobilize a fracture or to restrict movement of a part.

Spontaneous pneumothorax: a rupture of the lung parenchyma resulting in the accumulation of air in the pleural space without trauma.

Spores: the reproductive element of one of the lower organisms.

Sprains: a trauma to a joint causing injury to the ligaments.

    first-degree (mild) sprain: characterized by pain with mild disability, some point tenderness, no abnormal motion, but frequently considerable swelling.

    second-degree (moderate) sprain: sprain with pain, moderate disability, point tenderness, moderately abnormal motion, swelling, and hemorrhage.

    third-degree (severe) sprain: sprain with pain, disability, loss of function, severely abnormal motion, and possible deformity, also tenderness, swelling, hemorrhage, and usually a torn ligament.

Staphylococcus: a bacteria that causes boils and other infections.

Sterile: free from living organisms, such as bacteria.

Stimulants: any agent that increases the level of bodily activity.

Stoma: a small opening, especially an artificially created opening such as made by tracheostomy.

Stomach: the part of the digestive tract between the esophagus (food pipe) and the duodenum. The stomach churns food and starts the process of digestion.

Straddle injury: an injury that usually occurs to the genital area from an object between the legs.

Strain: a muscle pull; a stretched or torn muscle.

Strangling injury: an injury in which an object constricts an extremity and cuts off circulation.

Street drugs: drugs acquired "on the street" by addicts from pushers or other addicts, not prescribed by a physician.

Stroke: cerebrovascular accident.

Stroke volume: the amount of blood pumped forward by the heart each time the ventricles contract.

Strychnine: an extremely poisonous alkaloid.

Subcutaneous emphysema: a condition in which trauma to the lung or airway results in the escape of air into body tissues, especially the chest wall, neck, and face; a crackling sensation will be felt on palpation of the skin.

Subdiaphragmatic abdominal thrust: *see* Heimlich maneuver.

Substernal notch: the point where the ribs meet the sternum.

Sucking chest wound: open pneumothorax.

Sudden infant death syndrome (SIDS): crib death; death of an infant after the first few weeks of life where the cause cannot be established by careful autopsy.

Suffocation: the act of having one's breathing blocked; suffering from lack of oxygen.

Supine: on the back.

Swathe: a cravat tied around the body to decrease movement of a part.

Sympathetic nervous system: a part of the autonomic nervous system that causes blood vessels to constrict, stimulates sweating, increases the heart rate, causes the sphincter muscles to constrict, and prepares the body to respond to stress.

Symptom: a subjective sensation or awareness of disturbance of bodily function.

Syrup of Ipecac: preparation of the dried root of a shrub found in Brazil and other parts of South America that can cause vomiting.

T

Temporal artery: the artery located on either side of the face that supplies the scalp; it can be palpated just anterior to the ear at the temporomandibular joint.

Tendon: a tough band of dense, fibrous, connective tissue that attaches muscles to bone and other parts.

tendon of insertion: the tendon connecting a muscle's point of action to the bone.

tendon of origin: a tendon lying at the base of a muscle and attaching it to a bone.

Tension of pneumothorax: situation in which air enters the pleural space through a one-way valve defect in the lung, causing progressive increase in intrapleural pressure, with lung collapse and impairment of circulation.

Testis (pl. testes): the male reproductive gland that produces spermatozoa.

Tetanus: an infectious disease caused by an exotoxin of a bacteria, Clostridium tetani, that is usually introduced through a wound, characterized by extreme body rigidity and spasms, trismus, or opisthotonos, of voluntary body muscles.

Thermal burns: burns caused by heat; the most common type of burn.

Thoracic vertebrae: the 12 vertebrae that lie between the cervical vertebrae and the lumbar vertebrae.

Thorax: the part of the body between the neck and the diaphragm, encased by the ribs.

Thready pulse: a pulse that is weak or scarcely audible, characteristic of a person in shock.

Thrombus: a blood clot which forms inside a blood vessel.

Tibia: the larger of the two bones in the leg; the shin bone.

Tolerance: the state of enduring, or of less susceptibility to the effects of a drug or poison after repeated doses.

Tonsil: either of two small, lymph tissue organs at the back of the throat.

Torsion: twisting.

Tourniquet: constrictive device used on the extremities to impede venous blood return to the heart or obstruct arterial blood flow to the extremity.

Toxemia of pregnancy: a condition sometimes occurring during the second half of pregnancy manifested by symptoms of eclampsia.

Trachea: the cartilaginous tube extending from the larynx to its division into the primary bronchi; windpipe.

Tracheostomy tube: a surgical opening made through the anterior neck, entering into the trachea.

Traction: pulling or exerting force to straighten the alignment of a part of the body.

Traction splint: a splint designed to apply tension to fractured bones and hold them in alignment while they heal.

Transfusion: an injection of blood, saline solution, or other liquid into a vein.

Transient ischemic attack (TIA): a recurrent episode of neurologic deficit, often a warning sign of an impending stroke.

Transverse: across from side to side.

Trauma: surgical definition, physical injury; psychiatric definition, emotional distress relation to a specific incident.

Trauma packs: one of many names for large, thick-layered bulky pads used for quick application to stem profuse bleeding.

Triangular bandage: a piece of cloth cut in the shape of a right-angled triangle; used as a sling, or folded for a cravat bandage.

Type A personality: a hard driving, competitive, often hostile individual.

U

Ulcer: an open lesion of the skin or mucous membrane.

Ulnar artery: a major artery of the forearm; pulse is palpable on the medial wrist at the base of the fifth finger.

Ultraviolet light burns: burns resulting from the rays of the sun.

Umbilical cord: the flexible, cordlike structure connecting the fetus at the navel with the placenta and containing two umbilical arteries and one vein that nourish the fetus and remove its waste.

Umbilicus: the navel.

Universal dressing: a large (9 x 36 inches) dressing of multilayered material that can be used open, folded, or rolled to cover most wounds, to pad splints, or to form a cervical collar.

Urethra: the canal that leads urine from the bladder to the urethral orifice.

Uterus: the muscular organ that hold and nourishes the fetus, opening into the vagina through the cervix; the womb.

V

Vagina: genital canal in the female extending from the uterus to the vulva; the birth canal.

Vascular: relating to, or containing blood vessels.

Vasoconstriction: the diminution of the caliber of vessels, especially constriction of arterioles leading to decreased blood flow to a part.

Vein: any blood vessel that carries blood from the tissues to the heart.

Ventilation: supplying air to the lungs.

Ventricles: the thick-walled, muscular chambers in the heart that receive blood from the atrium and force blood into the arteries; also any small cavities; cerebral chambers containing cerebrospinal fluid.

Vial of Life Program: an emergency medical information system, similar to Medic Alert, which uses a small bottle or vial kept in the refrigerator which contains victim's medical information; sign or card near front entrance tell First Aiders that the vial is present.

Vital signs: in basic EMT-level care, pulse rate and character, breathing rate and character, blood pressure, and relative skin temperature.

Voluntary muscle: muscle under direct voluntary control of the brain, which can be contracted or relaxed at will; skeletal muscle.

W

White blood cells: also called leukocytes and WBCs. Blood cells involved with destroying microorganisms and producing antibodies to fight off infection.

Windpipe: the trachea.

Withdrawal: physical or psychological removal of oneself from a situation.

Wound: a bodily injury caused by physical means, with disruption of the normal continuity of structures.

X

Xiphoid process: one of three components of the sternum; the narrow, cartilaginous lower tip of the sternum.

INDEX